MW01064855

S A U N D E R S

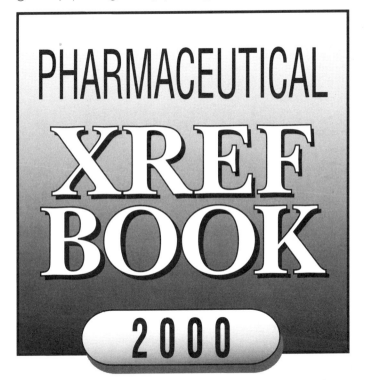

PHARMACEUTICAL

XREF
BOOK

2000

RANDY DRAKE, BS
ELLEN DRAKE, CMT

S A U N D E R S

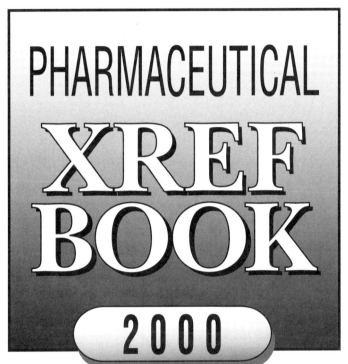

PHARMACEUTICAL
XREF
BOOK

2000

**W.B. SAUNDERS COMPANY**
*A Harcourt Health Sciences Company*
Philadelphia London Toronto Montreal Sydney Tokyo

**W.B. SAUNDERS COMPANY**
*A Harcourt Health Sciences Company*

The Curtis Center
Independence Square West
Philadelphia, Pennsylvania 19106

www.wbsaunders.com

SAUNDERS PHARMACEUTICAL XREF BOOK 2000 ISBN 0–7216–8412–2

ISSN 1527–0696

Printed in the United States of America.

Last digit is the print number:   9   8   7   6   5   4   3   2   1

# To the Lord Jesus

Oh, that my words were written!
Oh, that they were inscribed in a book!
That with an iron stylus and lead
They were engraved in the rock forever!

As for me, I know that my Redeemer lives,
And in the end He will take His stand on the earth.
I myself shall behold Him with my own eyes.
How my heart yearns within me!

— Job 19:23–25, 27

# Contents

# Preface

This is the first edition of *Saunders Pharmaceutical Xref Book*. It is designed to be a companion to our main reference book, *Saunders Pharmaceutical Word Book*, and provide new ways to access the information it contains. This book has been written in response to numerous requests for a cross-reference between generic drugs and the brands that contain them, and a listing of drugs by indication (also known as the drug's "designated use," "approved use," or "therapeutic action").

Our new companion book contains both of these cross-references, plus a comprehensive listing of over 3000 hazardous materials and their potential adverse effects. The Investigational Codes and Street Drug Slang appendices have been moved from our original book to this *Xref Book*.

We urge you to take a moment to study the contents page and read "Notes on Using the Text" and "How the Book is Arranged" on the following pages. It will be well worth your time to help make the most of this valuable tool.

As you use the book, you may have suggestions for changes or additions that would make the book more complete or easier to use. In particular, you may find that Section 2 should have more, less, or different indications listed. The categorization of drugs by indications is not an exact science, and there are several different schemes to accomplish it. We have chosen a scheme, then modified it slightly, to present the information in a form we feel is most intuitive to our readers. The indications listing will be refined in future editions, and we welcome your input. We also welcome your comments regarding additions, inconsistencies, or inaccuracies in either book. Please send them to us via e-mail at the address below, or via regular mail to W.B. Saunders Company, The Curtis Center, Independence Square West, Philadelphia, PA 19106-3399.

Authors' e-mail address:
PharmaceuticalWordBook@Saunders.net

RANDY DRAKE, BS
ELLEN DRAKE, CMT
Orlando, Florida

# Acknowledgments

We would like to acknowledge Maureen Pfeifer who has been unheralded since her appointment as our editor a couple of years ago. She has ably filled the position formerly held by Margaret Biblis, our original editor and the one who conceived the original idea for what became *Saunders Pharmaceutical Word Book*. After a couple of editorial changes and a period without an editor, we were a bit apprehensive at Maureen's appointment, but we are happy to say there was no need for apprehension. She and her capable assistant, Toral Patel, have been wonderful to work with. We appreciate the support, patience, attention to detail, and certainty of follow-through that both of them have provided for the last two editions of *Saunders Pharmaceutical Word Book* and throughout the conception, proposal, approval, and production of this book, the first edition of the *Saunders Pharmaceutical Xref Book*. We truly appreciate both Maureen and Toral.

We would also like to thank the many people on the production staff at W.B. Saunders Co. with whom we have worked closely and who have provided valuable assistance in editing and proofreading our books.

Finally and very importantly, we would like to thank the many users of the *Pharmaceutical Word Book* who have sent us corrections, omissions, clarifications, and suggestions for improvements and additions to the book. Thanks to you all!

RANDY DRAKE, BS
ELLEN DRAKE, CMT

# Notes on Using the Text

The purpose of the *Saunders Pharmaceutical Xref Book* is to provide medical transcriptionists (as well as medical record administrators and technicians, coders, nurses, ward clerks, court reporters, legal secretaries, medical assistants, allied health students, physicians, and even pharmacists) a quick, easy-to-use cross-reference to the information contained in our main reference book, *Saunders Pharmaceutical Word Book*. Specifically, *Saunders Pharmaceutical Xref Book 2000* is a cross-reference to the entries contained in *Saunders Pharmaceutical Word Book 2000*. As such, it is not intended to be used as a stand-alone reference book.

## How the Book Is Arranged

This book is arranged in five sections. Section markings in the right margin make it easy to quickly turn to the needed section.

**Section 1** is a cross-reference between generic drugs and the ℞ brand name drugs that contain those generics. The drug names in bold are the generic ingredients; the indented list that follows are the brands which contain that ingredient. *Every* generic contained in *every* ℞ brand name drug appearing in *Saunders Pharmaceutical Word Book* is included in the list of generics. A brand name drug with more than one active ingredient is listed under each ingredient, with an asterisk denoting it as a combination product. For example, Ser-Ap-Es* appears three times —under hydrochlorothiazide, under reserpine, and under hydralazine HCl.

**Section 2** is a cross-reference between a drug's indication (also known as the drug's "designated use," "approved use," or "therapeutic action") and generic or ℞ brand name drugs. In effect, all drugs used for a particular indication are listed together under the indication heading. For example, all beta-blockers appear under the heading, "Antihypertensives, β-Blockers."

Combination brands may be listed under multiple indications, according to the generic ingredients they contain. Hyzaar, for example, will be listed under both "Antihypertensives, Angiotensin II Inhibitors" (due to its losartan content) and under "Antihypertensives, Diuretics" (due to its hydrochlorothiazide content). Not all combination brands are listed under multiple categories, however. The combination product Ortho-Novum appears only under "Sex Hormones, Oral Contraceptives," for example. Both generic drugs and single-ingredient brands may appear under more than one category, if they're used for multiple purposes. The generic bupropion HCl, for example, appears under "Psychotherapeutics, Antidepressants" (along with the Wellbutrin brand), and also under "Smoking Cessation Agents" (along with the Zyban brand). Valium (diazepam) appears in four categories, reflecting its use as an anticonvulsant, anxiolytic, sedative/hypnotic, and muscle relaxant.

**Section 3** is a listing of investigational code names, cross-referenced to the subsequently assigned generic name, if any. A code name is a temporary identification assigned to a substance by its manufacturer. The number or letter-number combination is used while it is undergoing testing. The generic names shown in this section may be found in the main list of *Saunders Pharmaceutical Word Book*. If no name has been assigned, the code itself can be found in *Saunders Pharmaceutical Word Book*, along with its investigational use.

**Section 4** has over 1500 "street slang" terms for illegally abused drugs. Each slang term cross-references to the official name of the substance, which can be found in the main list of *Saunders Pharmaceutical Word Book*. For example, "magic mushroom" shows a cross-reference to psilocybin and psilocin, which can be found in the main list.

**Section 5** lists over 3000 hazardous materials (HazMat) and their potential adverse effects. These industrial chemicals, poisons, flammable materials, radioactive substances, petroleum products, and biological agents produce a wide variety of adverse effects in the human body. While this section has no cross-reference to the main book, the information can be of great use to those who work in or with emergency departments.

# Xref: Generic Names to Brand-Name ℞ Drugs

Each brand name drug entry in the *Saunders Pharmaceutical Word Book* shows the generic name for each of the active ingredients it contains. It is often helpful, however, to cross-reference the generic ingredients back to the brand name drugs. Listed below is every active ingredient contained in every ℞ brand name entry in *Saunders Pharmaceutical Word Book 2000*. Following each generic name is a list of every ℞ brand name drug which contains that generic. Brands with multiple active ingredients are listed under each ingredient and noted with an asterisk.

**abacavir sulfate**
  Ziagen
**abciximab**
  ReoPro
**absorbable collagen sponge**
  Helistat
**absorbable gelatin film**
  Gelfilm; Gelfilm Ophthalmic
**absorbable gelatin powder**
  Gelfoam
**absorbable gelatin sponge**
  Gelfoam
**acarbose**
  Prandase ⓒᴬᴺ
  Precose
**acebutolol HCl**
  Sectral
**acecarbromal**
  Paxarel
**acemannan**
  Carrisyn
**acetaminophen**
  Aceta with Codeine*
  Aclophen*
  Alumadrine*
  Amacodone*
  Amaphen*
  Amaphen with Codeine #3*
  Anatuss*
  Anexsia 5/500; Anexsia 7.5/650;
    Anexsia 10/660*
  Anoquan*

**acetaminophen (cont.)**
  Arcet*
  Axocet*
  Bancap HC*
  Bucet*
  Bupap*
  Capital with Codeine*
  Ceta Plus*
  Co-Gesic*
  Darvocet-N 50; Darvocet-N 100*
  DHC Plus*
  Dolacet*
  Dolene*
  Dolfen*
  Duocet*
  E-Lor*
  Endocet*
  Endolor*
  Esgic*
  Esgic-Plus*
  Femcet*
  Fioricet*
  Fioricet with Codeine*
  Fiorpap*
  Flexaphen*
  Genagesic*
  Hy-Phen*
  Hycomine Compound*
  Hydrocet*
  Hydrogesic*

*This brand is a combination product.

**acetaminophen (cont.)**
Isocet*
Isocom*
Isopap*
Lobac*
Lorcet*
Lorcet-HD*
Lorcet Plus; Lorcet 10/650*
Lortab*
Lortab 2.5/500; Lortab 5/500; Lortab 7.5/500; Lortab 10/500*
Margesic*
Margesic H*
Margesic No. 3*
Marten-Tab*
Medigesic*
Medipain 5*
Midchlor*
Midrin*
Migratine*
Mus-Lax*
Myapap
Norcet*
Norco*
Norel Plus*
Oncet*
Panacet 5/500*
Papadeine #3*
Percocet*
Phenaphen-650 with Codeine*
Phenaphen with Codeine No. 3 & No. 4*
Phenate*
Phrenilin*
Phrenilin Forte*
Prominol*
Propacet 100*
Proxy 65*
Repan*
Repan CF*
Rid-A-Pain with Codeine*
Roxicet*
Roxicet 5/500*
Roxilox*
Sedapap*
Stagesic*
T-Gesic*
Talacen*
Tencet*
Tencon*

**acetaminophen (cont.)**
Triad*
Triaprin*
Two-Dyne*
Tylenol with Codeine*
Tylenol with Codeine No. 2, No. 3, and No. 4*
Tylox*
Vicodin; Vicodin ES; Vicodin HP*
Wygesic*
Zydone*
**acetazolamide**
Dazamide
Diamox
**acetazolamide sodium**
Diamox
**acetic acid**
AA-HC Otic*
Acetasol
Acetasol HC*
Borofair Otic*
Otic Domeboro*
Otic Tridesilon*
Otomycet-HC*
VōSol HC Otic*
VōSol Otic
Vasotate HC*
**acetohexamide**
Dymelor
**acetohydroxamic acid**
Lithostat
**acetophenazine maleate**
Tindal
**acetylcholine chloride**
Miochol
Miochol-E
**acetylcysteine**
Fluimucil
Mucomyst 10
**acetylcysteine sodium**
Mucomyst
Mucosil-10; Mucosil-20
**acidulated phosphate fluoride**
Minute-Gel
Phos-Flur
**acitretin**
Soriatane

*This brand is a combination product.

**Generic ◆ Brands**

**acrivastine**
 Semprex-D*
**acyclovir**
 Apo-Acyclovir Ⓒ
 Genvir
 Zovirax
**acyclovir sodium**
 Zovirax
**adapalene**
 Differin
**adefovir dipivoxil**
 Preveon
**adenosine**
 Adenocard
 Adenoscan
**adenosine phosphate**
 Kaysine
**AIDS vaccine gp160 MN**
 ALVAC-HIV 1
**alatrofloxacin mesylate**
 Trovan
**albendazole**
 Albenza
**albuterol**
 Proventil
 Ventolin
**albuterol sulfate**
 Airet
 Combivent*
 Proventil
 Proventil HFA
 Ventolin
 Volmax
**alclometasone dipropionate**
 Aclovate
**alcohol**
 Accurbron*
 Actifed with Codeine Cough*
 5% Alcohol and 5% Dextrose in
  Water; 10% Alcohol and 5%
  Dextrose in Water*
 Ambenyl Cough*
 Ana-Kit*
 Bromanate DC Cough*
 Bromarest DX Cough*
 Bromphen DX Cough*
 Brompheniramine DC Cough*
 Bronkotuss Expectorant*
 Calcidrine*
 Cheracol Cough*

**alcohol (cont.)**
 Codehist DH*
 Contuss*
 Cophene XP*
 Cresylate*
 Cyclofed Pediatric*
 Cycofed Pediatric*
 Decohistine DH*
 Decongestant Expectorant*
 Deconsal Pediatric*
 Deproist Expectorant with Codeine*
 Detussin*
 Detussin Expectorant*
 Dexacort Phosphate*
 Dihistine Expectorant*
 Dilaudid Cough*
 Dimetane-DC Cough*
 Dimetane-DX Cough*
 Endal Expectorant*
 Entuss-D Jr.*
 Erygel*
 Guiatuss AC*
 Guiatuss DAC*
 Guiatussin DAC*
 Guiatussin with Codeine Expecto-
  rant*
 H-Tuss-D*
 Histor-D*
 Hycotuss Expectorant*
 Hydramyn*
 Hyphed*
 Isoclor Expectorant*
 Kaochlor 10%; Kaochlor S-F*
 Kaon-Cl 20%*
 Kaylixir*
 Levsin-PB*
 Levsin PB*
 Liquid Pred*
 Myphetane DC Cough*
 Myphetane DX Cough*
 Mytussin AC Cough*
 Mytussin DAC*
 Neoral*
 Norisodrine with Calcium Iodide*
 Novagest Expectorant with
  Codeine*
 Novahistine DH*
 Novahistine Expectorant*

*This brand is a combination product.

**alcohol (cont.)**
  Nucofed Expectorant; Nucofed
    Pediatric Expectorant*
  P-V-Tussin*
  Pancof-HC*
  Pediacof*
  Peridex*
  PerioGard*
  Phenameth DM*
  Phenergan Fortis*
  Phenergan VC*
  Phenergan VC with Codeine*
  Phenergan with Codeine*
  Phenergan with Dextromethorphan*
  Phenhist DH with Codeine*
  Phenhist Expectorant*
  Pherazine DM*
  Pherazine VC with Codeine*
  Pherazine with Codeine*
  Point-Two*
  Polaramine Expectorant*
  Potasalan*
  Prelone*
  Prometh*
  Prometh VC with Codeine*
  Prometh with Dextromethorphan*
  Promethazine DM*
  Promethazine VC Plain*
  Promethazine VC with Codeine*
  Promethist with Codeine*
  Robafen AC Cough*
  Robafen DAC*
  Robitussin A-C*
  Robitussin-DAC*
  Rolatuss Expectorant*
  Ru-Tuss with Hydrocodone*
  SangCya*
  Septisol*
  Sil-Tex*
  SRC Expectorant*
  Statuss Expectorant*
  Statuss Green*
  Synophylate-GG*
  Theomax DF*
  Theostat 80*
  Tinver*
  Toposar*
  Triacin-C Cough*
  Triaminic Expectorant DH*

**alcohol (cont.)**
  Triaminic Expectorant with
    Codeine*
  Trifed-C Cough*
  Tusquelin*
  Tussafin Expectorant*
  Tussanil DH*
  Tussanil Plain*
  Tussar SF; Tussar-2*
  Tussend*
  Tussgen*
  Tusstat*
  Tyrodone*
  Vanex Expectorant*
  Versiclear*
  Vetuss HC*
  Xerac AC*
**aldesleukin**
  Maxamine
  Proleukin
**alendronate sodium**
  Fosamax
**alfentanil HCl**
  Alfenta
**alglucerase**
  Ceredase
**alitretinoin**
  Panretin
**allantoin**
  Alasulf*
  D.I.T.I.-2*
  Deltavac*
**allergenic extracts**
  Allpyral
  Center-Al
**allopurinol**
  Purinol (CAN)
  Zurinol
  Zyloprim
**allopurinol sodium**
  Zyloprim
**alpha-galactosidase A**
  CC-Galactosidase
  FABRase
**alpha$_1$-proteinase inhibitor**
  Prolastin
**alprazolam**
  Xanax

*This brand is a combination product.

**alprostadil**
Alprox-TD
Caverject
Edex
Muse
Prostin VR Pediatric
Topiglan
Vasoprost
**alteplase**
Activase
**altretamine**
Hexalen
**aluminum acetate**
Borofair Otic*
Otic Domeboro*
**aluminum chloride**
Drysol
Xerac AC*
**aluminum hydroxide gel**
Dialume
**amantadine HCl**
Symadine
Symmetrel
**ambenonium chloride**
Mytelase
**amcinonide**
Cyclocort
**amifostine**
Ethyol
**amikacin**
MiKasome
**amikacin sulfate**
Amikin
**amiloride HCl**
Midamor
Moduretic*
**aminacrine HCl**
Alasulf*
D.I.T.I.-2*
Deltavac*
Vagisec Plus
**amino acids, multiple**
Aminess 5.2%*
Aminosyn 3.5% (5%, 7%, 8.5%, 10%); Aminosyn (pH6) 10%; Aminosyn II 3.5% (5%, 7%, 8.5%, 10%, 15%); Aminosyn-PF 7% (10%)*
Aminosyn 3.5% M; Aminosyn II 3.5% M*

**amino acids, multiple (cont.)**
Aminosyn 7% (8.5%) with Electrolytes; Aminosyn II 7% (8.5%, 10%) with Electrolytes*
Aminosyn-HBC 7%*
Aminosyn II 3.5% in 5% (25%) Dextrose; Aminosyn II 4.25% in 10% (20%, 25%) Dextrose; Aminosyn II 5% in 25% Dextrose*
Aminosyn II 3.5% M in 5% Dextrose; Aminosyn II 4.25% M in 10% Dextrose*
Aminosyn-RF 5.2%*
BranchAmin 4%*
FreAmine HBC 6.9%*
FreAmine III 3% (8.5%) with Electrolytes*
FreAmine III 8.5%; FreAmine III 10%*
HepatAmine*
NephrAmine 5.4%*
Novamine; Novamine 15%*
ProcalAmine*
ProSol 20%*
RenAmin*
Travasol 2.75% in 5% (10%, 25%) Dextrose; Travasol 4.25% in 5% (10%, 25%) Dextrose*
Travasol 3.5% (5.5%, 8.5%) with Electrolytes*
Travasol 5.5% (8.5%, 10%)*
TrophAmine 6%; TrophAmine 10%*
**aminobenzoate potassium**
Pabalate-SF*
Potaba
**aminocaproic acid**
Amicar
Caprogel
**aminoglutethimide**
Cytadren
**aminolevulinic acid HCl**
Levulan
**aminophylline**
Mudrane*
Mudrane-2*
Phyllocontin
Truphylline

*This brand is a combination product.

**aminosalicylate sodium**
Sodium P.A.S.
**aminosalicylic acid**
Pamisyl
Paser
Rezipas
**aminosidine**
Gabbromicina
Paromomycin
**amiodarone HCl**
Amio-Aqueous
Cordarone
Pacerone
**amiprilose HCl**
Therafectin
**amitriptyline HCl**
Elavil
Endep
Enovil
Etrafon; Etrafon 2–10; Etrafon-A;
    Etrafon-Forte*
Limbitrol DS 10-25*
Triavil 2-10; Triavil 2-25; Triavil 4-
    10; Triavil 4-25; Triavil 4-50*
**amlexanox**
Aphthasol
**amlodipine**
Norvasc
**amlodipine besylate**
Lotrel*
**ammoniated mercury**
Emersal*
Unguentum Bossi*
**ammonium chloride**
Rolatuss Expectorant*
**ammonium lactate**
Lac-Hydrin
**ammonium molybdate tetrahydrate**
Molypen
**amobarbital sodium**
Amytal Sodium
Tuinal*
**amoxapine**
Asendin
**amoxicillin**
Amoxil
Augmentin*
Biomox
Polymox
Prevpac*

**amoxicillin (cont.)**
Trimox
Wymox
**amoxicillin sodium**
Augmentin*
**amphetamine aspartate**
Adderall*
**amphetamine sulfate**
Adderall*
**amphotericin B**
Fungizone
**amphotericin B cholesteryl sulfate**
Amphotec
**amphotericin B deoxycholate**
Fungizone
**amphotericin B lipid complex (ABLC)**
Abelcet
AmBisome
TLC ABLC
**ampicillin**
D-Amp
Marcillin
Omnipen
Polycillin
Polycillin-PRB*
Principen
Probampacin*
Totacillin
**ampicillin sodium**
Omnipen-N
Polycillin-N
Totacillin-N
Unasyn*
**ampicillin trihydrate**
Principen with Probenecid*
**amprenavir**
Agenerase
**amrinone lactate**
Inocor
**amsacrine**
Amsidyl
**amyl nitrite inhalant**
Cyanide Antidote Package*
**amylase**
Arco-Lase Plus*
Bilezyme*
Cotazym*

*This brand is a combination product.

**amylase (cont.)**
Cotazym-S*
Creon*
Creon 10; Creon 20*
Donnazyme*
Gustase Plus*
Ilozyme*
Ku-Zyme*
Ku-Zyme HP*
Kutrase*
Pancrease; Pancrease MT 4; Pancrease MT 10; Pancrease MT 16; Pancrease MT 20*
Pancrecarb MS-8*
Protilase*
Ultrase MT 12; Ultrase MT 20*
Viokase*
Zymase*
**anagrelide HCl**
Agrylin
**anakinra**
Antril
**ananain**
Vianain*
**anastrozole**
Arimidex
**ancestim**
Stemgen
**ancrod**
Arvin
Viprinex (CAN)
**anisindione**
Miradon
**anistreplase**
Eminase
**antazoline phosphate**
Antazoline-V*
Vasocon-A*
**anthralin**
Anthra-Derm
Drithocreme; Drithocreme HP 1%; Dritho-Scalp
Lasan
Lasan HP-1
Miconal
**anti-B4-blocked ricin MAb**
Oncolysin B
**anti-human thymocyte immuno-globulin**
Thymoglobulin

**anti-inhibitor coagulant complex**
Autoplex T
Feiba VH Immuno
**antihemophilic factor VIII**
Bioclate
Helixate
Hemofil M
Humate-P
Koāte-DVI
Koāte-HP
KoGENate
KoGENate SF
Recombinate
**antihemophilic factor VIII:C**
Alphanate
Antihemophilic Factor Hyate:C
Monoclate
Monoclate P
Profilate HP
Profilate OSD
**antipyrine**
Allergen Ear Drops*
Auralgan Otic*
Auroto Otic*
Otocalm*
Tympagesic*
**antithrombin III**
ATnativ
Kybernin
Thrombate III
**antivenin (Crotalidae) polyvalent Fab**
CroTab
**apomorphine HCl**
Apokinon
Zydis
**apraclonidine HCl**
Iopidine
**aprobarbital**
Alurate
**aprotinin**
Trasylol
**aptiganel HCl**
Cerestat
**arbutamine HCl**
GenESA
**arcitumomab**
CEA-Scan

*This brand is a combination product.

**ardeparin sodium**
  Normiflo
**argatroban**
  Novastan
**arginine HCl**
  R-gene 10
**articaine HCl**
  Astracaine; Astracaine Forte ⓒⒶⓃ*
**ascorbic acid**
  Cevalin
  Cevi-Fer*
  Chromagen*
  Contrin*
  Fergon Plus*
  Fero-Folic-500*
  Ferotrinsic*
  Foltrin*
  Fumatinic*
  Hem Fe*
  Livitamin with Intrinsic Factor*
  Livitrinsic-f*
  Nephlex Rx*
  Nephro-Vite Rx + Fe*
  Nephron FA*
  Pronemia Hematinic*
  TriHemic 600*
  Trinsicon*
**asparaginase**
  Elspar
**aspirin**
  Aggrenox*
  Alor 5/500*
  Aspirin with Codeine No. 2, No. 3, and No. 4*
  Axotal*
  Azdone*
  Butalbital Compound*
  Damason-P*
  Darvon Compound-65*
  Easprin
  Empirin with Codeine No. 3 & No. 4*
  Epromate*
  Equagesic*
  Equazine M*
  Fiorgen PF*
  Fiorinal*
  Fiorinal with Codeine*
  Fiortal*
  Isollyl Improved*

**aspirin (cont.)**
  Lanorinal*
  Lortab ASA*
  Marnal*
  Meprogesic Q*
  Micrainin*
  Norgesic; Norgesic Forte*
  Orphengesic; Orphengesic Forte*
  Panasal 5/500*
  Percodan; Percodan-Demi*
  Rid-A-Pain with Codeine*
  Robaxisal*
  Roxiprin*
  Sodol Compound*
  Soma Compound*
  Soma Compound with Codeine*
  Synalgos-DC*
  Talwin Compound*
  ZORprin
**astemizole**
  Hismanal
**atenolol**
  Tenoretic 50; Tenoretic 100*
  Tenormin
**atorvastatin calcium**
  Lipitor
**atovaquone**
  Malarone ⓒⒶⓃ*
  Mepron
**atracurium besylate**
  Tracrium
**atropine sulfate**
  Antispasmodic*
  Antrocol*
  Arco-Lase Plus*
  Atrohist Plus*
  AtroPen
  Atropine Care
  Atropine-1
  Atropisol
  Atrosept*
  Barbidonna*
  Barbidonna; Barbidonna No. 2*
  Barophen*
  Bellacane*
  Deconhist L.A.*
  Dolsed*
  Donna-Sed*

*This brand is a combination product.

**atropine sulfate (cont.)**
    Donnamor*
    Donnapine*
    Donnatal*
    Donnatal No. 2*
    Enlon Plus*
    Hyosophen*
    Isopto Atropine
    Kinesed*
    Logen*
    Lomanate*
    Lomotil*
    Lonox*
    Malatal*
    Motofen*
    Phenahist-TR*
    Phenchlor S.H.A.*
    Prosed/DS*
    Relaxadon*
    Ru-Tuss*
    Sal-Tropine
    Spasmolin*
    Spasmophen*
    Spasquid*
    Stahist*
    Susano*
    Trac Tabs 2X*
    UAA*
    Uridon Modified*
    Urinary Antiseptic No. 2*
    Urised*
    Uritin*
**auranofin**
    Ridaura
**aurothioglucose**
    Solganal
**azatadine maleate**
    Optimine
    Rynatan*
    Trinalin*
**azathioprine**
    Imuran
**azathioprine sodium**
    Imuran
**azelaic acid**
    Azelex
**azelastine HCl**
    Astelin
**azithromycin**
    Trovan/Zithromax Compliance Pak*

**azithromycin (cont.)**
    Zithromax
    Zithromax ⓒᴬᴺ
**aztreonam**
    Azactam
**bacampicillin HCl**
    Spectrobid
**bacitracin**
    AK-Tracin
    Baci-IM
**bacitracin zinc**
    AK-Poly-Bac*
    AK-Spore*
    AK-Spore H.C.*
    Coracin*
    Cortisporin*
    Neosporin*
    Neotal*
    Neotricin HC*
    Ocutricin*
    Triple Antibiotic*
**baclofen**
    Lioresal
**bactericidal and permeability-increasing protein**
    Neuprex
**balsalazide disodium**
    Colazide
**barium sulfate**
    Anatrast
    Baricon
    Baro-cat
    Barobag
    Baroflave
    Barosperse
    Barosperse, Liquid
    Bear-E-Bag Pediatric
    Bear-E-Yum CT
    Bear-E-Yum GI
    Enecat
    Enhancer
    Entrobar*
    Epi-C
    Flo-Coat
    HD 200 Plus
    HD 85
    Imager ac
    Intropaste

*This brand is a combination product.

Generic ◆ Brands

**barium sulfate (cont.)**
  Liqui-Coat HD
  Liquipake
  Medebar Plus
  Medescan
  Novopaque
  Prepcat
  Quick AC Enema Kit
  Tomocat
  Tonopaque
**basic fuchsin**
  Castellani Paint Modified*
**BCG vaccine**
  ImmuCyst ⓒⓐⓝ
  OncoTICE ⓒⓐⓝ
  Pacis ⓒⓐⓝ
  TheraCys
  Tice BCG
**becaplermin**
  Regranex
**beclomethasone dipropionate**
  Becloforte Inhaler ⓒⓐⓝ
  Beclovent
  Beclovent Inhaler ⓒⓐⓝ
  Beconase
  Beconase AQ
  Vancenase
  Vancenase AQ
  Vanceril; Vanceril Double Strength
**belladonna alkaloids**
  Bel-Phen-Ergot SR*
  Bellacane SR*
  Folergot-DF*
  Phenerbel-S*
**belladonna extract**
  B & O Supprettes No. 15A; B & O
    Supprettes No. 16A*
  Bellafoline
  Bellergal-S*
  Butibel*
  Cafatine-PB*
  Chardonna-2*
**benactyzine HCl**
  Deprol*
**benazepril HCl**
  Lotensin
  Lotensin HCT 5/6.25; Lotensin
    HCT 10/12.5; Lotensin HCT
    20/12.5; Lotensin HCT 20/25*
  Lotrel*

**bendroflumethiazide**
  Corzide 40/5; Corzide 80/5*
  Naturetin
  Rauzide*
**benoxinate HCl**
  Flu-Oxinate*
  Flurate*
  Fluress*
**bentiromide**
  Chymex
**benzocaine**
  Allergen Ear Drops*
  Americaine Anesthetic Lubricant
  Americaine Otic
  Auralgan Otic*
  Auroto Otic*
  Cetacaine*
  Otocain
  Otocalm*
  Triban; Pediatric Triban*
  Tympagesic*
**benzoic acid**
  Atrosept*
  Bensal HP*
  Cystex*
  Dolsed*
  Prosed/DS*
  Trac Tabs 2X*
  UAA*
  Uridon Modified*
  Urinary Antiseptic No. 2*
  Urised*
  Uritin*
**benzonatate**
  Tessalon
**benzoyl peroxide**
  Benzac AC 2½; Benzac W 2½; Benzac 5; Benzac AC 5; Benzac W 5; Benzac 10; Benzac AC 10; Benzac W 10
  Benzac AC Wash 2½; Benzac AC Wash 5; Benzac W Wash 5; Benzac AC Wash 10; Benzac W Wash 10
  5 Benzagel; 10 Benzagel
  10 Benzagel; 5 Benzagel
  Benzamycin*
  Benzashave
  Benzox-10

*This brand is a combination product.

**benzoyl peroxide (cont.)**
Brevoxyl
Del Aqua-5; Del Aqua-10
Desquam-E; Desquam-E 5;
  Desquam-E 10
Desquam-X 2.5
Desquam-X 5 Wash; Desquam-X 10
  Wash
Desquam-X 5; Desquam-X 10
Panoxyl
Panoxyl AQ 2½; Panoxyl 5; Panoxyl
  AQ 5; Panoxyl 10; Panoxyl AQ 10
Peroxin A 5; Peroxin A 10
Persa-Gel; Persa-Gel W 5%; Persa-
  Gel W 10%
Sulfoxyl Regular; Sulfoxyl Strong*
Triaz
Vanoxide-HC*
**benzphetamine HCl**
Didrex
**benzthiazide**
Exna
**benztropine mesylate**
Cogentin
**benzydamine HCl**
Tantrum
**benzylpenicillin**
Pre-Pen/MDM
**benzylpenicilloyl polylysine**
Pre-Pen
**bepridil HCl**
Vascor
**beractant**
Survanta
**beta carotene**
Solatene
**betaine HCl**
Cystadane
**betamethasone acetate**
Celestone Soluspan*
**betamethasone benzoate**
Uticort
**betamethasone dipropionate**
Alphatrex
Diprosone
Lotrisone*
Maxivate
Psorion
Teladar

**betamethasone dipropionate, augmented**
Diprolene
Diprolene AF
**betamethasone sodium phosphate**
Cel-U-Jec
Celestone Phosphate
Celestone Soluspan*
Selestoject
**betamethasone valerate**
Beta-Val
Betatrex
Dermabet
Luxiq
Valisone
Valisone Reduced Strength
**betaxolol HCl**
Betoptic; Betoptic S
Kerlone
**bethanechol chloride**
Duvoid
Myotonachol
PMS-Bethanechol Chloride 🄲
Urecholine
**bexarotene**
Targretin
**bicalutamide**
Casodex
**bile salts**
Digepepsin*
**biotin**
B-C with Folic Acid Plus*
Bacmin*
Berocca Parenteral Nutrition*
Berocca Plus*
Berplex Plus*
Cernevit-12*
Formula B Plus*
M.V.C. 9+3*
M.V.C. 9+4 Pediatric*
M.V.I. Pediatric*
M.V.I.-12*
Materna*
Mynatal*
Mynatal FC*
Mynatal Rx*
Natalins Rx*
Natarex Prenatal*

*This brand is a combination product.

Generic ◆ Brands

**biotin (cont.)**
  Nephlex Rx*
  Nephro-Vite Rx + Fe*
  Nephro-Vite Rx*
  Nephrocaps*
  Nephron FA*
  Prenatal Maternal*
  Prenatal Rx with Betacarotene*
  Strovite Plus; Strovite Forte*
  Zodeac-100*
**biperiden HCl**
  Akineton
**biperiden lactate**
  Akineton
**biricodar dicitrate**
  Incel
**bisacodyl tannex**
  Clysodrast
**bismuth subsalicylate**
  Helidac*
**bisoprolol fumarate**
  Zebeta
  Ziac*
**bithionol**
  Bitin
  Lorothidol
**bitolterol mesylate**
  Tornalate
**bivalirudin**
  Hirulog
**bleomycin sulfate**
  Blenoxane
**blood mononuclear cells**
  CytoImplant
**boric acid**
  Succus Cineraria Maritima*
**botulinum toxin**
  Botox
  Dysport
  Neurobloc
  Ortholinum
**bovine myelin**
  Myloral
**bretylium tosylate**
  Bretylol
**brimonidine tartrate**
  Alphagan
**brinzolamide**
  Azopt

**brofaromine**
  Consonar
**bromelains**
  Vianain*
**bromfenac sodium**
  Duract
**bromocriptine mesylate**
  Ergoset
  Parlodel
**bromodiphenhydramine HCl**
  Ambenyl Cough*
  Amgenal Cough*
  Bromanyl*
  Bromotuss with Codeine*
**brompheniramine maleate**
  Allent*
  Brofed*
  Bromadine-DM*
  Bromadine-DX*
  Bromanate DC Cough*
  Bromarest DX Cough*
  Bromatane DX Cough*
  Bromfed*
  Bromfed-DM Cough*
  Bromfed-PD*
  Bromfenex*
  Bromfenex PD*
  Bromophen T.D.*
  Bromphen DC with Codeine Cough*
  Bromphen DX Cough*
  Brompheniramine DC Cough*
  Brotane DX Cough*
  Cophene-B
  Dallergy-JR*
  Dehist
  Diamine T.D.
  Dimetane-DC Cough*
  Dimetane-DX Cough*
  E.N.T.*
  Endafed*
  Histaject
  Histine DM*
  Iofed*
  Iofed PD*
  Iohist DM*
  Liqui-Histine DM*
  Lodrane LD*
  Myphetane DC Cough*

*This brand is a combination product.

**brompheniramine maleate (cont.)**
  Myphetane DX Cough*
  Nasahist B
  ND Stat
  Oraminic II
  Partapp TD*
  Poly-Histine CS*
  Poly-Histine DM*
  Respahist*
  Rondec*
  Siltapp with Dextromethorphan
    HBr Cold & Cough*
  Sinusol-B
  Tamine S.R.*
  Touro A & H*
  UltraBrom*
  UltraBrom PD*
  Veltane
**broxuridine**
  Broxine
  Neomark
**budesonide**
  Entocort (CAN)
  Pulmicort
  Rhinocort
  Rhinocort Aqua (CAN)
  Rhinocort Turbuhaler (CAN)
**bumetanide**
  Bumex
**bupivacaine HCl**
  Marcaine HCl
  Marcaine HCl*
  Marcaine Spinal
  Marcaine with Epinephrine*
  Sensorcaine
  Sensorcaine*
  Sensorcaine MPF
  Sensorcaine MPF*
  Sensorcaine MPF Spinal
**buprenorphine HCl**
  Buprenex
**bupropion HCl**
  Wellbutrin
  Wellbutrin SR
  Zyban
**buserelin acetate**
  Suprefact (CAN)
  Suprefact; Suprefact Depot (CAN)
**buspirone HCl**
  BuSpar

**busulfan**
  Busulfex
  Myleran
**butabarbital**
  Pyridium Plus*
**butabarbital sodium**
  Butibel*
  Butisol Sodium
**butalbital**
  Amaphen*
  Amaphen with Codeine #3*
  Anoquan*
  Arcet*
  Axocet*
  Axotal*
  Bucet*
  Bupap*
  Butalbital Compound*
  Endolor*
  Esgic*
  Esgic-Plus*
  Femcet*
  Fiorgen PF*
  Fioricet*
  Fioricet with Codeine*
  Fiorinal*
  Fiorinal with Codeine*
  Fiorpap*
  Fiortal*
  Isocet*
  Isollyl Improved*
  Lanorinal*
  Margesic*
  Marnal*
  Marten-Tab*
  Medigesic*
  Phrenilin*
  Phrenilin Forte*
  Prominol*
  Repan*
  Repan CF*
  Sedapap*
  Tencet*
  Tencon*
  Triad*
  Triaprin*
  Two-Dyne*

*This brand is a combination product.

**Generic ◆ Brands**

**butamben**
  Cetacaine*
**butenafine HCl**
  Mentax
**butoconazole nitrate**
  Femstat
**butorphanol tartrate**
  Stadol
  Stadol NS
**C1-esterase-inhibitor**
  Berinert-P
**cabergoline**
  Dostinex
**caffeine**
  Amaphen*
  Amaphen with Codeine #3*
  Anoquan*
  Arcet*
  Butalbital Compound*
  Cafatine*
  Cafatine-PB*
  Cafergot*
  Cafetrate*
  Darvon Compound-65*
  DHC Plus*
  Endolor*
  Ercaf*
  Esgic*
  Esgic-Plus*
  Femcet*
  Fiorgen PF*
  Fioricet*
  Fioricet with Codeine*
  Fiorinal*
  Fiorinal with Codeine*
  Fiorpap*
  Fiortal*
  Hycomine Compound*
  Isocet*
  Isollyl Improved*
  Lanorinal*
  Margesic*
  Marnal*
  Medigesic*
  Neocaf
  Norgesic; Norgesic Forte*
  Orphengesic; Orphengesic Forte*
  Repan*
  Rid-A-Pain with Codeine*
  Synalgos-DC*

**caffeine (cont.)**
  Tencet*
  Triad*
  Two-Dyne*
  Wigraine*
**caffeine citrate**
  Tussirex*
**calcifediol**
  Calderol
**calcipotriene**
  Dovonex
**calcitonin**
  Calcimar
  Cibacalcin
  Fortical
  Macritonin
  Miacalcin
  Osteocalcin
  Salmonine
**calcitriol**
  Calcijex
  Rocaltrol
**calcium**
  Adeflor M*
  Filibon F.A.; Filibon Forte*
  Lactocal-F*
  Marnatal-F*
  Materna*
  Mission Prenatal Rx*
  Mynatal*
  Mynatal FC*
  Mynatal P.N.*
  Mynatal P.N. Forte*
  Mynatal Rx*
  Mynate 90 Plus*
  Natabec Rx*
  Natafort*
  NatalCare Plus*
  Natalins Rx*
  Natarex Prenatal*
  Nestabs FA*
  Niferex-PN Forte*
  Norlac Rx*
  O-Cal f.a.*
  Par-F*
  Par-Natal Plus 1 Improved*
  Pramet FA*
  Pramilet FA*

*This brand is a combination product.

**Generic ♦ Brands**

**calcium (cont.)**
Pre-H Cal*
Prenatal H.P.*
Prenatal Maternal*
Prenatal MR 90*
Prenatal One*
Prenatal Plus Iron*
Prenatal Plus with Betacarotene*
Prenatal Plus; Prenatal Plus
   Improved*
Prenatal Rx*
Prenatal Rx with Betacarotene*
Prenatal Z*
Prenatal-1 + Iron*
Prenate 90; Prenate Ultra*
Secran Prenatal*
Stuartnatal Plus*
**calcium acetate**
PhosLo
**calcium alginate fiber**
Sorbsan
**calcium carbonate**
Cotazym*
R & D Calcium Carbonate/600
**calcium chloride**
Plegisol*
**calcium gluconate**
Calgonate
H-F Gel
**calcium glycerophosphate**
Calphosan*
**calcium iodide**
Calcidrine*
Norisodrine with Calcium Iodide*
**calcium lactate**
Calphosan*
**calfactant**
Infasurf
**candesartan cilexetil**
Atacand
***Candida albicans* skin test antigen**
Candin
Dermatophytin "O"
**cantharidin**
Verr-Canth
Verrusol*
**capecitabine**
Xeloda
**capreomycin sulfate**
Capastat Sulfate

**capromab pendetide**
ProstaScint
**captopril**
Capoten
Capozide 25/15; Capozide 25/25;
   Capozide 50/15; Capozide 50/25*
**caramiphen edisylate**
Ordrine AT*
Rescaps-D S.R.*
Tuss-Allergine Modified T.D.*
Tuss-Genade Modified*
Tuss-Ornade*
Tussogest*
**carbachol**
Carbastat
Carboptic
Isopto Carbachol
Miostat
**carbamazepine**
Atretol
Carbatrol
Depitol
Epitol
Tegretol
Tegretol-XR
**carbenicillin indanyl sodium**
Geocillin
**carbetapentane citrate**
Cophene-X*
**carbetapentane tannate**
Rentamine Pediatric*
Rynatuss*
Tri-Tannate Plus Pediatric*
Tussi-12*
**carbidopa**
Lodosyn
Sinemet 10/100; Sinemet 25/100;
   Sinemet 25/250*
Sinemet CR*
**carbinoxamine maleate**
Biohist-LA*
Carbinoxamine Compound*
Carbiset*
Carbiset-TR*
Carbodec*
Carbodec DM*
Carbodec TR*
Cardec-DM*

*This brand is a combination product.

**carbinoxamine maleate (cont.)**
  Cardec-S*
  Pseudo-Car DM*
  Rondamine-DM*
  Rondec*
  Rondec-DM*
  Rondec-TR*
  Sildec-DM*
  Tussafed*
**carbohydrate polymer gel**
  Adcon-L
**carbon C 14 urea**
  PYtest
**carboplatin**
  Paraplatin
**carboprost tromethamine**
  Hemabate
**carisoprodol**
  Sodol
  Sodol Compound*
  Soma
  Soma Compound*
  Soma Compound with Codeine*
**carmustine**
  BiCNU
  Gliadel
**carprofen**
  Rimadyl
**carteolol HCl**
  Ocupress
**carvedilol**
  Coreg
**CD4, human truncated 369 AA polypeptide**
  Soluble T4
**CD4, recombinant soluble human**
  Receptin
**cefaclor**
  Apo-Cefaclor ⒸⒶⓃ
  Ceclor
  Ceclor CD
**cefadroxil**
  Duricef
  Ultracef
**cefamandole nafate**
  Mandol
**cefazolin sodium**
  Ancef
  Kefzol
  Zolicef

**cefdinir**
  Omnicef
**cefepime HCl**
  Maxipime
**cefixime**
  Suprax
**cefmetazole sodium**
  Zefazone
**cefodizime**
  Modivid
**cefonicid sodium**
  Monocid
**cefoperazone sodium**
  Cefobid
**cefotaxime sodium**
  Claforan
**cefotetan disodium**
  Cefotan
**cefoxitin sodium**
  Mefoxin
**cefpodoxime proxetil**
  Vantin
**cefprozil**
  Cefzil
**ceftazidime**
  Fortaz
  Pentacef
  Tazicef
  Tazidime
**ceftazidime pentahydrate**
  Ceptaz
**ceftibuten**
  Cedax
**ceftizoxime sodium**
  Cefizox
**ceftriaxone sodium**
  Rocephin
**cefuroxime axetil**
  Ceftin
**cefuroxime sodium**
  Kefurox
  Zinacef
**celecoxib**
  Celebrex
**celgosivir HCl**
  Bucast
**celiprolol HCl**
  Selecor

*This brand is a combination product.

**Generic ◆ Brands**

**cellulase**
 Arco-Lase Plus*
 Gustase Plus*
 Ku-Zyme*
 Kutrase*
**cellulose, oxidized**
 Oxycel
 Surgicel
**cellulose sodium phosphate**
 Calcibind
**cephalexin**
 Biocef
 Cefanex
 Keflex
 Zartan
**cephalexin HCl**
 Keftab
**cephalothin sodium**
 Keflin, Neutral
**cephapirin sodium**
 Cefadyl
**cephradine**
 Velosef
**cerivastatin sodium**
 Baycol
**cetirizine HCl**
 Reactine ⒸⒶⓃ
 Zyrtec
**chenodiol**
 Chenix
**chloral hydrate**
 Aquachloral
**chlorambucil**
 Leukeran
**chloramphenicol**
 AK-Chlor
 Chloromycetin
 Chloromycetin Hydrocortisone*
 Chloromycetin Otic
 Chloroptic
 Chloroptic S.O.P.
 Elase-Chloromycetin*
 Ophthocort*
**chloramphenicol sodium succinate**
 Chloromycetin Sodium Succinate
**chlorazepate dipotassium**
 Gen-Xene
**chlorcyclizine HCl**
 Mantadil*

**chlordiazepoxide**
 Libritabs
 Limbitrol DS 10-25*
 Menrium 5-2; Menrium 5-4; Menrium 10-4*
**chlordiazepoxide HCl**
 Clindex*
 Clinoxide*
 Clipoxide*
 Librax*
 Librium
 Lidox*
 Mitran
 Reposans-10
**chlorhexidine gluconate**
 Peridex*
 PerioChip
 PerioGard*
**chlormezanone**
 Trancopal
**chlorobutanol**
 Cresylate*
 Pontocaine HCl*
 Pred-G S.O.P.*
 TobraDex*
**chlorophyllin copper complex**
 Panafil*
**chloroprocaine HCl**
 Nesacaine; Nesacaine MPF
**chloroquine HCl**
 Aralen HCl
**chloroquine phosphate**
 Aralen Phosphate
 Aralen Phosphate with Primaquine Phosphate*
**chlorothiazide**
 Aldoclor-150; Aldoclor-250*
 Chloroserpine*
 Diupres-250; Diupres-500*
 Diurigen
 Diuril
 Sodium Diuril
**chlorotrianisene**
 Tace
**chloroxine**
 Capitrol
**chloroxylenol**
 Cortic*

*This brand is a combination product.

**chloroxylenol (cont.)**
  Gordochom*
  Oti-Med*
  Otomar-HC*
  Tri-Otic*
  Zoto-HC*
**chlorphenesin carbamate**
  Maolate
**chlorpheniramine maleate**
  Aclophen*
  AH-chew*
  Alersule*
  Alumadrine*
  Ana-Kit*
  Anamine*
  Anamine T.D.*
  Anaplex*
  Anaplex HD*
  Anaplex SR*
  Atrohist Pediatric*
  Atrohist Plus*
  Atuss DM*
  Atuss HD*
  Brexin-L.A.*
  Bronkotuss Expectorant*
  Chlor-Pro
  Chlor-100
  Chlor-Trimeton
  Chlorafed; Chlorafed HS*
  Chlordrine S.R.*
  Chlorgest-HD*
  Chlorphedrine SR*
  Chlorspan-12
  Chlortab-4
  Chlortab-8
  Codehist DH*
  Codimal-L.A.; Codimal-L.A. Half*
  Colfed-A*
  Comhist*
  Comhist LA*
  Condrin-LA*
  Cophene No. 2*
  D.A.*
  D.A. II*
  Dallergy*
  Decohistine DH*
  Deconamine*
  Deconamine SR*
  Decongestabs*
  Decongestant*

**chlorpheniramine maleate (cont.)**
  Decongestant S.R.*
  Deconhist L.A.*
  Deconomed SR*
  Donatussin*
  Drize*
  Dura-Vent/A*
  Dura-Vent/DA*
  Dura-Tap/PD*
  Duralex*
  Ed A-Hist*
  ED-TLC; ED Tuss HC*
  Endagen-HD*
  Endal-HD; Endal-HD Plus*
  Ex-Histine*
  Extendryl*
  Extendryl JR*
  Extendryl SR*
  Fedahist*
  Hista-Vadrin*
  Histalet*
  Histalet Forte*
  Histamic*
  Histinex HC*
  Histinex PV*
  Histor-D*
  Histussin HC*
  Hycomine Compound*
  Hydrocodone CP; Hydrocodone HD*
  Hyphed*
  Iodal HD*
  Iotussin HC*
  Klerist-D*
  Kronofed-A*
  Kronofed-A Jr.*
  Mescolor*
  Naldec Pediatric*
  Naldecon*
  Naldelate*
  Nalgest*
  ND Clear*
  Nolamine*
  Norel Plus*
  Novafed A*
  Novahistine DH*
  OMNIhist L.A.*
  Ordrine S.R.*
  Ornade*

*This brand is a combination product.

**chlorpheniramine maleate (cont.)**
P-V-Tussin*
Pancof-HC*
Pannaz*
Para-Hist HD*
Parhist SR*
Pediacof*
Pedituss Cough*
Phenahist-TR*
Phenate*
Phenchlor S.H.A.*
Phenetron
Phenhist DH with Codeine*
Prehist*
Prehist D*
Pseudo-Chlor*
Quadra-Hist*
Quadra-Hist Pediatric*
Resaid*
Rescon*
Rescon-ED*
Rescon JR*
Rhinolar*
Rhinolar-EX; Rhinolar-EX 12*
Rinade B.I.D.*
Rolatuss Expectorant*
Ru-Tuss*
Ru-Tuss II*
Ryna-C*
S-T Forte 2*
Stahist*
T-Koff*
Telachlor
Time-Hist*
Tri-Phen-Chlor*
Tri-Phen-Chlor T.R.*
Tri-Phen-Mine*
Tri-Phen-Mine S.R.*
Tusquelin*
Tussanil DH*
Tussanil Plain*
Tussend*
Uni-Decon*
Unituss HC*
Vanex Forte*
Vanex Forte-R*
Vanex-HD*
**chlorpheniramine polistirex**
Tussionex Pennkinetic*

**chlorpheniramine tannate**
Atrohist Pediatric*
R-Tannamine*
R-Tannate*
Rentamine Pediatric*
Rhinatate*
Rynatan*
Rynatan-S*
Rynatuss*
Tanafed*
Tanoral*
Tri-Tannate*
Tri-Tannate Plus Pediatric*
Triotann*
Tritan*
Tritann Pediatric*
Tussi-12*
**chlorpromazine**
Thorazine
**chlorpromazine HCl**
Ormazine
**chlorpropamide**
Diabinese
**chlortetracycline HCl**
Aureomycin
**chlorthalidone**
Combipres 0.1; Combipres 0.2;
Combipres 0.3*
Demi-Regroton*
Hygroton
Regroton*
Tenoretic 50; Tenoretic 100*
Thalitone
**chlorzoxazone**
Flexaphen*
Mus-Lax*
Paraflex
Parafon Forte DSC
Remular-S
**cholestyramine resin**
LoCholest; LoCholest Light
Prevalite
Questran; Questran Light
**choline bitartrate**
Ilopan-Choline*
**choline chloride**
Intrachol

*This brand is a combination product.

**choline magnesium trisalicylate**
  Tricosal
**choline salicylate**
  Arthropan
  Trilisate*
**chondrocytes, cultured autologous**
  Carticel
**chondroitin sulfate sodium**
  Viscoat*
**chorionic gonadotropin**
  A.P.L.
  Chorex-5; Chorex-10
  Chorigon
  Choron-10
  Follutein
  Glukor
  Gonic
  Pregnyl
  Profasi
**chromic chloride hexahydrate**
  Chroma-Pak
  Chromium Chloride
**chromic phosphate P 32**
  Phosphocol P 32
**chymopapain**
  Chymodiactin
**chymotrypsin**
  Catarase 1:5000
**ciclopirox olamine**
  Loprox
**cidofovir**
  Vistide
**cifenline succinate**
  Cipralan
**cilastatin sodium**
  Primaxin I.M.*
  Primaxin I.V.*
**cilazapril**
  Inhibace
**cilmostim**
  Macstim
**cilostazol**
  Pletal
**cimetidine**
  Tagamet
**cimetidine HCl**
  Tagamet
**cinoxacin**
  Cinobac

**ciprofloxacin**
  Cipro
  Cipro HC Otic*
**ciprofloxacin HCl**
  Ciloxan
**cisapride**
  Prepulsid ⓒⓐⓝ
  Propulsid
**cisatracurium besylate**
  Nimbex
**cisplatin**
  IntraDose*
  Platinol
  Platinol-AQ
**citalopram hydrobromide**
  Celexa
**citicoline sodium**
  CerAxon
  Interquim
**citric acid**
  Bicitra*
  Cytra-2*
  Cytra-3*
  Cytra-K*
  Cytra-LC*
  Oracit*
  PMS-Dicitrate ⓒⓐⓝ
  Polycitra*
  Polycitra-K*
  Polycitra-LC*
  Renacidin*
  Renacidin Irrigation*
**cladribine**
  Leustatin
**clarithromycin**
  Biaxin
  Prevpac*
**clavulanate potassium**
  Augmentin*
  Timentin*
**clemastine fumarate**
  Tavist
**clidinium bromide**
  Clindex*
  Clinoxide*
  Clipoxide*
  Librax*
  Lidox*

*This brand is a combination product.

*This brand is a combination product.

**Generic ♦ Brands**

## codeine phosphate
- Aceta with Codeine*
- Actagen-C Cough*
- Actifed with Codeine Cough*
- Allerfrin with Codeine*
- Amaphen with Codeine #3*
- Ambenyl Cough*
- Amgenal Cough*
- Aprodine with Codeine*
- Aspirin with Codeine No. 2, No. 3, and No. 4*
- Bromanate DC Cough*
- Bromanyl*
- Bromotuss with Codeine*
- Bromphen DC with Codeine Cough*
- Brompheniramine DC Cough*
- Brontex*
- Calcidrine*
- Calmylin Codeine (CAN)*
- Capital with Codeine*
- Cheracol Cough*
- Codegest Expectorant*
- Codehist DH*
- Conex with Codeine*
- Cotridin (CAN)*
- Cotridin Expectorant (CAN)*
- Cyclofed Pediatric*
- Cycofed Pediatric*
- Decohistine DH*
- Decongestant Expectorant*
- Deconsal Pediatric*
- Deproist Expectorant with Codeine*
- Dihistine Expectorant*
- Dimetane-DC Cough*
- Empirin with Codeine No. 3 & No. 4*
- Endal Expectorant*
- Fioricet with Codeine*
- Fiorinal with Codeine*
- Guiatuss AC*
- Guiatuss DAC*
- Guiatussin DAC*
- Guiatussin with Codeine Expectorant*
- Iophen-C*
- Isoclor Expectorant*
- Margesic No. 3*
- Myphetane DC Cough*
- Mytussin AC Cough*
- Mytussin DAC*

## codeine phosphate (cont.)
- Naldecon CX Adult*
- Novagest Expectorant with Codeine*
- Novahistine DH*
- Novahistine Expectorant*
- Nucofed*
- Nucofed Expectorant; Nucofed Pediatric Expectorant*
- Papadeine #3*
- Pediacof*
- Pedituss Cough*
- Pentazine VC with Codeine*
- Phenaphen-650 with Codeine*
- Phenaphen with Codeine No. 3 & No. 4*
- Phenergan VC with Codeine*
- Phenergan with Codeine*
- Phenhist DH with Codeine*
- Phenhist Expectorant*
- Pherazine VC with Codeine*
- Pherazine with Codeine*
- Poly-Histine CS*
- Prometh VC with Codeine*
- Prometh with Codeine*
- Promethazine VC with Codeine*
- Promethist with Codeine*
- Rid-A-Pain with Codeine*
- Robafen AC Cough*
- Robafen DAC*
- Robitussin A-C*
- Robitussin-DAC*
- Rolatuss Expectorant*
- Ryna-C*
- Ryna-CX*
- Soma Compound with Codeine*
- Statuss Expectorant*
- T-Koff*
- Triacin-C Cough*
- Triafed with Codeine*
- Triaminic Expectorant with Codeine*
- Tricodene Cough and Cold*
- Trifed-C Cough*
- Tussar SF; Tussar-2*
- Tussi-Organidin NR; Tussi-Organidin-S NR*
- Tussirex*

*This brand is a combination product.

**codeine phosphate (cont.)**
   Tylenol with Codeine*
   Tylenol with Codeine No. 2, No. 3,
      and No. 4*
**colchicine**
   Col-Probenecid*
   Colabid*
   ColBenemid*
   Proben-C*
**colesevelam HCl**
   CholestaGel
**colestipol HCl**
   Colestid
**colfosceril palmitate**
   Alec*
   Exosurf
   Exosurf Neonatal
**colistimethate sodium**
   Coly-Mycin M
**colistin sulfate**
   Coly-Mycin S
   Coly-Mycin S Otic*
   Cortisporin-TC*
**collagen implant, purified**
   Contigen
**collagenase**
   Cordase
   Plaquase
   Santyl
**comosain**
   Vianain*
**conjugated estrogens**
   Cenestin
   PMB 200; PMB 400*
   Premarin
   Premarin Intravenous
   Premarin with Methyltestosterone*
   Premphase*
   Prempro*
**corticorelin ovine triflutate**
   Acthrel
**corticotropin**
   ACTH
   ACTH-80
   Acthar
   H.P. Acthar Gel
**cortisone acetate**
   Cortone Acetate
**cosyntropin**
   Cortrosyn

**coumarin**
   Oncostate
   Onkolox
*m*-**cresyl acetate**
   Cresylate*
**cromolyn sodium**
   Apo-Cromolyn Ⓒ
   Crolom
   Gastrocrom
   Intal
   Opticrom 4%
**crotamiton**
   Eurax
*Cryptosporidium parvum* **bovine**
   **colostrum IgG concentrate**
   BACI
   Immuno-C
   Sporidin-G
**cyanocobalamin**
   Chromagen*
   Contrin*
   Crystamine
   Crysti 1000
   Cyanoject
   Cyomin
   Ferotrinsic*
   Foltrin*
   Fumatinic*
   Hem Fe*
   Livitrinsic-f*
   Nascobal
   Niferex Forte*
   Niferex-150 Forte*
   Nu-Iron Plus*
   Pronemia Hematinic*
   Rubesol-1000
   Rubramin PC
   TriHemic 600*
   Trinsicon*
**cyclandelate**
   Cyclan
   Cyclospasmol
   Cyclospasmol Ⓒ
**cyclobenzaprine HCl**
   Flexeril
**cyclopentolate HCl**
   AK-Pentolate
   Cyclogyl

*This brand is a combination product.

**cyclopentolate HCl (cont.)**
  Cyclomydril*
  Pentolair
**cyclophosphamide**
  Cytoxan
  Neosar
**cycloserine**
  Seromycin
**cyclosporine**
  Neoral*
  Optimmune
  Sandimmune
  Sandimmune Neoral ⒸⒶⒷ
  SangCya*
**cyproheptadine HCl**
  Periactin
**cyproterone acetate**
  Diane-35 ⒸⒶⒷ*
  Novo-Cyproterone ⒸⒶⒷ
**cysteamine bitartrate**
  Cystagon
**cystine**
  Amino-Cerv pH 5.5*
**cytarabine**
  Cytosar-U
  DepoCyt
  Tarabine PFS
**cytomegalovirus immune globulin**
  CytoGam
**dacarbazine**
  DTIC-Dome
**dacliximab**
  Zenapax
**dactinomycin**
  Cosmegen
**dalfopristin**
  Synercid*
**dalteparin sodium**
  Fragmin
**danaparoid sodium**
  Orgaran
**danazol**
  Danocrine
**dantrolene sodium**
  Dantrium
**dapiprazole HCl**
  Rēv-Eyes
**daunorubicin citrate**
  DaunoXome

**daunorubicin HCl**
  Cerubidine
**deferoxamine**
  Bio-Rescue*
**deferoxamine mesylate**
  Desferal
**dehydrocholic acid**
  Bilezyme*
  Digestozyme*
**dehydroemetine**
  Mebadin
**delavirdine mesylate**
  Rescriptor
**demecarium bromide**
  Humorsol
**demeclocycline HCl**
  Declomycin
**denileukin diftitox**
  Ontak
**depreotide**
  NeoTect
**deserpidine**
  Enduronyl; Enduronyl Forte*
**desflurane**
  Suprane
**desipramine HCl**
  Norpramin
  Pertofrane
**desirudin**
  Revasc
**deslorelin**
  Somagard
**desmopressin acetate**
  DDAVP
  Stimate
**desogestrel**
  Desogen*
  Mircette*
  Ortho-Cept*
**desonide**
  DesOwen
  Otic Tridesilon*
  Tridesilon
**desoximetasone**
  Topicort
  Topicort LP
**desoxycholic acid**
  Bilezyme*

*This brand is a combination product.

**desoxyribonuclease**
  Elase*
  Elase-Chloromycetin*
**dexamethasone**
  Aeroseb-Dex
  AK-Trol*
  Decadron
  Decaspray
  Dexacidin*
  Dexameth
  Dexasporin*
  Dexone
  Hexadrol
  Maxidex
  Maxitrol*
  Storz-N-P-D*
  Surodex
  TobraDex*
**dexamethasone acetate**
  Dalalone D.P.
  Dalalone L.A.
  Decadron-LA
  Decaject-L.A.
  Dexasone L.A.
  Dexone LA
  Solurex LA
**dexamethasone sodium phosphate**
  AK-Dex
  AK-Neo-Dex*
  Dalalone
  Decadron Phosphate
  Decadron with Xylocaine*
  Decaject
  Dexacort Phosphate
  Dexacort Phosphate*
  Dexasone
  Dexone
  Diodex ⒸⒶⓃ
  Hexadrol Phosphate
  Neo-Dexair*
  Neo-Dexameth*
  NeoDecadron*
  R.O.-Dexsone ⒸⒶⓃ
  Solurex
  Spersadex ⒸⒶⓃ
  Storz-N-D*
**dexbrompheniramine maleate**
  Ami-Drix*
  Dexaphen S.A.*
  Disobrom*

**dexbrompheniramine maleate (cont.)**
  Drixomed*
**dexchlorpheniramine maleate**
  Dexchlor
  Poladex
  Polaramine
  Polaramine Expectorant*
**dexfenfluramine HCl**
  Redux
**dexpanthenol**
  Ilopan
  Ilopan-Choline*
**dexrazoxane**
  Zinecard
**dextran**
  Bio-Rescue*
  Gendex 75
  Gentran 40
  Gentran 70
  Gentran 75
  Hyskon*
  10% LMD
  Macrodex
  Promit
  Rheomacrodex
**dextran sulfate**
  Uendex
**dextranomer**
  Debrisan
**dextroamphetamine saccharate**
  Adderall*
**dextroamphetamine sulfate**
  Adderall*
  Dexedrine
  Dextrostat
  Oxydess II
  Spancap No. 1
**dextromethorphan**
  MorphiDex*
**dextromethorphan hydrobromide**
  Anatuss*
  Atuss DM*
  Bromadine-DM*
  Bromadine-DX*
  Bromarest DX Cough*
  Bromatane DX Cough*
  Bromfed-DM Cough*

*This brand is a combination product.

**dextromethorphan hydrobromide (cont.)**
- Bromphen DX Cough*
- Brotane DX Cough*
- Carbinoxamine Compound*
- Carbodec DM*
- Cardec-DM*
- Dimetane-DX Cough*
- Donatussin*
- Fenesin DM*
- Guaifenex DM*
- Histine DM*
- Humibid DM*
- Humibid DM Sprinkle*
- Iobid DM*
- Iohist DM*
- Iophen-DM*
- Liqui-Histine DM*
- MED-Rx DM*
- Monafed DM*
- Muco-Fen-DM*
- Myphetane DX Cough*
- Phenameth DM*
- Phenergan with Dextromethorphan*
- Pherazine DM*
- Poly-Histine DM*
- Profen II DM*
- Prometh with Dextromethorphan*
- Promethazine DM*
- Protuss DM*
- Pseudo-Car DM*
- Respa-DM*
- Rondamine-DM*
- Rondec-DM*
- Sildec-DM*
- Siltapp with Dextromethorphan HBr Cold & Cough*
- Tusquelin*
- Tussafed*
- Tussi-Organidin DM NR; Tussi-Organidin DM-S NR*
- Tusso-DM*

**dextrose**
- 5% Alcohol and 5% Dextrose in Water; 10% Alcohol and 5% Dextrose in Water*
- Aminosyn II 3.5% in 5% (25%) Dextrose; Aminosyn II 4.25% in 10% (20%, 25%) Dextrose; Aminosyn II 5% in 25% Dextrose*

**dextrose (cont.)**
- Aminosyn II 3.5% M in 5% Dextrose; Aminosyn II 4.25% M in 10% Dextrose*
- D-2.5-W; D-5-W; D-10-W; D-20-W; D-25-W; D-30-W; D-40-W; D-50-W; D-60-W; D-70-W
- 5% Dextrose and Electrolyte #48; 5% Dextrose and Electrolyte #75; 10% Dextrose and Electrolyte #48*
- 50% Dextrose with Electrolyte Pattern A (or N)*
- Dialyte Pattern LM*
- Hyskon*
- Inpersol; Inpersol-LM*
- Isolyte E (G; H; M; P; R; S) with 5% Dextrose*
- Normosol-M and 5% Dextrose; Normosol-R and 5% Dextrose*
- Plasma-Lyte M (R; 56; 148) and 5% Dextrose*
- Primacor in 5% Dextrose*
- Travasol 2.75% in 5% (10%, 25%) Dextrose; Travasol 4.25% in 5% (10%, 25%) Dextrose*
- Xylocaine HCl*

**dextrothyroxine sodium**
- Choloxin

**dezocine**
- Dalgan

**diatrizoate meglumine**
- Angiovist 282
- Angiovist 292; Angiovist 370*
- Cystografin; Cystografin Dilute
- Gastrografin*
- Hypaque-76*
- Hypaque-Cysto
- Hypaque-M 75; Hypaque-M 90*
- Hypaque Meglumine 30%; Hypaque Meglumine 60%
- MD-60; MD-76*
- MD-76 R*
- MD-Gastroview*
- Reno-30
- Reno-Dip; Reno-60
- RenoCal-76*
- Renografin-60*
- Renografin-76*

*This brand is a combination product.

**diatrizoate meglumine (cont.)**
Renovist; Renovist II*
Sinografin*
Urovist Cysto
Urovist Meglumine DIU/CT
**diatrizoate sodium**
Angiovist 292; Angiovist 370*
Gastrografin*
Hypaque-76*
Hypaque-M 75; Hypaque-M 90*
Hypaque Sodium
Hypaque Sodium 20%
Hypaque Sodium 25%; Hypaque Sodium 50%
MD-60; MD-76*
MD-76 R*
MD-Gastroview*
RenoCal-76*
Renografin-60*
Renografin-76*
Renovist; Renovist II*
Urovist Sodium 300
**diazepam**
Diastat
Diazemuls ⓒⒶⓃ
Dizac
Valium
Valium Roche Oral ⓒⒶⓃ
Valrelease
Zetran
**diazoxide**
Hyperstat
Proglycem
**dichloralphenazone**
Isocom*
Isopap*
Midchlor*
Midrin*
Migratine*
**dichloroacetic acid**
Bichloracetic Acid
**dichlorodifluoromethane**
Fluori-Methane*
**dichlorotetrafluoroethane**
Fluro-Ethyl*
**dichlorphenamide**
Daranide
**diclofenac potassium**
Cataflam
Hyanalgese-D*

**diclofenac potassium (cont.)**
Pennsaid
Solarase*
Voltaren Rapide ⓒⒶⓃ
**diclofenac sodium**
Arthrotec*
Diclotec ⓒⒶⓃ
Voltaren
Voltaren ⓒⒶⓃ
Voltaren SR ⓒⒶⓃ
Voltaren XR
**dicloxacillin sodium**
Dycill
Dynapen
Pathocil
**dicyclomine HCl**
Antispas
Bentyl
Byclomine
Di-Spaz
Dibent
Spasmoject
**didanosine**
Scriptene*
Videx
**dienestrol**
DV
Ortho Dienestrol
**diethylcarbamazine citrate**
Hetrazan
**diethyldithiocarbamate**
Imuthiol
**diethylpropion HCl**
Tenuate
Tepanil
**diethylstilbestrol diphosphate**
Stilphostrol
**difenoxin HCl**
Motofen*
**diflorasone diacetate**
Florone
Florone E
Maxiflor
Psorcon
**diflunisal**
Dolobid
**digitoxin**
Crystodigin

*This brand is a combination product.

Generic ♦ Brands

**digoxin**
 Lanoxicaps
 Lanoxin
**digoxin immune Fab**
 Digibind
 Digidote
**dihydrocodeine bitartrate**
 DHC Plus*
 Synalgos-DC*
**dihydroergotamine mesylate**
 D.H.E. 45
 Migranal
**dihydrotachysterol**
 DHT
 Hytakerol
**dihydrotestosterone**
 Androgel-DHT
**diloxanide furoate**
 Furamide
**diltiazem HCl**
 Cardizem
 Cardizem SR; Cardizem CD
 Dilacor XR
 Tiazac
**diltiazem maleate**
 Teczem*
 Tiamate
**dimenhydrinate**
 Dimetabs
 Dinate
 Dramamine
 Dramanate
 Dramilin
 Dramoject
 Dymenate
 Hydrate
 Marmine
**dimercaprol**
 BAL in Oil
**dimethyl sulfoxide (DMSO)**
 Kemsol ⓒⒶⓃ
 Rimso-50
**dinoprostone**
 Cervidil
 Prepidil
 Prostin E2
**dioxybenzone**
 Nuquin HP*
 Solaquin Forte*
 Viquin Forte*

**diphenhydramine HCl**
 Ben-Allergin-50
 Bena-D 10; Bena-D 50
 Benadryl
 Benadryl Allergy
 Benahist 10; Benahist 50
 Benoject-10; Benoject-50
 Genahist
 Hydramyn*
 Hyrexin-50
 Tusstat*
 Wehdryl
**diphenidol HCl**
 Vontrol
**diphenoxylate HCl**
 Logen*
 Lomanate*
 Lomotil*
 Lonox*
**diphtheria & tetanus toxoids & acellular pertussis (DTaP) vaccine**
 Acel-Imune
 ActHIB/Tripedia*
 Certiva
 Infanrix
 TriHIBit
 Tripedia
**diphtheria & tetanus toxoids & whole-cell pertussis (DTwP) vaccine**
 Tetramune*
 Tri-Immunol
**dipivefrin HCl**
 AKPro
 Propine
**dipyridamole**
 Aggrenox*
 Persantine
 Persantine IV
**dirithromycin**
 Dynabac
**disaccharide tripeptide glycerol dipalmitoyl**
 ImmTher
**disodium clodronate tetrahydrate**
 Bonefos
**disopyramide phosphate**
 Napamide

---

*This brand is a combination product.

**Generic ♦ Brands**

**disopyramide phosphate (cont.)**
  Norpace
  Norpace CR
**disulfiram**
  Antabuse
**divalproex sodium**
  Depakote
  Epival ⓒ
**dobutamine HCl**
  Dobutrex
**docetaxel**
  Taxotere
*n*-docosanol
  Lidakol
**docusate sodium**
  Hem Fe*
  Nephron FA*
  Tabron*
  TriHemic 600*
**dolasetron mesylate**
  Anzemet
**domperidone maleate**
  Apo-Domperidone ⓒ
  Motilium ⓒ
  Novo-Domperidone ⓒ
**donepezil HCl**
  Aricept
**dopamine HCl**
  Intropin
**dornase alfa**
  Pulmozyme
**dorzolamide HCl**
  Cosopt*
  Trusopt
**dothiepin HCl**
  Prothiaden
**doxacurium chloride**
  Nuromax
**doxapram HCl**
  Dopram
**doxazosin mesylate**
  Cardura
**doxepin HCl**
  Adapin
  Sinequan
  Zonalon
**doxercalciferol**
  Hectorol
**doxorubicin**
  Evacet

**doxorubicin HCl**
  Adriamycin PFS
  Adriamycin RDF
  Doxil
  Rubex
**doxycycline**
  Monodox
  Vibramycin
**doxycycline calcium**
  Vibramycin
**doxycycline hyclate**
  Atridox
  Bio-Tab
  Doryx
  Doxy 100; Doxy 200
  Doxy Caps
  Doxychel Hyclate
  Periostat
  Vibra-Tabs
  Vibramycin
**dronabinol**
  Marinol
**droperidol**
  Inapsine
  Innovar*
**dyclonine HCl**
  Dyclone
**dyphylline**
  Dilor
  Dilor 400
  Dilor-G*
  Dy-G*
  Dyflex-200
  Dyflex-G*
  Dyline-GG*
  Lufyllin
  Lufyllin 400
  Lufyllin-EPG*
  Lufyllin-GG*
  Neothylline
  Neothylline-GG*
  Thylline-GG*
**echothiophate iodide**
  Phospholine Iodide
**econazole nitrate**
  Spectazole
**edetate calcium disodium**
  Calcium Disodium Versenate

*This brand is a combination product.

**edetate disodium**
  Disotate
  Endrate
**edrecolomab**
  Panorex
**edrophonium chloride**
  Enlon
  Enlon Plus*
  Reversol
  Tensilon
**efavirenz**
  Sustiva
**eflornithine HCl**
  Ornidyl
**electrolytes**
  Aminosyn 3.5% M; Aminosyn II
    3.5% M*
  Aminosyn 7% (8.5%) with Electro-
    lytes; Aminosyn II 7% (8.5%,
    10%) with Electrolytes*
  Aminosyn-HBC 7%*
  Aminosyn II 3.5% M in 5% Dex-
    trose; Aminosyn II 4.25% M in
    10% Dextrose*
  Co-Lav*
  5% Dextrose and Electrolyte #48; 5%
    Dextrose and Electrolyte #75; 10%
    Dextrose and Electrolyte #48*
  50% Dextrose with Electrolyte Pat-
    tern A (or N)*
  FreAmine HBC 6.9%*
  FreAmine III 3% (8.5%) with Elec-
    trolytes*
  Go-Evac*
  HepatAmine*
  Hyperlyte; Hyperlyte CR; Hyperlyte R
  Isolyte E (G; H; M; P; R; S) with
    5% Dextrose*
  Isolyte E; Isolyte S; Isolyte S pH 7.4
  Isolyte S pH 7.4
  Lypholyte; Lypholyte II
  Multilyte-20; Multilyte-40
  NephrAmine 5.4%*
  Normosol-M and 5% Dextrose; Nor-
    mosol-R and 5% Dextrose*
  Normosol-R; Normosol-R pH 7.4
  Nutrilyte; Nutrilyte II
  Plasma-Lyte A pH 7.4; Plasma-Lyte
    R; Plasma-Lyte 56; Plasma-Lyte 148

**electrolytes (cont.)**
  Plasma-Lyte M (R; 56; 148) and 5%
    Dextrose*
  ProcalAmine*
  RenAmin*
  TPN Electrolytes; TPN Electrolytes
    II; TPN Electrolytes III
  Tracelyte; Tracelyte II; Tracelyte
    with Double Electrolytes; Trace-
    lyte II with Double Electrolytes*
  Travasol 3.5% (5.5%, 8.5%) with
    Electrolytes*
  5% Travert and Electrolyte No. 2;
    10% Travert and Electrolyte No. 2*
**ELISA assay**
  OraSure HIV-1*
**embutramide**
  Embutane
  T-61
**emedastine difumarate**
  Emadine
**emtricitabine**
  Coviracil
**enalapril maleate**
  Lexxel*
  Teczem*
  Vaseretic 5-12.5; Vaseretic 10-25*
  Vasotec
**enalaprilat**
  Vasotec I.V.
**enflurane**
  Ethrane
**enoxacin**
  Penetrex
**enoxaparin sodium**
  Lovenox
**enprostil**
  Gardrin
**entacapone**
  Comtan
**ephedrine HCl**
  Broncholate*
  KIE*
  Lufyllin-EPG*
  Mudrane*
  Mudrane GG*
  Quadrinal*

*This brand is a combination product.

**Generic ◆ Brands**

**ephedrine sulfate**
Bronkotuss Expectorant*
Hydrophed*
Marax*
Marax-DF*
Theomax DF*
**ephedrine tannate**
Rentamine Pediatric*
Rynatuss*
Tri-Tannate Plus Pediatric*
**epinephrine**
AccuSite*
Ana-Guard
Ana-Kit*
Astracaine; Astracaine Forte (CAN)*
Citanest Forte*
Duranest; Duranest MPF*
EpiPen; EpiPen Jr.
IntraDose*
Marcaine with Epinephrine*
Octocaine HCl*
Sensorcaine*
Sensorcaine MPF*
Sus-Phrine
Xylocaine HCl*
Xylocaine MPF*
**epinephrine bitartrate**
E-Pilo-3*
E-Pilo-1; E-Pilo-2; E-Pilo-4; E-Pilo-6*
Marcaine HCl*
$P_1E_1$; $P_2E_1$; $P_4E_1$; $P_6E_1$*
$P_3E_1$*
**epinephrine borate**
Eppy/N 1%; Eppy/N 2%
**epinephrine HCl**
Adrenalin Chloride
Epifrin
Epinephrine Pediatric
Glaucon
**epinephryl borate**
Epinal
**epirubicin HCl**
Pharmorubicin PFS; Pharmorubicin RDF (CAN)
**epoetin alfa**
Epogen
Procrit
**epoetin beta**
Marogen

**epoprostenol**
Cyclo-Prostin
Flolan
**eptifibatide**
Integrilin
**ergocalciferol**
Calciferol
Drisdol
**ergoloid mesylates**
Gerimal
Hydergine
Hydergine LC
**ergonovine maleate**
Ergotrate Maleate
**ergotamine tartrate**
Bel-Phen-Ergot SR*
Bellacane SR*
Bellergal-S*
Cafatine*
Cafatine-PB*
Cafergot*
Cafetrate*
Ercaf*
Ergomar
Ergostat
Folergot-DF*
Phenerbel-S*
Wigraine*
**ersofermin**
Ossigel*
**erwinia L-asparaginase**
Erwinase
**erythrityl tetranitrate**
Cardilate
**erythromycin**
A/T/S
AK-Mycin
Akne-mycin
Benzamycin*
Del-Mycin
E-Base
E-Mycin
Emgel
Ery-Sol
Ery-Tab
ERYC
Erycette
EryDerm 2%

*This brand is a combination product.

**erythromycin (cont.)**
Erygel*
Erymax
Erythra-Derm
Ilotycin
PCE
Robimycin
Romycin
Staticin
T-Stat
Theramycin Z
**erythromycin estolate**
Ilosone
**erythromycin ethylsuccinate**
E.E.S.
E.E.S. 200
E.E.S. 400
EryPed
EryPed 200; EryPed 400
Eryzole*
Pediazole*
**erythromycin gluceptate**
Ilotycin Gluceptate
**erythromycin lactobionate**
Erythrocin
**erythromycin stearate**
Eramycin
Erythrocin Stearate
**esmolol HCl**
Brevibloc
**estazolam**
ProSom
**esterified estrogens**
Estratab
Estratest; Estratest H.S.*
Menest
Menogen; Menogen H.S.*
Menrium 5-2; Menrium 5-4; Menrium 10-4*
**estradiol**
Activelle*
Alora
Climara
CombiPatch*
Esclim
Estrace
Estraderm
Estring
FemPatch
Menorest

**estradiol (cont.)**
TheraDerm-MTX*
Vivelle; Vivelle-Dot
**estradiol cypionate**
Andro/Fem*
depAndrogyn*
depGynogen
Depo-Estradiol Cypionate
Depo-Testadiol*
DepoGen
Depotestogen*
Duo-Cyp*
Dura-Estrin
Duratestrin*
Estra-D
Estro-Cyp
Estroject-L.A.
Test-Estro Cypionates*
**estradiol hemihydrate**
Vagifem
**estradiol valerate**
Deladiol-40
Deladumone*
Delestrogen
Dioval XX; Dioval 40
Duragen-20; Duragen-40
Estra-L 20
Estra-L 40
Estra-Testrin*
Gynogen L.A. 20
Gynogen L.A. 40
Valergen 10
Valergen 20; Valergen 40
Valertest No. 1*
**estramustine phosphate sodium**
Emcyt
**estrogen**
E2III
Estrasorb
**estrone**
Aquest
Estrogenic Substance Aqueous
Estrone 5
Estrone Aqueous
Kestrone 5
Ogen
Ortho-Est
Theelin Aqueous

*This brand is a combination product.

**estrone (cont.)**
Wehgen
**estropipate**
Ogen
**etanercept**
Enbrel
**ethacrynate sodium**
Edecrin Sodium
**ethacrynic acid**
Edecrin
**ethambutol HCl**
Myambutol
**ethanolamine oleate**
Ethamolin
**ethaverine HCl**
Ethaquin
Ethatab
Ethavex-100
Isovex
**ethchlorvynol**
Placidyl
**ethinyl estradiol**
Alesse*
Brevicon*
Demulen 1/35; Demulen 1/50*
Desogen*
Diane-35 ⓒⒶⓃ*
Estinyl
Estrostep 21*
Estrostep Fe*
Genora 0.5/35; Genora 1/35*
Jenest-28*
Levlen*
Levlite 21; Levlite 28*
Levora*
Lo/Ovral*
Loestrin 21 1/20; Loestrin 21 1.5/30*
Loestrin Fe 1/20; Loestrin Fe 1.5/30*
Minesse*
Mircette*
Modicon*
N.E.E. 1/35*
Necon 0.5/35-21; Necon 0.5/35-28*
Necon 1/35-21; Necon 1/35-28*
Necon 10/11-21; Necon 10/11-28*
Nelova 1/35E; Nelova 0.5/35E*
Nelova 10/11*
Nordette*
Norethin 1/35E*
Norinyl 1 + 35*

**ethinyl estradiol (cont.)**
Ortho-Cept*
Ortho-Cyclen*
Ortho-Novum 1/35*
Ortho-Novum 10/11*
Ortho-Novum 7/7/7*
Ortho Tri-Cyclen*
Ovcon-35; Ovcon-50*
Ovral*
Preven*
Tri-Levlen*
Tri-Norinyl*
Triphasil*
Trivora-28*
Zovia*
**ethiodized oil**
Ethiodol
**ethionamide**
Trecator-SC
**ethopropazine HCl**
Parsidol
**ethosuximide**
Zarontin
**ethotoin**
Peganone
**ethyl chloride**
Fluro-Ethyl*
**ethyl dihydroxypropyl PABA**
Solaquin Forte*
**ethylnorepinephrine HCl**
Bronkephrine
**ethynodiol diacetate**
Demulen 1/35; Demulen 1/50*
Zovia*
**etidocaine**
Duranest; Duranest MPF*
**etidocaine HCl**
Duranest; Duranest MPF
**etidronate disodium**
Didronel
**etodolac**
Apo-Etodolac ⓒⒶⓃ
Lodine
Lodine XL
**etomidate**
Amidate
**etoposide**
Toposar*

*This brand is a combination product.

**etoposide (cont.)**
  VePesid
**etoposide phosphate diethanolate**
  Etopophos
**etretinate**
  Tegison
**exisulind**
  Prevatac
**extracts of honeybee, yellow
  jacket, yellow hornet, white-
  faced hornet, mixed vespid, and
  wasp venom**
  Albay
  Pharmalgen
  Venomil
**factor VIIa**
  NovoSeven
**factor XIII**
  Fibrogammin P
**famciclovir**
  Famvir
**famotidine**
  Pepcid
  Pepcid RPD
**fat emulsion**
  Intralipid 10%; Intralipid 20%
  Liposyn II 10%; Liposyn III 10%
  Liposyn II 20%; Liposyn III 20%
**felbamate**
  Felbatol
**felodipine**
  Lexxel*
  Plendil
**fenfluramine HCl**
  Pondimin
**fenleuton**
  LoFrin
**fenofibrate**
  Tricor
**fenoldopam mesylate**
  Corlopam
**fenoprofen calcium**
  Nalfon
**fenoterol hydrobromide**
  Berotec
**fentanyl**
  Duragesic-25; Duragesic-50; Dura-
    gesic-75; Duragesic-100
**fentanyl citrate**
  Actiq

**fentanyl citrate (cont.)**
  Fentanyl Oralet
  Innovar*
  Sublimaze
**ferric pyrophosphate**
  Senilezol*
  Vitafōl*
**ferristene**
  Dynospheres M-035
**ferrous fumarate**
  B-C with Folic Acid Plus*
  Berocca Plus*
  Berplex Plus*
  Cevi-Fer*
  Chromagen*
  Contrin*
  Estrostep Fe*
  Feocyte*
  Ferotrinsic*
  Foltrin*
  Formula B Plus*
  Fumatinic*
  Hem Fe*
  Hemocyte-F*
  Hemocyte Plus*
  Livitamin with Intrinsic Factor*
  Livitrinsic-f*
  Loestrin Fe 1/20; Loestrin Fe 1.5/30*
  Nephro-Fer Rx*
  Nephro-Vite Rx + Fe*
  Nephron FA*
  Nestabs FA*
  Pronemia Hematinic*
  Tabron*
  Theragran Hematinic*
  Tri-Tinic*
  TriHemic 600*
  Trinsicon*
  Vitafōl; Vitafōl-PN*
  Zodeac-100*
**ferrous gluconate**
  Co Tinic*
  Feocyte*
  Fergon Plus*
  Forte L.I.V.*
  Hemocyte*
  Hemocyte-V*
  Hytinic*

*This brand is a combination product.

**ferrous gluconate (cont.)**
  Licoplex DS*
**ferrous sulfate**
  Feocyte*
  Fero-Folic-500*
  Florvite + Iron*
  Florvite + Iron; Half Strength
    Florvite + Iron*
  Heptuna Plus*
  Iberet-Folic-500*
  Multibret-500 Hematinic*
  Multibret-Folic-500*
  Vi-Daylin/F ADC + Iron*
  Vi-Daylin/F Multivitamin + Iron*
**ferucarbotran**
  Resovist
**ferumoxides**
  Feridex
**ferumoxsil**
  GastroMARK
**ferumoxtran-10**
  Combidex
**fexofenadine HCl**
  Allegra
  Allegra-D*
**fibrinolysin**
  Elase*
  Elase-Chloromycetin*
**filgrastim**
  Neupogen
**finasteride**
  Propecia
  Proscar
**flavoxate HCl**
  Urispas
**flecainide acetate**
  Tambocor
**floxuridine**
  FUDR
**fluconazole**
  Diflucan
**flucytosine**
  Ancobon
**fludarabine phosphate**
  Fludara
**fludrocortisone acetate**
  Florinef Acetate
**flumazenil**
  Romazicon

**flumecinol**
  Zixoryn
**flunarizine HCl**
  Sibelium
**flunisolide**
  AeroBid; AeroBid-M
  Bronalide ⓒⒶⓃ
  Nasalide
  Nasarel
**fluocinolone acetonide**
  Derma-Smoothe/FS
  Fluonid
  Flurosyn
  FS Shampoo
  Neo-Synalar*
  Synalar
  Synalar-HP
  Synemol
**fluocinonide**
  Fluonex
  Lidex
  Lidex-E
  Vasoderm; Vasoderm-E
**fluorescein**
  AK-Fluor
**fluorescein sodium**
  Flu-Oxinate*
  Fluor-I-Strip; Fluor-I-Strip A.T.
  Fluoracaine*
  Fluorescite
  Flurate*
  Fluress*
  Ful-Glo
  Funduscein-10; Funduscein-25
  Healon Yellow*
  Ophthifluor
**fluorexon**
  Fluoresoft
**fluoride**
  ADC with Fluoride*
  Adeflor M*
  Apatate with Fluoride*
  Chewable Multivitamins with Fluoride*
  Chewable Triple Vitamins with Fluoride*
  Multivitamin with Fluoride*
  Mulvidren-F*

---

*This brand is a combination product.

**fluoride (cont.)**
Polytabs-F*
Polyvitamin Fluoride*
Polyvitamin Fluoride with Iron*
Polyvitamins with Iron and Fluoride*
Polyvitamins with Fluoride and Iron*
Soluvite C.T.*
Soluvite-f*
Tri-A-Vite F*
Tri-Flor-Vite with Fluoride*
Tri Vit with Fluoride*
Tri-Vitamin with Fluoride*
Triple Vitamin ADC with Fluoride*
Triple Vitamins with Fluoride*
Trivitamin Fluoride*
**fluorometholone**
Fluor-Op
FML-S*
FML S.O.P.
FML; FML Forte
**fluorometholone acetate**
Eflone
Flarex
**fluorouracil**
AccuSite*
Adrucil
Efudex
Fluoroplex
**fluoxetine HCl**
Prozac
**fluoxymesterone**
Halotestin
**fluphenazine decanoate**
Modecate (CAN)
PMS-Fluphenazine (CAN)
Prolixin Decanoate
Rho-Fluphenazine (CAN)
**fluphenazine enanthate**
Moditen Enanthate (CAN)
Prolixin Enanthate
**fluphenazine HCl**
Apo-Fluphenazine (CAN)
Moditen HCl (CAN)
Permitil
Prolixin
**flurandrenolide**
Cordran
Cordran SP
**flurazepam HCl**
Dalmane

**flurbiprofen**
Ansaid
**flurbiprofen sodium**
Ocufen
**flutamide**
Euflex (CAN)
Eulexin
**fluticasone propionate**
Advair*
Cutivate
Flonase
Flovent
**fluvastatin sodium**
Lescol
**fluvoxamine maleate**
Luvox
**folic acid**
B-C with Folic Acid*
B-C with Folic Acid Plus*
B-Plex*
Bacmin*
Berocca*
Berocca Parenteral Nutrition*
Berocca Plus*
Berplex Plus*
Cefol*
Cernevit-12*
Cevi-Fer*
Cezin-S*
Chewable Multivitamins with Fluo-ride*
Contrin*
Eldercaps*
Feocyte*
Fero-Folic-500*
Ferotrinsic*
Filibon F.A.; Filibon Forte*
Florvite + Iron; Half Strength Florvite + Iron*
Florvite; Florvite Half Strength*
Foltrin*
Folvite
Formula B*
Formula B Plus*
Fumatinic*
Hemocyte-F*
Hemocyte Plus*
Iberet-Folic-500*

*This brand is a combination product.

**folic acid (cont.)**
Lactocal-F*
Liver Combo No. 5*
Livitrinsic-f*
M.V.C. 9+3*
M.V.C. 9+4 Pediatric*
M.V.I. Pediatric*
M.V.I.-12*
Marnatal-F*
Materna*
May-Vita*
Megaton*
Mission Prenatal Rx*
Multibret-Folic-500*
Mynatal*
Mynatal FC*
Mynatal P.N.*
Mynatal P.N. Forte*
Mynatal Rx*
Mynate 90 Plus*
Natabec Rx*
Natafort*
NatalCare Plus*
Natalins Rx*
Natarex Prenatal*
Nephlex Rx*
Nephro-Fer Rx*
Nephro-Vite Rx + Fe*
Nephro-Vite Rx*
Nephrocaps*
Nephron FA*
Nestabs FA*
Niferex Forte*
Niferex-PN*
Niferex-PN Forte*
Niferex-150 Forte*
Norlac Rx*
Nu-Iron Plus*
Nu-Iron V*
O-Cal f.a.*
Par-F*
Par-Natal Plus 1 Improved*
Poly-Vi-Flor*
Poly-Vi-Flor with Iron*
Polytabs-F*
Polyvitamin Fluoride*
Polyvitamin Fluoride with Iron*
Polyvitamins with Fluoride and Iron*
Pramet FA*
Pramilet FA*

**folic acid (cont.)**
Pre-H Cal*
Prenatal H.P.*
Prenatal Maternal*
Prenatal MR 90*
Prenatal One*
Prenatal Plus Iron*
Prenatal Plus with Betacarotene*
Prenatal Plus; Prenatal Plus
    Improved*
Prenatal Rx*
Prenatal Rx with Betacarotene*
Prenatal Z*
Prenatal-1 + Iron*
Prenate 90; Prenate Ultra*
Pronemia Hematinic*
Secran Prenatal*
Soluvite C.T.*
Strovite*
Strovite Plus; Strovite Forte*
Stuartnatal Plus*
Tabron*
Theragran Hematinic*
Tri-Tinic*
TriHemic 600*
Trinsicon*
Vi-Daylin/F Multivitamin + Iron*
Vi-Daylin/F Multivitamin*
Vicon Forte*
Vitafōl*
Vitafōl; Vitafōl-PN*
Zenate, Advanced Formula*
Zincvit*
Zodeac-100*
**follitropin alfa**
Gonal-F
**follitropin beta**
Follistim
Puregon (CAN)
**fomepizole**
Antizol
**fomivirsen sodium**
Vitravene
**formaldehyde**
Formalyde-10
Lazer Formalyde
**formoterol fumarate**
Foradil (CAN)

*This brand is a combination product.

**formoterol fumarate (cont.)**
Oxeze (CAN)
**foscarnet sodium**
Foscavir
**fosfomycin tromethamine**
Monurol
**fosinopril sodium**
Monopril
**fosphenytoin sodium**
Cerebyx
**frovatriptan succinate**
Miguard
**fructose-1,6-diphosphate**
Cordox
**furazolidone**
Furoxone
**furosemide**
Lasix
**gabapentin**
Neurontin
**gadodiamide**
Omniscan
**gadopentetate dimeglumine**
Magnevist
**gadoteridol**
ProHance
**galactose**
Echovist (CAN)
Levovist (CAN)
**galantamine**
Reminyl
**gallamine triethiodide**
Flaxedil
**gallium nitrate**
Ganite
**ganciclovir**
Cytovene
Vitrasert
**ganciclovir sodium**
Cytovene
**gatifloxacin**
Tequin
**gemcitabine HCl**
Gemzar
**gemfibrozil**
Apo-Gemfibrozil (CAN)
Gemcor
Lopid
Novo-Gemfibrozil (CAN)

**gentamicin sulfate**
G-myticin
Garamycin
Garamycin Pediatric
Genoptic
Genoptic S.O.P.
Gentacidin
Gentak
Jenamicin
Maitec
Pred-G*
Pred-G S.O.P.*
Septopal
**gestodene**
Minesse*
**glatiramer acetate**
Copaxone
**glimepiride**
Amaryl
**glipizide**
Glucotrol
Glucotrol XL
**glucagon**
GlucaGen Diagnostic Kit
GlucaGen Emergency Kit
Glucagon Diagnostic Kit
Glucagon Emergency Kit
**D-gluconic acid lactone**
Renacidin*
**glucono-delta-lactone**
Renacidin Irrigation*
**glucose**
Glucose-40
Xylocaine MPF*
**L-glutathione**
Cachexon
**glyburide**
Diaβeta (or DiaBeta)
Euglucon (CAN)
Glynase
Micronase
Micronized Glyburide
**glycerin**
Ophthalgan
Osmoglyn
**glycopyrrolate**
Robinul
Robinul Forte

---

*This brand is a combination product.

**gold sodium thiomalate**
Aurolate
Myochrysine
**gonadorelin acetate**
Lutrepulse
**gonadorelin HCl**
Factrel
**goserelin acetate**
Zoladex
**gp160 antigens**
VaxSyn HIV-1
**graftskin**
Apligraf
**gramicidin**
AK-Spore*
Neosporin*
Ocutricin*
**granisetron HCl**
Kytril
**grepafloxacin HCl**
Raxar
**griseofulvin**
Fulvicin P/G
Fulvicin U/F
Grifulvin V
Gris-PEG
Grisactin 500
Grisactin Ultra
Grisactin; Grisactin 250
**guaifenesin**
Ami-Tex LA*
Anatuss*
Anatuss LA*
Asbron-G*
Atuss EX*
Atuss G*
Banex*
Bronchial*
Broncholate*
Brondelate*
Bronkotuss Expectorant*
Brontex*
Calmylin Codeine ⓒ*
Cheracol Cough*
Co-Tuss V*
Codegest Expectorant*
Codiclear DH*
Coldloc*
Coldloc-LA*
Conex with Codeine*

**Generic ◆ Brands**

**guaifenesin (cont.)**
Congess JR*
Congess SR*
Contuss*
Cophene XP*
Cotridin Expectorant ⓒ*
Cyclofed Pediatric*
Cycofed Pediatric*
Deconamine CX*
Decongestant Expectorant*
Deconsal II*
Deconsal Pediatric*
Deconsal Sprinkle*
Defen-LA*
Deproist Expectorant with Codeine*
Despec*
Detussin Expectorant*
Dihistine Expectorant*
Dilaudid Cough*
Dilor-G*
Donatussin*
Donatussin DC*
Dura-Gest*
Dura-Vent*
Duratuss*
Duratuss-G
Duratuss HD*
Dy-G*
Dyflex-G*
Dyline-GG*
Elixophyllin GG*
Endal*
Endal Expectorant*
Enomine*
Entex*
Entex LA*
Entex PSE*
Entuss-D*
Entuss-D Jr.*
Entuss Expectorant*
Eudal-SR*
Exgest LA*
Fenesin
Fenesin DM*
Glyceryl-T*
GP-500*
Guai-Vent/PSE*
Guaifed*

*This brand is a combination product.

**guaifenesin (cont.)**
 Guaifed-PD*
 Guaifenex*
 Guaifenex DM*
 Guaifenex LA
 Guaifenex PPA 75*
 Guaifenex PSE 60; Guaifenex PSE
    120; Guaifenex Rx DM*
 Guaifenex Rx*
 GuaiMAX-D*
 Guaipax*
 Guaitex*
 Guaitex LA*
 Guaitex PSE*
 Guaivent*
 Guaivent PD*
 Guiatex LA*
 Guiatex PSE*
 Guiatuss AC*
 Guiatuss DAC*
 Guiatussin DAC*
 Guiatussin with Codeine Expecto-
    rant*
 Guipax*
 Histalet X*
 Humibid DM*
 Humibid DM Sprinkle*
 Humibid L.A.
 Humibid Sprinkle
 HycoClear Tuss*
 Hycotuss Expectorant*
 Hydrocodone GF*
 Iobid DM*
 Iosal II*
 Isoclor Expectorant*
 Kwelcof*
 Liquibid-D*
 Liquibid; Liquibid-1200
 Lufyllin-EPG*
 Lufyllin-GG*
 MED-Rx*
 MED-Rx DM*
 Monafed
 Monafed DM*
 Muco-Fen-DM*
 Muco-Fen-LA
 Mudrane GG*
 Mudrane GG-2*
 Mytussin AC Cough*
 Mytussin DAC*

**guaifenesin (cont.)**
 Naldecon CX Adult*
 Nasabid*
 Nasabid SR*
 Nasatab LA*
 Neothylline-GG*
 Norel*
 Novagest Expectorant with
    Codeine*
 Novahistine Expectorant*
 Nucofed Expectorant; Nucofed
    Pediatric Expectorant*
 Organidin NR
 P-V-Tussin*
 Panmist JR*
 Partuss LA*
 Phenhist Expectorant*
 Phenylfenesin L.A.*
 Pneumomist
 Pneumotussin HC*
 Polaramine Expectorant*
 Profen II DM*
 Profen II; Profen LA*
 Protuss DM*
 Quibron; Quibron-300*
 Respa-DM*
 Respa-GF
 Respa-1st*
 Respaire-60; Respaire-120*
 Robafen AC Cough*
 Robafen DAC*
 Robitussin A-C*
 Robitussin-DAC*
 Ru-Tuss DE*
 Rymed*
 Rymed-TR*
 Ryna-CX*
 Sil-Tex*
 Sinufed*
 Sinumist-SR
 Sinupan*
 SinuVent*
 Slo-phyllin GG*
 SRC Expectorant*
 Stamoist E*
 Stamoist LA*
 Statuss Expectorant*
 Sudal 120/600*

*This brand is a combination product.

**guaifenesin (cont.)**
Sudal 60/500*
Sudex*
Syn-Rx*
Synophylate-GG*
Theolate*
Thylline-GG*
Touro Ex
Touro LA*
Triaminic Expectorant DH*
Triaminic Expectorant with
    Codeine*
Tuss-LA*
Tussafed HC*
Tussafin Expectorant*
Tussanil DH*
Tussar SF; Tussar-2*
Tussi-Organidin DM NR; Tussi-
    Organidin DM-S NR*
Tussi-Organidin NR; Tussi-Organi-
    din-S NR*
ULR-LA*
V-Dec-M*
Vanex Expectorant*
Vanex-LA*
Versacaps*
Vicodin Tuss*
Zephrex*
Zephrex LA*
**guanabenz acetate**
Wytensin
**guanadrel sulfate**
Hylorel
**guanethidine monosulfate**
Esimil*
Ismelin
**guanfacine HCl**
Tenex
**halazepam**
Paxipam
**halcinonide**
Halog
Halog-E
**halobetasol propionate**
Ultravate
**halofantrine HCl**
Halfan
**haloperidol**
Haldol

**haloperidol decanoate**
Haldol Decanoate 50; Haldol Deca-
    noate 100
Haloperidol LA ⓒⒶⓃ
**haloperidol lactate**
Haldol
PMS-Haloperidol; PMS-Haloperidol
    LA ⓒⒶⓃ
**haloprogin**
Halotex
**halothane**
Fluothane
**hamamelis water**
Succus Cineraria Maritima*
**heme arginate**
Normosang
**hemin**
Hemex*
Panhematin
**Hemophilus b conjugate vaccine**
ActHIB*
ActHIB/Tripedia*
HibTITER
OmniHIB*
PedvaxHIB
ProHIBiT
Tetramune*
**Hemophilus b purified capsular
    polysaccharide**
Comvax*
**heparin, 2-0-desulfated**
Aeropin
**heparin calcium**
Calciparine
**heparin sodium**
Hep-Lock; Hep-Lock U/P
Heparin Lock Flush
Liquaemin Sodium
**hepatitis A vaccine**
Havrix
Vaqta
**hepatitis B immune globulin**
H-BIG
Hep-B-Gammagee
HyperHep
Nabi-HB
**hepatitis B virus vaccine**
Comvax*

*This brand is a combination product.

**hepatitis B virus vaccine (cont.)**
  Engerix-B
  Recombivax HB
**hetastarch**
  Hespan
**hexachlorophene**
  pHisoHex
  Septisol*
**hexoprenaline sulfate**
  Delaprem
**histoplasmin**
  Histolyn-CYL
**histrelin acetate**
  Supprelin
**HIV-1 immunogen, gp120-depleted**
  Remune
**HIV immune globulin**
  HIV-IG
**HIV immunotherapeutic**
  Retrovector
**homatropine hydrobromide**
  AK-Homatropine
  Hydrocodone Compound*
  Isopto Homatropine
**homatropine methylbromide**
  Gustase Plus*
  Hycodan*
  Hydromet*
  Tussigon*
**human albumin**
  Albuminar-5; Albuminar-25
  Albutein 5%; Albutein 25%
  Buminate 5%; Buminate 25%
  Plasbumin-5; Plasbumin-25
**human albumin, sonicated**
  Albunex
**human hemoglobin**
  Optro
  PolyHeme
**hyaluronate sodium**
  AMO Vitrax
  Amvisc; Amvisc Plus
  Healon Yellow*
  Healon; Healon GV
  Hyalgan
  Hyanalgese-D*
  Ossigel*
  Solarase*
  Staarvisc
  Viscoat*

**hyaluronidase**
  Wydase
**hydralazine HCl**
  Apresazide 25/25; Apresazide 50/50;
    Apresazide 100/50*
  Apresoline
  Aprozide 25/25; Aprozide 50/50;
    Aprozide 100/50*
  Cam-Ap-Es*
  Hydrap-ES*
  Hydrazide 25/25; Hydrazide 50/50*
  Marpres*
  Ser-Ap-Es*
  Serpazide*
  Tri-Hydroserpine*
  Unipres*
**hydriodic acid**
  Bronkotuss Expectorant*
**hydrochlorothiazide**
  Accuretic ⒸⒶⓃ*
  Aldactazide*
  Aldoril 15; Aldoril 25; Aldoril D30;
    Aldoril D50*
  Alodopa-15; Alodopa-25*
  Apresazide 25/25; Apresazide 50/50;
    Apresazide 100/50*
  Aprozide 25/25; Aprozide 50/50;
    Aprozide 100/50*
  Avalide*
  Cam-Ap-Es*
  Capozide 25/15; Capozide 25/25;
    Capozide 50/15; Capozide 50/25*
  Diovan HCT*
  Dyazide*
  Esidrix
  Esimil*
  Ezide
  Hydrap-ES*
  Hydrazide 25/25; Hydrazide 50/50*
  Hydro-Par
  Hydro-Serp*
  HydroDIURIL
  Hydropres-25*
  Hydropres-50*
  Hydroserpine #1; Hydroserpine #2*
  Hydrosine 25, Hydrosine 50*
  Hyzaar*
  Inderide 40/25; Inderide 80/25*

*This brand is a combination product.

## hydrochlorothiazide (cont.)

Inderide LA 80/50; Inderide LA 120/50; Inderide LA 160/50*
Lopressor HCT 50/25; Lopressor HCT 100/25; Lopressor HCT 100/50*
Lotensin HCT 5/6.25; Lotensin HCT 10/12.5; Lotensin HCT 20/12.5; Lotensin HCT 20/25*
Marpres*
Maxzide*
Microzide
Moduretic*
Oretic
Prinzide*
Prinzide 12.5; Prinzide 25*
Ser-Ap-Es*
Serpazide*
Timolide 10-25*
Tri-Hydroserpine*
Unipres*
Uniretic*
Vaseretic 5-12.5; Vaseretic 10-25*
Zestoretic*
Ziac*

## hydrocodone bitartrate

Alor 5/500*
Amacodone*
Anaplex HD*
Anexsia 5/500; Anexsia 7.5/650; Anexsia 10/660*
Atuss EX*
Atuss G*
Atuss HD*
Azdone*
Bancap HC*
Ceta Plus*
Chlorgest-HD*
Co-Gesic*
Co-Tuss V*
Codamine*
Codiclear DH*
Codimal DH*
Cophene XP*
Damason-P*
Deconamine CX*
Detussin*
Detussin Expectorant*
Dolacet*
Dolfen*
Donatussin DC*

## hydrocodone bitartrate (cont.)

Duocet*
Duratuss HD*
ED-TLC; ED Tuss HC*
Endagen-HD*
Endal-HD; Endal-HD Plus*
Entuss-D*
Entuss-D Jr.*
Entuss Expectorant*
H-Tuss-D*
Histinex HC*
Histinex PV*
Histussin D*
Histussin HC*
Hy-Phen*
HycoClear Tuss*
Hycodan*
Hycomine*
Hycomine Compound*
Hycotuss Expectorant*
Hydrocet*
Hydrocodone Compound*
Hydrocodone CP; Hydrocodone HD*
Hydrocodone GF*
Hydrocodone PA*
Hydrogesic*
Hydromet*
Hyphed*
Iodal HD*
Iotussin HC*
Kwelcof*
Lorcet*
Lorcet-HD*
Lorcet Plus; Lorcet 10/650*
Lortab*
Lortab 2.5/500; Lortab 5/500; Lortab 7.5/500; Lortab 10/500*
Lortab ASA*
Marcof Expectorant*
Margesic H*
Medipain 5*
Norcet*
Norco*
Oncet*
P-V-Tussin*
Panacet 5/500*
Panasal 5/500*
Pancof-HC*

*This brand is a combination product.

**hydrocodone bitartrate (cont.)**
    Para-Hist HD*
    Pneumotussin HC*
    Protuss*
    Protuss-D*
    Rolatuss with Hydrocodone*
    Ru-Tuss with Hydrocodone*
    S-T Forte 2*
    SRC Expectorant*
    Stagesic*
    Statuss Green*
    T-Gesic*
    Triaminic Expectorant DH*
    Tussafed HC*
    Tussafin Expectorant*
    Tussanil DH*
    Tussend*
    Tussgen*
    Tussigon*
    Unituss HC*
    Vanex Expectorant*
    Vanex-HD*
    Vetuss HC*
    Vicodin Tuss*
    Vicodin; Vicodin ES; Vicodin HP*
    Vicoprofen*
    Zydone*
**hydrocodone polistirex**
    Tussionex Pennkinetic*
**hydrocortisone**
    AA-HC Otic*
    Acetasol HC*
    Acticort 100
    Aeroseb-HC
    AK-Spore H.C.*
    Ala-Cort
    Ala-Quin*
    Ala-Scalp
    AntibiŌtic*
    Antibiotic Ear Solution*
    Antibiotic Ear Suspension*
    Anusol-HC
    Bacticort*
    Cetacort
    Cipro HC Otic*
    Corque*
    Cort-Dome
    Cortatrigen Modified*
    Cortef
    Cortenema

**hydrocortisone (cont.)**
    Cortic*
    Cortin*
    Cortisporin*
    Cortisporin Otic*
    Dermacort
    Dermol HC
    Drotic*
    Ear-Eze*
    Eldecort
    1+1-F Creme*
    Fungoid-HC*
    1% HC
    Hi-Cor 1.0; Hi-Cor 2.5
    Hycort
    HydroTex
    Hydrocort
    Hydrocortone
    Hytone
    Hytone 1%
    LactiCare-HC
    LazerSporin-C*
    Neo-Cortef*
    Nutracort
    Octicare*
    Oti-Med*
    Otic-Care*
    OtiTricin*
    Otobiotic Otic*
    Otocort*
    Otomar-HC*
    Otomycet-HC*
    Otomycin-HPN Otic*
    Otosporin*
    Pedi-Cort V Creme*
    Pediotic*
    Pedotic*
    Penecort
    Proctocort
    S-T Cort
    Synacort
    Texacort
    Tri-Otic*
    UAD*
    UAD Otic*
    VōSol HC Otic*
    Vanoxide-HC*
    Vasotate HC*

*This brand is a combination product.

**hydrocortisone (cont.)**
Vytone*
Zoto-HC*
**hydrocortisone acetate**
Analpram-HC*
Anucort HC
Anumed HC
Anuprep HC
Anusol-HC
Anusol-HC 1
Carmol HC*
Chloromycetin Hydrocortisone*
Coly-Mycin S Otic*
Coracin*
Cort-Dome High Potency
Cortifoam
Cortisporin*
Cortisporin-TC*
Enzone*
Epifoam*
Hemorrhoidal HC
Hemril-HC
Hydrocortone Acetate
Lida-Mantle-HC*
Mantadil*
Neotricin HC*
Ophthocort*
Orabase HCA
Pramosone*
Pramoxine HC*
ProctoCream-HC
ProctoCream-HC*
Proctofoam-HC*
Rectacort
Terra-Cortril*
U-Cort
Zone-A Forte*
**hydrocortisone butyrate**
Locoid
**hydrocortisone probutate**
Pandel
**hydrocortisone sodium phosphate**
Hydrocortone Phosphate
**hydrocortisone sodium succinate**
A-Hydrocort
Solu-Cortef
**hydrocortisone valerate**
Westcort
**hydrodocone bitartrate**
Tyrodone*

**hydroflumethiazide**
Diucardin
Salazide; Salazide-Demi*
Saluron
Salutensin; Salutensin-Demi*
**hydromorphone HCl**
Dilaudid
Dilaudid Cough*
Dilaudid-HP
HydroStat IR
**hydroquinone**
Lustra
Melanex
Melpaque HP
Melquin HP
Nuquin HP*
Solaquin Forte*
Viquin Forte*
**hydroxocobalamin**
Hydro Cobex
Hydro-Crysti 12
Hydrobexan
LA-12
**hydroxyamphetamine hydrobro-**
**mide**
Paredrine
Paremyd*
**hydroxychloroquine sulfate**
Plaquenil Sulfate
**hydroxyprogesterone caproate**
Duralutin
Hylutin
Hyprogest 250
**hydroxypropyl methylcellulose**
Occucoat
**hydroxyurea**
Hydrea
**hydroxyzine HCl**
Anxanil
Atarax
Atarax 100
E-Vista
Hydrophed*
Hyzine-50
Marax-DF*
Quiess
Rezine
Theomax DF*

*This brand is a combination product.

**hydroxyzine HCl (cont.)**
  Vistacon
  Vistaject-25; Vistaject-50
  Vistaquel 50
  Vistaril
  Vistazine 50
**hydroxyzine pamoate**
  Vistaril
**hylan G-F 20**
  Synvisc
**hyoscyamine**
  Urisedamine*
**hyoscyamine hydrobromide**
  Barbidonna*
  Barbidonna; Barbidonna No. 2*
  Donna-Sed*
  Donnamor*
  Donnapine*
  Hyosophen*
  Kinesed*
  Malatal*
  Pyridium Plus*
  Relaxadon*
  Spasmolin*
  Spasmophen*
  Spasquid*
  Susano*
**hyoscyamine sulfate**
  A-Spas S/L
  Anaspaz
  Antispasmodic*
  Arco-Lase Plus*
  Atrohist Plus*
  Atrosept*
  Barophen*
  Bellacane*
  Cystospaz
  Cystospaz-M
  Deconhist L.A.*
  Dolsed*
  Donnamar
  Donnatal*
  Donnatal No. 2*
  Ed-Spaz
  Gastrosed
  Kutrase*
  Levbid
  Levsin
  Levsin PB*
  Levsin-PB*

**hyoscyamine sulfate (cont.)**
  Levsin with Phenobarbital*
  Levsin/SL
  Levsinex
  Phenahist-TR*
  Phenchlor S.H.A.*
  Prosed/DS*
  Ru-Tuss*
  Stahist*
  Trac Tabs 2X*
  UAA*
  Uridon Modified*
  Urimar-T*
  Urinary Antiseptic No. 2*
  Urised*
  Uritin*
  Urogesic Blue*
**hypericin**
  VIMRxyn
**ibandronate sodium**
  Bondronat
  Bonviva
**ibuprofen**
  Ibu
  Ibu-Tab
  Ibuprohm
  Motrin
  Rufen
  Saleto-400; Saleto-600; Saleto-800
  Salprofen
  Vicoprofen*
**ibutilide fumarate**
  Corvert
**icodextrin**
  Extraneal Peritoneal Dialysis Solution
**idarubicin HCl**
  Idamycin
  Idamycin PFS
**idoxuridine**
  Herplex
**ifosfamide**
  Ifex
**IGF-BP3 complex**
  SomatoKine
**ilomastat**
  Galardin
**iloperidone**
  Zomaril

*This brand is a combination product.

**Generic ♦ Brands**

**imciromab pentetate**
  Myoscint
**imiglucerase**
  Cerezyme
**imipenem**
  Primaxin I.M.*
  Primaxin I.V.*
**imipramine HCl**
  Janimine
  Tofranil
**imipramine pamoate**
  Tofranil-PM
**imiquimod**
  Aldara
**immune globulin**
  Gamastan
  Gamimune N
  Gammagard S/D
  Gammar
  Gammar-IV
  Gammar-P IV
  Iveegam
  Polygam
  Polygam S/D
  Sandoglobulin
  Venoglobulin-I
  Venoglobulin-S
**indapamide**
  Lozol
**indinavir sulfate**
  Crixivan
**indium In 111 IGIV pentetate**
  Macroscint
**indium In 111 pentetreotide**
  OctreoScan 111
**indium In 111 satumomab pende-tide**
  OncoScint CR/OV
**indocyanine green**
  Cardio-Green (CG)
**indomethacin**
  Indochron E-R
  Indocin
  Indocin SR
**indomethacin sodium trihydrate**
  Indocin I.V.
**infliximab**
  Remicade
**influenza vaccine**
  Fluogen

**influenza vaccine (cont.)**
  FluShield
  Fluvirin
  Fluzone
  Vaxigrip (CAN)
**inosine pranobex**
  Isoprinosine
**inositol**
  Amino-Cerv pH 5.5*
**insulin**
  Regular Iletin II U-500 (concentrated)
**insulin aspart**
  NovoRapid
**insulin lispro**
  Humalog
**interferon alfa**
  Omniferon
  Veldona
**interferon alfa-2a**
  Roferon-A
**interferon alfa-2b**
  Intron A
  Rebetron*
**interferon alfa-n1**
  Wellferon
  Wellferon (CAN)
**interferon alfa-n3**
  Alferon LDO
  Alferon N
**interferon alfacon-1**
  Infergen
**interferon beta**
  r-IFN-beta
**interferon beta-1a**
  Avonex
  R-Frone
  Rebif (CAN)
**interferon beta-1b**
  Betaseron
**interferon gamma-1b**
  Actimmune
**interleukin**
  MultiKine*
**interleukin-4 receptor**
  Nuvance

*This brand is a combination product.

**intravascular perfluorochemical (PFC) emulsion**
Fluosol
**intrinsic factor concentrate**
Chromagen*
Contrin*
Fergon Plus*
Ferotrinsic*
Foltrin*
Heptuna Plus*
Livitamin with Intrinsic Factor*
Livitrinsic-f*
Pronemia Hematinic*
Tri-Tinic*
TriHemic 600*
Trinsicon*
**invert sugar**
Travert
5% Travert and Electrolyte No. 2;
10% Travert and Electrolyte No. 2*
**iocetamic acid**
Cholebrine
**iodamide meglumine**
Renovue-Dip; Renovue-65
**iodinated glycerol**
Iophen
Iophen-C*
Iophen-DM*
Iophylline*
Par Glycerol
R-Gen
Theo-Organidin*
Tusso-DM*
**iodine**
Lugol*
Strong Iodine*
**iodine I 131 Lym-1 MAb**
Oncolym
**iodine I 131 murine MAb IgG$_2$a to B cell**
ImmuRAIT-LL2
**iodine I 131 tositumomab**
Bexxar
**iodipamide meglumine**
Cholografin Meglumine
Sinografin*
**iodixanol**
Visipaque
**iodoquinol**
Vytone*

**iodoquinol (cont.)**
Yodoxin
**iohexol**
Omnipaque
**iopamidol**
Isovue-M 200; Isovue-M 300
Isovue-128; Isovue-200; Isovue-250;
Isovue-300; Isovue-370
**iopanoic acid**
Telepaque
**iopromide**
Ultravist
**iothalamate meglumine**
Conray; Conray 30; Conray 43
Cysto-Conray; Cysto-Conray II
Vascoray*
**iothalamate sodium**
Angio-Conray
Conray 325
Conray 400
Vascoray*
**iotrolan**
Osmovist
**ioversol**
Optiray 160; Optiray 240; Optiray
300; Optiray 320; Optiray 350
**ioxaglate meglumine**
Hexabrix*
**ioxaglate sodium**
Hexabrix*
**ipodate calcium**
Oragrafin Calcium
**ipodate sodium**
Bilivist
Oragrafin Sodium
**ipratropium bromide**
Apo-Ipravent ⓒᴬᴺ
Atrovent
Combivent*
**irbesartan**
Avalide*
Avapro
**irinotecan HCl**
Camptosar
**iron**
Adeflor M*
Bacmin*
Filibon F.A.; Filibon Forte*

*This brand is a combination product.

**iron (cont.)**
Lactocal-F*
Marnatal-F*
Materna*
Mission Prenatal Rx*
Mynatal*
Mynatal FC*
Mynatal P.N.*
Mynatal P.N. Forte*
Mynatal Rx*
Mynate 90 Plus*
Natabec Rx*
Natafort*
NatalCare Plus*
Natalins Rx*
Natarex Prenatal*
Norlac Rx*
O-Cal f.a.*
Par-F*
Par-Natal Plus 1 Improved*
Poly-Vi-Flor with Iron*
Polyvitamin Fluoride with Iron*
Polyvitamin with Iron and Fluoride*
Polyvitamins with Fluoride and Iron*
Pramet FA*
Pramilet FA*
Pre-H Cal*
Prenatal H.P.*
Prenatal Maternal*
Prenatal MR 90*
Prenatal One*
Prenatal Plus Iron*
Prenatal Plus with Betacarotene*
Prenatal Plus; Prenatal Plus
    Improved*
Prenatal Rx*
Prenatal Rx with Betacarotene*
Prenatal Z*
Prenatal-1 + Iron*
Prenate 90; Prenate Ultra*
Secran Prenatal*
Stuartnatal Plus*
Tri-Vi-Flor with Iron*
Zenate, Advanced Formula*
**iron dextran**
DexFerrum
Dexiron ⒸⒶⓃ
InFeD
Infurfer ⒸⒶⓃ

**isocarboxazid**
Marplan
**isoetharine HCl**
Beta-2
Bronkosol
**isoetharine mesylate**
Bronkometer
**isoflurane**
Forane
**isoflurophate**
Floropryl
**isoleucine**
VIL*
**isometheptene mucate**
Isocom*
Isopap*
Midchlor*
Midrin*
Migratine*
**isoniazid**
Laniazid
Laniazid C.T.
Nydrazid
Rifamate*
Rifater*
Rimactane/INH*
**isopropyl alcohol**
Ovide*
**isopropyl unoprostone**
Rescula
**isoproterenol HCl**
Duo-Medihaler*
Isuprel
Norisodrine
**isoproterenol sulfate**
Medihaler-Iso
Norisodrine with Calcium Iodide*
**isosorbide**
Ismotic
**isosorbide dinitrate**
Dilatrate-SR
Iso-Bid
Isordil
Isotrate
Isotrate ER
Sorbitrate
Sorbitrate SA

*This brand is a combination product.

**isosorbide mononitrate**
  Imdur
  Ismo
  Monoket
**isosulfan blue**
  Lymphazurin 1%
**isotretinoin**
  Accutane
**isoxicam**
  Maxicam
**isoxsuprine HCl**
  Vasodilan
  Voxsuprine
**isradipine**
  DynaCirc
  DynaCirc CR
**itraconazole**
  Sporanox
**ivermectin**
  Stromectol
**Japanese encephalitis virus vaccine**
  JE-VAX
**kanamycin sulfate**
  Kantrex
**ketamine HCl**
  Ketalar
**ketoconazole**
  Apo-Ketoconazole (CAN)
  Nizoral
**ketoprofen**
  Orudis
  Oruvail
**ketorolac tromethamine**
  Acular; Acular PF
  Toradol
**ketotifen fumarate**
  Zaditen
  Zaditor
**KL4 surfactant**
  Surfaxin
**labetalol HCl**
  Normodyne
  Trandate
**lacidipine**
  Lacipil
**lactic acid**
  Lactinol
  Lactinol-E*
**lactulose**
  Cephulac

**lactulose (cont.)**
  Cholac
  Chronulac
  Constilac
  Constulose
  Duphalac
  Enulose
  Evalose
  Heptalac
**lamivudine**
  Combivir*
  Epivir
  Epivir-HBV
  Heptovir (CAN)
  Zeffix
**lamotrigine**
  Lamictal
**lansoprazole**
  Prevacid
  Prevpac*
**latanoprost**
  Xalatan
**latex agglutination test**
  Bactigen N meningitidis
**leflunomide**
  Arava
**leteprinim potassium**
  Neotrofin
**letrozole**
  Femara
**leucine**
  VIL*
**L-leucovorin**
  Isovorin
**leucovorin calcium**
  Wellcovorin
**leukocyte**
  MultiKine*
**leuprolide acetate**
  DUROS
  Lupron Depot
  Lupron Depot-Ped
  Lupron Depot<b.75>—>3 month;
    Lupron Depot<b.75>—>4 month
  Lupron; Lupron Pediatric
**levalbuterol**
  Contramid

*This brand is a combination product.

**levalbuterol HCl**
  Xopenex
**levamisole HCl**
  Ergamisol
**levobunolol HCl**
  AKBeta
  Betagan Liquifilm
**levobupivacaine**
  Chirocaine
**levocabastine HCl**
  Livostin
  Livostin ⒸⒶⓃ
**levocarnitine**
  Carnitor
  VitaCarn
**levodopa**
  Dopar
  Larodopa
  Sinemet 10/100; Sinemet 25/100;
    Sinemet 25/250*
  Sinemet CR*
**levofloxacin**
  Levaquin
**levomethadyl acetate HCl**
  Orlaam
**levonordefrin**
  Carbocaine with Neo-Cobefrin*
  Isocaine HCl*
  Polocaine*
  Ravocaine & Novocaine with Neo-
    Cobefrin*
**levonorgestrel**
  Alesse*
  Levlen*
  Levlite 21; Levlite 28*
  Levora*
  Nordette*
  Norplant
  Plan B
  Preven*
  Tri-Levlen*
  Triphasil*
  Trivora-28*
**levorphanol tartrate**
  Levo-Dromoran
**levothyroxine sodium**
  Eltroxin
  Levo-T
  Levothroid

**levothyroxine sodium (cont.)**
  Levothroid ⒸⒶⓃ
  Levoxyl
  Synthroid
  Triacana*
**lexipafant**
  Zacutex
**lidocaine**
  EMLA*
  Lida-Mantle-HC*
  Lidoderm
  Terramycin IM*
**lidocaine HCl**
  Anestacon
  Baylocaine 2% Viscous; Baylocaine
    4%
  Decadron with Xylocaine*
  Dentipatch
  Dilocaine
  Duo-Trach Kit
  L-Caine
  Lidoject-1; Lidoject-2
  LidoPen
  Nervocaine 1%
  Nervocaine 2%
  Nulicaine
  Octocaine HCl*
  Xylocaine
  Xylocaine 10% Oral
  Xylocaine HCl*
  Xylocaine HCl IV for Cardiac
    Arrhythmias
  Xylocaine MPF
  Xylocaine MPF*
  Xylocaine Viscous
**lincomycin HCl**
  Lincocin
  Lincorex
**lindane**
  G-Well
  Kwell
  Kwildane
  Scabene
**linezolid**
  Zyvox
**liothyronine sodium**
  Cytomel
  Triostat

*This brand is a combination product.

**liotrix**
 Thyrolar-0.25; -0.5; -1; -2; -3
**lipase**
 Arco-Lase Plus*
 Cotazym*
 Cotazym-S*
 Creon*
 Creon 10; Creon 20*
 Donnazyme*
 Ilozyme*
 Ku-Zyme*
 Ku-Zyme HP*
 Kutrase*
 Pancrease; Pancrease MT 4; Pancrease MT 10; Pancrease MT 16; Pancrease MT 20*
 Pancrecarb MS-8*
 Protilase*
 Ultrase MT 12; Ultrase MT 20*
 Viokase*
 Zymase*
**lipoprotein OspA**
 LYMErix
**lisinopril**
 Prinivil
 Prinzide*
 Prinzide 12.5; Prinzide 25*
 Zestoretic*
 Zestril
**lisofylline**
 ProTec
**lithium carbonate**
 Carbolith ⓒⒶⓃ
 Duralith ⓒⒶⓃ
 Eskalith
 Eskalith CR
 Lithane ⓒⒶⓃ
 Lithobid
 Lithonate
 Lithotabs
 PMS-Lithium Carbonate ⓒⒶⓃ
**lithium citrate**
 PMS-Lithium Citrate ⓒⒶⓃ
**liver derivative complex**
 Kutapressin
**liver, desiccated**
 Feocyte*
 Livitamin with Intrinsic Factor*
**liver extracts**
 Liver Combo No. 5*

**lobeline sulfate**
 NicErase-SL
**lodoxamide tromethamine**
 Alomide
**lomefloxacin HCl**
 Maxaquin; Maxaquin-3
**lomustine**
 CeeNu
**loperamide HCl**
 Imodium
**loracarbef**
 Lorabid
**loratadine**
 Claritin
 Claritin-D; Claritin-D 12 Hour; Claritin-D 24 Hour*
**lorazepam**
 Ativan
**losartan potassium**
 Cozaar
 Hyzaar*
**loteprednol etabonate**
 Alrex
 Lotemax
**lovastatin**
 Mevacor
**loxapine**
 Loxapac ⓒⒶⓃ
**loxapine HCl**
 Loxapac ⓒⒶⓃ
 Loxitane C
 Loxitane IM
**loxapine succinate**
 Apo-Loxapine ⓒⒶⓃ
 Loxitane
**lutetium texaphyrin**
 Lu-Tex
**lymphocyte immune globulin, antithymocyte**
 Atgam
 Nashville Rabbit Antithymocyte Serum
**lypressin**
 Diapid
**mafenide acetate**
 Sulfamylon
**magnesium carbonate**
 Renacidin Irrigation*

*This brand is a combination product.

**magnesium chloride**
Plegisol*
**magnesium hydroxycarbonate**
Renacidin*
**magnesium salicylate**
Magan
Magsal*
Mobidin
Trilisate*
**malathion**
Ovide*
**mangofodipir trisodium**
Teslascan
**mannitol**
Osmitrol
Resectisol
**maprotiline HCl**
Ludiomil
**masoprocol**
Actinex
**mazindol**
Mazanor
Sanorex
**measles and rubella virus vaccine**
M-R-Vax II
**measles, mumps, and rubella virus vaccine**
M-M-R II
Priorix
**measles virus vaccine**
Attenuvax
**mebendazole**
Vermox
**mecamylamine HCl**
Inversine
**mecasermin**
Myotrophin
**mechlorethamine HCl**
Mustargen
**meclizine HCl**
Antivert; Antivert/25; Antivert/50
Antivert/25
Antrizine
Meni-D
Nico-Vert
Ru-Vert-M
**meclocycline sulfosalicylate**
Meclan
**meclofenamate sodium**
Meclomen

**medroxyprogesterone acetate**
Amen
Curretab
Cycrin
Depo-Provera
Premphase*
Prempro*
Provera
**medrysone**
HMS
**mefenamic acid**
Ponstel
**mefloquine HCl**
Lariam
Mephaquin
**megakaryocyte growth and development factor, pegylated**
Megagen
**megestrol acetate**
Megace
**melanoma vaccine**
Melacine
**melarsoprol**
Arsobal
**meloxicam**
Mobic
**melphalan**
Alkeran
**meningococcal polysaccharide vaccine**
Menomune-A/C/Y/W-135
**menotropins**
Humegon
Pergonal
Repronex
**menthol**
Tussafed*
**mepenzolate bromide**
Cantil
**meperidine HCl**
Demerol HCl
Mepergan*
Mepergan Fortis*
**mephentermine sulfate**
Wyamine Sulfate
**mephenytoin**
Mesantoin

*This brand is a combination product.

**mephobarbital**
  Mebaral
**mepivacaine HCl**
  Carbocaine
  Carbocaine with Neo-Cobefrin*
  Isocaine HCl
  Isocaine HCl*
  Polocaine
  Polocaine*
  Polocaine MPF
**meprobamate**
  Deprol*
  Epromate*
  Equagesic*
  Equanil
  Equazine M*
  Meprogesic Q*
  Meprospan
  Micrainin*
  Miltown; Miltown-600
  Neuramate
  PMB 200; PMB 400*
**mercaptopurine**
  Purinethol
**meropenem**
  Merrem
**mesalamine**
  Asacol
  Pentasa
  Rowasa
  Salofalk ⒸⒶⓃ
**mesna**
  Mesnex
**mesoridazine besylate**
  Serentil
**mestranol**
  Enovid*
  Genora 1/50*
  Necon 1/50-21; Necon 1/50-28*
  Nelova 1/50M*
  Norethin 1/50M*
  Norinyl 1 + 50*
  Ortho-Novum 1/50*
**metaproterenol sulfate**
  Alupent
  Metaprel
  Prometa
**metaraminol bitartrate**
  Aramine

**metaxalone**
  Skelaxin
**metformin HCl**
  Glucophage
**methacholine chloride**
  Provocholine
**methadone HCl**
  Dolophine HCl
  Methadose
**methamphetamine HCl**
  Desoxyn
**methantheline bromide**
  Banthīne
**methazolamide**
  GlaucTabs
  MZM
  Neptazane
**methdilazine HCl**
  Tacaryl
**methenamine**
  Atrosept*
  Cystex*
  Dolsed*
  Prosed/DS*
  Trac Tabs 2X*
  UAA*
  Uridon Modified*
  Urimar-T*
  Urinary Antiseptic No. 2*
  Urised*
  Uritin*
  Uro-Phosphate*
  Urogesic Blue*
**methenamine hippurate**
  Hiprex
  Urex
**methenamine mandelate**
  Mandameth
  Mandelamine
  Urisedamine*
  Uroqid-Acid No. 2*
**methenamine sulfosalicylate**
  Unguentum Bossi*
**methicillin sodium**
  Staphcillin
**methimazole**
  Tapazole

*This brand is a combination product.

**Generic ⬆ Brands**

**methionine**
  Amino-Cerv pH 5.5*
**methocarbamol**
  Robaxin
  Robaxisal*
**methohexital sodium**
  Brevital Sodium
  Brietal Sodium ⒸⒶⓃ
**methotrexate sodium**
  Abitrexate
  Folex PFS
  Methotrexate LPF Sodium
  Rheumatrex
**methotrimeprazine HCl**
  Levoprome
**methoxamine HCl**
  Vasoxyl
**methoxsalen**
  8-MOP
  Oxsoralen
  Oxsoralen-Ultra
  Uvadex
**8-methoxycarbonyloctyl oligosac-
  charides**
  Synsorb-Pk
**methoxyflurane**
  Penthrane
**methscopolamine bromide**
  Ex-Histine*
  Pamine
  Pannaz*
**methscopolamine nitrate**
  AH-chew*
  D.A.*
  D.A. II*
  Dallergy*
  Dura-Vent/DA*
  Extendryl*
  Extendryl JR*
  Extendryl SR*
  Histor-D*
  Mescolor*
  OMNIhist L.A.*
  Prehist D*
  Rhinolar*
**methsuximide**
  Celontin
**methyclothiazide**
  Aquatensen
  Diutensen-R*

**methyclothiazide (cont.)**
  Enduron
  Enduronyl; Enduronyl Forte*
**methyldopa**
  Aldoclor-150; Aldoclor-250*
  Aldomet
  Aldoril 15; Aldoril 25; Aldoril D30;
    Aldoril D50*
  Alodopa-15; Alodopa-25*
  Amodopa
**methyldopate HCl**
  Aldomet; Aldomet Ester HCl
**methylene blue**
  Atrosept*
  Dolsed*
  Methblue 65
  Prosed/DS*
  Trac Tabs 2X*
  UAA*
  Uridon Modified*
  Urimar-T*
  Urinary Antiseptic No. 2*
  Urised*
  Uritin*
  Urogesic Blue*
  Urolene Blue
**methylergonovine maleate**
  Methergine
**methylphenidate HCl**
  Methylin
  Ritalin
  Ritalin-SR
**methylprednisolone**
  Medrol
**methylprednisolone acetate**
  Adlone
  depMedalone 40; depMedalone 80
  Depo-Medrol
  Depoject
  Depopred-40; Depopred-80
  Duralone-40; Duralone-80
  M-Prednisol-40; M-Prednisol-80
  Medralone 40; Medralone 80
**methylprednisolone sodium succi-
  nate**
  A-Methapred
  Solu-Medrol

*This brand is a combination product.

**methyltestosterone**
Android-10; Android-25
Estratest; Estratest H.S.*
Menogen; Menogen H.S.*
Oreton Methyl
Premarin with Methyltestosterone*
Testred
Virilon
**methysergide maleate**
Sansert
**metipranolol HCl**
OptiPranolol
**metoclopramide HCl**
Clopra
Emitasol
Maxolon
Octamide PFS
Pramidin
Reclomide
Reglan
Sensamide
**metocurine iodide**
Metubine Iodide
**metolazone**
Mykrox
Zaroxolyn
**metoprolol succinate**
Toprol XL
**metoprolol tartrate**
Lopressor
Lopressor HCT 50/25; Lopressor HCT
    100/25; Lopressor HCT 100/50*
**metrizamide**
Amipaque
**metronidazole**
Flagyl
Flagyl ER
Flagyl IV RTU
Helidac*
Metric 21
Metro I.V.
MetroCream
MetroGel Vaginal
MetroGel; MetroLotion
Nidagel ⒸⒶⓃ
Noritate
Protostat
**metronidazole HCl**
Flagyl IV

**metyrapone**
Metopirone
**metyrosine**
Demser
**mexiletine HCl**
Mexitil
**mezlocillin sodium**
Mezlin
**mibefradil dihydrochloride**
Posicor
**miconazole**
Monistat i.v.
**miconazole nitrate**
Fungoid-HC*
Monistat-Derm
Monistat Dual-Pak
Ony-Clear
**microbubble contrast agent**
Filmix
**microfibrillar collagen hemostat**
Avitene Hemostat
Hemopad
Hemotene
**midazolam HCl**
Versed
**midodrine HCl**
ProAmatine
**mifepristone**
Mifegyne
**miglitol**
Glyset
**milodistim**
Pixykine
**milrinone lactate**
Primacor
Primacor in 5% Dextrose*
**minerals, multiple**
B-C with Folic Acid Plus*
Bacmin*
Berocca Plus*
Berplex Plus*
Cezin-S*
Eldercaps*
Florvite + Iron*
Florvite + Iron; Half Strength
    Florvite + Iron*
Formula B Plus*
Hemocyte Plus*

*This brand is a combination product.

**minerals, multiple (cont.)**
Heptuna Plus*
Lactocal-F*
Marnatal-F*
Materna*
Megaton*
Mynatal*
Mynatal FC*
Mynatal P.N. Forte*
Mynatal Rx*
NatalCare Plus*
Niferex-PN*
Niferex-PN Forte*
Norlac Rx*
O-Cal f.a.*
Par-F*
Poly-Vi-Flor with Iron*
Polyvitamin Fluoride with Iron*
Pramilet FA*
Prenatal Maternal*
Strovite Plus; Strovite Forte*
Theragran Hematinic*
Vicon Forte*
Zincvit*
Zodeac-100*
**minocycline HCl**
Dynacin
Minocin
Vectrin
**minoxidil**
Loniten
**mirtazapine**
Remeron
**misoprostol**
Arthrotec*
Cytotec
**mitomycin**
Mutamycin
**mitotane**
Lysodren
**mitoxantrone HCl**
Novantrone
**mivacurium chloride**
Mivacron
**mixed respiratory vaccine**
MRV
**moclobemide**
Apo-Moclobemide (CAN)
Manerex (CAN)

**modafinil**
Alertec (CAN)
Provigil
**moexipril HCl**
Uniretic*
Univasc
**molgramostim**
Leucomax
**molindone HCl**
Moban
**mometasone furoate**
Elocon
Nasonex
**monobenzone**
Benoquin
**monochloroacetic acid**
Mono-Chlor
Monocete
**monoclonal antibodies**
Ceprate SC
Osteomark
**monoclonal antibody B43.13**
BrevaRex
OvaRex
**monoclonal antibody CD22 antigen on B-cells**
LymphoCide
**monoclonal antibody to CEA, humanized**
CEA-Cide
**monoctanoin**
Moctanin
**monolaurin**
Glylorin
**montelukast sodium**
Singulair
**moricizine HCl**
Ethmozine
**morphine sulfate**
AERx
Astramorph PF
DepoMorphine
Duramorph
Infumorph
Kadian
MorphiDex*
MS Contin
MS/L; MS/L Concentrate

*This brand is a combination product.

**morphine sulfate (cont.)**
  MS/S
  MSIR
  OMS Concentrate
  Oramorph SR
  RMS
  Roxanol
  Roxanol; Roxanol 100; Roxanol Res-
    cudose; Roxanol T; Roxanol UD
  UltraJect
**morrhuate sodium**
  Scleromate
**multiple amino acids**
  Aminess 5.2%*
  Aminosyn 3.5% (5%, 7%, 8.5%,
    10%); Aminosyn (pH6) 10%;
    Aminosyn II 3.5% (5%, 7%,
    8.5%, 10%, 15%); Aminosyn-PF
    7% (10%)*
  Aminosyn 3.5% M; Aminosyn II
    3.5% M*
  Aminosyn 7% (8.5%) with Electro-
    lytes; Aminosyn II 7% (8.5%,
    10%) with Electrolytes*
  Aminosyn-HBC 7%*
  Aminosyn II 3.5% in 5% (25%) Dex-
    trose; Aminosyn II 4.25% in 10%
    (20%, 25%) Dextrose; Aminosyn
    II 5% in 25% Dextrose*
  Aminosyn II 3.5% M in 5% Dex-
    trose; Aminosyn II 4.25% M in
    10% Dextrose*
  Aminosyn-RF 5.2%*
  BranchAmin 4%*
  FreAmine HBC 6.9%*
  FreAmine III 3% (8.5%) with Elec-
    trolytes*
  FreAmine III 8.5%; FreAmine III
    10%*
  HepatAmine*
  NephrAmine 5.4%*
  Novamine; Novamine 15%*
  ProcalAmine*
  ProSol 20%*
  RenAmin*
  Travasol 2.75% in 5% (10%, 25%)
    Dextrose; Travasol 4.25% in 5%
    (10%, 25%) Dextrose*
  Travasol 3.5% (5.5%, 8.5%) with
    Electrolytes*

**multiple amino acids (cont.)**
  Travasol 5.5% (8.5%, 10%)*
  TrophAmine 6%; TrophAmine 10%*
**multiple B vitamins**
  B-C with Folic Acid*
  B-Ject-100*
  B-Plex*
  Becomject-100*
  Berocca*
  Co Tinic*
  Formula B*
  Forte L.I.V.*
  Hemocyte*
  Hemocyte Plus*
  Hemocyte-V*
  Hytinic*
  Iberet-Folic-500*
  Key-Plex*
  Licoplex DS*
  Livitamin with Intrinsic Factor*
  Lypholized Vitamin B Complex &
    Vitamin C with $B_{12}$*
  May-Vita*
  Megaton*
  Multibret-500 Hematinic*
  Multibret-Folic-500*
  Nephlex Rx*
  Nephro-Vite Rx + Fe*
  Nephro-Vite Rx*
  Nephrocaps*
  Nephron FA*
  Neurodep*
  Senilezol*
  Strovite*
  Tabron*
  Vicam*
  Vitafōl*
  Vitamin B Complex 100*
**multiple electrolytes**
  Dialyte Pattern LM*
  Inpersol; Inpersol-LM*
**multiple minerals**
  B-C with Folic Acid Plus*
  Bacmin*
  Berocca Plus*
  Berplex Plus*
  Cezin-S*
  Eldercaps*

*This brand is a combination product.

## multiple minerals (cont.)

Florvite + Iron*
Florvite + Iron; Half Strength
  Florvite + Iron*
Formula B Plus*
Hemocyte Plus*
Heptuna Plus*
Lactocal-F*
Marnatal-F*
Materna*
Megaton*
Mynatal*
Mynatal FC*
Mynatal P.N. Forte*
Mynatal Rx*
NatalCare Plus*
Niferex-PN*
Niferex-PN Forte*
Norlac Rx*
O-Cal f.a.*
Par-F*
Poly-Vi-Flor with Iron*
Polyvitamin Fluoride with Iron*
Pramilet FA*
Prenatal Maternal*
Strovite Plus; Strovite Forte*
Theragran Hematinic*
Vicon Forte*
Zincvit*
Zodeac-100*

## multiple trace elements (metals)

ConTE-Pak-4
M.T.E.-4; M.T.E.-5; M.T.E.-6;
  M.T.E.-7; M.T.E.-4 Concentrated;
  M.T.E.-5 Concentrated; M.T.E.-6
  Concentrated
MulTE-Pak-4; MulTE-Pak-5
Multiple Trace Element with Sele-
  nium; Multiple Trace Element
  with Selenium Concentrated
Multiple Trace Element; Multiple
  Trace Element Concentrated;
  Multiple Trace Element Neonatal;
  Multiple Trace Element Pediatric
Multitrace-5 Concentrate
Neotrace-4
P.T.E.-4; P.T.E.-5
PedTE-Pak-4
Pedtrace-4
Trace Metals Additive in 0.9% NaCl

## multiple trace elements (metals) (cont.)

Tracelyte; Tracelyte II; Tracelyte
  with Double Electrolytes; Tracelyte II with Double Electrolytes*

## multiple vitamins

Adeflor M*
B Complex with C and B-12*
B-C with Folic Acid Plus*
Bacmin*
Berocca Parenteral Nutrition*
Berocca Plus*
Berplex Plus*
Cefol*
Cernevit-12*
Cezin-S*
Chewable Multivitamins with Fluo-
  ride*
Eldercaps*
Filibon F.A.; Filibon Forte*
Florvite + Iron*
Florvite + Iron; Half Strength
  Florvite + Iron*
Florvite*
Florvite; Florvite Half Strength*
Formula B Plus*
Heptuna Plus*
Lactocal-F*
Lipo-Nicin/100*
Lipo-Nicin/300*
M.V.C. 9+3*
M.V.C. 9+4 Pediatric*
M.V.I. Neonatal*
M.V.I. Pediatric*
M.V.I.-12*
Marnatal-F*
Materna*
Mission Prenatal Rx*
Multi Vitamin Concentrate*
Multivitamin with Fluoride*
Mulvidren-F*
Mynatal*
Mynatal FC*
Mynatal P.N.*
Mynatal P.N. Forte*
Mynatal Rx*
Mynate 90 Plus*
Natabec Rx*

*This brand is a combination product.

**multiple vitamins (cont.)**
Natafort*
NatalCare Plus*
Natalins Rx*
Natarex Prenatal*
Nestabs FA*
Niferex-PN*
Niferex-PN Forte*
Norlac Rx*
Nu-Iron V*
O-Cal f.a.*
Par-F*
Par-Natal Plus 1 Improved*
Poly-Vi-Flor*
Poly-Vi-Flor with Iron*
Polytabs-F*
Polyvitamin Fluoride*
Polyvitamin Fluoride with Iron*
Polyvitamin with Iron and Fluoride*
Polyvitamins with Fluoride and Iron*
Pramet FA*
Pramilet FA*
Pre-H Cal*
Prenatal H.P.*
Prenatal Maternal*
Prenatal MR 90*
Prenatal One*
Prenatal Plus Iron*
Prenatal Plus with Betacarotene*
Prenatal Plus; Prenatal Plus
    Improved*
Prenatal Rx*
Prenatal Rx with Betacarotene*
Prenatal Z*
Prenatal-1 + Iron*
Prenate 90; Prenate Ultra*
Secran Prenatal*
Soluvite C.T.*
Strovite Plus; Strovite Forte*
Stuartnatal Plus*
Theragran Hematinic*
Vi-Daylin/F Multivitamin + Iron*
Vi-Daylin/F Multivitamin*
Vicon Forte*
Vitafōl; Vitafōl-PN*
Zenate, Advanced Formula*
Zincvit*
Zodeac-100*
**mumps and rubella virus vaccine**
Biavax II

**mumps skin test antigen**
MSTA (Mumps Skin Test Antigen)
**mumps virus vaccine**
Mumpsvax
**mupirocin**
Bactroban
**mupirocin calcium**
Bactroban
Bactroban Nasal
**muromonab-CD3**
Orthoclone OKT3
**mycophenolate mofetil**
CellCept
**mycophenolate mofetil HCl**
CellCept
**nabumetone**
Relafen
**nadolol**
Corgard
Corzide 40/5; Corzide 80/5*
**nadroparin calcium**
Fraxiparine Ⓒ
**nafarelin acetate**
Synarel
**nafcillin sodium**
Nafcil
Nallpen
Unipen
**naftifine HCl**
Naftin
**nalbuphine HCl**
Nubain
**nalidixic acid**
NegGram
**nalmefene**
Revex
**naloxone HCl**
Narcan
Talwin NX*
**naltrexone HCl**
Depade
ReVia
**nandrolone decanoate**
Androlone-D 200
Deca-Durabolin
Hybolin Decanoate-50; Hybolin
    Decanoate-100
Neo-Durabolic

*This brand is a combination product.

**nandrolone phenpropionate**
  Durabolin
  Hybolin Improved
**naphazoline HCl**
  AK-Con
  AK-Con-A*
  Albalon*
  Antazoline-V*
  Muro's Opcon
  Nafazair
  Nafazair A*
  Naphazole-A*
  Naphcon Forte
  Naphoptic-A*
  Vasocon-A*
  Vasocon Regular
**naproxen**
  Anaprox; Anaprox DS
  EC-Naprosyn
  Naprelan
  Napron X
  Naprosyn
**naratriptan HCl**
  Amerge
**natamycin**
  Natacyn
**nebacumab**
  Centoxin
**nedocromil sodium**
  Mireze (CAN)
  Tilade
**nefazodone HCl**
  Serzone
*Neisseria meningitidis* **OMPC**
  Comvax*
**nelfinavir mesylate**
  Viracept
**neomycin sulfate**
  AK-Neo-Dex*
  AK-Spore*
  AK-Spore H.C.*
  AK-Trol*
  AntibiŌtic*
  Antibiotic Ear Solution*
  Antibiotic Ear Suspension*
  Bacticort*
  Coly-Mycin S Otic*
  Coracin*
  Cortatrigen Modified*
  Cortisporin*

**neomycin sulfate (cont.)**
  Cortisporin Otic*
  Cortisporin-TC*
  Dexacidin*
  Dexasporin*
  Drotic*
  Ear-Eze*
  LazerSporin-C*
  Maxitrol*
  Mycifradin Sulfate
  Myco-Biotic II*
  Neo-Cortef*
  Neo-Dexair*
  Neo-Dexameth*
  Neo-fradin
  Neo-Synalar*
  Neo-Tabs
  NeoDecadron*
  Neosporin*
  Neosporin G.U. Irrigant*
  Neotal*
  Neotricin HC*
  Octicare*
  Ocutricin*
  Otic-Care*
  OtiTricin*
  Otocort*
  Otomycin-HPN Otic*
  Otosporin*
  Pediotic*
  Pedotic*
  Poly-Pred*
  Storz-N-D*
  Storz-N-P-D*
  Triple Antibiotic*
  UAD Otic*
**neostigmine bromide**
  Prostigmin
**neostigmine methylsulfate**
  Prostigmin
**nesiritide**
  Natrecor
**netilmicin sulfate**
  Netromycin
**neural dopaminergic cells**
  NeuroCell-PD
**neural gabaergic cells**
  NeuroCell-HD

*This brand is a combination product.

**nevirapine**
Viramune
**niacin**
Lipo-Nicin/100*
Lipo-Nicin/300*
Niacor
Niaspan
Nicolar
**niacinamide**
Lipo-Nicin/100*
**nicardipine HCl**
Cardene
Cardene I.V.
Cardene SR
**niclosamide**
Niclocide
**nicotine**
Habitrol
Nicoderm
Nicotrol
Nicotrol NS
ProStep
**nicotine polacrilex**
Nicorette DS
**nifedipine**
Adalat
Adalat CC; Adalat Oros
Procardia
Procardia XL
**nifurtimox**
Lampit
**nilutamide**
Anandron ⒸⒶⓃ
Nilandron
**nimodipine**
Nimotop
**nisoldipine**
Sular
**nitazoxanide**
Cryptaz
**nitrazepam**
Mogadon
**nitrendipine**
Baypress
**nitrofurantoin**
Furadantin
Furalan
Macrobid*
Macrodantin

**nitrofurantoin monohydrate**
Macrobid*
**nitrofurazone**
Furacin
Furacin Soluble Dressing
**nitroglycerin**
Anogesic
Deponit
Minitran
Nitrek
Nitro-Bid
Nitro-Bid IV
Nitro-Derm
Nitro-Dur
Nitro-Time
Nitrocine
Nitrodisc
Nitrogard
Nitroglyn
Nitrol
Nitrolingual Pumpspray ⒸⒶⓃ
Nitrong
NitroQuick
Nitrostat
NTS
Transderm-Nitro
Tridil
Trinipatch ⒸⒶⓃ
**nizatidine**
Axid
**nofetumomab merpentan**
Verluma
**norepinephrine bitartrate**
Levophed
Ravocaine & Novocaine with
Levophed*
**norethindrone**
Brevicon*
Genora 0.5/35; Genora 1/35*
Genora 1/50*
Jenest-28*
Micronor
Modicon*
N.E.E. 1/35*
Necon 0.5/35-21; Necon 0.5/35-28*
Necon 1/35-21; Necon 1/35-28*
Necon 1/50-21; Necon 1/50-28*
Necon 10/11-21; Necon 10/11-28*

*This brand is a combination product.

**norethindrone (cont.)**
Nelova 1/35E; Nelova 0.5/35E*
Nelova 1/50M*
Nelova 10/11*
Nor-Q.D.
Norethin 1/35E*
Norethin 1/50M*
Norinyl 1 + 35*
Norinyl 1 + 50*
Norlutin
Ortho-Novum 1/35*
Ortho-Novum 1/50*
Ortho-Novum 10/11*
Ortho-Novum 7/7/7*
Ovcon-35; Ovcon-50*
Tri-Norinyl*
**norethindrone acetate**
Activelle*
Aygestin
CombiPatch*
Estrostep 21*
Estrostep Fe*
Loestrin 21 1/20; Loestrin 21 1.5/30*
Loestrin Fe 1/20; Loestrin Fe 1.5/30*
Norlutate
**norethynodrel**
Enovid*
**norfloxacin**
Chibroxin
Noroxin
**norgestimate**
Ortho-Cyclen*
Ortho Tri-Cyclen*
**norgestrel**
Lo/Ovral*
Ovral*
Ovrette
**nortriptyline HCl**
Aventyl HCl
Pamelor
**novobiocin sodium**
Albamycin
**nystatin**
Derma Comb*
Myco-Biotic II*
Myco-Triacet II*
Mycogen II*
Mycolog-II*
Myconel*
Mycostatin

**nystatin (cont.)**
Mykinac
Mytrex*
N.G.T.*
Nilstat
Nyotran
Nystatin-LF
Nystex
Pedi-Dri
Tri-Statin II*
**octreotide acetate**
Sandostatin
Sandostatin LAR Depot
**ofloxacin**
Apo-Oflox ⒸⒶⒷ
Floxin
Floxin Otic
Ocuflox
**olanzapine**
Zyprexa
**old tuberculin**
Mono-Vacc Test (O.T.)
Tuberculin Tine Test, Old
**olopatadine HCl**
Patanol
**olsalazine sodium**
Dipentum
**omeprazole**
Losec ⒸⒶⒷ
Prilosec
**ondansetron HCl**
Zofran
Zofran ODT
**opium**
B & O Supprettes No. 15A; B & O Supprettes No. 16A*
**oprelvekin**
Neumega
**orgotein**
OxSODrol
**orlistat**
Xenical
**orphenadrine citrate**
Banflex
Flexoject
Flexon
Myolin
Norflex

*This brand is a combination product.

**orphenadrine citrate (cont.)**
  Norgesic; Norgesic Forte*
  Orphengesic; Orphengesic Forte*
**orphenadrine HCl**
  Disipal ⒸⒶⓃ
**oxacillin sodium**
  Bactocill
  Prostaphlin
**oxaliplatin**
  Dacplat
  Eloxatin
  Foloxatine
  Transplatin
**oxamniquine**
  Vansil
**oxandrolone**
  Hepandrin
  Oxandrin
**oxaprozin**
  Daypro
**oxazepam**
  Serax
**oxcarbazepine**
  Trileptal
**oxiconazole nitrate**
  Oxistat
  Oxizole ⒸⒶⓃ
**oxidronate sodium**
  OctreoScan
**oxothiazolidine carboxylate**
  Procysteine
**oxtriphylline**
  Choledyl
  Choledyl SA
**oxybenzone**
  Solaquin Forte*
  Viquin Forte*
**oxybutynin chloride**
  Ditropan
  Ditropan XL
**oxycodone HCl**
  Endocet*
  OxyContin
  OxyFast
  OxyIR
  Percocet*
  Percodan; Percodan-Demi*
  Percolone
  Roxicet*
  Roxicet 5/500*

**oxycodone HCl (cont.)**
  Roxicodone
  Roxilox*
  Roxiprin*
  Tylox*
**oxycodone terephthalate**
  Percodan; Percodan-Demi*
  Roxiprin*
**oxymetholone**
  Anadrol-50
**oxymorphone HCl**
  Numorphan
**oxyphencyclimine HCl**
  Daricon
**oxytetracycline**
  Terramycin IM*
**oxytetracycline HCl**
  Terak*
  Terra-Cortril*
  Terramycin
  Terramycin with Polymyxin B*
  Uri-Tet
  Urobiotic-250*
**oxytocin**
  Pitocin
  Syntocinon
**p30 protein**
  Onconase
**paclitaxel**
  Paxene
  Taxol
**padimate O**
  Viquin Forte*
**palivizumab**
  Synagis
**pamidronate disodium**
  Aredia
**pancreatin**
  Creon*
  Digepepsin*
  Digestozyme*
  Donnazyme*
**pancuronium bromide**
  Pavulon
**pantoprazole**
  Pantozol
**papain**
  Accuzyme*

*This brand is a combination product.

**papain (cont.)**
Panafil*
Panafil White*
**papaverine HCl**
Cerespan
Genabid
Pavabid
Pavabid HP
Pavagen TD
Pavarine
Pavased
Pavatine
Paverolan
**paraldehyde**
Paral
**parathyroid hormone (1-84)**
Allelix
**paricalcitol**
Zemplar
**paromomycin sulfate**
Humatin
**paroxetine HCl**
Paxil
Paxil CR
**PEG-camptothecin**
Prothecan
**PEG-glucocerebrosidase**
Lysodase
**pegademase bovine**
Adagen
**pegaspargase**
Oncaspar
**pemetrexed disodium**
Rolazar
Tifolar
**pemoline**
Cylert
**penbutolol sulfate**
Levatol
**penciclovir**
Denavir
**penicillamine**
Cuprimine
Depen
**penicillin G benzathine**
Bicillin C-R; Bicillin C-R 900/300*
Bicillin L-A
Permapen
**penicillin G potassium**
Pfizerpen

**penicillin G procaine**
Bicillin C-R; Bicillin C-R 900/300*
Crysticillin 300 A.S.; Crysticillin
600 A.S.
Pfizerpen-AS
Wycillin
**penicillin V potassium**
Beepen-VK
Betapen-VK
Ledercillin VK
Pen-V
Pen-Vee K
Penicillin VK
Robicillin VK
V-Cillin K
Veetids
Veetids '125'; Veetids '250'
**pentaerythritol tetranitrate**
Duotrate; Duotrate 45
Pentylan
Peritrate
Peritrate SA
**pentagastrin**
Peptavlon
**pentamidine isethionate**
NebuPent
Pentacarinat
Pentam 300
Pneumopent
**pentastarch**
Pentaspan
**pentazocine HCl**
Talacen*
Talwin Compound*
Talwin NX*
**pentazocine lactate**
Talwin
**pentobarbital**
Nembutal
**pentobarbital sodium**
Cafatine-PB*
Nembutal Sodium
**pentosan polysulfate sodium**
Elmiron
**pentostatin**
Nipent
**pentoxifylline**
Trental

*This brand is a combination product.

**pepsin**
  Digepepsin*
  Digestozyme*
**perflenapent**
  EchoGen*
**perflisopent**
  EchoGen*
**perflubron**
  Imagent GI
  LiquiVent
  Oxygent
**perflutren**
  Definity
**perfosfamide**
  Pergamid
**pergolide mesylate**
  Permax
**permethrin**
  Acticin
  Elimite
**perphenazine**
  Apo-Perphenazine ⓒ
  Etrafon; Etrafon 2–10; Etrafon-A;
    Etrafon-Forte*
  Triavil 2-10; Triavil 2-25; Triavil 4-
    10; Triavil 4-25; Triavil 4-50*
  Trilafon
**pertussis vaccine**
  Acel-P ⓒ
**peruvian balsam**
  Dermuspray*
  Granulderm*
  Granulex*
  GranuMed*
**pexiganan acetate**
  Cytolex
**PGG glucan**
  Betafectin
**phenacemide**
  Phenurone
**phenazopyridine HCl**
  Azo Gantanol*
  Azo Gantrisin*
  Azo-Sulfisoxazole*
  Baridium
  Eridium
  Geridium
  Phenazo ⓒ
  Phenazodine
  Pyridiate; Pyridate No. 2

**phenazopyridine HCl (cont.)**
  Pyridium
  Pyridium Plus*
  Uristat
  Urobiotic-250*
  Urodine
  Urogesic
**phendimetrazine tartrate**
  Adipost
  Anorex
  Bontril
  Bontril PDM
  Ditel
  Dyrexan-OD
  Melfiat-105
  Obalan
  Plegine
  Prelu-2
  Rexigen Forte
  Trimstat
  Wehless
  Weightrol
**phenelzine sulfate**
  Nardil
**phenindamine tartrate**
  Nolamine*
  P-V-Tussin*
**pheniramine maleate**
  AK-Con-A*
  Iohist D*
  Liqui-Histine-D*
  Nafazair A*
  Naphazole-A*
  Naphoptic-A*
  Poly-Histine*
  Poly-Histine-D*
  Poly-Histine-D Ped Caps*
  Rolatuss with Hydrocodone*
  Ru-Tuss with Hydrocodone*
  Statuss Green*
  Tri-P*
  Triaminic*
  Triaminic Expectorant DH*
  Tussirex*
  Vetuss HC*
**phenobarbital**
  Antispasmodic*
  Antrocol*

*This brand is a combination product.

**phenobarbital (cont.)**
  Arco-Lase Plus*
  Barbidonna*
  Barbidonna; Barbidonna No. 2*
  Barophen*
  Bel-Phen-Ergot SR*
  Bellacane*
  Bellacane SR*
  Bellatal
  Bellergal-S*
  Chardonna-2*
  Dilantin with Phenobarbital*
  Donna-Sed*
  Donnamor*
  Donnapine*
  Donnatal*
  Donnatal No. 2*
  Folergot-DF*
  Gustase Plus*
  Hyosophen*
  Kinesed*
  Levsin-PB*
  Levsin PB*
  Levsin with Phenobarbital*
  Lufyllin-EPG*
  Malatal*
  Mudrane*
  Mudrane GG*
  Phenerbel-S*
  Quadrinal*
  Relaxadon*
  Solfoton
  Spasmolin*
  Spasmophen*
  Spasquid*
  Susano*
**phenobarbital sodium**
  Luminal Sodium
**phenol**
  Castellani Paint Modified*
**phenoxybenzamine HCl**
  Dibenzyline
**phensuximide**
  Milontin
**phentermine HCl**
  Adipex-P
  Fastin
  Ionamin
  Obenix
  Obephen

**phentermine HCl (cont.)**
  Oby-Cap
  Phentrol
  Phentrol 2; Phentrol 4; Phentrol 5
  Zantryl
**phentolamine mesylate**
  Invicorp*
  Regitine
  Vasomax
**phenyl salicylate**
  Atrosept*
  Dolsed*
  Prosed/DS*
  Trac Tabs 2X*
  UAA*
  Uridon Modified*
  Urimar-T*
  Urinary Antiseptic No. 2*
  Urised*
  Uritin*
  Urogesic Blue*
**phenylephrine bitartrate**
  Duo-Medihaler*
**phenylephrine HCl**
  Aclophen*
  AH-chew*
  AH-chew D
  AK-Dilate
  Alersule*
  Anaplex HD*
  Atrohist Plus*
  Atuss DM*
  Atuss G*
  Atuss HD*
  Banex*
  Bromophen T.D.*
  Chlorgest-HD*
  Codimal DH*
  Coldloc*
  Comhist*
  Comhist LA*
  Contuss*
  Cophene-X*
  Cyclomydril*
  D.A.*
  D.A. II*
  Dallergy*
  Decongestabs*

*This brand is a combination product.

**phenylephrine HCl (cont.)**
  Decongestant*
  Decongestant S.R.*
  Deconhist L.A.*
  Deconsal Sprinkle*
  Despec*
  Donatussin*
  Donatussin DC*
  Dura-Gest*
  Dura-Vent/DA*
  Ed A-Hist*
  ED-TLC; ED Tuss HC*
  Endagen-HD*
  Endal*
  Endal-HD; Endal-HD Plus*
  Enomine*
  Entex*
  Ex-Histine*
  Extendryl*
  Extendryl JR*
  Extendryl SR*
  Guaifenex*
  Guaitex*
  Hista-Vadrin*
  Histalet Forte*
  Histamic*
  Histinex HC*
  Histor-D*
  Histussin HC*
  Hycomine Compound*
  Hydrocodone CP; Hydrocodone HD*
  Iodal HD*
  Iotussin HC*
  Liquibid-D*
  Murocoll-2*
  Mydfrin 2.5%
  Naldec Pediatric*
  Naldecon*
  Naldelate*
  Nalgest*
  Neo-Synephrine
  No-Hist*
  Norel*
  OMNIhist L.A.*
  Para-Hist HD*
  Partapp TD*
  Pediacof*
  Pedituss Cough*
  Phenahist-TR*
  Phenchlor S.H.A.*

**phenylephrine HCl (cont.)**
  Phenergan VC*
  Phenergan VC with Codeine*
  Phenoptic
  Pherazine VC with Codeine*
  Prehist*
  Prehist D*
  Prometh VC Plain*
  Prometh VC with Codeine*
  Promethazine VC*
  Promethazine VC Plain*
  Promethazine VC with Codeine*
  Promethist with Codeine*
  Quadra-Hist*
  Quadra-Hist Pediatric*
  Rolatuss Expectorant*
  Rolatuss with Hydrocodone*
  Ru-Tuss*
  Ru-Tuss with Hydrocodone*
  Sil-Tex*
  Sinupan*
  Stahist*
  Statuss Green*
  Storzfen
  T-Koff*
  Tamine S.R.*
  Tri-Phen-Chlor*
  Tri-Phen-Chlor T.R.*
  Tri-Phen-Mine*
  Tri-Phen-Mine S.R.*
  Tusquelin*
  Tussafed HC*
  Tussanil DH*
  Tussanil Plain*
  Tussirex*
  Tympagesic*
  Uni-Decon*
  Unituss HC*
  Vanex Forte*
  Vanex-HD*
  Vasosulf*
  Vetuss HC*
**phenylephrine tannate**
  Atrohist Pediatric*
  R-Tannamine*
  R-Tannate*
  Rentamine Pediatric*
  Rhinatate*

*This brand is a combination product.

**phenylephrine tannate (cont.)**
Rynatan*
Rynatan-S*
Rynatuss*
Tanoral*
Tri-Tannate*
Tri-Tannate Plus Pediatric*
Triotann*
Tritan*
Tritann Pediatric*
Tussi-12*

**phenylpropanolamine HCl**
Alumadrine*
Ami-Tex LA*
Anatuss*
Atrohist Plus*
Banex*
Bromanate DC Cough*
Bromophen T.D.*
Bromphen DC with Codeine Cough*
Brompheniramine DC Cough*
Codamine*
Codegest Expectorant*
Coldloc*
Coldloc-LA*
Condrin-LA*
Conex with Codeine*
Contuss*
Cophene-X*
Decongestabs*
Decongestant*
Decongestant S.R.*
Deconhist L.A.*
Despec*
Dimetane-DC Cough*
Drize*
Dura-Gest*
Dura-Vent*
Dura-Vent/A*
E.N.T.*
Endal Expectorant*
Enomine*
Entex*
Entex LA*
Exgest LA*
Guaifenex*
Guaifenex PPA 75*
Guaipax*
Guaitex*
Guaitex LA*

**phenylpropanolamine HCl (cont.)**
Guiatex LA*
Guipax*
Hista-Vadrin*
Histalet Forte*
Histamic*
Histine DM*
Hycomine*
Hydrocodone PA*
Iohist D*
Iohist DM*
Liqui-Histine-D*
Liqui-Histine DM*
Myphetane DC Cough*
Naldec Pediatric*
Naldecon*
Naldecon CX Adult*
Naldelate*
Nalgest*
No-Hist*
Nolamine*
Norel*
Norel Plus*
Ordrine AT*
Ordrine S.R.*
Ornade*
Pannaz*
Parhist SR*
Partapp TD*
Partuss LA*
Phenahist-TR*
Phenate*
Phenchlor S.H.A.*
Phenylfenesin L.A.*
Poly-Histine CS*
Poly-Histine-D*
Poly-Histine-D Ped Caps*
Poly-Histine DM*
Profen II DM*
Profen II; Profen LA*
Quadra-Hist*
Quadra-Hist Pediatric*
Resaid*
Rescaps-D S.R.*
Rhinolar*
Rhinolar-EX; Rhinolar-EX 12*
Rolatuss with Hydrocodone*
Ru-Tuss*

*This brand is a combination product.

Generic ♦ Brands

**phenylpropanolamine HCl (cont.)**
Ru-Tuss II*
Ru-Tuss with Hydrocodone*
Rymed-TR*
Sil-Tex*
Siltapp with Dextromethorphan
   HBr Cold & Cough*
SinuVent*
Stahist*
Stamoist LA*
Statuss Expectorant*
Statuss Green*
T-Koff*
Tamine S.R.*
Tri-P*
Tri-Phen-Chlor*
Tri-Phen-Chlor T.R.*
Tri-Phen-Mine*
Tri-Phen-Mine S.R.*
Triaminic*
Triaminic Expectorant DH*
Triaminic Expectorant with
   Codeine*
Tusquelin*
Tuss-Allergine Modified T.D.*
Tuss-Genade Modified*
Tuss-Ornade*
Tussanil DH*
Tussogest*
ULR-LA*
Uni-Decon*
Vanex Forte*
Vanex Forte-R*
Vanex-LA*
Vetuss HC*
**phenyltoloxamine**
Lobac*
**phenyltoloxamine citrate**
Comhist*
Comhist LA*
Decongestabs*
Decongestant*
Decongestant S.R.*
Histamic*
Iohist D*
Kutrase*
Liqui-Histine-D*
Magsal*
Naldec Pediatric*
Naldecon*

**phenyltoloxamine citrate (cont.)**
Naldelate*
Nalgest*
Poly-Histine*
Poly-Histine-D*
Poly-Histine-D Ped Caps*
Quadra-Hist*
Quadra-Hist Pediatric*
Tri-Phen-Chlor*
Tri-Phen-Chlor T.R.*
Tri-Phen-Mine*
Tri-Phen-Mine S.R.*
Uni-Decon*
**phenyltoloxamine dihydrogen citrate**
Norel Plus*
**phenytoin**
Dilantin
Dilantin-30 Pediatric
Dilantin-125
**phenytoin sodium**
Dilantin
Dilantin with Phenobarbital*
Diphenylan Sodium
**phosphatidylglycerol**
Alec*
**physiological irrigating solution**
Cytosol
Physiolyte
PhysioSol
Tis-U-Sol
**physostigmine**
Synapton SR
**physostigmine salicylate**
Antilirium
Eserine Salicylate
**physostigmine sulfate**
Eserine Sulfate
**phytonadione**
AquaMEPHYTON
Konakion
Mephyton
**pilocarpine**
Ocusert Pilo-20; Ocusert Pilo-40
**pilocarpine HCl**
Adsorbocarpine
Akarpine
E-Pilo-3*

*This brand is a combination product.

**pilocarpine HCl (cont.)**
E-Pilo-1; E-Pilo-2; E-Pilo-4; E-Pilo-6*
Isopto Carpine
Ocu-Carpine
$P_1E_1$; $P_2E_1$; $P_4E_1$; $P_6E_1$*
$P_3E_1$*
Pilocar
Pilopine HS
Piloptic-½; Piloptic-1; Piloptic-2;
    Piloptic-3; Piloptic-4; Piloptic-6
Pilopto-Carpine
Pilostat
Salagen
Storzine 2
**pilocarpine nitrate**
Pilagan
**pimozide**
Orap
**pinacidil**
Pindac
**pindolol**
Visken
**pioglitazone HCl**
Actos
**pipecuronium bromide**
Arduan
**piperacillin sodium**
Pipracil
Zosyn*
**piracetam**
Nootropil
**pirbuterol acetate**
Maxair
**pirenzepine HCl**
Gastrozepine
**piroxicam**
Feldene
Fexicam (CAN)
**piroxicam betadex**
Brexidol
**plasma protein fraction**
Plasma-Plex
Plasmanate
Plasmatein
Protenate
**plicamycin**
Mithracin
**pneumococcal polysaccharide vaccine**
Pneumo 23 (CAN)

**pneumococcal vaccine, polyvalent**
Pneumovax 23
Pnu-Imune 23
**podofilox**
Condylox
Wartec (CAN)
**podophyllum**
Verrex*
Verrusol*
**podophyllum resin**
Podocon-25
Podofin
**poliovirus vaccine**
IPOL
Orimune
**poloxamer 331**
Protox
**poly I: poly C12U**
Ampligen
**polydimethylsiloxane**
AdatoSil 5000
**polyethylene glycol 3350**
MiraLax
**polyethylene glycol-electrolyte solution**
Co-Lav*
Colovage
Colyte
Go-Evac*
GoLYTELY
NuLytely
OCL
**polymyxin B sulfate**
Aerosporin
AK-Poly-Bac*
AK-Spore*
AK-Spore H.C.*
AK-Trol*
AntibiŌtic*
Antibiotic Ear Solution*
Antibiotic Ear Suspension*
Bacticort*
Coracin*
Cortatrigen Modified*
Cortisporin*
Cortisporin Otic*
Dexacidin*
Dexasporin*

*This brand is a combination product.

**polymyxin B sulfate (cont.)**
Drotic*
Ear-Eze*
LazerSporin-C*
Maxitrol*
Neosporin*
Neosporin G.U. Irrigant*
Neotal*
Neotricin HC*
Octicare*
Ocutricin*
Ophthocort*
Otic-Care*
OtiTricin*
Otobiotic Otic*
Otocort*
Otomycin-HPN Otic*
Otosporin*
Pediotic*
Pedotic*
Poly-Pred*
Polytrim*
Storz-N-P-D*
Terak*
Terramycin with Polymyxin B*
Triple Antibiotic*
UAD Otic*
**polysaccharide-iron complex**
Hemocyte Plus*
Niferex Forte*
Niferex-PN*
Niferex-PN Forte*
Niferex-150 Forte*
Nu-Iron Plus*
Nu-Iron V*
**polythiazide**
Minizide 1; Minizide 2; Minizide 5*
Renese
Renese-R*
**polyvinyl alcohol**
Albalon*
**polyvinyl chloride**
Sitzmarks
**porfimer sodium**
Photofrin
**potassium acetate**
Tri-K*
**potassium acid phosphate**
K-Phos M.F.*
K-Phos No. 2*

**potassium acid phosphate (cont.)**
K-Phos Original
**potassium bicarbonate**
Effer-K*
Effervescent Potassium*
K+ Care ET
K-Lyte; K-Lyte DS*
Klor-Con/EF*
Tri-K*
**potassium chloride**
Cena-K
Gen-K
K-vescent
K+ 8; K+ 10
K+ Care
K-Tab
K-Dur 10; K-Dur 20
K-Lease
K-Lor
K-Lyte/Cl
K-Lyte/Cl; K-Lyte/Cl 50
K-Norm
Kaochlor 10%; Kaochlor S-F*
Kaon-Cl 20%*
Kaon-Cl; Kaon-Cl 10
Kato
Kay Ciel
Klor-Con 8; Klor-Con 10
Klor-Con; Klor-Con/25
Klorvess
Klotrix
Kolyum*
Micro-K LS
Micro-K; Micro-K 10
Plegisol*
Potasalan*
Rum-K
Slow-K
Ten-K
**potassium citrate**
Citrolith*
Cytra-3*
Cytra-K*
Cytra-LC*
Effer-K*
Effervescent Potassium*
K-Lyte; K-Lyte DS*
K-Lyte Ⓐⁿ

---

*This brand is a combination product.

**potassium citrate (cont.)**
 Klor-Con/EF*
 Polycitra*
 Polycitra-K*
 Polycitra-LC*
 Tri-K*
 Twin-K*
 Urocit-K
**potassium gluconate**
 K-G Elixir
 Kaon
 Kaylixir*
 Kolyum*
 Twin-K*
**potassium guaiacolsulfonate**
 Cophene-X*
 Entuss Expectorant*
 Marcof Expectorant*
 Protuss*
 Protuss-D*
**potassium iodide**
 Elixophyllin-KI*
 KIE*
 Lugol*
 Mudrane*
 Mudrane-2*
 Pediacof*
 Pedituss Cough*
 Pima
 Quadrinal*
 SSKI
 Strong Iodine*
 Theophyllin KI*
 Thyro-Block
**potassium perchlorate**
 Perchloracap
**potassium phosphate**
 K-Phos Neutral*
 Uro-KP-Neutral*
**potassium salicylate**
 Pabalate-SF*
**povidone-iodine**
 Betadine 5% Sterile Ophthalmic Prep
**pralidoxime chloride**
 Protopam Chloride
**pramipexole dihydrochloride**
 Mirapex
**pramlintide acetate**
 Symlin

**pramoxine**
 Analpram-HC*
 Epifoam*
 1+1-F Creme*
 Pramosone*
 Zone-A Forte*
**pramoxine HCl**
 Cortic*
 Enzone*
 Oti-Med*
 Otomar-HC*
 Pramoxine HC*
 ProctoCream-HC*
 Proctofoam-HC*
 Tri-Otic*
 Zoto-HC*
**pravastatin sodium**
 Pravachol
**prazepam**
 Centrax
**praziquantel**
 Biltricide
**prazosin HCl**
 Minipress
 Minizide 1; Minizide 2; Minizide 5*
**prednicarbate**
 Dermatop
**prednimustine**
 Sterecyt
**prednisolone**
 Delta-Cortef
 Prelone*
**prednisolone acetate**
 Articulose-50
 Blephamide*
 Cetapred*
 Econopred; Econopred Plus
 Isopto Cetapred*
 Key-Pred 25; Key-Pred 50
 Metimyd*
 Poly-Pred*
 Pred-G*
 Pred-G S.O.P.*
 Pred Mild; Pred Forte
 Predaject-50
 Predalone 50
 Predcor-50
 Sulpred*

*This brand is a combination product.

**prednisolone acetate (cont.)**
  Vasocidin*
  Vasocine*
**prednisolone sodium phosphate**
  AK-Pred
  Hydeltrasol
  Inflamase Mild; Inflamase Forte
  Key-Pred-SP
  Optimyd*
  Pediapred
  Sulster*
  Vasocidin*
**prednisolone tebutate**
  Hydeltra-T.B.A.
  Prednisol TBA
**prednisone**
  Deltasone
  Liquid Pred*
  Meticorten
  Orasone
  Panasol-S
  Prednicen-M
  Sterapred
  Sterapred DS
**prezatide copper acetate**
  Iamin
**priliximab**
  Centara
**prilocaine**
  EMLA*
**prilocaine HCl**
  Citanest Forte*
  Citanest Plain
**primaquine phosphate**
  Aralen Phosphate with Primaquine
    Phosphate*
**primidone**
  Mysoline
**probenecid**
  Benemid ⒸⒶⓃ
  Benuryl ⒸⒶⓃ
  Col-Probenecid*
  Colabid*
  ColBenemid*
  Polycillin-PRB*
  Principen with Probenecid*
  Probalan
  Probampacin*
  Proben-C*

**probucol**
  Lorelco
  Panavir
**procainamide HCl**
  Procan SR
  Procanbid
  Promine
  Pronestyl
  Pronestyl-SR
  Rhythmin
**procaine**
  Co Tinic*
  Forte L.I.V.*
  Ravocaine & Novocaine with
    Levophed*
  Ravocaine & Novocaine with Neo-
    Cobefrin*
**procaine HCl**
  Hemocyte*
  Hytinic*
  Licoplex DS*
  Novocain
**procarbazine HCl**
  Matulane
**prochlorperazine**
  Compazine
  Stemetil ⒸⒶⓃ
**prochlorperazine bimaleate**
  Nu-Prochlor ⒸⒶⓃ
  Stemetil ⒸⒶⓃ
**prochlorperazine edisylate**
  Compazine
**prochlorperazine maleate**
  Compazine
**prochlorperazine mesylate**
  Stemetil ⒸⒶⓃ
**procyclidine HCl**
  Kemadrin
**progesterone**
  Crinone
  Progestasert
  Prometrium
**proguanil HCl**
  Malarone ⒸⒶⓃ*
**promazine HCl**
  Prozine-50
  Sparine

*This brand is a combination product.

**promethazine HCl**
Anergan 25
Anergan 50
K-Phen-50
Mepergan*
Mepergan Fortis*
Pentazine
Pentazine VC with Codeine*
Phenameth
Phenameth DM*
Phenazine 25
Phenazine 50
Phenergan
Phenergan Fortis*
Phenergan Plain
Phenergan VC*
Phenergan VC with Codeine*
Phenergan with Codeine*
Phenergan with Dextromethorphan*
Phenoject-50
Pherazine DM*
Pherazine VC with Codeine*
Pherazine with Codeine*
Pro-50
Prometh*
Prometh-50
Prometh VC Plain*
Prometh VC with Codeine*
Prometh with Codeine*
Prometh with Dextromethorphan*
Promethazine DM*
Promethazine VC*
Promethazine VC Plain*
Promethazine VC with Codeine*
Promethist with Codeine*
Prorex-25; Prorex-50
Prothazine
Prothazine Plain
V-Gan 25; V-Gan 50
**propafenone HCl**
Rythmol
**propantheline bromide**
Pro-Banthīne
**proparacaine HCl**
AK-Taine
Alcaine
Fluoracaine*
Ophthaine
Ophthetic

**propiomazine HCl**
Largon
**propiram fumarate**
Dirame
**propofol**
Diprivan
**propoxycaine HCl**
Ravocaine & Novocaine with Levophed*
Ravocaine & Novocaine with Neo-Cobefrin*
**propoxyphene HCl**
Darvon
Darvon Compound-65*
Dolene*
E-Lor*
Genagesic*
Proxy 65*
Wygesic*
**propoxyphene napsylate**
Darvocet-N 50; Darvocet-N 100*
Darvon-N
Propacet 100*
**propranolol HCl**
Betachron E-R
Inderal
Inderal LA
Inderide 40/25; Inderide 80/25*
Inderide LA 80/50; Inderide LA 120/50; Inderide LA 160/50*
Ipran
**propylhexedrine**
Benzedrex
**propyliodone**
Dionosil Oily
**protease**
Arco-Lase Plus*
Bilezyme*
Cotazym*
Cotazym-S*
Creon*
Creon 10; Creon 20*
Donnazyme*
Gustase Plus*
Ilozyme*
Ku-Zyme*
Ku-Zyme HP*
Kutrase*

*This brand is a combination product.

**protease (cont.)**
Pancrease; Pancrease MT 4; Pancrease MT 10; Pancrease MT 16; Pancrease MT 20*
Pancrecarb MS-8*
Protilase*
Ultrase MT 12; Ultrase MT 20*
Viokase*
Zymase*

**protein A**
Prosorba Column

**protirelin**
Thymone
Thypinone
Thyrel-TRH

**protriptyline HCl**
Vivactil

**pseudoephedrine HCl**
Actagen-C Cough*
Actifed with Codeine Cough*
Allegra-D*
Allent*
Allerfrin with Codeine*
Anamine*
Anamine T.D.*
Anaplex*
Anaplex SR*
Anatuss LA*
Aprodine with Codeine*
Atrohist Pediatric*
Biohist-LA*
Brexin-L.A.*
Brofed*
Bromadine-DM*
Bromadine-DX*
Bromarest DX Cough*
Bromatane DX Cough*
Bromfed*
Bromfed-DM Cough*
Bromfed-PD*
Bromfenex*
Bromfenex PD*
Bromphen DX Cough*
Brotane DX Cough*
Calmylin Codeine ⓒᴬᴺ*
Carbinoxamine Compound*
Carbiset*
Carbiset-TR*
Carbodec*
Carbodec DM*

**pseudoephedrine HCl (cont.)**
Carbodec TR*
Cardec-DM*
Cardec-S*
Chlorafed; Chlorafed HS*
Chlordrine S.R.*
Chlorphedrine SR*
Codehist DH*
Codimal-L.A.; Codimal-L.A. Half*
Colfed-A*
Congess JR*
Congess SR*
Cophene No. 2*
Cophene XP*
Cotridin ⓒᴬᴺ*
Cotridin Expectorant ⓒᴬᴺ*
Cyclofed Pediatric*
Cycofed Pediatric*
Dallergy-JR*
Decohistine DH*
Deconamine*
Deconamine CX*
Deconamine SR*
Decongestant Expectorant*
Deconomed SR*
Deconsal II*
Deconsal Pediatric*
Defen-LA*
Deproist Expectorant with Codeine*
Detussin*
Detussin Expectorant*
Dihistine Expectorant*
Dimetane-DX Cough*
Dura-Tap/PD*
Duralex*
Duratuss*
Duratuss HD*
Endafed*
Entex PSE*
Entuss-D*
Entuss-D Jr.*
Eudal-SR*
Fedahist*
GP-500*
Guai-Vent/PSE*
Guaifed*
Guaifed-PD*

*This brand is a combination product.

**Generic ♦ Brands**

**pseudoephedrine HCl (cont.)**

Guaifenex PSE 60; Guaifenex PSE 120; Guaifenex Rx DM*
Guaifenex Rx*
GuaiMAX-D*
Guaitex PSE*
Guaivent*
Guaivent PD*
Guiatex PSE*
Guiatuss DAC*
Guiatussin DAC*
H-Tuss-D*
Histalet*
Histalet X*
Histinex PV*
Histussin D*
Hyphed*
Iofed*
Iofed PD*
Iosal II*
Isoclor Expectorant*
Klerist-D*
Kronofed-A*
Kronofed-A Jr.*
Lodrane LD*
MED-Rx*
MED-Rx DM*
Mescolor*
Myphetane DX Cough*
Mytussin DAC*
Nasabid*
Nasabid SR*
Nasatab LA*
ND Clear*
No-Hist*
Novafed
Novafed A*
Novagest Expectorant with Codeine*
Novahistine DH*
Novahistine Expectorant*
Nucofed*
Nucofed Expectorant; Nucofed Pediatric Expectorant*
P-V-Tussin*
Pancof-HC*
Panmist JR*
Phenhist DH with Codeine*
Phenhist Expectorant*

**pseudoephedrine HCl (cont.)**

Protuss-D*
Protuss DM*
Pseudo-Car DM*
Pseudo-Chlor*
Rescon*
Rescon-ED*
Rescon JR*
Respa-1st*
Respahist*
Respaire-60; Respaire-120*
Rinade B.I.D.*
Robafen DAC*
Robitussin-DAC*
Rondamine-DM*
Rondec*
Rondec-DM*
Rondec-TR*
Ru-Tuss DE*
Rymed*
Ryna-C*
Ryna-CX*
Seldane-D*
Semprex-D*
Sildec-DM*
Sinufed*
SRC Expectorant*
Stamoist E*
Sudal 120/600*
Sudal 60/500*
Sudex*
Syn-Rx*
Time-Hist*
Touro A & H*
Touro LA*
Triacin-C Cough*
Triafed with Codeine*
Trifed*
Trifed-C Cough*
Tuss-LA*
Tussafed*
Tussafin Expectorant*
Tussar SF; Tussar-2*
Tussend*
Tussgen*
Tyrodone*
UltraBrom*
UltraBrom PD*

*This brand is a combination product.

**pseudoephedrine HCl (cont.)**
V-Dec-M*
Vanex Expectorant*
Versacaps*
Zephrex*
Zephrex LA*
**pseudoephedrine sulfate**
Ami-Drix*
Claritin-D; Claritin-D 12 Hour;
    Claritin-D 24 Hour*
Dexaphen S.A.*
Disobrom*
Drixomed*
Polaramine Expectorant*
Rynatan*
Trinalin*
**pseudoephedrine tannate**
Tanafed*
**pulmonary surfactant replacement**
Curosurf
**pyrazinamide**
Rifater*
**pyridostigmine bromide**
Mestinon
Regonol
**pyrilamine maleate**
Codimal DH*
Histalet Forte*
Iohist D*
Liqui-Histine-D*
Poly-Histine*
Poly-Histine-D*
Poly-Histine-D Ped Caps*
Rolatuss with Hydrocodone*
Ru-Tuss with Hydrocodone*
Statuss Green*
Tri-P*
Triaminic*
Triaminic Expectorant DH*
Tricodene Cough and Cold*
Vanex Forte*
Vetuss HC*
**pyrilamine tannate**
Atrohist Pediatric*
R-Tannamine*
R-Tannate*
Rhinatate*
Rynatan*
Rynatan-S*
Tanoral*

**pyrilamine tannate (cont.)**
Tri-Tannate*
Triotann*
Tritan*
Tritann Pediatric*
**pyrimethamine**
Daraprim
Fansidar*
**quazepam**
Doral
**quetiapine fumarate**
Seroquel
**quinapril HCl**
Accupril
Accuretic ⒸⒶⓃ*
**quinestrol**
Estrovis
**quinethazone**
Hydromox
**quinidine gluconate**
Quin-Release
Quinaglute
Quinalan
**quinidine polygalacturonate**
Cardioquin
**quinidine sulfate**
Quinidex
Quinora
**quinine sulfate**
Quinamm
Quiphile
**quinupristin**
Synercid*
**rabeprazole sodium**
Aciphex
**rabies immune globulin**
Hyperab
Imogam
**rabies vaccine**
Imovax
RabAvert
**racemethionine**
M-Caps
Pedameth
Uracid
**raloxifene HCl**
Evista

*This brand is a combination product.

**Generic ◆ Brands**

**raltitrexed**
Tomudex
**ramipril**
Altace
**ranitidine bismuth citrate**
Pylorid ⓒᴬᴺ
Tritec
**ranitidine HCl**
Zantac
Zantac EFFERdose
Zantac GELdose
**rapid immunoassay (RIA)**
BTA Stat Test
**rauwolfia serpentina**
Raudixin
Rauverid
Rauzide*
**reboxetine**
Edronax
**regramostim**
Leucotropin
**remifentanil HCl**
Ultiva
**repaglinide**
Prandin
**rescinnamine**
Moderil
**reserpine**
Cam-Ap-Es*
Chloroserpine*
Demi-Regroton*
Diupres-250; Diupres-500*
Diutensen-R*
Hydrap-ES*
Hydro-Serp*
Hydropres-25*
Hydropres-50*
Hydroserpine #1; Hydroserpine #2*
Hydrosine 25, Hydrosine 50*
Marpres*
Metatensin #2; Metatensin #4*
Regroton*
Renese-R*
Salazide; Salazide-Demi*
Salutensin; Salutensin-Demi*
Ser-Ap-Es*
Serpalan
Serpazide*
Tri-Hydroserpine*
Unipres*

**resorcinol**
Castellani Paint Modified*
**respiratory syncytial virus immune globulin (RSV-IG)**
Hypermune RSV
RespiGam
**reteplase**
Retavase
**$Rh_0$(D) immune globulin**
Gamulin Rh
HypRho-D; HypRho-D Mini-Dose
MICRhoGAM
Mini-Gamulin Rh
Rhesonativ
RhoGAM
WinRho SD; WinRho SDF
**ribavirin**
Rebetol
Virazole
**ribavirin capsules**
Rebetron*
**rifabutin**
Mycobutin
**rifampin**
Rifadin
Rifamate*
Rifater*
Rimactane
Rimactane/INH*
**rifapentine**
Priftin
**rifaximin**
Normix
**riluzole**
Rilutek
**rimantadine HCl**
Flumadine
**rimexolone**
Vexol
**risedronate sodium**
Actonel
**risperidone**
Risperdal
**ritodrine HCl**
Yutopar
**ritonavir**
Norvir

*This brand is a combination product.

**rituximab**
  Rituxan
**rivastigmine tartrate**
  Exelon
**rizatriptan benzoate**
  Maxalt
  Maxalt-MLT
**rocuronium bromide**
  Zemuron
**rofecoxib**
  Vioxx
**ropinirole HCl**
  Requip
**ropivacaine HCl**
  Naropin
**roquinimex**
  Linomide
**rosiglitazone maleate**
  Avandia
**rotavirus vaccine**
  RotaShield
**roxatidine acetate HCl**
  Roxin
**rubella virus vaccine**
  Meruvax II
**sacrosidase**
  Sucraid
**salicylamide**
  Lobac*
  Rid-A-Pain with Codeine*
  Tussanil DH*
**salicylic acid**
  Bensal HP*
  DuoPlant
  Emersal*
  Gordofilm
  Paplex Ultra
  PROPApH Foaming Face Wash
  Sal-Oil-T*
  Tinver*
  Verrex*
  Verrusol*
  Versiclear*
**salmeterol xinafoate**
  Advair*
  Serevent
**salsalate**
  Amigesic
  Argesic-SA
  Disalcid

**salsalate (cont.)**
  Marthritic
  Mono-Gesic
  Salsitab
**samarium Sm 153 lexidronam**
  Quadramet
**saquinavir**
  Fortovase
**saquinavir mesylate**
  Invirase
**sargramostim**
  Leukine
**saruplase**
  r-ProUK
**scarlet red**
  Scarlet Red Ointment Dressings
**scopolamine hydrobromide**
  Antispasmodic*
  Atrohist Plus*
  Barbidonna*
  Barbidonna; Barbidonna No. 2*
  Barophen*
  Bellacane*
  Deconhist L.A.*
  Donna-Sed*
  Donnamor*
  Donnapine*
  Donnatal*
  Donnatal No. 2*
  Hyosophen*
  Isopto Hyoscine
  Kinesed*
  Malatal*
  Murocoll-2*
  Phenahist-TR*
  Phenchlor S.H.A.*
  Relaxadon*
  Ru-Tuss*
  Scopace
  Spasmolin*
  Spasmophen*
  Spasquid*
  Stahist*
  Susano*
  Transderm Scōp
**secalciferol**
  Osteo-D

*This brand is a combination product.

**secobarbital sodium**
  Seconal Sodium
  Tuinal*
**secretin**
  Secretin Ferring
**selegiline HCl**
  Carbex
  Eldepryl
**selenious acid**
  Sele-Pak
  Selepen
**selenium sulfide**
  Exsel
  Selsun
**senecio compositae**
  Succus Cineraria Maritima*
**sermorelin acetate**
  Geref
*Serratia marcescens* **extract**
  Imuvert
**Sertoli cells**
  N-Graft
**sertraline HCl**
  Zoloft
  Zoloft ⒸⒶⓃ
**sevelamer HCl**
  Renagel
**sevirumab**
  Protovir
**sevoflurane**
  Ultane
**short chain fatty acids**
  Colomed
**sibutramine HCl**
  Meridia
**sildenafil citrate**
  Viagra
**silicone plug**
  Herrick Lacrimal Plug
  Punctum Plug
**silver protein, mild**
  Argyrol S.S. 20%
**silver sulfadiazine**
  Silvadene
  SSD; SSD AF
  Thermazene
**simethicone**
  Baros*
**simethicone-coated cellulose**
  SonoRx

**simvastatin**
  Zocor
**sincalide**
  Kinevac
**sirolimus**
  Rapamune
**skin test antigens**
  Multitest CMI*
  T.R.U.E. Test
**sodium acid phosphate**
  K-Phos M.F.*
  K-Phos No. 2*
  Uroqid-Acid No. 2*
**sodium ascorbate**
  Cenolate
  Hemocyte Plus*
  Iberet-Folic-500*
  Multibret-500 Hematinic*
  Multibret-Folic-500*
**sodium benzoate**
  Ucephan*
**sodium bicarbonate**
  Baros*
  Neut
**sodium biphosphate**
  Urimar-T*
  Uro-Phosphate*
  Urogesic Blue*
**sodium chloride**
  AMO Endosol; AMO Endosol Extra
  B-Salt Forte
  Bacteriostatic Sodium Chloride
    Injection
  BSS; BSS Plus
  Dey-Pak Sodium Chloride 3% & 10%
  Plegisol*
**sodium citrate**
  Bicitra*
  Citrolith*
  Cytra-2*
  Cytra-3*
  Cytra-LC*
  Oracit*
  PMS-Dicitrate ⒸⒶⓃ
  Polycitra*
  Polycitra-LC*
  Tussirex*

*This brand is a combination product.

Generic ♦ Brands

**sodium ferric gluconate**
  Ferrlecit
**sodium fluoride**
  Florvite + Iron*
  Florvite + Iron; Half Strength
    Florvite + Iron*
  Florvite*
  Florvite; Florvite Half Strength*
  Fluoride Loz
  Fluorinse
  Fluoritab
  Flura
  Flura-Drops
  Flura-Loz
  Karidium
  Karigel; Karigel-N
  Luride
  Luride SF
  O-Cal f.a.*
  Osteo-F
  Pediaflor
  Pharmaflur; Pharmaflur df; Phar-
    maflur 1.1
  Point-Two*
  Poly-Vi-Flor*
  Poly-Vi-Flor with Iron*
  PreviDent
  PreviDent Rinse
  Slow Fluoride
  Thera-Flur; Thera-Flur-N
  Tri-Vi-Flor*
  Tri-Vi-Flor with Iron*
  Vi-Daylin/F ADC + Iron*
  Vi-Daylin/F ADC*
  Vi-Daylin/F Multivitamin + Iron*
  Vi-Daylin/F Multivitamin*
**sodium iodide**
  Iodo-Pak
  Iodopen
**sodium iodide I 131**
  Iodotope
**sodium monomercaptoundecahy-
  dro-closo-dodecaborate**
  Borocell
**sodium nitrite**
  Cyanide Antidote Package*
**sodium nitroprusside**
  Nitropress
**sodium oxybate**
  Xyrem

**sodium phenylacetate**
  Ucephan*
**sodium phenylbutyrate**
  Buphenyl
**sodium phosphate**
  K-Phos Neutral*
  Uro-KP-Neutral*
**sodium polystyrene sulfonate**
  Kayexalate
  SPS
**sodium propionate**
  Amino-Cerv pH 5.5*
**sodium salicylate**
  Cystex*
  Tussirex*
**sodium stibogluconate**
  Pentostam
**sodium tetradecyl sulfate**
  Sotradecol
**sodium thiosalicylate**
  Rexolate
**sodium thiosulfate**
  Cyanide Antidote Package*
  Tinver*
  Versiclear*
**somatostatin**
  Reducin
  Zecnil
**somatrem**
  Protropin
**somatropin**
  Genotropin
  Humatrope
  Norditropin
  Nutropin
  Nutropin AQ
  Nutropin Depot
  Protropin II
  Saizen
  Serostim
**sorivudine**
  Bravavir
**sotalol HCl**
  Betapace
**sparfloxacin**
  Zagam
**spectinomycin HCl**
  Trobicin

*This brand is a combination product.

**spirapril HCl**
  Renormax
**spironolactone**
  Aldactazide*
  Aldactone
**squalamine**
  BeneFin
**stannous fluoride**
  Gel-Kam
  Stop
**stanozolol**
  Winstrol
**staphage lysate**
  SPL-Serologic types I and III*
*Staphylococcus aureus* **vaccine**
  SPL-Serologic types I and III*
**Staphylococcus bacteriophage plaque-forming units**
  SPL-Serologic types I and III*
**stavudine**
  Zerit
**streptokinase**
  Kabikinase
  Streptase
**streptozocin**
  Zanosar
**strontium chloride Sr 89**
  Metastron
**succimer**
  Chemet
**succinylcholine chloride**
  Anectine
  Quelicin
  Sucostrin
**sucralfate**
  Carafate
**sufentanil citrate**
  Sufenta
**sulbactam sodium**
  Unasyn*
**sulconazole nitrate**
  Exelderm
**sulfabenzamide**
  Dayto Sulf*
  Gyne-Sulf*
  Sultrin Triple Sulfa*
  Triple Sulfa*
  Trysul*
  V.V.S.*

**sulfacetamide**
  Dayto Sulf*
  Gyne-Sulf*
  Sultrin Triple Sulfa*
  Triple Sulfa*
  Trysul*
  V.V.S.*
**sulfacetamide sodium**
  AK-Sulf
  Bleph-10
  Blephamide*
  Cetamide
  Cetapred*
  FML-S*
  Isopto Cetamide
  Isopto Cetapred*
  Klaron
  Metimyd*
  Novacet*
  Ocusulf-10
  Optimyd*
  Sebizon
  Sodium Sulamyd
  Storz-Sulf
  Sulf-10
  Sulf-15
  Sulfacet-R*
  Sulpred*
  Sulster*
  Vasocidin*
  Vasocine*
  Vasosulf*
**sulfacytine**
  Renoquid
**sulfadoxine**
  Fansidar*
**sulfamethizole**
  Thiosulfil Forte
  Urobiotic-250*
**sulfamethoxazole**
  Azo Gantanol*
  Bactrim IV*
  Bactrim Pediatric*
  Bactrim; Bactrim DS*
  Cotrim Pediatric*
  Cotrim; Cotrim D.S.*
  Gantanol
  Septra*

*This brand is a combination product.

**sulfamethoxazole (cont.)**
Septra DS*
Septra IV*
Sulfatrim*
Urobak
**sulfanilamide**
Alasulf*
AVC
D.I.T.I.-2*
Deltavac*
**sulfasalazine**
Azulfidine
Azulfidine EN-tabs
**sulfathiazole**
Dayto Sulf*
Gyne-Sulf*
Sultrin Triple Sulfa*
Triple Sulfa*
Trysul*
V.V.S.*
**sulfinpyrazone**
Anturane
Aprazone
**sulfisoxazole**
Azo Gantrisin*
Azo-Sulfisoxazole*
Gantrisin
**sulfisoxazole acetyl**
Eryzole*
Gantrisin
Pediazole*
**sulfisoxazole diolamine**
Gantrisin
**sulfur**
Novacet*
Sulfacet-R*
Sulfoxyl Regular; Sulfoxyl Strong*
**sulindac**
Clinoril
**sumatriptan succinate**
Imitrex
**suprofen**
Profenal
**suramin hexasodium**
Metaret
**suramin sodium**
Antrypol
Belganyl
Fourneau 309
Germanin

**suramin sodium (cont.)**
Moranyl
Naganol
Naphuride
**sutilains**
Travase
**tacrine HCl**
Cognex
**tacrolimus**
Prograf
**talc, sterile**
Sclerosol
**tamoxifen citrate**
Nolvadex
**tamsulosin HCl**
Flomax
**tartaric acid**
Baros*
Wigraine*
**tasosartan**
Verdia
**tazarotene**
Tazorac
**tazobactam sodium**
Zosyn*
**technetium Tc 99m antimelanoma murine MAb**
OncoTrac
**technetium Tc 99m apcitide**
AcuTect
**technetium Tc 99m bectumomab**
LymphoScan
**technetium Tc 99m bicisate**
Neurolite
**technetium Tc 99m murine MAb to human alpha-fetoprotein (AFP)**
ImmuRAID-AFP
**technetium Tc 99m murine MAb to human chorionic gonadotropin (hCG)**
ImmuRAID-hCG
**technetium Tc 99m sestamibi**
Cardiolite
Miraluma
**tegafur**
UFT*
**teicoplanin**
Targocid

*This brand is a combination product.

**telmisartan**
Micardis
**temazepam**
Restoril
**temozolomide**
Temodar
**tenidap**
Enable
**teniposide**
Vumon
**terazosin HCl**
Apo-Terazosin Ⓒ
Hytrin
Hytrin Ⓒ
Novo-Terazosin Ⓒ
**terbinafine HCl**
Lamisil
Lamisil DermGel
**terbutaline sulfate**
Brethaire
Brethine
Bricanyl
**terconazole**
Terazol 3
Terazol 7
**terfenadine**
Seldane
Seldane-D*
**teriparatide acetate**
Parathar
**terlipressin**
Glypressin
**testolactone**
Teslac
**testosterone**
Androderm
Androtest-SL
Histerone 100
Tesamone
Testandro
Testoderm TTS
Testoderm; Testoderm with Adhesive
Testopel
Testosterone Aqueous
TheraDerm
TheraDerm-MTX*
**testosterone cypionate**
Andro/Fem*
depAndro 100; depAndro 200
depAndrogyn*

**testosterone cypionate (cont.)**
Depo-Testadiol*
Depo-Testosterone
Depotest 100; Depotest 200
Depotestogen*
Duo-Cyp*
Duratest 100; Duratest 200
Duratestrin*
Test-Estro Cypionates*
**testosterone enanthate**
Andro L.A. 200
Andropository-200
Deladumone*
Delatestryl
Durathate-200
Estra-Testrin*
Everone 200
Valertest No. 1*
**tetanus immune globulin**
Hyper-Tet
**tetanus toxoid**
ActHIB*
OmniHIB*
**tetracaine HCl**
Cetacaine*
Pontocaine HCl
Pontocaine HCl*
**tetracycline**
Actisite
**tetracycline HCl**
Achromycin
Achromycin V
Helidac*
Nor-Tet
Panmycin
Robitet
Sumycin
Sumycin '250'; Sumycin '500'
Teline; Teline-500
Tetracap
Tetracyn; Tetracyn 500
Tetralan
Tetralan "250"; Tetralan-500
Tetram
Topicycline
**tetrahydrozoline HCl**
Tyzine

*This brand is a combination product.

**thalidomide**
  Thalomid
**theophylline**
  Accurbron*
  Aerolate Sr.; Aerolate Jr.; Aerolate III
  Aquaphyllin
  Asbron-G*
  Asmalix
  Bronchial*
  Brondelate*
  Bronkodyl
  Elixomin
  Elixophyllin
  Elixophyllin GG*
  Elixophyllin-KI*
  Glyceryl-T*
  Hydrophed*
  Iophylline*
  Lanophyllin
  Marax*
  Marax-DF*
  Mudrane GG*
  Mudrane GG-2*
  Quadrinal*
  Quibron; Quibron-300*
  Quibron-T
  Quibron-T/SR
  Respbid
  Slo-bid
  Slo-phyllin
  Slo-phyllin GG*
  Sustaire
  Synophylate-GG*
  T-Phyl
  Theo-24
  Theo-Dur
  Theo-Dur Sprinkle
  Theo-Organidin*
  Theo-Sav
  Theo-X
  Theobid
  Theobid Jr.
  Theochron
  Theoclear-80
  Theoclear L.A.
  Theolair
  Theolair-SR
  Theolate*
  Theomax DF*
  Theophyllin KI*

**theophylline (cont.)**
  Theospan-SR
  Theostat 80*
  Theovent
  Uni-Dur
  Uniphyl
**thiabendazole**
  Mintezol
**thiethylperazine maleate**
  Norzine
  Torecan
**thiopental sodium**
  Pentothal
**thioridazine HCl**
  Apo-Thioridazine ⓒᴬᴺ
  Mellaril
  Mellaril-S
**thiotepa**
  Thioplex
**thiothixene**
  Navane
**thiothixene HCl**
  Navane
**thonzonium bromide**
  Cortisporin-TC*
**L-threonine**
  Threostat
**thrombin**
  Thrombin-JMI
  Thrombinar
  Thrombogen
  Thrombostat
**thymalfasin**
  Zadaxin
**thymopentin**
  Timunox
**thyroid, desiccated**
  Armour Thyroid
  S-P-T
  Thyrar
  Thyroid Strong
**thyrotropin**
  Thytropar
**thyrotropin alfa**
  Thyrogen
**tiagabine HCl**
  Gabitril

*This brand is a combination product.

**ticarcillin disodium**
  Ticar
  Timentin*
**ticlopidine HCl**
  Apo-Ticlopidine (CAN)
  Ticlid
**tiludronate disodium**
  Skelid
**timolol hemihydrate**
  Betimol
**timolol maleate**
  Beta-Tim (CAN)
  Blocadren
  Cosopt*
  Med Timolol (CAN)
  Novo-Timol (CAN)
  Nu-Timolol (CAN)
  Timodal (CAN)
  Timolide 10-25*
  Timoptic
  Timoptic-XE
**tin etiopurpurin dichloride**
  PhotoPoint
**tinzaparin sodium**
  Innohep
**tiopronin**
  Thiola
**tiratricol**
  Triacana*
**tirilazad mesylate**
  Freedox
**tirofiban HCl**
  Aggrastat
**tizanidine HCl**
  Zanaflex
**tobramycin**
  AKTob
  Defy
  TOBI
  TobraDex*
  Tobrex
**tobramycin sulfate**
  Nebcin
  Scheinpharm Tobramycin (CAN)
**tocainide HCl**
  Tonocard
**tolazamide**
  Tolinase
**tolazoline HCl**
  Priscoline HCl

**tolbutamide**
  Oramide
  Orinase
**tolbutamide sodium**
  Orinase Diagnostic
**tolcapone**
  Tasmar
**tolmetin sodium**
  Tolectin 200; Tolectin 600
  Tolectin DS
**tolrestat**
  Alredase
**tolterodine tartrate**
  Detrol
**topiramate**
  Topamax
**topotecan HCl**
  Hycamtin
**toremifene citrate**
  Fareston
**torsemide**
  Demadex
**tourniquet**
  Ana-Kit*
**trafermin**
  Fiblast
**tramadol HCl**
  Ultram
**trandolapril**
  Mavik
  Mavik (CAN)
  Tarka*
**tranexamic acid**
  Cyklokapron
**tranylcypromine sulfate**
  Parnate
**trastuzumab**
  Herceptin
**trazodone HCl**
  Desyrel
**treosulfan**
  Ovastat
**tretinoin**
  Atragen
  Avita
  Rejuva-A (CAN)
  Renova
  Retin-A

*This brand is a combination product.

**tretinoin (cont.)**
  Retin-A Micro
  Vesanoid
  Vitinoin (CAN)
**triamcinolone**
  Aristocort
  Atolone
  Kenacort
**triamcinolone acetonide**
  Aristocort
  Aristocort A
  Azmacort
  Delta-Tritex
  Derma Comb*
  Flutex
  Kenaject-40
  Kenalog
  Kenalog-H
  Kenalog in Orabase
  Kenalog-10; Kenalog-40
  Kenonel
  Myco-Biotic II*
  Myco-Triacet II*
  Mycogen II*
  Mycolog-II*
  Myconel*
  Mytrex*
  N.G.T.*
  Nasacort
  Nasacort AQ
  Oralone Dental
  Tac-3
  Tac-40
  Tri-Kort
  Tri-Statin II*
  Triacet
  Triam-A
  Triamonide 40
  Triderm
  Trilog
**triamcinolone diacetate**
  Amcort
  Aristocort Forte
  Aristocort Intralesional
  Articulose L.A.
  Triam Forte
  Triamolone 40
  Trilone
  Tristoject

**triamcinolone hexacetonide**
  Aristospan Intra-articular
  Aristospan Intralesional
**triamterene**
  Dyazide*
  Dyrenium
  Maxzide*
**triazolam**
  Halcion
**trichlormethiazide**
  Diurese
  Metahydrin
  Metatensin #2; Metatensin #4*
  Naqua
**trichloroacetic acid**
  Tri-Chlor
**trichloromonofluoromethane**
  Fluori-Methane*
**Trichophyton extract**
  Dermatophytin
**triclosan**
  Septi-Soft
  Septisol
**tridihexethyl chloride**
  Pathilon
**trientine HCl**
  Syprine
**trifluoperazine HCl**
  Apo-Trifluoperazine (CAN)
  Stelazine
**triflupromazine HCl**
  Vesprin
**trifluridine**
  Viroptic
**trihexyphenidyl HCl**
  Artane
  Trihexy-2; Trihexy-5
**trilostane**
  Modrastane
**trimeprazine tartrate**
  Temaril
**trimethadione**
  Tridione
**trimethaphan camsylate**
  Arfonad
**trimethobenzamide HCl**
  Arrestin
  T-Gen

*This brand is a combination product.

**trimethobenzamide HCl (cont.)**
Tebamide
Ticon
Tigan
Triban; Pediatric Triban*
Trimazide
**trimethoprim**
Bactrim IV*
Bactrim Pediatric*
Bactrim; Bactrim DS*
Cotrim Pediatric*
Cotrim; Cotrim D.S.*
Polytrim*
Proloprim
Septra*
Septra DS*
Septra IV*
Sulfatrim*
Trimpex
**trimetrexate glucuronate**
NeuTrexin
**trimipramine maleate**
Surmontil
**trioxsalen**
Trisoralen
**tripelennamine HCl**
PBZ
PBZ-SR
Pelamine
**triprolidine HCl**
Actagen-C Cough*
Actifed with Codeine Cough*
Allerfrin with Codeine*
Aprodine with Codeine*
Cotridin ⓒ*
Cotridin Expectorant ⓒ*
Myidyl
Triacin-C Cough*
Triafed with Codeine*
Trifed*
Trifed-C Cough*
**triptorelin pamoate**
Decapeptyl
**trisaccharides A and B**
Biosynject
**trisulfapyrimidines**
Triple Sulfa No. 2
**troglitazone**
Rezulin

**trolamine polypeptide oleate-condensate**
Cerumenex
**troleandomycin**
Tao
**tromethamine**
Tham
**tropicamide**
Mydriacyl
Opticyl
Paremyd*
Tropi-Storz
Tropicacyl
**trospectomycin**
Spexil
**trovafloxacin mesylate**
Trovan
Trovan/Zithromax Compliance Pak*
**trypsin**
Dermuspray*
Granulderm*
Granulex*
GranuMed*
**tuberculin purified protein derivative**
Aplisol
Aplitest
Sclavo PPD Solution
Sclavo Test-PPD
Tine Test PPD
Tubersol
**tuvirumab**
Ostavir
**typhoid vaccine**
Typhim Vi
Typhoid Vaccine (AKD)
Typhoid Vaccine (H-P)
Vivotif Berna
**tyropanoate sodium**
Bilopaque
**undecylenic acid**
Fungoid
Gordochom*
**uracil**
UFT*
**urea**
Accuzyme*
Amino-Cerv pH 5.5*

*This brand is a combination product.

**Generic ◆ Brands**

**urea (cont.)**
Carmol HC*
Gordon's Urea 40%
Panafil*
Panafil White*
Ureacin-40
Ureaphil
**urofollitropin**
Fertinex
Metrodin
**urokinase**
Abbokinase
Abbokinase Open-Cath
**ursodiol**
Actigall
Urso
**vaccinia virus vaccine for human papillomavirus (HPV)**
TA-HPV
**valacyclovir HCl**
Valtrex
**valine**
VIL*
**valproate sodium**
Depacon
Depakene
Epiject ⒸⒶⓃ
**valproic acid**
Depakene
Deproic ⒸⒶⓃ
**valrubicin**
Valstar
**valsartan**
Diovan
Diovan HCT*
**vancomycin HCl**
Lyphocin
Vancocin
Vancoled
**varicella virus vaccine**
Varivax
**vasoactive intestinal polypeptide**
Invicorp*
**vasopressin**
Pitressin Synthetic
**vecuronium bromide**
Norcuron
**velnacrine**
Mentane

**venlafaxine HCl**
Effexor
Effexor XR
**verapamil HCl**
Calan
Calan SR
Chronovera ⒸⒶⓃ
Covera-HS
Isoptin
Isoptin SR
Tarka*
Verelan
Verelan PM
**verteporfin**
Visudyne
**vesnarinone**
Arkin Z
**vidarabine**
Vira-A
**vigabatrin**
Sabril
**viloxazine**
Catatrol
**vinblastine sulfate**
Alkaban-AQ
Velban
**vincristine sulfate**
Oncovin
Vincasar PFS
**vindesine sulfate**
Eldisine
**vinorelbine tartrate**
Navelbine
**vitamin A**
ADC with Fluoride*
Aquasol A
Chewable Triple Vitamins with Fluoride*
Del-Vi-A
Soluvite-f*
Tri-A-Vite F*
Tri-Flor-Vite with Fluoride*
Tri-Vi-Flor*
Tri-Vi-Flor with Iron*
Tri Vit with Fluoride*
Tri-Vitamin with Fluoride*
Triple Vitamin ADC with Fluoride*
Triple Vitamins with Fluoride*

*This brand is a combination product.

**vitamin A (cont.)**
  Trivitamin Fluoride*
  Vi-Daylin/F ADC + Iron*
  Vi-Daylin/F ADC*
**vitamin B₁**
  Apatate with Fluoride*
**vitamin B₆**
  Apatate with Fluoride*
  Feocyte*
**vitamin B₁₂**
  Apatate with Fluoride*
  Feocyte*
  Fergon Plus*
  Liver Combo No. 5*
  Tri-Tinic*
**vitamin B complex**
  B-C with Folic Acid*
  B-Ject-100*
  B-Plex*
  Becomject-100*
  Berocca*
  Co Tinic*
  Formula B*
  Forte L.I.V.*
  Hemocyte*
  Hemocyte Plus*
  Hemocyte-V*
  Hytinic*
  Iberet-Folic-500*
  Key-Plex*
  Licoplex DS*
  Livitamin with Intrinsic Factor*
  Lypholized Vitamin B Complex &
    Vitamin C with B₁₂*
  May-Vita*
  Megaton*
  Multibret-500 Hematinic*
  Multibret-Folic-500*
  Nephlex Rx*
  Nephro-Vite Rx + Fe*
  Nephro-Vite Rx*
  Nephrocaps*
  Nephron FA*
  Neurodep*
  Senilezol*
  Strovite*
  Tabron*
  Vicam*
  Vitafōl*
  Vitamin B Complex 100*

**vitamin C**
  ADC with Fluoride*
  B-C with Folic Acid*
  B-Plex*
  Berocca*
  Chewable Triple Vitamins with Fluoride*
  Feocyte*
  Formula B*
  Key-Plex*
  Lypholized Vitamin B Complex &
    Vitamin C with B₁₂*
  Nephro-Vite Rx*
  Nephrocaps*
  Neurodep*
  Soluvite-f*
  Strovite*
  Tabron*
  Tri-A-Vite F*
  Tri-Flor-Vite with Fluoride*
  Tri-Vi-Flor*
  Tri-Vi-Flor with Iron*
  Tri Vit with Fluoride*
  Tri-Vitamin with Fluoride*
  Tri-Tinic*
  Triple Vitamin ADC with Fluoride*
  Triple Vitamins with Fluoride*
  Trivitamin Fluoride*
  Vi-Daylin/F ADC + Iron*
  Vi-Daylin/F ADC*
  Vicam*
**vitamin D**
  ADC with Fluoride*
  Chewable Triple Vitamins with Fluoride*
  Soluvite-f*
  Tri-A-Vite F*
  Tri-Flor-Vite with Fluoride*
  Tri-Vi-Flor*
  Tri-Vi-Flor with Iron*
  Tri Vit with Fluoride*
  Tri-Vitamin with Fluoride*
  Triple Vitamin ADC with Fluoride*
  Triple Vitamins with Fluoride*
  Trivitamin Fluoride*
  Vi-Daylin/F ADC + Iron*
  Vi-Daylin/F ADC*

*This brand is a combination product.

**vitamin E**
  Aquavit-E
  Lactinol-E*
  Tabron*
  TriHemic 600*
**vitamins, multiple**
  Adeflor M*
  B Complex with C and B-12*
  B-C with Folic Acid Plus*
  Bacmin*
  Berocca Parenteral Nutrition*
  Berocca Plus*
  Berplex Plus*
  Cefol*
  Cernevit-12*
  Cezin-S*
  Chewable Multivitamins with Fluoride*
  Eldercaps*
  Filibon F.A.; Filibon Forte*
  Florvite + Iron*
  Florvite + Iron; Half Strength
    Florvite + Iron*
  Florvite*
  Florvite; Florvite Half Strength*
  Formula B Plus*
  Heptuna Plus*
  Lactocal-F*
  Lipo-Nicin/100*
  Lipo-Nicin/300*
  M.V.C. 9+3*
  M.V.C. 9+4 Pediatric*
  M.V.I. Neonatal*
  M.V.I. Pediatric*
  M.V.I.-12*
  Marnatal-F*
  Materna*
  Mission Prenatal Rx*
  Multi Vitamin Concentrate*
  Multivitamin with Fluoride*
  Mulvidren-F*
  Mynatal*
  Mynatal FC*
  Mynatal P.N.*
  Mynatal P.N. Forte*
  Mynatal Rx*
  Mynate 90 Plus*
  Natabec Rx*
  Natafort*
  NatalCare Plus*

**vitamins, multiple (cont.)**
  Natalins Rx*
  Natarex Prenatal*
  Nestabs FA*
  Niferex-PN*
  Niferex-PN Forte*
  Norlac Rx*
  Nu-Iron V*
  O-Cal f.a.*
  Par-F*
  Par-Natal Plus 1 Improved*
  Poly-Vi-Flor*
  Poly-Vi-Flor with Iron*
  Polytabs-F*
  Polyvitamin Fluoride*
  Polyvitamin Fluoride with Iron*
  Polyvitamin with Iron and Fluoride*
  Polyvitamins with Fluoride and Iron*
  Pramet FA*
  Pramilet FA*
  Pre-H Cal*
  Prenatal H.P.*
  Prenatal Maternal*
  Prenatal MR 90*
  Prenatal One*
  Prenatal Plus Iron*
  Prenatal Plus with Betacarotene*
  Prenatal Plus; Prenatal Plus
    Improved*
  Prenatal Rx*
  Prenatal Rx with Betacarotene*
  Prenatal Z*
  Prenatal-1 + Iron*
  Prenate 90; Prenate Ultra*
  Secran Prenatal*
  Soluvite C.T.*
  Strovite Plus; Strovite Forte*
  Stuartnatal Plus*
  Theragran Hematinic*
  Vi-Daylin/F Multivitamin + Iron*
  Vi-Daylin/F Multivitamin*
  Vicon Forte*
  Vitafōl; Vitafōl-PN*
  Zenate, Advanced Formula*
  Zincvit*
  Zodeac-100*
**warfarin sodium**
  Carfin

*This brand is a combination product.

**warfarin sodium (cont.)**
  Coumadin
  Sofarin
**Western Blot assay**
  OraSure HIV-1*
**yellow fever vaccine**
  YF-Vax
**yohimbine HCl**
  Aphrodyne
  Dayto Himbin
  Yocon
  Yohimex
**zafirlukast**
  Accolate
**zalcitabine**
  Hivid
**zaleplon**
  Sonata
**zidovudine**
  Aztec
  Combivir*

**zidovudine (cont.)**
  Retrovir
  Scriptene*
**zileuton**
  Zyflo
**zinc acetate**
  Galzin
**zinc mesoporphyrin**
  Hemex*
**zinc sulfate**
  Zinca-Pak
  Zincate
**ziprasidone HCl**
  Zeldox
**zolmitriptan**
  Zomig
**zolpidem tartrate**
  Ambien
**zonisamide**
  Zonegran
**zopiclone**
  Imovane ⒸⒶⓃ

**Generic ♦ Brands**

*This brand is a combination product.

SECTION **2**

# Xref: Indications to Generic & Brand-Name ℞ Drugs

The "indications" for a drug—also called its "designated use," "approved use," or "therapeutic action"—is the reason a drug is prescribed. We can categorize drugs by their indications, grouping together drugs used for a similar purpose. The indications shown below are broad categories of therapeutic action. Individual drugs may be placed in subcategories or have specifically targeted diseases beyond the scope of this listing. Such nuances of use are shown in each individual drug's entry in *Saunders Pharmaceutical Word Book*.

**Indications**

**Abortifacients** [*see: Gynecological Agents, Labor Stimulants*]
**Acne Preparations** [*see: Dermatological Preparations, Acne Products*]
**Adhesion Prevention Agents** [*see: Wound Treatment*]
**AIDS** [*see: HIV Infections*]

## Alcoholism Agents
[*see also: Psychotherapeutics, Antidepressants*]
Antabuse
Depade
disulfiram
naltrexone HCl
ReVia

## Allergy and Anaphylaxis Agents
[*see also: Corticosteroids, Systemic; Dermatological Preparations, Antiinflammatory Agents; Nasal Preparations; Ophthalmologicals*]
Albay
allergenic extracts (aqueous, glycerinated, or alum-precipitated)
Allpyral
Ana-Guard
Ana-Kit

**Allergy and Anaphylaxis Agents (cont.)**
Center-Al
cromolyn sodium
dextran 1
epinephrine
EpiPen; EpiPen Jr.
Gastrocrom
Intal
Pharmalgen
Promit
Sus-Phrine
Venomil

## Alzheimer's Disease Agents
AD7C
Aricept
Celexa
citalopram hydrobromide
Cognex
donepezil HCl
ergoloid mesylates
Exelon
galantamine
Gerimal
Hydergine
Hydergine LC
lecithin
leteprinim potassium
memantine
Mentane

## Alzheimer's Disease Agents (cont.)
Neotrofin
nimodipine
Nimotop
Nootropil
physostigmine
piracetam
Reminyl
rivastigmine tartrate
Synapton SR
tacrine HCl
velnacrine maleate

**Anabolic Steroids** [see: Sex Hormones, Androgenic/Anabolic Steroids]

---

# Analgesics
[see also: Gout Agents; Rheumatic Disease Agents]

## Analgesics, Antimigraine
Amaphen
Amaphen with Codeine #3
Amerge
Anoquan
Arcet
Axocet
Axotal
Betachron E-R
Bucet
Bupap
butalbital
Butalbital Compound
Cafatine
Cafatine-PB
Cafergot
Cafetrate
D.H.E. 45
dihydroergotamine mesylate
Endolor
Ercaf
Ergomar
Ergostat
ergotamine tartrate
Esgic
Esgic-Plus
Femcet
feverfew (Chrysanthemum parthenium; Leucanthemum parthenium; Pyrethrum parthenium; Tanacetum parthenium)

## Analgesics, Antimigraine (cont.)
Fiorgen PF
Fioricet
Fioricet with Codeine
Fiorinal
Fiorinal with Codeine
Fiorpap
Fiortal
frovatriptan succinate
Imitrex
Inderal
Inderal LA
Ipran
Isocet
Isocom
Isollyl Improved
isometheptene mucate
Isopap
Lanorinal
Margesic
Marnal
Marten-Tab
Maxalt
Maxalt-MLT
Medigesic
methysergide maleate
Midchlor
Midrin
Migranal
Migratine
Miguard
naratriptan HCl
Phrenilin
Phrenilin Forte
Prominol
propranolol HCl
Repan
Repan CF
rizatriptan benzoate
Sansert
Sedapap
sumatriptan succinate
Tencet
Tencon
Triad
Triaprin
Two-Dyne
Wigraine
zolmitriptan
Zomig

# Analgesics, Narcotic

Aceta with Codeine
Actiq
AERx
Alfenta
alfentanil HCl
Alor 5/500
Amacodone
Amaphen with Codeine #3
Anexsia 5/500; Anexsia 7.5/650; Anexsia 10/660
Aspirin with Codeine No. 2, No. 3, and No. 4
Astramorph PF
Azdone
B & O Supprettes No. 15A; B & O Supprettes No. 16A
Bancap HC
Buprenex
buprenorphine HCl
butorphanol tartrate
Capital with Codeine
Ceta Plus
Co-Gesic
codeine phosphate
Dalgan
Damason-P
Darvocet-N 50; Darvocet-N 100
Darvon
Darvon Compound-65
Darvon-N
Demerol HCl
DepoMorphine
dezocine
DHC Plus
dihydrocodeine bitartrate
Dilaudid
Dilaudid Cough
Dilaudid-HP
Dirame
Dolacet
Dolene
Dolfen
Dolophine HCl
Duocet
Duragesic-25; Duragesic-50; Duragesic-75; Duragesic-100
Duramorph
E-Lor
Empirin with Codeine No. 3 & No. 4

# Analgesics, Narcotic (cont.)

fentanyl
fentanyl citrate
Fentanyl Oralet
Fioricet with Codeine
Fiorinal with Codeine
Genagesic
Hy-Phen
Hydrocet
hydrocodone bitartrate
Hydrogesic
hydromorphone HCl
HydroStat IR
Infumorph
Innovar
Kadian
Levo-Dromoran
levomethadyl acetate
levorphanol tartrate
Lorcet
Lorcet-HD
Lorcet Plus; Lorcet 10/650
Lortab
Lortab 2.5/500; Lortab 5/500; Lortab 7.5/500; Lortab 10/500
Lortab ASA
Margesic H
Margesic No. 3
Medipain 5
Mepergan
Mepergan Fortis
meperidine HCl
methadone HCl
Methadose
MorphiDex
morphine HCl
morphine sulfate (MS)
MS Contin
MS/L; MS/L Concentrate
MS/S
MSIR
nalbuphine HCl
Norcet
Norco
Nubain
Numorphan
OMS Concentrate
opium
Oramorph SR
Orlaam

Indications

**Analgesics, Narcotic (cont.)**
oxycodone HCl
oxycodone terephthalate
OxyContin
OxyFast
OxyIR
oxymorphone HCl
Panacet 5/500
Panasal 5/500
Papadeine #3
paregoric (PG)
pentazocine HCl
pentazocine lactate
Percocet
Percodan; Percodan-Demi
Percolone
Phenaphen-650 with Codeine
Phenaphen with Codeine No. 3 &
    No. 4
Propacet 100
propiram fumarate
propoxyphene HCl
propoxyphene napsylate
Proxy 65
Rid-A-Pain with Codeine
RMS
Roxanol
Roxanol; Roxanol 100; Roxanol Res-
    cudose; Roxanol T; Roxanol UD
Roxicet
Roxicet 5/500
Roxicodone
Roxilox
Roxiprin
Soma Compound with Codeine
Stadol
Stadol NS
Stagesic
Sublimaze
Sufenta
sufentanil citrate
Synalgos-DC
T-Gesic
Talacen
Talwin
Talwin Compound
Talwin NX
Tylenol with Codeine
Tylenol with Codeine No. 2, No. 3,
    and No. 4

**Analgesics, Narcotic (cont.)**
Tylox
UltraJect
Vicodin; Vicodin ES; Vicodin HP
Vicoprofen
Wygesic
Zydone
**Analgesics, Neuralgia**
Atretol
carbamazepine
Carbatrol
Depitol
Epitol
Tegretol
**Analgesics, Nonsteroidal (NSAIDs)**
acetaminophen
Aclophen
Alumadrine
Amaphen
Amigesic
aminobenzoate potassium
Anaprox; Anaprox DS
Anatuss
Anoquan
Ansaid
Apo-Etodolac (CAN)
Arcet
Argesic-SA
Arthropan
Arthrotec
aspirin
aspirin, buffered
Axocet
Axotal
Brexidol
bromfenac sodium
Bucet
Bupap
Butalbital Compound
carprofen
Cataflam
Celebrex
celecoxib
choline magnesium trisalicylate
    (choline salicylate + magnesium
    salicylate)
choline salicylate
Clinoril
Daypro
diclofenac potassium

## Analgesics, Nonsteroidal (NSAIDs) (cont.)

diclofenac sodium
Diclotec Ⓒᴬᴺ
diflunisal
Disalcid
Dolobid
Duract
Easprin
EC-Naprosyn
Enable
Endolor
Epromate
Equagesic
Equazine M
Esgic
Esgic-Plus
etodolac
Feldene
Femcet
fenoprofen calcium
Fexicam Ⓒᴬᴺ
Fiorgen PF
Fioricet
Fiorinal
Fiorpap
Fiortal
Flexaphen
flurbiprofen
Hyanalgese-D
Hycomine Compound
Ibu
Ibu-Tab
ibuprofen
Ibuprohm
Indochron E-R
Indocin
Indocin SR
indomethacin
Isocet
Isocom
Isollyl Improved
Isopap
isoxicam
ketoprofen
ketorolac tromethamine
Lanorinal
Lobac
Lodine
Lodine XL

## Analgesics, Nonsteroidal (NSAIDs) (cont.)

Magan
magnesium salicylate
Magsal
Margesic
Marnal
Marten-Tab
Marthritic
Maxicam
meclofenamate sodium
Meclomen
Medigesic
mefenamic acid
meloxicam
Meprogesic Q
Micrainin
Midchlor
Midrin
Migratine
Mobic
Mobidin
Mono-Gesic
Motrin
Mus-Lax
Myapap
nabumetone
Nalfon
Naprelan
Napron X
Naprosyn
naproxen
naproxen sodium
Norel Plus
Norgesic; Norgesic Forte
Orphengesic; Orphengesic Forte
Orudis
Oruvail
oxaprozin
Pabalate-SF
Pennsaid
Phenate
Phrenilin
Phrenilin Forte
piroxicam
piroxicam betadex
Ponstel
Prominol
Relafen
Repan

## Analgesics, Nonsteroidal (NSAIDs) (cont.)
Repan CF
Rexolate
Rid-A-Pain with Codeine
Rimadyl
Robaxisal
rofecoxib
Rufen
Saleto-400; Saleto-600; Saleto-800
salicylamide
Salprofen
salsalate
Salsitab
Sedapap
sodium salicylate (SS)
sodium thiosalicylate
Sodol Compound
Soma Compound
Soma Compound with Codeine
sulindac
Tencet
Tencon
tenidap
Tolectin 200; Tolectin 600
Tolectin DS
tolmetin sodium
Toradol
Triad
Triaprin
Tricosal
Trilisate
Tussanil DH
Tussirex
Two-Dyne
Vioxx
Voltaren
Voltaren ⒸⒶⓃ
Voltaren Rapide ⒸⒶⓃ
Voltaren SR ⒸⒶⓃ
Voltaren XR
ZORprin

## Analgesics, Topical
[see also: Dermatological Preparations]
capsaicin
diclofenac potassium
menthol
Pennsaid
Solarase

## Analgesics, Other
CereCRIB
clonidine
Duraclon
Levoprome
Metastron
methotrimeprazine
Oralease
Quadramet
samarium Sm 153 lexidronam
strontium chloride Sr 89
tramadol HCl
Ultram

# Anemia Agents
## Anemia Agents, B Vitamins
[see also: Vitamin Replacement, B Vitamins]
B Complex with C and B-12
B-Ject-100
Becomject-100
Cevi-Fer
Chromagen
Co Tinic
Contrin
Crystamine
Crysti 1000
cyanocobalamin
Cyanoject
Cyomin
Feocyte
Fergon Plus
Fero-Folic-500
Ferotrinsic
folic acid
Foltrin
Folvite
Forte L.I.V.
Fumatinic
Hem Fe
Hemocyte
Hemocyte-F
Hemocyte Plus
Hemocyte-V
Heptuna Plus
Hydro Cobex
Hydro-Crysti 12
Hydrobexan
hydroxocobalamin

**Anemia Agents, B Vitamins (cont.)**
Hytinic
Iberet-Folic-500
intrinsic factor concentrate
Key-Plex
LA-12
Licoplex DS
Liver Combo No. 5
Livitamin with Intrinsic Factor
Livitrinsic-f
Lypholized Vitamin B Complex &
    Vitamin C with $B_{12}$
May-Vita
Megaton
Multibret-500 Hematinic
Multibret-Folic-500
Nascobal
Nephlex Rx
Nephro-Fer Rx
Nephro-Vite Rx
Nephro-Vite Rx + Fe
Nephrocaps
Nephron FA
Neurodep
Niferex Forte
Niferex-150 Forte
Nu-Iron Plus
Pronemia Hematinic
Rubesol-1000
Rubramin PC
Senilezol
Strovite
Tabron
Theragran Hematinic
Tri-Tinic
TriHemic 600
Trinsicon
Vicam
Vitafōl
Vitafōl; Vitafōl-PN
Vitamin B Complex 100
Zodeac-100
**Anemia Agents, Iron**
[see also: Mineral Replacement, Iron]
Cevi-Fer
Chromagen
Co Tinic
Contrin
DexFerrum

**Anemia Agents, Iron (cont.)**
Dexiron ⓒⒶⓃ
Feocyte
Fergon Plus
Fero-Folic-500
Ferotrinsic
Ferrlecit
ferrous fumarate
ferrous gluconate
ferrous sulfate
ferrous sulfate, dried
Foltrin
Forte L.I.V.
Fumatinic
Hem Fe
Hemocyte
Hemocyte-F
Hemocyte Plus
Hemocyte-V
Heptuna Plus
Hytinic
Iberet-Folic-500
InFeD
Infurfer ⓒⒶⓃ
iron
iron dextran
Licoplex DS
Livitamin with Intrinsic Factor
Livitrinsic-f
Multibret-500 Hematinic
Multibret-Folic-500
Nephro-Fer Rx
Nephro-Vite Rx + Fe
Nephron FA
Niferex Forte
Niferex-150 Forte
Nu-Iron Plus
polysaccharide-iron complex
Pronemia Hematinic
Senilezol
Tabron
Theragran Hematinic
Tri-Tinic
TriHemic 600
Trinsicon
Vitafōl
Vitafōl; Vitafōl-PN
Zodeac-100
**Anemia Agents, Other**
Androlone-D 200

**Indications**

**Anemia Agents, Other (cont.)**
Deca-Durabolin
epoetin alfa (EPO)
epoetin beta
Epogen
hemoglobin, recombinant human
(rHb1.1)
Hybolin Decanoate-50; Hybolin
Decanoate-100
Marogen
nandrolone decanoate
Neo-Durabolic
Optro
Procrit

---

# Anesthetics
**Anesthetics, General**
Alfenta
alfentanil HCl
Amidate
Brevital Sodium
Brietal Sodium 🇨🇦
desflurane
Diprivan
enflurane
Ethrane
etomidate
fentanyl citrate
Fluothane
Forane
halothane
Innovar
isoflurane
Ketalar
ketamine HCl
methohexital sodium
methoxyflurane
midazolam HCl
Penthrane
Pentothal
propofol
remifentanil HCl
sevoflurane
Sublimaze
Sufenta
sufentanil citrate
Suprane
thiopental sodium
Ultane

**Anesthetics, General (cont.)**
Ultiva
Versed
**Anesthetics, Local**
[see also: Hemorrhoidal Agents; Ophthalmologicals, Local Anesthetics]
articaine
Baylocaine 2% Viscous; Baylocaine
4%
benzocaine
bupivacaine HCl
butamben
butamben picrate
Carbocaine
Carbocaine with Neo-Cobefrin
Cetacaine
Chirocaine
chloroprocaine HCl
Citanest Plain
cocaine
cocaine HCl
Cocaine Viscous
Decadron with Xylocaine
Dentipatch
dibucaine
dibucaine HCl
dichlorodifluoromethane
dichlorotetrafluoroethane
Dilocaine
diperodon
Duranest; Duranest MPF
Dyclone
dyclonine HCl
EMLA
Enzone
Epifoam
ethyl chloride
etidocaine
1+1-F Creme
Fluori-Methane
Fluro-Ethyl
Isocaine HCl
L-Caine
levobupivacaine HCl
Lida-Mantle-HC
lidocaine
lidocaine HCl
Lidoderm
Lidoject-1; Lidoject-2
Marcaine HCl

**Anesthetics, Local (cont.)**
Marcaine Spinal
Marcaine with Epinephrine
mepivacaine HCl
Naropin
Nervocaine 1%
Nervocaine 2%
Nesacaine; Nesacaine MPF
Novocain
Nulicaine
Octocaine HCl
Polocaine
Polocaine MPF
Pontocaine HCl
Pramosone
pramoxine
pramoxine HCl
prilocaine
prilocaine HCl
procaine HCl
propoxycaine HCl
Ravocaine & Novocaine with Neo-
    Cobefrin
ropivacaine HCl
RSD-921
Sensorcaine
Sensorcaine MPF
Sensorcaine MPF Spinal
tetracaine HCl
Triban; Pediatric Triban
trichloromonofluoromethane
Xylocaine
Xylocaine HCl
Xylocaine MPF
Zone-A Forte
**Angina** [see: Cardiac Agents, Antiangi-
    nals]
**Anorexiants** [see: Weight Reduction
    Agents, CNS Modifiers]

# Antacids
[see also: Peptic Ulcer and Gastric
    Reflux Agents]
aluminum hydroxide gel
calcium carbonate
Cotazym
Dialume
magaldrate
magnesia, milk of

**Antacids (cont.)**
magnesium carbonate
magnesium hydroxide
magnesium oxide
sodium bicarbonate
sodium citrate

# Anthelmintics
albendazole
Albenza
Biltricide
bithionol
Bitin
diethylcarbamazine citrate
Hetrazan
ivermectin
Lorothidol
mebendazole
Mintezol
Niclocide
niclosamide
oxamniquine
piperazine citrate
praziquantel
pyrantel pamoate
Stromectol
thiabendazole (TBZ)
Vansil
Vermox
**Antiarrhythmics** [see: Cardiac Agents,
    Antiarrhythmics]

# Antiarthritics
[see also: Analgesics; Rheumatic Dis-
    ease Agents]
Hyalgan
hyaluronate sodium
hylan G-F 20
Synvisc

# Antibiotics
[see also: Antidiarrheal Agents, Intesti-
    nal Antibacterials; Antiprotozoals;
    Antituberculosis Agents; Dermato-
    logical Preparations, Acne Products;
    Ophthalmologicals, Antibiotics; Oto-

**Indications**

logicals; *Urinary Tract Agents,
Antibacterials; Vaginal Preparations,
Antibacterial; Wound Treatment,
Medicated Dressings*]

## Antibiotics, Aminoglycosides
amikacin
amikacin sulfate
Amikin
Garamycin
Garamycin Pediatric
gentamicin sulfate
Humatin
Jenamicin
kanamycin sulfate
Kantrex
MiKasome
Mycifradin Sulfate
Nebcin
Neo-fradin
Neo-Tabs
neomycin sulfate
netilmicin sulfate
Netromycin
paromomycin sulfate
Scheinpharm Tobramycin ⓒⒶⓃ
Septopal
streptomycin sulfate
TOBI
tobramycin
tobramycin sulfate

## Antibiotics, Carbapenems
imipenem
Lorabid
loracarbef
meropenem
Merrem
Primaxin I.M.
Primaxin I.V.

## Antibiotics, Cephalosporins
Ancef
Apo-Cefaclor ⓒⒶⓃ
Biocef
Ceclor
Ceclor CD
Cedax
cefaclor
cefadroxil
Cefadyl
cefamandole nafate
Cefanex

## Antibiotics, Cephalosporins (cont.)
cefazolin sodium
cefdinir
cefepime HCl
cefixime
Cefizox
cefmetazole sodium
Cefobid
cefodizime
cefonicid sodium
cefoperazone sodium
Cefotan
cefotaxime sodium
cefotetan disodium
cefoxitin sodium
cefpodoxime proxetil
cefprozil
ceftazidime
ceftibuten
Ceftin
ceftizoxime sodium
ceftriaxone sodium
cefuroxime axetil
cefuroxime sodium
Cefzil
cephalexin
cephalexin HCl
cephalothin sodium
cephapirin sodium
cephradine
Ceptaz
Claforan
Duricef
Fortaz
Keflex
Keflin, Neutral
Keftab
Kefurox
Kefzol
Mandol
Maxipime
Mefoxin
Modivid
Monocid
Omnicef
Pentacef
Rocephin
Suprax
Tazicef
Tazidime

**Antibiotics, Cephalosporins (cont.)**
Ultracef
Vantin
Velosef
Zartan
Zefazone
Zinacef
Zolicef
**Antibiotics, Fluoroquinolones**
alatrofloxacin mesylate
Apo-Oflox ⓒ
Cipro
ciprofloxacin
enoxacin
Floxin
gatifloxacin
grepafloxacin HCl
Levaquin
levofloxacin
lomefloxacin HCl
Maxaquin; Maxaquin-3
norfloxacin
Noroxin
ofloxacin
Penetrex
Raxar
sparfloxacin
Tequin
trovafloxacin mesylate
Trovan
Trovan/Zithromax Compliance Pak
Zagam
**Antibiotics, Glycopeptides**
Lyphocin
Targocid
teicoplanin
Vancocin
Vancoled
vancomycin HCl
**Antibiotics, Lincosamides**
Cleocin
Cleocin Pediatric
Cleocin Phosphate
clindamycin
clindamycin HCl
clindamycin palmitate HCl
clindamycin phosphate
Dalacin C ⓒ
Dalacin C Phosphate ⓒ
HyClinda

**Antibiotics, Lincosamides (cont.)**
Lincocin
lincomycin HCl
Lincorex
**Antibiotics, Macrolides**
azithromycin
Biaxin
clarithromycin
dirithromycin
Dynabac
E.E.S.
E.E.S. 200
E.E.S. 400
Eramycin
Ery-Tab
EryPed
EryPed 200; EryPed 400
Erythrocin
Erythrocin Stearate
erythromycin
erythromycin estolate
erythromycin ethylsuccinate (EES)
erythromycin gluceptate
erythromycin lactobionate
erythromycin stearate
Eryzole
Ilosone
Ilotycin Gluceptate
PCE
Pediazole
Prevpac
Robimycin
Tao
troleandomycin
Trovan/Zithromax Compliance Pak
Zithromax
Zithromax ⓒ
**Antibiotics, Penicillins**
amoxicillin
amoxicillin sodium
Amoxil
ampicillin
ampicillin sodium
Augmentin
bacampicillin HCl
Bactocill
Beepen-VK
Betapen-VK
Bicillin C-R; Bicillin C-R 900/300
Bicillin L-A

Indications

## Antibiotics, Penicillins (cont.)
Biomox
carbenicillin indanyl sodium
cloxacillin sodium
Cloxapen
Crysticillin 300 A.S.; Crysticillin
   600 A.S.
D-Amp
dicloxacillin sodium
Dycill
Dynapen
Geocillin
Ledercillin VK
Marcillin
methicillin sodium
Mezlin
mezlocillin
Nafcil
nafcillin sodium
Nallpen
Omnipen
Omnipen-N
oxacillin sodium
Pathocil
Pen-V
Pen-Vee K
penicillin G benzathine
penicillin G potassium
penicillin G procaine
penicillin G sodium
penicillin V potassium
Penicillin VK
Permapen
Pfizerpen
Pfizerpen-AS
piperacillin sodium
Pipracil
Polycillin
Polycillin-N
Polycillin-PRB
Polymox
Principen
Principen with Probenecid
Probampacin
Prostaphlin
Robicillin VK
Spectrobid
Staphcillin
Tegopen
Ticar

## Antibiotics, Penicillins (cont.)
ticarcillin disodium
Timentin
Totacillin
Totacillin-N
Trimox
Unasyn
Unipen
V-Cillin K
Veetids
Veetids '125'; Veetids '250'
Wycillin
Wymox
Zosyn

## Antibiotics, Sulfonamides
Bactrim IV
Bactrim Pediatric
Bactrim; Bactrim DS
Cotrim Pediatric
Cotrim; Cotrim D.S.
Eryzole
Gantanol
Gantrisin
Pediazole
Septra
Septra DS
Septra IV
sulfacytine
sulfadoxine
sulfamethizole
sulfamethoxazole (SMX; SMZ)
Sulfatrim
sulfisoxazole
sulfisoxazole acetyl
Thiosulfil Forte
Triple Sulfa No. 2
trisulfapyrimidines

## Antibiotics, Tetracyclines
Achromycin V
Bio-Tab
Declomycin
demeclocycline HCl
Doryx
Doxy 100; Doxy 200
Doxy Caps
Doxychel Hyclate
doxycycline
doxycycline calcium
doxycycline hyclate
Dynacin

## Antibiotics, Tetracyclines (cont.)

Helidac
Minocin
minocycline HCl
Monodox
Nor-Tet
oxytetracycline
oxytetracycline HCl
Panmycin
Periostat
Robitet
Sumycin
Sumycin '250'; Sumycin '500'
Teline; Teline-500
Terramycin
Terramycin IM
Tetracap
tetracycline HCl
Tetracyn; Tetracyn 500
Tetralan
Tetralan "250"; Tetralan-500
Tetram
Uri-Tet
Vectrin
Vibra-Tabs
Vibramycin

## Antibiotics, Topical

[see also: Dermatological Preparations, Acne Products]

A/T/S
AK-Neo-Dex
AK-Tracin
Akne-mycin
Ala-Quin
Atridox
bacitracin
bacitracin zinc
Bactroban
Bactroban Nasal
Benzamycin
C/T/S
Castellani Paint Modified
chloramphenicol
chloramphenicol palmitate
chlorhexidine gluconate
chlortetracycline HCl
ciprofloxacin
Cleocin T
Clinda-Derm
clindamycin phosphate

## Antibiotics, Topical (cont.)

Clindets
clioquinol
Corque
Cortin
Cortisporin
Cytolex
Dalacin T (CAN)
Del-Mycin
doxycycline hyclate
Elase-Chloromycetin
Emgel
Ery-Sol
Erycette
EryDerm 2%
Erygel
Erymax
Erythra-Derm
erythromycin
1+1-F Creme
Floxin Otic
fuchsin, basic
Furacin
G-myticin
Garamycin
gentamicin sulfate
Klaron
mafenide
mafenide acetate
MetroCream
MetroGel; MetroLotion
mupirocin
mupirocin calcium
Myco-Biotic II
Neo-Cortef
Neo-Dexair
Neo-Dexameth
Neo-Synalar
NeoDecadron
neomycin sulfate
Neosporin G.U. Irrigant
nitrofurazone
Noritate
Novacet
oxytetracycline HCl
Pedi-Cort V Creme
pexiganan acetate
polymyxin B sulfate
Romycin
Sebizon

Indications

## Antibiotics, Topical (cont.)
Silvadene
silver sulfadiazine (SSD)
SSD; SSD AF
Staticin
Storz-N-D
Sulfacet-R
sulfacetamide sodium
Sulfamylon
T-Stat
tetracycline HCl
Theramycin Z
Thermazene
Topicycline
UAD

## Antibiotics, Other (including Synergists)
Aerosporin
Albamycin
Altracin
Azactam
aztreonam
Baci-IM
bacitracin
bactericidal and permeability-increasing (BPI) protein, recombinant
Bactrim IV
Bactrim Pediatric
Bactrim; Bactrim DS
Centoxin
chloramphenicol
chloramphenicol sodium succinate
Chloromycetin
Chloromycetin Sodium Succinate
clavulanate potassium
clofazimine
colistimethate sodium
colistin sulfate
Coly-Mycin M
Coly-Mycin S
Cotrim Pediatric
Cotrim; Cotrim D.S.
dalfopristin
Flagyl
Flagyl ER
Flagyl IV
Flagyl IV RTU
furazolidone
Furoxone
Helidac

## Antibiotics, Other (including Synergists) (cont.)
Lamprene
linezolid
Metaret
Metric 21
Metro I.V.
metronidazole
metronidazole HCl
Mycobutin
nebacumab
Neuprex
Normix
novobiocin calcium
polymyxin B sulfate
Proloprim
Protostat
quinupristin
Renoquid
rifabutin
rifaximin
Rituxan
rituximab
Septra
Septra DS
Septra IV
spectinomycin HCl
Spexil
sulbactam sodium
Sulfatrim
suramin hexasodium
Synercid
trimethoprim (TMP)
Trimpex
Trobicin
trospectomycin sulfate
Unasyn
Zyvox

# Anticoagulants
ancrod
anisindione
antithrombin III (AT-III)
ardeparin sodium
Arvin
ATnativ
bivalirudin
Calciparine
Carfin

**Anticoagulants (cont.)**

Coumadin
coumarin
dalteparin sodium
danaparoid sodium
desirudin
dicumarol
enoxaparin sodium
Flocor
Fragmin
Fraxiparine Ⓒᴬᴺ
Hep-Lock; Hep-Lock U/P
heparin calcium
heparin sodium
Heparin Lock Flush
Hirulog
Innohep
Kybernin
Liquaemin Sodium
Lovenox
Miradon
nadroparin calcium
Normiflo
Orgaran
Revasc
Sofarin
Thrombate III
tinzaparin sodium
Vasoflux
Viprinex Ⓒᴬᴺ
warfarin
warfarin sodium

## Anticonvulsants

[see also: Psychotherapeutics, Anxiolytics; Sedatives and Hypnotics]
acetazolamide
acetazolamide sodium
Ativan
Atretol
Bellatal
carbamazepine
Carbatrol
Celontin
Cerebyx
clonazepam
Depacon
Depakene
Depakote

**Anticonvulsants (cont.)**

Depitol
Deproic Ⓒᴬᴺ
Diamox
Diastat
Diazemuls Ⓒᴬᴺ
diazepam
Dilantin
Dilantin-30 Pediatric
Dilantin with Phenobarbital
Dilantin-125
Diphenylan Sodium
divalproex sodium
Dizac
Epiject Ⓒᴬᴺ
Epitol
Epival Ⓒᴬᴺ
ethosuximide
ethotoin
felbamate
Felbatol
fosphenytoin sodium
gabapentin
Gabitril
Klonopin
Lamictal
lamotrigine
levetiracetam
lorazepam
Luminal Sodium
magnesium sulfate
Mebaral
mephenytoin
mephobarbital
Mesantoin
methsuximide
Milontin
Mogadon
Mysoline
neural gabaergic cells (or precursors), porcine fetal
NeuroCell-HD
Neurontin
nitrazepam
oxcarbazepine
Paral
paraldehyde
Peganone
phenacemide
phenobarbital

Indications

**Anticonvulsants (cont.)**
 phenobarbital sodium
 phensuximide
 Phenurone
 phenytoin
 phenytoin sodium
 primidone
 Sabril
 Solfoton
 Tegretol
 Tegretol-XR
 tiagabine HCl
 Topamax
 topiramate
 Tridione
 Trileptal
 trimethadione
 Valium
 Valium Roche Oral ⓒᴬᴺ
 valproate sodium
 valproic acid
 Valrelease
 vigabatrin
 Zarontin
 Zetran
 Zonegran
 zonisamide
**Antidepressants** [see: Psychotherapeutics, Antidepressants]

# Antidiarrheal Agents
**Antidiarrheal Agents, Antiflatulents**
 charcoal
 simethicone
**Antidiarrheal Agents, Antiperistaltics**
 Antispasmodic
 Antrocol
 Arco-Lase Plus
 atropine sulfate
 Barbidonna
 Barbidonna; Barbidonna No. 2
 Barophen
 Bellacane
 difenoxin HCl
 diphenoxylate HCl
 Donna-Sed
 Donnamor
 Donnapine
 Donnatal

**Antidiarrheal Agents, Antiperistaltics (cont.)**
 Donnatal No. 2
 Hyosophen
 Imodium
 Kinesed
 Logen
 Lomanate
 Lomotil
 Lonox
 loperamide HCl
 Malatal
 Motofen
 Relaxadon
 Sal-Tropine
 Spasmolin
 Spasmophen
 Spasquid
 Susano
**Antidiarrheal Agents, Intestinal Antibacterials**
 [see also: Antibiotics; Antifungals, Systemic]
 Bactrim Pediatric
 Bactrim; Bactrim DS
 Bio-Tab
 Cipro
 ciprofloxacin
 Cotrim Pediatric
 Cotrim; Cotrim D.S.
 Cryptosporidium parvum bovine colostrum IgG concentrate
 Doryx
 Doxy Caps
 Doxychel Hyclate
 doxycycline hyclate
 Flagyl
 Helidac
 Immuno-C
 Metric 21
 metronidazole
 Monodox
 Mycostatin
 Neo-fradin
 neomycin sulfate
 Nilstat
 nystatin
 Nystex
 Protostat
 Septra

**Antidiarrheal Agents, Intestinal Antibacterials (cont.)**
Septra DS
Sporidin-G
Sulfatrim
Synsorb-Pk
Vancocin
vancomycin HCl
Vibra-Tabs
Vibramycin
**Antidiarrheal Agents, Other**
attapulgite, activated
bismuth subsalicylate (BSS)
dehydroemetine
*Lactobacillus acidophilus*
Mebadin
8-methoxycarbonyloctyl oligosac-
    charides

# Antidotes
**Antidotes, Acetaminophen**
acetylcysteine (*N*-acetylcysteine)
acetylcysteine sodium
Mucomyst
Mucomyst 10
**Antidotes, Benzodiazepine**
flumazenil
Romazicon
**Antidotes, Chelating Agents**
BAL in Oil
Bio-Rescue
Calcium Disodium Versenate
Chemet
deferoxamine
deferoxamine mesylate
Desferal
dimercaprol
Disotate
edetate calcium disodium
edetate disodium
Endrate
succimer
Syprine
trientine HCl
**Antidotes, Cyanide**
amyl nitrite
Cyanide Antidote Package
Methblue 65
methylene blue (MB)

**Antidotes, Cyanide (cont.)**
sodium nitrite
sodium thiosulfate
Urolene Blue
**Antidotes, Digoxin**
Digibind
Digidote
digoxin immune Fab (ovine)
**Antidotes, Heparin**
protamine sulfate
**Antidotes, Insecticide**
AtroPen
atropine sulfate
pralidoxime chloride
Protopam Chloride
**Antidotes, Narcotic**
buprenorphine HCl
Depade
nalmefene
naloxone HCl
naltrexone HCl
Narcan
ReVia
Revex
**Antidotes, Other**
Antilirium
Antizol
charcoal, activated
cupric sulfate
edrophonium chloride
Enlon
fomepizole
ipecac
physostigmine salicylate
Reversol
Tensilon
Universal Antidote

# Antiemetics and Antinauseants
[*see also: Peptic Ulcer and Gastric
    Reflux Agents*]
Anergan 25
Anergan 50
Antivert; Antivert/25; Antivert/50
Antivert/25
Antrizine
Anzemet
Apo-Domperidone ⒸⒶⓃ

**Indications**

## Antiemetics and Antinauseants (cont.)

Apo-Perphenazine ⒸⒶⓃ
Apo-Trifluoperazine ⒸⒶⓃ
Arrestin
chlorpromazine
chlorpromazine HCl
Clopra
Compazine
dimenhydrinate
Dimetabs
Dinate
diphenidol HCl
dolasetron mesylate
domperidone
Dramamine
Dramanate
Dramilin
Dramoject
dronabinol
droperidol
Dymenate
E-Vista
Emitasol
granisetron HCl
Hydrate
hydroxyzine HCl
Hyzine-50
Inapsine
K-Phen-50
Kytril
Marinol
Marmine
Maxolon
meclizine HCl
Meni-D
metoclopramide HCl
metoclopramide monohydrochloride monohydrate
MK-869
Motilium ⒸⒶⓃ
Nico-Vert
Norzine
Novo-Domperidone ⒸⒶⓃ
Nu-Prochlor ⒸⒶⓃ
Octamide PFS
ondansetron HCl
Ormazine
Pentazine
perphenazine

## Antiemetics and Antinauseants (cont.)

Phenameth
Phenazine 25
Phenazine 50
Phenergan
Phenergan Fortis
Phenergan Plain
Phenoject-50
Pramidin
Pro-50
prochlorperazine
prochlorperazine bimaleate
prochlorperazine edisylate
prochlorperazine maleate
prochlorperazine mesylate
Prometh
Prometh-50
promethazine HCl
Prorex-25; Prorex-50
Prothazine
Prothazine Plain
Quiess
Reclomide
Reglan
Ru-Vert-M
Scopace
scopolamine hydrobromide
Stelazine
Stemetil ⒸⒶⓃ
T-Gen
Tebamide
thiethylperazine
thiethylperazine malate
Thorazine
Ticon
Tigan
Torecan
Transderm Scōp
Triban; Pediatric Triban
trifluoperazine HCl
Trilafon
Trimazide
trimethobenzamide HCl
V-Gan 25; V-Gan 50
Vistacon
Vistaject-25; Vistaject-50
Vistaril
Vistazine 50
Vontrol

## Antiemetics and Antinauseants (cont.)
Zofran
Zofran ODT

---

# Antifungals
## Antifungals, Systemic
[see also: Antidiarrheal Agents]
Abelcet
AmBisome
Amphotec
amphotericin B
amphotericin B cholesteryl sulfate
Ancobon
Apo-Ketoconazole Ⓒ
Diflucan
fluconazole
flucytosine
Fulvicin P/G
Fulvicin U/F
Fungizone
Grifulvin V
Gris-PEG
Grisactin 500
Grisactin Ultra
Grisactin; Grisactin 250
griseofulvin
itraconazole
ketoconazole
Lamisil
miconazole
Monistat i.v.
Mycostatin
Nilstat
Nizoral
Nyotran
nystatin
Nystatin-LF
Nystex
Sporanox
terbinafine HCl
TLC ABLC
## Antifungals, Topical
[see also: Dermatological Preparations; Mouth and Throat Preparations; Vaginal Preparations, Antifungal]
Ala-Quin
amphotericin B
amphotericin B deoxycholate

## Antifungals, Topical (cont.)
amphotericin B lipid complex (ABLC)
Bensal HP
benzoic acid
butenafine HCl
Castellani Paint Modified
ciclopirox olamine
clioquinol
clotrimazole (CLT)
Corque
Cortin
Derma Comb
econazole nitrate
Exelderm
Exsel
1+1-F Creme
fuchsin, basic
Fungizone
Fungoid
Fungoid-HC
Gordochom
haloprogin
Halotex
ketoconazole
Lamisil
Lamisil DermGel
Loprox
Lotrimin
Lotrisone
Mentax
miconazole nitrate
Monistat-Derm
Mycelex
Myco-Biotic II
Myco-Triacet II
Mycogen II
Mycolog-II
Myconel
Mycostatin
Mykinac
Mytrex
N.G.T.
naftifine HCl
Naftin
Nilstat
Nizoral
nystatin
Nystex
Ony-Clear

## Antifungals, Topical (cont.)
oxiconazole nitrate
Oxistat
Oxizole ⒸⒶⓃ
Pedi-Cort V Creme
Pedi-Dri
resorcinol
selenium sulfide
Selsun
Spectazole
sulconazole nitrate
terbinafine HCl
tolnaftate
Tri-Statin II
UAD
undecylenic acid

---

# Antihistamines
## Antihistamines, Systemic
[see also: Allergy and Anaphylaxis Agents]
Aclophen
acrivastine
Actagen-C Cough
Actifed with Codeine Cough
AH-chew
Alersule
Allegra
Allegra-D
Allent
Allerfrin with Codeine
Alumadrine
Ambenyl Cough
Amgenal Cough
Ami-Drix
Ana-Kit
Anamine
Anamine T.D.
Anaplex
Anaplex HD
Anaplex SR
Anergan 25
Anergan 50
Aprodine with Codeine
astemizole
Atarax
Atarax 100
Atrohist Pediatric
Atrohist Plus

## Antihistamines, Systemic (cont.)
Atuss DM
Atuss HD
azatadine maleate
Ben-Allergin-50
Bena-D 10; Bena-D 50
Benadryl
Benadryl Allergy
Benahist 10; Benahist 50
Benoject-10; Benoject-50
Biohist-LA
Brexin-L.A.
Brofed
Bromadine-DM
Bromadine-DX
Bromanate DC Cough
Bromanyl
Bromarest DX Cough
Bromatane DX Cough
Bromfed
Bromfed-DM Cough
Bromfed-PD
Bromfenex
Bromfenex PD
Bromophen T.D.
Bromotuss with Codeine
Bromphen DC with Codeine Cough
Bromphen DX Cough
brompheniramine maleate
Brompheniramine DC Cough
Bronkotuss Expectorant
Brotane DX Cough
carbinoxamine maleate
Carbinoxamine Compound
Carbiset
Carbiset-TR
Carbodec
Carbodec DM
Carbodec TR
Cardec-DM
Cardec-S
cetirizine HCl
Chlor-Pro
Chlor-100
Chlor-Trimeton
Chlorafed; Chlorafed HS
Chlordrine S.R.
Chlorgest-HD
Chlorphedrine SR
chlorphenamine maleate

**Antihistamines, Systemic (cont.)**
chlorpheniramine maleate
chlorpheniramine polistirex
Chlorspan-12
Chlortab-4
Chlortab-8
Claritin
Claritin-D; Claritin-D 12 Hour;
    Claritin-D 24 Hour
clemastine fumarate
Codehist DH
Codimal DH
Codimal-L.A.; Codimal-L.A. Half
Colfed-A
Comhist
Comhist LA
Condrin-LA
Cophene-B
Cophene No. 2
Cotridin (CAN)
Cotridin Expectorant (CAN)
cyproheptadine HCl
D.A.
D.A. II
Dallergy
Dallergy-JR
Decohistine DH
Deconamine
Deconamine SR
Decongestabs
Decongestant
Decongestant S.R.
Deconhist L.A.
Deconomed SR
Dehist
Dexaphen S.A.
dexbrompheniramine maleate
Dexchlor
dexchlorpheniramine maleate
Diamine T.D.
Dimetane-DC Cough
Dimetane-DX Cough
diphenhydramine HCl
Disobrom
Donatussin
Drixomed
Drize
Dura-Vent/A
Dura-Vent/DA
Dura-Tap/PD

**Antihistamines, Systemic (cont.)**
Duralex
E.N.T.
Ed A-Hist
ED-TLC; ED Tuss HC
Endafed
Endagen-HD
Endal-HD; Endal-HD Plus
Ex-Histine
Extendryl
Extendryl JR
Extendryl SR
Fedahist
fexofenadine HCl
Genahist
Hismanal
Hista-Vadrin
Histaject
Histalet
Histalet Forte
Histamic
Histine DM
Histinex HC
Histinex PV
Histor-D
Histussin HC
Hycomine Compound
Hydramyn
Hydrocodone CP; Hydrocodone HD
Hydrophed
hydroxyzine HCl
hydroxyzine pamoate
Hyphed
Hyrexin-50
Iodal HD
Iofed
Iofed PD
Iohist D
Iohist DM
Iotussin HC
K-Phen-50
ketotifen fumarate
Klerist-D
Kronofed-A
Kronofed-A Jr.
Kutrase
Liqui-Histine-D
Liqui-Histine DM
Lodrane LD
loratadine

## Antihistamines, Systemic (cont.)

Magsal
Marax-DF
Mescolor
methdilazine HCl
Myidyl
Myphetane DC Cough
Myphetane DX Cough
Naldec Pediatric
Naldecon
Naldelate
Nalgest
Nasahist B
ND Clear
ND Stat
Nolamine
Norel Plus
Novafed A
Novahistine DH
OMNIhist L.A.
Optimine
Oraminic II
Ordrine S.R.
Ornade
P-V-Tussin
Pancof-HC
Pannaz
Para-Hist HD
Parhist SR
Partapp TD
PBZ
PBZ-SR
Pediacof
Pedituss Cough
Pelamine
Pentazine
Pentazine VC with Codeine
Periactin
Phenahist-TR
Phenameth
Phenameth DM
Phenate
Phenazine 25
Phenazine 50
Phenchlor S.H.A.
Phenergan
Phenergan Fortis
Phenergan Plain
Phenergan VC
Phenergan VC with Codeine

## Antihistamines, Systemic (cont.)

Phenergan with Codeine
Phenergan with Dextromethorphan
Phenetron
Phenhist DH with Codeine
phenindamine tartrate
pheniramine maleate
Phenoject-50
phenyltoloxamine citrate
Pherazine DM
Pherazine VC with Codeine
Pherazine with Codeine
Poladex
Polaramine
Polaramine Expectorant
Poly-Histine
Poly-Histine CS
Poly-Histine-D
Poly-Histine-D Ped Caps
Poly-Histine DM
Prehist
Prehist D
Pro-50
Prometh
Prometh-50
Prometh VC Plain
Prometh VC with Codeine
Prometh with Codeine
Prometh with Dextromethorphan
promethazine HCl
Promethazine DM
Promethazine VC
Promethazine VC Plain
Promethazine VC with Codeine
Promethist with Codeine
Prorex-25; Prorex-50
Prothazine
Prothazine Plain
Pseudo-Car DM
Pseudo-Chlor
pyrilamine maleate
Quadra-Hist
Quadra-Hist Pediatric
R-Tannamine
R-Tannate
Reactine (CAN)
Rentamine Pediatric
Resaid
Rescon
Rescon-ED

**Antihistamines, Systemic (cont.)**
Rescon JR
Respahist
Rhinatate
Rhinolar
Rhinolar-EX; Rhinolar-EX 12
Rinade B.I.D.
Rolatuss Expectorant
Rolatuss with Hydrocodone
Rondamine-DM
Rondec
Rondec-DM
Rondec-TR
Ru-Tuss
Ru-Tuss II
Ru-Tuss with Hydrocodone
Ryna-C
Rynatan
Rynatan-S
Rynatuss
S-T Forte 2
Seldane
Seldane-D
Semprex-D
Sildec-DM
Siltapp with Dextromethorphan
    HBr Cold & Cough
Sinusol-B
Stahist
Statuss Green
T-Koff
Tacaryl
Tamine S.R.
Tanafed
Tanoral
Tavist
Telachlor
Temaril
terfenadine
Theomax DF
Time-Hist
Touro A & H
Tri-P
Tri-Phen-Chlor
Tri-Phen-Chlor T.R.
Tri-Phen-Mine
Tri-Phen-Mine S.R.
Tri-Tannate
Tri-Tannate Plus Pediatric
Triacin-C Cough

**Antihistamines, Systemic (cont.)**
Triafed with Codeine
Triaminic
Triaminic Expectorant DH
Tricodene Cough and Cold
Trifed
Trifed-C Cough
trimeprazine tartrate
Trinalin
Triotann
tripelennamine HCl
triprolidine HCl
Tritan
Tritann Pediatric
Tusquelin
Tussafed
Tussanil DH
Tussanil Plain
Tussend
Tussi-12
Tussionex Pennkinetic
Tussirex
Tusstat
UltraBrom
UltraBrom PD
Uni-Decon
Unituss HC
V-Gan 25; V-Gan 50
Vanex Forte
Vanex Forte-R
Vanex-HD
Veltane
Vetuss HC
Vistaril
Vistazine 50
Wehdryl
Zyrtec

**Antihistamines, Topical**
[see also: Dermatological Preparations;
    Nasal Preparations, Antiallergic;
    Ophthalmologicals, Antiallergic]
chlorcyclizine HCl
diphenhydramine HCl
doxepin HCl
Mantadil
phenyltoloxamine citrate
pyrilamine maleate
tripelennamine HCl
Zonalon

**Indications**

# Antihypertensives
[see also: Cardiac Agents]
## Antihypertensives, α-Blockers
Apo-Terazosin ⓒ
Cardura
doxazosin mesylate
Hytrin
Hytrin ⓒ
labetalol HCl
Minipress
Minizide 1; Minizide 2; Minizide 5
Normodyne
Novo-Terazosin ⓒ
phentolamine mesylate
prazosin HCl
Regitine
terazosin HCl
Trandate

## Antihypertensives, ACE Inhibitors
Accupril
Accuretic ⓒ
Altace
benazepril HCl
Capoten
Capozide 25/15; Capozide 25/25;
    Capozide 50/15; Capozide 50/25
captopril
cilazapril
enalapril maleate
enalaprilat
fosinopril sodium
Inhibace
Lexxel
lisinopril
Lotensin
Lotensin HCT 5/6.25; Lotensin
    HCT 10/12.5; Lotensin HCT
    20/12.5; Lotensin HCT 20/25
Lotrel
Mavik
Mavik ⓒ
moexipril HCl
Monopril
Prinivil
Prinzide
Prinzide 12.5; Prinzide 25
quinapril HCl
ramipril
Renormax
spirapril HCl

## Antihypertensives, ACE Inhibitors (cont.)
Tarka
Teczem
trandolapril
Uniretic
Univasc
Vaseretic 5-12.5; Vaseretic 10-25
Vasotec
Vasotec I.V.
Zestoretic
Zestril

## Antihypertensives, Angiotensin II Inhibitors
Atacand
Avalide
Avapro
candesartan cilexetil
Cozaar
Diovan
Diovan HCT
Hyzaar
irbesartan
losartan potassium
Micardis
tasosartan
telmisartan
valsartan
Verdia

## Antihypertensives, β-Blockers
acebutolol HCl
atenolol
Betachron E-R
betaxolol HCl
bisoprolol fumarate
Blocadren
celiprolol HCl
Corgard
Corzide 40/5; Corzide 80/5
Inderal
Inderal LA
Inderide 40/25; Inderide 80/25
Inderide LA 80/50; Inderide LA
    120/50; Inderide LA 160/50
Ipran
Kerlone
labetalol HCl
Levatol
Lopressor

## Antihypertensives, β-Blockers (cont.)

Lopressor HCT 50/25; Lopressor HCT 100/25; Lopressor HCT 100/50
metoprolol succinate
metoprolol tartrate
nadolol
Normodyne
penbutolol sulfate
pindolol
propranolol HCl
Sectral
Selecor
Tenoretic 50; Tenoretic 100
Tenormin
Timolide 10-25
timolol maleate
Toprol XL
Trandate
Visken
Zebeta
Ziac

## Antihypertensives, Calcium Channel Blockers

Adalat
Adalat CC; Adalat Oros
amlodipine
amlodipine besylate
Baypress
Calan
Calan SR
Cardene
Cardene I.V.
Cardene SR
Cardizem
Cardizem SR; Cardizem CD
Chronovera ⓒⒶⓃ
Covera-HS
Dilacor XR
diltiazem HCl
diltiazem malate
DynaCirc
DynaCirc CR
felodipine
Isoptin
Isoptin SR
isradipine
lacidipine
Lacipil
Lexxel

## Antihypertensives, Calcium Channel Blockers (cont.)

Lotrel
mibefradil dihydrochloride
nicardipine HCl
nifedipine
nimodipine
Nimotop
nisoldipine
nitrendipine
Norvasc
Plendil
Posicor
Procardia
Procardia XL
Sular
Tarka
Teczem
Tiamate
Tiazac
verapamil HCl
Verelan
Verelan PM

## Antihypertensives, Diuretics

[see also: Diuretics]
Accuretic ⓒⒶⓃ
Aldactazide
Aldactone
Aldoclor-150; Aldoclor-250
Aldoril 15; Aldoril 25; Aldoril D30; Aldoril D50
Alodopa-15; Alodopa-25
amiloride HCl
Apresazide 25/25; Apresazide 50/50; Apresazide 100/50
Aprozide 25/25; Aprozide 50/50; Aprozide 100/50
Aquatensen
Avalide
bendroflumethiazide
benzthiazide
bumetanide
Bumex
Cam-Ap-Es
Capozide 25/15; Capozide 25/25; Capozide 50/15; Capozide 50/25
Chloroserpine
chlorothiazide
chlorthalidone

## Antihypertensives, Diuretics (cont.)

Combipres 0.1; Combipres 0.2; Combipres 0.3
Corzide 40/5; Corzide 80/5
Demadex
Demi-Regroton
Diovan HCT
Diucardin
Diupres-250; Diupres-500
Diurese
Diurigen
Diuril
Diutensen-R
Dyazide
Dyrenium
Edecrin
Edecrin Sodium
Enduron
Enduronyl; Enduronyl Forte
Esidrix
Esimil
ethacrynate sodium
ethacrynic acid
Exna
Ezide
furosemide
Hydrap-ES
Hydrazide 25/25; Hydrazide 50/50
Hydro-Par
Hydro-Serp
hydrochlorothiazide (HCT; HCTZ)
HydroDIURIL
hydroflumethiazide
Hydromox
Hydropres-25
Hydropres-50
Hydroserpine #1; Hydroserpine #2
Hydrosine 25, Hydrosine 50
Hygroton
Hyzaar
indapamide
Inderide 40/25; Inderide 80/25
Inderide LA 80/50; Inderide LA 120/50; Inderide LA 160/50
Lasix
Lopressor HCT 50/25; Lopressor HCT 100/25; Lopressor HCT 100/50
Lotensin HCT 5/6.25; Lotensin HCT 10/12.5; Lotensin HCT 20/12.5; Lotensin HCT 20/25

## Antihypertensives, Diuretics (cont.)

Lozol
mannitol (D-mannitol)
Marpres
Maxzide
Metahydrin
Metatensin #2; Metatensin #4
methyclothiazide
metolazone
Microzide
Midamor
Minizide 1; Minizide 2; Minizide 5
Moduretic
Mykrox
Naqua
Naturetin
Oretic
Osmitrol
polythiazide
Prinzide
Prinzide 12.5; Prinzide 25
quinethazone
Rauzide
Regroton
Renese
Renese-R
Salazide; Salazide-Demi
Saluron
Salutensin; Salutensin-Demi
Ser-Ap-Es
Serpazide
Sodium Diuril
spironolactone
Tenoretic 50; Tenoretic 100
Thalitone
Timolide 10-25
torsemide
Tri-Hydroserpine
triamterene
trichlormethiazide
Unipres
Uniretic
Vaseretic 5-12.5; Vaseretic 10-25
Zaroxolyn
Zestoretic
Ziac

## Antihypertensives, Vasodilators

Apresazide 25/25; Apresazide 50/50; Apresazide 100/50
Apresoline

**Antihypertensives, Vasodilators (cont.)**
Aprozide 25/25; Aprozide 50/50; Aprozide 100/50
Arfonad
Cam-Ap-Es
Corlopam
Cyclo-Prostin
diazoxide
epoprostenol
fenoldopam mesylate
Flolan
hydralazine HCl
Hydrap-ES
Hydrazide 25/25; Hydrazide 50/50
Hyperstat
Loniten
Marpres
minoxidil
Nitro-Bid IV
nitroglycerin
Nitropress
Proglycem
Ser-Ap-Es
Serpazide
sodium nitroprusside
Tri-Hydroserpine
Tridil
trimethaphan camsylate
Unipres

**Antihypertensives, Other**
Aldomet
Aldomet; Aldomet Ester HCl
Amodopa
Catapres
Catapres-TTS-1; Catapres-TTS-2; Catapres-TTS-3
clonidine HCl
Demser
deserpidine
Dibenzyline
guanabenz acetate
guanadrel sulfate
guanethidine monosulfate
guanfacine HCl
Hylorel
Inversine
Ismelin
mecamylamine HCl
methyldopa

**Antihypertensives, Other (cont.)**
methyldopate HCl
metyrosine
Moderil
phenoxybenzamine HCl
pinacidil
Pindac
Raudixin
Rauverid
rauwolfia serpentina
rescinnamine
reserpine
Serpalan
Tenex
Wytensin

# Antineoplastics
[see also: Immunostimulants; Immuno-suppressants; Urinary Tract Agents, Antineoplastics]
**Antineoplastics, Alkylating**
Alkeran
BiCNU
busulfan
Busulfex
carboplatin
carmustine
CeeNu
chlorambucil
cisplatin
cyclophosphamide
Cytoxan
Dacplat
Eloxatin
Emcyt
estramustine phosphate sodium
Foloxatine
Gliadel
Ifex
ifosfamide
IntraDose
Leukeran
lomustine
mechlorethamine HCl
melphalan (MPL)
Mustargen
Myleran
Neosar
oxaliplatin

**Antineoplastics, Alkylating (cont.)**
Paraplatin
Platinol
Platinol-AQ
streptozocin
Temodar
temozolomide
Thioplex
thiotepa
Transplatin
Triapine
Zanosar
**Antineoplastics, Angiogenesis Inhibitors**
AE-941
BeneFin
Neovastat
squalamine
SU-5416
Vitaxin
**Antineoplastics, Antibiotics**
Adriamycin PFS
Adriamycin RDF
Blenoxane
bleomycin sulfate
Cerubidine
Cosmegen
dactinomycin
DaunoXome
daunorubicin citrate, liposomal
daunorubicin HCl
Doxil
doxorubicin HCl
epirubicin HCl
Evacet
Idamycin
Idamycin PFS
idarubicin HCl
Lysodren
Mithracin
mitomycin
mitotane
mitoxantrone HCl
Mutamycin
Nipent
Novantrone
pentostatin
Pharmorubicin PFS; Pharmorubicin RDF ⒸⒶⓃ
plicamycin

**Antineoplastics, Antibiotics (cont.)**
Rubex
valrubicin
Valstar
**Antineoplastics, Antimetabolites**
Abitrexate
Adrucil
capecitabine
cladribine
cytarabine
cytarabine, liposomal
Cytosar-U
DepoCyt
Efudex
floxuridine
Fluoroplex
fluorouracil (5-FU)
Folex PFS
FUDR
gemcitabine
Gemzar
Hydrea
hydroxyurea
Leustatin
mercaptopurine (6-MP)
methotrexate (MTX)
methotrexate sodium
Methotrexate LPF Sodium
Purinethol
raltitrexed
Rheumatrex
Tarabine PFS
tegafur
thioguanine (6-TG)
Tomudex
UFT
Xeloda
**Antineoplastics, Hormones**
Andro L.A. 200
Android-10; Android-25
Andropository-200
Aquest
buserelin acetate
chlorotrianisene
Deladiol-40
Delatestryl
Delestrogen
depAndro 100; depAndro 200
Depo-Provera
Depo-Testosterone

**Antineoplastics, Hormones (cont.)**
Depotest 100; Depotest 200
diethylstilbestrol (DES)
diethylstilbestrol diphosphate
Dioval XX; Dioval 40
Durabolin
Duragen-20; Duragen-40
Duratest 100; Duratest 200
Durathate-200
DUROS
Estinyl
Estra-L 20
Estra-L 40
Estrace
estradiol
estradiol valerate
Estratab
Estrogenic Substance Aqueous
estrogens, conjugated
estrogens, esterified
estrone
Estrone 5
Estrone Aqueous
ethinyl estradiol
Everone 200
fluoxymesterone
goserelin acetate
Gynogen L.A. 20
Gynogen L.A. 40
Halotestin
Histerone 100
Hybolin Improved
Kestrone 5
leuprolide acetate
Lupron Depot
Lupron Depot–3 month; Lupron
    Depot–4 month
Lupron; Lupron Pediatric
medroxyprogesterone acetate
Megace
megestrol acetate
Menest
methyltestosterone
nandrolone phenpropionate
Oreton Methyl
PEG-camptothecin
Premarin
ProMaxx-100
Prothecan
Stilphostrol

**Antineoplastics, Hormones (cont.)**
Suprefact ⒸⒶⓃ
Suprefact; Suprefact Depot ⒸⒶⓃ
Tace
Tesamone
Teslac
Testandro
testolactone
testosterone
testosterone cypionate
testosterone enanthate
Testosterone Aqueous
Testred
Theelin Aqueous
Valergen 10
Valergen 20; Valergen 40
Virilon
Wehgen
Zoladex

**Antineoplastics, Hormone Antagonists**
aminoglutethimide
Anandron ⒸⒶⓃ
anastrozole
Arimidex
bicalutamide
Casodex
cyproterone acetate
Cytadren
Euflex ⒸⒶⓃ
Eulexin
Fareston
Femara
flutamide
letrozole
MGI-114
Modrastane
Nilandron
nilutamide
Nolvadex
Novo-Cyproterone ⒸⒶⓃ
tamoxifen citrate
toremifene citrate
trilostane

**Antineoplastics, Plant Alkaloids and Other Natural Products**
Alkaban-AQ
Camptosar
docetaxel
Eldisine

**Indications**

## Antineoplastics, Plant Alkaloids and Other Natural Products (cont.)

Etopophos
etoposide
etoposide phosphate
irinotecan HCl
Navelbine
Oncovin
paclitaxel
Paxene
Taxol
Taxotere
teniposide
Toposar
Velban
VePesid
vinblastine sulfate
Vincasar PFS
vincristine sulfate
vindesine sulfate
vinorelbine tartrate
Vumon

## Antineoplastics, Protective and Rescue Agents

amifostine
dexrazoxane
Ethyol
Isovorin
L-leucovorin
leucovorin calcium
mesna
Mesnex
pilocarpine HCl
Salagen
sucralfate
Wellcovorin
Zinecard

## Antineoplastics, Therapeutic Vaccines (Theraccines)

AdjuVax-100a
Avicine
BrevaRex
Gastrimmune
GVAX
M-Vax
Melacine
melanoma vaccine
monoclonal antibody B43.13
O-Vax
OncoVax-CL

## Antineoplastics, Therapeutic Vaccines (Theraccines) (cont.)

OncoVax-P
OvaRex
TA-HPV
Theratope-STn
vaccinia virus vaccine for human papillomavirus (HPV), recombinant

## Antineoplastics, Unclassified and Adjuncts

AdjuVax-100a
allopurinol sodium
Allovectin-7
altretamine
amsacrine
Amsidyl
Armour Thyroid
asparaginase (L-asparaginase)
Atragen
Avicidin
bexarotene
Bexxar
biricodar dicitrate
blood mononuclear cells, allogenic peripheral
Bondronat
Bonefos
Bonviva
Broxine
broxuridine
C-225
CEA-Cide
Ceprate SC
chromic phosphate P 32
coumarin
CYT-103-Y-90
CytoImplant
dacarbazine
Decapeptyl
denileukin diftitox
disaccharide tripeptide glycerol dipalmitoyl
disodium clodronate tetrahydrate
DTIC-Dome
edrecolomab
Elspar
EpiLeukin
Ergamisol
Erwinase

## Antineoplastics, Unclassified and Adjuncts (cont.)

erwinia L-asparaginase
Fludara
fludarabine phosphate
Herceptin
Hexalen
Hycamtin
ibandronate sodium
ImmTher
ImmuRAIT-LL2
Imuvert
Incel
iodine I 131 Lym-1 MAb
iodine I 131 murine MAb IgG$_2$a to B cell
iodine I 131 murine MAb to alpha-fetoprotein (AFP)
iodine I 131 murine MAb to human chorionic gonadotropin (hCG)
iodine I 131 radiolabeled B1 MAb
iodine I 131 tositumomab
Iodotope
Leucotropin
Leuvectin
levamisole HCl
Lu-Tex
lutetium texaphyrin
LymphoCide
Matulane
MDX-210
Metastat
methoxsalen (8-methoxsalen)
metoclopramide HCl
monoclonal antibody to CD22 antigen on B-cells, radiolabeled
monoclonal antibody to CEA, humanized
MultiKine
Neomark
9-nitrocamptothecin
Oncaspar
Onco-TCS
Oncocine-HspE7
Oncolym
Oncolysin B
Onconase
OncoRad OV103
Oncostate
Onkolox

## Antineoplastics, Unclassified and Adjuncts (cont.)

Ontak
ONYX-015
Orzel
Ovastat
p30 protein
Pan-HER
Panorex
pegaspargase (PEG-L-asparaginase)
pemetrexed disodium
perfosfamide
Pergamid
Phosphocol P 32
Photofrin
Pivanex
porfimer sodium
prednimustine
Prevatac
procarbazine HCl
Regressin
ricin (blocked) conjugated murine MAb (anti-B4)
Rolazar
S-P-T
Sensamide
*Serratia marcescens* extract (polyribosomes)
sodium iodide ($^{131}$I)
sodium iodide I 131
sodium phosphate P 32
Sterecyt
Targretin
Theragyn
Thyrar
Thyrogen
thyroid
thyrotropin alfa
Tifolar
topotecan HCl
trastuzumab
treosulfan
tretinoin
Tretinoin LF
Triacana
triptorelin pamoate
uracil
Uvadex
Vesanoid
Zyloprim

## Antineoplastics, Chemotherapy Protocols

5 + 2 protocol (cytarabine, daunorubicin)

5 + 2 protocol (cytarabine, mitoxantrone)

7 + 3 protocol (cytarabine, daunorubicin)

7 + 3 protocol (cytarabine, idarubicin)

7 + 3 protocol (cytarabine, mitoxantrone)

8 in 1 (Medrol, vincristine, CCNU, procarbazine, hydroxyurea, cisplatin, ara-C, cyclophosphamide)

8 in 1 (Medrol, vincristine, CCNU, procarbazine, hydroxyurea, cisplatin, ara-C, dacarbazine)

A + D (ara-C, daunorubicin)

A-DIC (Adriamycin, dacarbazine)

AA (ara-C, Adriamycin)

ABC (Adriamycin, BCNU, cyclophosphamide)

ABCM (Adriamycin, bleomycin, cyclophosphamide, mitomycin)

ABD (Adriamycin, bleomycin, DTIC)

ABDIC (Adriamycin, bleomycin, DIC, [CCNU, prednisone])

ABDV (Adriamycin, bleomycin, DTIC, vinblastine)

ABP (Adriamycin, bleomycin, prednisone)

ABV (actimomycin D, bleomycin, vincristine)

ABV (Adriamycin, bleomycin, vinblastine)

ABVD (Adriamycin, bleomycin, vinblastine, dacarbazine)

ABVD/MOPP (alternating cycles of ABVD and MOPP)

AC (Adriamycin, carmustine)

AC (Adriamycin, CCNU)

AC (Adriamycin, cisplatin)

AC; A-C (Adriamycin, cyclophosphamide)

ACe (Adriamycin, cyclophosphamide)

ACE (Adriamycin, cyclophosphamide, etoposide)

## Antineoplastics, Chemotherapy Protocols (cont.)

ACFUCY (actinomycin D, fluorouracil, cyclophosphamide)

ACM (Adriamycin, cyclophosphamide, methotrexate)

ACOP (Adriamycin, cyclophosphamide, Oncovin, prednisone)

ACOPP; A-COPP (Adriamycin, cyclophosphamide, Oncovin, procarbazine, prednisone)

ADBC (Adriamycin, DTIC, bleomycin, CCNU)

ADE (ara-C, daunorubicin, etoposide)

ADOAP (Adriamycin, Oncovin, ara-C, prednisone)

ADOP (Adriamycin, Oncovin, prednisone)

Adria + BCNU (Adriamycin, BCNU)

Adria-L-PAM (Adriamycin, L-phenylalanine mustard)

AFM (Adriamycin, fluorouracil, methotrexate [with leucovorin rescue])

ALOMAD (Adriamycin, Leukeran, Oncovin, methotrexate, actinomycin D, dacarbazine)

AOPA (ara-C, Oncovin, prednisone, asparaginase)

AOPE (Adriamycin, Oncovin, prednisone, etoposide)

AP (Adriamycin, Platinol)

APC (AMSA, prednisone, chlorambucil)

APE (Adriamycin, Platinol, etoposide)

APE (ara-C, Platinol, etoposide)

APO (Adriamycin, prednisone, Oncovin)

ara-C + 6-TG (ara-C, thioguanine)

ara-C + ADR (ara-C, Adriamycin)

ara-C + DNR + PRED + MP (ara-C, daunorubicin, prednisolone, mercaptopurine)

ara-C-HU (ara-C, hydroxyurea)

ASHAP; A-SHAP (Adriamycin, Solu-Medrol, high-dose ara-C, Platinol)

AV (Adriamycin, vincristine)

## Antineoplastics, Chemotherapy Protocols (cont.)

AVP (actinomycin D, vincristine, Platinol)

B-CHOP (bleomycin, Cytoxin, hydroxydaunomycin, Oncovin, prednisone)

B-DOPA (bleomycin, DTIC, Oncovin, prednisone, Adriamycin)

B-MOPP (bleomycin, nitrogen mustard, Oncovin, procarbazine, prednisone)

BAC (BCNU, ara-C, cyclophosphamide)

BACOD (bleomycin, Adriamycin, CCNU, Oncovin, dexamethasone)

BACON (bleomycin, Adriamycin, CCNU, Oncovin, nitrogen mustard)

BACOP (bleomycin, Adriamycin, cyclophosphamide, Oncovin, prednisone)

BACT (BCNU, ara-C, cyclophosphamide, thioguanine)

BAMON (bleomycin, Adriamycin, methotrexate, Oncovin, nitrogen mustard)

BAVIP (bleomycin, Adriamycin, vinblastine, imidazole carboxamide, prednisone)

BBVP-M (BCNU, bleomycin, VePesid, prednisone, methotrexate)

BCAP (BCNU, cyclophosphamide, Adriamycin, prednisone)

BCAVe; B-CAVe (bleomycin, CCNU, Adriamycin, Velban)

BCD (bleomycin, cyclophosphamide, dactinomycin)

BCMF (bleomycin, cyclophosphamide, methotrexate, fluorouracil)

BCOP (BCNU, cyclophosphamide, Oncovin, prednisone)

BCP (BCNU, cyclophosphamide, prednisone)

BCVP (BCNU, cyclophosphamide, vincristine, prednisone)

BCVPP (BCNU, cyclophosphamide, vinblastine, procarbazine, prednisone)

## Antineoplastics, Chemotherapy Protocols (cont.)

BEAC (BCNU, etoposide, ara-C, cyclophosphamide)

BEAM (BCNU, etoposide, ara-C, melphalan)

BEMP (bleomycin, Eldisine, mitomycin, Platinol)

BEP (bleomycin, etoposide, Platinol)

BHD (BCNU, hydroxyurea, dacarbazine)

BHDV; BHD-V (BCNU, hydroxyurea, dacarbazine, vincristine)

BIP (bleomycin, ifosfamide [with mesna rescue], Platinol)

BLEO-COMF (bleomycin, cyclophosphamide, Oncovin, methotrexate, fluorouracil)

BMP (BCNU, methotrexate, procarbazine)

BOAP (bleomycin, Oncovin, Adriamycin, prednisone)

BOLD (bleomycin, Oncovin, lomustine, dacarbazine)

BOMP (bleomycin, Oncovin, Matulane, prednisone)

BOMP (bleomycin, Oncovin, mitomycin, Platinol)

BOP (BCNU, Oncovin, prednisone)

BOPAM (bleomycin, Oncovin, prednisone, Adriamycin, mechlorethamine, methotrexate)

BOPP (BCNU, Oncovin, procarbazine, prednisone)

BVAP (BCNU, vincristine, Adriamycin, prednisone)

BVCPP (BCNU, vinblastine, cyclophosphamide, procarbazine, prednisone)

BVDS (bleomycin, Velban, doxorubicin, streptozocin)

BVPP (BCNU, vincristine, procarbazine, prednisone)

C-MOPP (cyclophosphamide, mechlorethamine, Oncovin, procarbazine, prednisone)

CA (cyclophosphamide, Adriamycin)

CABOP; CA-BOP (Cytoxin, Adriamycin, bleomycin, Oncovin, prednisone)

**Indications**

## Antineoplastics, Chemotherapy Protocols (cont.)

CABS (CCNU, Adriamycin bleomycin, streptozocin)

CAC (cisplatin, ara-C, caffeine)

CAD (cyclophosphamide, Adriamycin, dacarbazine)

CAD (cytarabine [and] daunorubicin)

CAE (cyclophosphamide, Adriamycin, etoposide)

CAF (cyclophosphamide, Adriamycin, fluorouracil)

CAFP (cyclophosphamide, Adriamycin, fluorouracil, prednisone)

CAFTH (cyclophosphamide, Adriamycin, fluorouracil, tamoxifen, Halotestin)

CAFVP (cyclophosphamide, Adriamycin, fluorouracil, vincristine, prednisone)

CALF (cyclophosphamide, Adriamycin, leucovorin [rescue], fluorouracil)

CALF-E (cyclophosphamide, Adriamycin, leucovorin [rescue], fluorouracil, ethinyl estradiol)

CAM (cyclophosphamide, Adriamycin, methotrexate)

CAMB (Cytoxin, Adriamycin, methotrexate, bleomycin)

CAMELEON (cytosine arabinoside, methotrexate, Leukovorin, Oncovin)

CAMEO (cyclophosphamide, Adriamycin, methotrexate, etoposide, Oncovin)

CAMF (cyclophosphamide, Adriamycin, methotrexate, folinic acid)

CAMP (cyclophosphamide, Adriamycin, methotrexate, procarbazine HCl)

CAO (cyclophosphamide, Adriamycin, Oncovin)

CAP (cyclophosphamide, Adriamycin, prednisone)

CAP; CAP-I (cyclophosphamide, Adriamycin, Platinol)

CAP-BOP (cyclophosphamide, Adriamycin, procarbazine, bleomycin, Oncovin, prednisone)

## Antineoplastics, Chemotherapy Protocols (cont.)

CAP-II (cyclophosphamide, Adriamycin, high-dose Platinol)

CAPPr (cyclophosphamide, Adriamycin, Platinol, prednisone)

CAT (cytarabine, Adriamycin, thioguanine)

CAV (cyclophosphamide, Adriamycin, vinblastine)

CAV (cyclophosphamide, Adriamycin, vincristine)

CAVE (cyclophosphamide, Adriamycin, vincristine, etoposide)

CAVe; CA-Ve (CCNU, Adriamycin, vinblastine)

CAVP16 (cyclophosphamide, Adriamycin, VP-16)

CBV (cyclophosphamide, BCNU, VePesid)

CBV (cyclophosphamide, BCNU, VP-16-213)

CC (carboplatin, cyclophosphamide)

CCM (cyclophosphamide, CCNU, methotrexate)

CCV-AV (CCNU, cyclophosphamide, vincristine [alternates with] Adriamycin, vincristine)

CCVPP (CCNU, cyclophosphamide, Velban, procarbazine, prednisone)

CD (cytarabine, daunorubicin)

CDC (carboplatin, doxorubicin, cyclophosphamide)

CDDP/VP (CDDP, VePesid)

CDE (cyclophosphamide, doxorubicin, etoposide)

CEB (carboplatin, etoposide, bleomycin)

CECA (cisplatin, etoposide, cyclophosphamide, Adriamycin)

CEF (cyclophosphamide, epirubicin, fluorouracil)

CEM (cytosine arabinoside, etoposide, methotrexate)

CEP (CCNU, etoposide, prednimustine)

CEV (cyclophosphamide, etoposide, vincristine)

CF (carboplatin, fluorouracil)

CF (cisplatin, fluorouracil)

## Antineoplastics, Chemotherapy Protocols (cont.)

CFL (cisplatin, fluorouracil, leucovorin [rescue])

CFM (cyclophosphamide, fluorouracil, mitoxantrone)

CFP (cyclophosphamide, fluorouracil, prednisone)

CFPT (cyclophosphamide, fluorouracil, prednisone, tamoxifen)

CH1VPP; Ch1VPP (chlorambucil, vinblastine, procarbazine, prednisone)

CHAD (cyclophosphamide, hexamethylmelamine, Adriamycin, DDP)

CHAMOCA (Cytoxan, hydroxyurea, actinomycin D, methotrexate, Oncovin, calcium folinate, Adriamycin)

CHAP (cyclophosphamide, Hexalen, Adriamycin, Platinol)

CHAP (cyclophosphamide, hexamethylmelamine, Adriamycin, Platinol)

ChexUP; Chex-Up; CHEX-UP (cyclophosphamide, hexamethylmelamine, fluorouracil, Platinol)

CHF (cyclophosphamide, hexamethylmelamine, fluorouracil)

CHL + PRED (chlorambucil, prednisone)

ChlVPP (chlorambucil, vinblastine, procarbazine, prednisone)

ChlVPP/EVA (chlorambucil, vinblastine, procarbazine, prednisone, etoposide, vincristine, Adriamycin)

CHO (cyclophosphamide, hydroxydaunomycin, Oncovin)

CHOB (cyclophosphamide, hydroxydaunomycin, Oncovin, bleomycin)

CHOD (cyclophosphamide, hydroxydaunomycin, Oncovin, dexamethasone)

CHOP (cyclophosphamide, hydroxydaunomycin, Oncovin, prednisone)

## Antineoplastics, Chemotherapy Protocols (cont.)

CHOP-BLEO (cyclophosphamide, hydroxydaunomycin, Oncovin, prednisone, bleomycin)

CHOPE (cyclophosphamide, hydroxydaunomycin, Oncovin, prednisone, etoposide)

CHOR (cyclophosphamide, hydroxydaunomycin, Oncovin, radiation therapy)

CHVP (cyclophosphamide, hydroxydaunomycin, VM-26, prednisone)

CISCA; CisCA (cisplatin, cyclophosphamide, Adriamycin)

$CISCA_{II}/VB_{IV}$ (cisplatin, cyclophosphamide, Adriamycin, vinblastine, bleomycin)

CIVPP (chlorambucil, vinblastine, procarbazine, prednisone)

CMC (cyclophosphamide, methotrexate, CCNU)

CMC-VAP (cyclophosphamide, methotrexate, CCNU, vincristine, Adriamycin, procarbazine)

CMF (cyclophosphamide, methotrexate, fluorouracil)

CMF/AV (cyclophosphamide, methotrexate, fluorouracil, Adriamycin, Oncovin)

CMFAVP (cyclophosphamide, methotrexate, fluorouracil, Adriamycin, vincristine, prednisone)

CMFP; CMF-P (cyclophosphamide, methotrexate, fluorouracil, prednisone)

CMFPT (cyclophosphamide, methotrexate, fluorouracil, prednisone, tamoxifen)

CMFPTH (cyclophosphamide, methotrexate, fluorouracil, prednisone, tamoxifen, Halotestin)

CMFT (cyclophosphamide, methotrexate, fluorouracil, tamoxifen)

CMFVAT (cyclophosphamide, methotrexate, fluorouracil, vincristine, Adriamycin, testosterone)

Indications

**Antineoplastics, Chemotherapy Protocols (cont.)**

CMFVP (cyclophosphamide, methotrexate, fluorouracil, vincristine, prednisone)

CMH (cyclophosphamide, *m*-AMSA, hydroxyurea)

CMV (cisplatin, methotrexate, vinblastine)

CNF (cyclophosphamide, Novantrone, fluorouracil)

CNOP (cyclophosphamide, Novantrone, Oncovin, prednisone)

COAP (cyclophosphamide, Oncovin, ara-C, prednisone)

COAP-BLEO (cyclophosphamide, Oncovin, ara-C, prednisone, bleomycin)

COB (cisplatin, Oncovin, bleomycin)

CODE (cisplatin, Oncovin, doxorubicin, etoposide)

COF/COM (cyclophosphamide, Oncovin, fluorouracil + cyclophosphamide, Oncovin, methotrexate)

COM (cyclophosphamide, Oncovin, MeCCNU)

COM (cyclophosphamide, Oncovin, methotrexate)

COMA-A (cyclophosphamide, Oncovin, methotrexate/citrovorum factor, Adriamycin, ara-C)

COMB (cyclophosphamide, Oncovin, MeCCNU, bleomycin)

COMB (Cytoxin, Oncovin, methotrexate, bleomycin)

COMe (Cytoxin, Oncovin, methotrexate)

COMF (cyclophosphamide, Oncovin, methotrexate, fluorouracil)

COMLA (cyclophosphamide, Oncovin, methotrexate, leucovorin [rescue], ara-C)

COMP (CCNU, Oncovin, methotrexate, procarbazine)

COMP (cyclophosphamide, Oncovin, methotrexate, prednisone)

CONPADRI; CONPADRI-I (cyclophosphamide, Oncovin, L-phenylalanine mustard, Adriamycin)

Cooper's regimen

**Antineoplastics, Chemotherapy Protocols (cont.)**

COP (cyclophosphamide, Oncovin, prednisone)

COP-BLAM (cyclophosphamide, Oncovin, prednisone, bleomycin, Adriamycin, Matulane)

COP-BLEO (cyclophosphamide, Oncovin, prednisone, bleomycin)

COPA (Cytoxin, Oncovin, prednisone, Adriamycin)

COPA-BLEO (cyclophosphamide, Oncovin, prednisone, Adriamycin, bleomycin)

COPAC (CCNU, Oncovin, prednisone, Adriamycin, cyclophosphamide)

COPB (cyclophosphamide, Oncovin, prednisone, bleomycin)

COPE (cyclophosphamide, Oncovin, Platinol, etoposide)

COPP (CCNU, Oncovin, procarbazine, prednisone)

COPP (cyclophosphamide, Oncovin, procarbazine, prednisone)

CP (chlorambucil, prednisone)

CP (cyclophosphamide, Platinol)

CP (cyclophosphamide, prednisone)

CPB (cyclophosphamide, Platinol, BCNU)

CPC (cyclophosphamide, Platinol, carboplatin)

CPM (CCNU, procarbazine, methotrexate)

CPOB (cyclophosphamide, prednisone, Oncovin, bleomycin)

CT (cisplatin, Taxol)

CT (cytarabine, thioguanine)

CTCb (cyclophosphamide, thiotepa, carboplatin)

Ctx-Plat (cyclophosphamide, Platinol)

CV (cisplatin, VePesid)

CVA (cyclophosphamide, vincristine, Adriamycin)

CVA-BMP; CVA + BMP (cyclophosphamide, vincristine, Adriamycin, BCNU, methotrexate, procarbazine)

**Antineoplastics, Chemotherapy Protocols (cont.)**

CVAD; C-VAD (cyclophosphamide, vincristine, Adriamycin, dexamethasone)

CVB (CCNU, vinblastine, bleomycin)

CVBD (CCNU, bleomycin, vinblastine, dexamethasone)

CVD (cisplatin, vinblastine, dacarbazine)

CVEB (cisplatin, vinblastine, etoposide, bleomycin)

CVI (carboplatin, VePesid, ifosfamide [with mesna rescue])

CVM (cyclophosphamide, vincristine, methotrexate)

CVP (cyclophosphamide, vincristine, prednisone)

CVPP (CCNU, vinblastine, procarbazine, prednisone)

CVPP (cyclophosphamide, Velban, procarbazine, prednisone)

CVPP-CCNU (cyclophosphamide, vinblastine, procarbazine, prednisone, CCNU)

CY-VA-DACT (Cytoxin, vincristine, Adriamycin, dactinomycin)

CyADIC (cyclophosphamide, Adriamycin, DIC)

CyHOP (cyclophosphamide, Halotestin, Oncovin, prednisone)

CYTABOM (cytarabine, bleomycin, Oncovin, mechlorethamine)

CYVADIC; CY-VA-DIC; CyVADIC (cyclophosphamide, vincristine, Adriamycin, DIC)

CYVMAD (cyclophosphamide, vincristine, methotrexate, Adriamycin, DTIC)

DA (daunorubicin, ara-C)

DAL (daunorubicin, ara-C, L-asparaginase)

DAT (daunorubicin, ara-C, thioguanine)

DATVP (daunorubicin, ara-C, thioguanine, vincristine, prednisone)

DAV (daunorubicin, ara-C, VePesid)

**Antineoplastics, Chemotherapy Protocols (cont.)**

DAVH (dibromodulcitol, Adriamycin, vincristine, Halotestin)

DC (daunorubicin, cytarabine)

DCMP (daunorubicin, cytarabine, mercaptopurine, prednisone)

DCPM (daunorubicin, cytarabine, prednisone, mercaptopurine)

DCT (daunorubicin, cytarabine, thioguanine)

DCV (DTIC, CCNU, vincristine)

DECAL (dexamethasone, etoposide, cisplatin, ara-C, L-asparaginase)

DFMO-MGBG (eflornithine, mitoguazone)

DFV (DDP, fluorouracil, VePesid)

DHAP (dexamethasone, high-dose ara-C, Platinol)

DI (doxorubicin, ifosfamide [with mesna rescue])

DMC (dactinomycin, methotrexate, cyclophosphamide)

DOAP (daunorubicin, Oncovin, ara-C, prednisone)

DTIC-ACTD; DTIC-ACT-D (DTIC, actinomycin D)

DVB (DDP, vindesine, bleomycin)

DVP (daunorubicin, vincristine, prednisone)

DVPL-ASP (daunorubicin, vincristine, prednisone, L-asparaginase)

DZAPO (daunorubicin, azacitidine, ara-C, prednisone, Oncovin)

E-VMAC (escalated methotrexate, vinblastine, Adriamycin, cisplatin)

E-VMAC (escalated methotrexate, vinblastine, Adriamycin, cyclophosphamide)

EAP (etoposide, Adriamycin, Platinol)

EC (etoposide, carboplatin)

ECHO (etoposide, cyclophosphamide, hydroxydaunomycin, Oncovin)

EDAP (etoposide, dexamethasone, ara-C, Platinol)

EFP (etoposide, fluorouracil, Platinol)

ELF (etoposide, leucovorin [rescue], fluorouracil)

**Antineoplastics, Chemotherapy Protocols (cont.)**

EMA 86 (etoposide, mitoxantrone, ara-C)

EMACO (etoposide, methotrexate, actinomycin D, cyclophosphamide, Oncovin)

EP (etoposide, Platinol)

EPOCH (etoposide, prednisone, Oncovin, cyclophosphamide, Halotestin)

ESHAP (etoposide, Solu-Medrol, high-dose ara-C, Platinol)

ESHAP-MINE (alternating cycles of ESHAP and MINE)

EVA (etoposide, vinblastine, Adriamycin)

F-CL (fluorouracil, leucovorin calcium [rescue])

FAC (fluorouracil, Adriamycin, cyclophosphamide)

FAC-LEV (fluorouracil, Adriamycin, Cytoxin, levamisole)

FAC-M (fluorouracil, Adriamycin, cyclophosphamide, methotrexate)

FAM (fluorouracil, Adriamycin, mitomycin)

FAM-CF (fluorouracil, Adriamycin, mitomycin, citrovorum factor)

FAM-S (fluorouracil, Adriamycin, mitomycin, streptozocin)

FAME; FAMe (fluorouracil, Adriamycin, MeCCNU)

FAMMe (fluorouracil, Adriamycin, mitomycin, MeCCNU)

FAMTX (fluorouracil, Adriamycin, methotrexate [with leucovorin rescue])

FAP (fluorouracil, Adriamycin, Platinol)

FCAP (fluorouracil, cyclophosphamide, Adriamycin, Platinol)

FCE (fluorouracil, cisplatin, etoposide)

FCP (fluorouracil, cyclophosphamide, prednisone)

FEC (fluorouracil, epirubicin, cyclophosphamide)

FED (fluorouracil, etoposide, DDP)

**Antineoplastics, Chemotherapy Protocols (cont.)**

FIME (fluorouracil, ICRF-159, MeCCNU)

FL (flutamide, leuprolide acetate)

FLAC (fluorouracil, leucovorin [rescue], Adriamycin, cyclophosphamide)

FLAP (fluorouracil, leucovorin [rescue], Adriamycin, Platinol)

FLe (fluorouracil, levamisole)

FLEP (fluorouracil, leucovorin, etoposide, Platinol)

FMS (fluorouracil, mitomycin, streptozocin)

FMV (fluorouracil, MeCCNU, vincristine)

FNC (fluorouracil, Novantrone, cyclophosphamide)

FNM (fluorouracil, Novantrone, methotrexate)

FOAM (fluorouracil, Oncovin, Adriamycin, mitomycin)

FOMI; FOMi (fluorouracil, Oncovin, mitomycin)

FU/LV (fluorouracil, leucovorin calcium [rescue])

FUM (fluorouracil, methotrexate)

FUVAC (5-FU, vinblastine, Adriamycin, cyclophosphamide)

FZ (flutamide, Zoladex)

H-CAP (hexamethylmelamine, cyclophosphamide, Adriamycin, Platinol)

HAD (hexamethylmelamine, Adriamycin, DDP)

HAM (hexamethylmelamine, Adriamycin, melphalan)

HAM (hexamethylmelamine, Adriamycin, methotrexate)

HD-VAC (high-dose [methotrexate], vinblastine, Adriamycin, cisplatin)

HDMTX (high-dose methotrexate [with leucovorin rescue])

HDMTX/LV (high-dose methotrexate, leucovorin [rescue])

HDMTX-CF (high-dose methotrexate, citrovorum factor)

HDPEB (high-dose PEB protocol)

## Antineoplastics, Chemotherapy Protocols (cont.)

HexaCAF; Hexa-CAF (hexamethyl-melamine, cyclophosphamide, amethopterin, fluorouracil)

HiDAC (high-dose ara-C)

HOAP-BLEO (hydroxydaunomycin, Oncovin, ara-C, prednisone, bleomycin)

HOP (hydroxydaunomycin, Oncovin, prednisone)

ICE (ifosfamide [with mesna rescue], carboplatin, etoposide)

IE (ifosfamide [with mesna rescue], etoposide)

IfoVP (ifosfamide [with mesna rescue], VePesid)

IMF (ifosfamide [with mesna rescue], methotrexate, fluorouracil)

L-VAM (leuprolide acetate, vinblastine, Adriamycin, mitomycin)

LAPOCA (L-asparaginase, Oncovin, cytarabine, Adriamycin)

LMF (Leukeran, methotrexate, fluorouracil)

LOMAC (leucovorin, Oncovin, methotrexate, Adriamycin, cyclophosphamide)

m-BACOD; M-BACOD (methotrexate, bleomycin, Adriamycin, cyclophosphamide, Oncovin, dexamethasone)

m-PFL (methotrexate, Platinol, fluorouracil, leucovorin [rescue])

M-2 protocol (vincristine, carmustine, cyclophosphamide, melphalan, prednisone)

M-BACOS (methotrexate, bleomycin, Adriamycin, cyclophosphamide, Oncovin, Solu-Medrol)

MABOP (Mustargen, Adriamycin, bleomycin, Oncovin, prednisone)

MAC (methotrexate, actinomycin D, chlorambucil)

MAC (mitomycin, Adriamycin, cyclophosphamide)

MAC; MAC III (methotrexate, actinomycin D, cyclophosphamide)

MACC (methotrexate, Adriamycin, cyclophosphamide, CCNU)

## Antineoplastics, Chemotherapy Protocols (cont.)

MACHO (methotrexate, asparaginase, cyclophosphamide, hydroxydaunomycin, Oncovin)

MACOP-B (methotrexate, Adriamycin, cyclophosphamide, Oncovin, prednisone, bleomycin)

MAD (MeCCNU, Adriamycin)

MADDOC (mechlorethamine, Adriamycin, dacarbazine, DDP, Oncovin, cyclophosphamide)

MAID (mesna [rescue], Adriamycin, ifosfamide, dacarbazine)

MAP (mitomycin, Adriamycin, Platinol)

MAZE (m-AMSA, azacitidine, etoposide)

MBC (methotrexate, bleomycin, cisplatin)

MBD (methotrexate, bleomycin, DDP)

MC (mitoxantrone, cytarabine)

MCBP (melphalan, cyclophosphamide, BCNU, prednisone)

MCP (melphalan, cyclophosphamide, prednisone)

MCV (methotrexate, cisplatin, vinblastine)

MECY (methotrexate, cyclophosphamide)

MF (methotrexate [with leucovorin rescue], fluorouracil)

MF (mitomycin, fluorouracil)

MFP (melphalan, fluorouracil, medroxyprogesterone acetate)

MICE (mesna [rescue], ifosfamide, carboplatin, etoposide)

MIFA (mitomycin, fluorouracil, Adriamycin)

MINE (mesna [rescue], ifosfamide, Novantrone, etoposide)

MINE-ESHAP (alternating cycles of MINE and ESHAP)

mini-BEAM (BCNU, etoposide, ara-C, melphalan)

mini-COAP (cyclophosphamide, Oncovin, ara-C, prednisone)

MIV (mitoxantrone, ifosfamide, VePesid)

**Indications**

## Antineoplastics, Chemotherapy Protocols (cont.)

MM (mercaptopurine, methotrexate)

MMOPP (methotrexate, mechlorethamine, Oncovin, procarbazine, prednisone)

MOB (mechlorethamine, Oncovin, bleomycin)

MOB-III (mitomycin, Oncovin, bleomycin, cisplatin)

MOF (MeCCNU, Oncovin, fluorouracil)

MOF-STREP; MOF-Strep (MeCCNU, Oncovin, fluorouracil, streptozocin)

MOMP (mechlorethamine, Oncovin, methotrexate, prednisone)

MOP (mechlorethamine, Oncovin, prednisone)

MOP (mechlorethamine, Oncovin, procarbazine)

MOP-BAP (mechlorethamine, Oncovin, procarbazine, bleomycin, Adriamycin, prednisone)

MOPP (mechlorethamine, Oncovin, procarbazine, prednisone)

MOPP (mustine HCl, Oncovin, procarbazine, prednisone)

MOPP/ABV (mechlorethamine, Oncovin, procarbazine, prednisone, Adriamycin, bleomycin, vinblastine)

MOPP/ABVD (alternating cycles of MOPP and ABVD)

MOPP-BLEO; MOPP-Bleo (mechlorethamine, Oncovin, procarbazine, prednisone, bleomycin)

MOPPHDB (mechlorethamine, Oncovin, procarbazine, prednisone, high-dose bleomycin)

MOPPLDB (mechlorethamine, Oncovin, procarbazine, prednisone, low-dose bleomycin)

MOPr (mechlorethamine, Oncovin, procarbazine)

MP (melphalan, prednisone)

MPL + PRED (melphalan, prednisone)

MTX + MP (methotrexate, mercaptopurine)

## Antineoplastics, Chemotherapy Protocols (cont.)

MTX + MP + CTX (methotrexate, mercaptopurine, cyclophosphamide)

MTXCP-PDAdr (methotrexate [with leucovorin rescue], cisplatin, doxorubicin)

MV (mitomycin, vinblastine)

MV (mitoxantrone, VePesid)

MVAC; M-VAC (methotrexate, vinblastine, Adriamycin, cisplatin)

MVF (mitoxantrone, vincristine, fluorouracil)

MVP (mitomycin, vinblastine, Platinol)

MVPP (mechlorethamine, vinblastine, procarbazine, prednisone)

MVT (mitoxantrone, VePesid, thiotepa)

MVVPP (mechlorethamine, vincristine, vinblastine, procarbazine, prednisone)

NAC (nitrogen mustard, Adriamycin, CCNU)

NFL (Novantrone, fluorouracil, leucovorin [rescue])

NOVP (Novantrone, Oncovin, vinblastine, prednisone)

OAP (Oncovin, ara-C, prednisone)

OMAD (Oncovin, methotrexate/citrovorum factor, Adriamycin, dactinomycin)

OPA (Oncovin, prednisone, Adriamycin)

OPAL (Oncovin, prednisone, L-asparaginase)

OPEN (Oncovin, prednisone, etoposide, Novantrone)

OPP (Oncovin, procarbazine, prednisone)

OPPA (Oncovin, prednisone, procarbazine, Adriamycin)

P-MVAC (Platinol, methotrexate, vinblastine, Adriamycin, carboplatin)

PAB-Esc-C (Platinol, Adriamycin, bleomycin, escalating doses of cyclophosphamide)

**Antineoplastics, Chemotherapy Protocols (cont.)**

PAC; PAC-I (Platinol, Adriamycin, cyclophosphamide)

PACE (Platinol, Adriamycin, cyclophosphamide, etoposide)

PATCO (prednisone, ara-C, thioguanine, cyclophosphamide, Oncovin)

PAVe (procarbazine, Alkeran, Velban)

PBV (Platinol, bleomycin, vinblastine)

PC (paclitaxel, carboplatin)

PCE (Platinol, cyclophosphamide, etoposide)

PCV (procarbazine, CCNU, vincristine)

PEB (Platinol, etoposide, bleomycin)

PFL (Platinol, fluorouracil, leucovorin [rescue])

PFT (L-phenylalanine mustard, fluorouracil, tamoxifen)

PHRT (procarbazine, hydroxyurea, radiotherapy)

PIA (Platinol, ifosfamide, Adriamycin)

POC (procarbazine, Oncovin, CCNU)

POCA (prednisone, Oncovin, cytarabine, Adriamycin)

POCC (procarbazine, Oncovin, cyclophosphamide, CCNU)

POMP (prednisone, Oncovin, methotrexate, Purinethol)

ProMACE (prednisone, methotrexate [with leucovorin rescue], Adriamycin, cyclophosphamide, etoposide)

ProMACE/cytaBOM (ProMACE [above], cytarabine, bleomycin, Oncovin, mitoxantrone)

ProMACE/MOPP (full course of ProMACE, followed by MOPP)

pulse VAC (vincristine, actinomycin D, cyclophosphamide)

pulse VAC (vincristine, Adriamycin, cyclophosphamide)

PVB (Platinol, vinblastine, bleomycin)

**Antineoplastics, Chemotherapy Protocols (cont.)**

PVDA (prednisone, vincristine, daunorubicin, asparaginase)

PVP; PVP-16 (Platinol, VP-16)

RIDD (recombinant interleukin-2, dacarbazine, DDP)

SMF (streptozocin, mitomycin, fluorouracil)

standard VAC

Stanford V (mechlorethamine, doxorubicin, vinblastine, vincristine, bleomycin, VePesid, prednisone)

STEAM (streptonigrin, thioguanine, cyclophosphamide, actinomycin, mitomycin)

T-2 protocol (dactinomycin, doxorubicin, vincristine, cyclophosphamide, radiation)

T-10 protocol (methotrexate, doxorubicin, cisplatin, bleomycin, cyclophosphamide, dactinomycin)

TAD (thioguanine, ara-C, daunorubicin)

TC (thioguanine, cytarabine)

TEC (thiotepa, etoposide, carboplatin)

TEMP (tamoxifen, etoposide, mitoxantrone, Platinol)

TOAP (thioguanine, Oncovin, [cytosine] arabinoside, prednisone)

TPCH (thioguanine, procarbazine, CCNU, hydroxyurea)

TPDCV (thioguanine, procarbazine, DCD, CCNU, vincristine)

V-CAP III (VP-16-213, cyclophosphamide, Adriamycin, Platinol)

V-TAD (VePesid, thioguanine, ara-C, daunorubicin)

VA (vincristine, actinomycin D)

VAAP (vincristine, asparaginase, Adriamycin, prednisone)

VAB; VAB-I (vinblastine, actinomycin D, bleomycin)

VAB-6 (vinblastine, actinomycin D, bleomycin, cyclophosphamide, cisplatin)

VAB-II (vinblastine, actinomycin D, bleomycin, cisplatin)

**Indications**

## Antineoplastics, Chemotherapy Protocols (cont.)

VAB-III (vinblastine, actinomycin D, bleomycin, cisplatin, chlorambucil, cyclophosphamide)

VAB-V (vinblastine, actinomycin D, bleomycin, cyclophosphamide, cisplatin)

VABCD (vinblastine, Adriamycin, bleomycin, CCNU, DTIC)

VAC (vincristine, Adriamycin, cisplatin)

VAC; VAC pulse; VAC standard (vincristine, actinomycin D, cyclophosphamide)

VAC; VAC pulse; VAC standard (vincristine, Adriamycin, cyclophosphamide)

VACA (vincristine, actinomycin D, cyclophosphamide, Adriamycin)

VACAD (vincristine, actinomycin D, cyclophosphamide, Adriamycin, dacarbazine)

VACAdr-IfoVP (vincristine, actinomycin D, cyclophosphamide, Adriamycin, ifosfamide, VePesid)

VACP (VePesid, Adriamycin, cyclophosphamide, Platinol)

VAD (vincristine, Adriamycin, dactinomycin)

VAD (vincristine, Adriamycin, dexamethasone)

VAD/V (vincristine, Adriamycin, dexamethasone, verapamil)

VAdrC (vincristine, Adriamycin, cyclophosphamide)

VAFAC (vincristine, amethopterin, fluorouracil, Adriamycin, cyclophosphamide)

VAI (vincristine, actinomycin D, ifosfamide)

VAM (vinblastine, Adriamycin, mitomycin)

VAM (VP-16-213, Adriamycin, methotrexate)

VAMP (vincristine, actinomycin, methotrexate, prednisone)

VAMP (vincristine, Adriamycin, methylprednisolone)

## Antineoplastics, Chemotherapy Protocols (cont.)

VAMP (vincristine, amethopterin, mercaptopurine, prednisone)

VAP (vinblastine, actinomycin D, Platinol)

VAP (vincristine, Adriamycin, prednisone)

VAP (vincristine, Adriamycin, procarbazine)

VAP (vincristine, asparaginase, prednisone)

VAT (vinblastine, Adriamycin, thiotepa)

VATD; VAT-D (vincristine, ara-C, thioguanine, daunorubicin)

VATH (vinblastine, Adriamycin, thiotepa, Halotestin)

VAV (VP-16-213, Adriamycin, vincristine)

VB (vinblastine, bleomycin)

VBA (vincristine, BCNU, Adriamycin)

VBAP (vincristine, BCNU, Adriamycin, prednisone)

VBC (VePesid, BCNU, cyclophosphamide)

VBC (vinblastine, bleomycin, cisplatin)

VBD (vinblastine, bleomycin, DDP)

VBM (vincristine, bleomycin, methotrexate)

VBMCP (vincristine, BCNU, melphalan, cyclophosphamide, prednisone)

VBMF (vincristine, bleomycin, methotrexate, fluorouracil)

VBP (vinblastine, bleomycin, Platinol)

VC (VePesid, carboplatin)

VC (vinorelbine, cisplatin)

VCAP (vincristine, cyclophosphamide, Adriamycin, prednisone)

VCF (vincristine, cyclophosphamide, fluorouracil)

VCMP (vincristine, cyclophosphamide, melphalan, prednisone)

VCP (vincristine, cyclophosphamide, prednisone)

**Antineoplastics, Chemotherapy Protocols (cont.)**

VDA (vincristine, daunorubicin, asparaginase)

VDP (vinblastine, dacarbazine, Platinol)

VDP (vincristine, daunorubicin, prednisone)

VeIP (Velban, ifosfamide, Platinol)

VIC (VePesid, ifosfamide [with mesna rescue], carboplatin)

VIC (vinblastine, ifosfamide, CCNU)

VIE (vincristine, ifosfamide, etoposide)

VIP (vinblastine, ifosfamide [with mesna rescue], Platinol)

VIP; VIP-1; VIP-2 (VePesid, ifosfamide [with mesna rescue], Platinol)

VIP-B (VP-16, ifosfamide, Platinol, bleomycin)

VLP (vincristine, L-asparaginase, prednisone)

VM (vinblastine, mitomycin)

VM-26PP (teniposide, procarbazine, prednisone)

VMAD (vincristine, methotrexate, Adriamycin, actinomycin D)

VMCP (vincristine, melphalan, cyclophosphamide, prednisone)

VMP (VePesid, mitoxantrone, prednimustine)

VOCAP (VP-16-213, Oncovin, cyclophosphamide, Adriamycin, Platinol)

VP (vincristine, prednisone)

VP + A (vincristine, prednisone, asparaginase)

VP-L-asparaginase (vincristine, prednisone, L-asparaginase)

VPB (vinblastine, Platinol, bleomycin)

VPBCPr (vincristine, prednisone, vinblastine, chlorambucil, procarbazine)

VPCA (vincristine, prednisone, cyclophosphamide, ara-C)

VPCMF (vincristine, prednisone, cyclophosphamide, methotrexate, fluorouracil)

VPP (VePesid, Platinol)

# Antiparkinsonian Agents
**Antiparkinsonian Agents, Anticholinergic Agents**

Akineton

Artane

belladonna extract

Bellafoline

benztropine mesylate

biperiden HCl

biperiden lactate

Cogentin

Disipal ⊛

ethopropazine HCl

Kemadrin

orphenadrine HCl

Parsidol

procyclidine HCl

Trihexy-2; Trihexy-5

trihexyphenidyl HCl

**Antiparkinsonian Agents, Dopaminergic Agents**

amantadine HCl

bromocriptine mesylate

cabergoline

Carbex

Dopar

Dostinex

Eldepryl

Larodopa

levodopa

Mirapex

N-Graft

neural dopaminergic cells (or precursors), porcine fetal

NeuroCell-PD

Parlodel

pergolide mesylate

Permax

pramipexole dihydrochloride

Requip

ropinirole HCl

selegiline HCl

Sertoli cells, porcine

Sinemet 10/100; Sinemet 25/100; Sinemet 25/250

Sinemet CR

Symadine

Symmetrel

**Antiparkinsonian Agents, Other**

Altropane

**Antiparkinsonian Agents, Other (cont.)**
Apokinon
apomorphine HCl
carbidopa
Comtan
entacapone
iodine I 123 murine MAb to alpha-fetoprotein (AFP)
Lodosyn
Rilutek
riluzole
Tasmar
tolcapone
Zydis

# Antiprotozoals
[see also: Antibiotics]
**Antiprotozoals, Amebicides**
dehydroemetine
diloxanide furoate
Flagyl
Flagyl IV
Flagyl IV RTU
Furamide
Humatin
iodoquinol
Mebadin
Metric 21
Metro I.V.
metronidazole
paromomycin sulfate
Protostat
Vytone
Yodoxin
**Antiprotozoals, Antimalarials**
Aralen HCl
Aralen Phosphate
Aralen Phosphate with Primaquine Phosphate
chloroguanide HCl
chloroquine HCl
chloroquine phosphate
Daraprim
Fansidar
Halfan
halofantrine HCl
hydroxychloroquine sulfate
Lariam

**Antiprotozoals, Antimalarials (cont.)**
Malarone ⒸⒶⓃ
mefloquine HCl
Mephaquin
Plaquenil Sulfate
primaquine phosphate
pyrimethamine
Quilimmune-M
Quinamm
quinidine gluconate
quinine sulfate
Quiphile
**Antiprotozoals, Other**
Antrypol
Arsobal
Belganyl
eflornithine HCl
Fourneau 309
Germanin
Lampit
melarsoprol
Moranyl
Naganol
Naphuride
nifurtimox
Ornidyl
Pentostam
sodium stibogluconate
suramin sodium
**Antipsychotics** [see: Psychotherapeutics, Antipsychotics]

# Antiseptics
[see also: Dermatological Preparations, Acne Products, Topical; Mouth and Throat Preparations; Ophthalmologicals, Contact Lens Preparations; Vaginal Preparations, Antiseptic Cleansers]
alcohol
benzalkonium chloride (BAC)
Castellani Paint Modified
chlorhexidine gluconate
chlorobutanol
chloroxylenol
Erygel
gentian violet
Gordochom
hexachlorophene

**Antiseptics (cont.)**
hexylresorcinol
ichthammol
iodine
isopropyl alcohol
Lugol
Ovide
phenol
pHisoHex
potassium iodide
povidone-iodine
Septi-Soft
Septisol
Strong Iodine
thimerosal
Tinver
triclosan
Versiclear
Xerac AC

## Antispasmodics

[see also: Urinary Tract Agents, Anti-
   spasmodics]
A-Spas S/L
Anaspaz
Antispas
Antispasmodic
Antrocol
Arco-Lase Plus
atropine sulfate
Barbidonna
Barbidonna; Barbidonna No. 2
Barophen
Bel-Phen-Ergot SR
Bellacane
Bellacane SR
belladonna extract
Bellafoline
Bellergal-S
Bentyl
Butibel
Byclomine
Cafatine-PB
Chardonna-2
clidinium bromide
Clindex
Clinoxide
Clipoxide
Cystospaz

**Antispasmodics (cont.)**
Cystospaz-M
dexpanthenol
Di-Spaz
Dibent
dicyclomine HCl
Donna-Sed
Donnamar
Donnamor
Donnapine
Donnatal
Donnatal No. 2
Ed-Spaz
Enlon Plus
Folergot-DF
Gastrosed
glycopyrrolate
hyoscyamine hydrobromide
hyoscyamine sulfate
Hyosophen
Ilopan
Ilopan-Choline
Kinesed
Kutrase
Levbid
Levsin
Levsin PB
Levsin-PB
Levsin with Phenobarbital
Levsin/SL
Levsinex
Librax
Lidox
Logen
Lomanate
Lomotil
Lonox
Malatal
methscopolamine bromide
Motofen
Pamine
Phenerbel-S
Pro-Banthīne
propantheline bromide
Quarzan
Relaxadon
Robinul
Robinul Forte
Sal-Tropine
Scopace

## Antispasmodics (cont.)
scopolamine hydrobromide
Spasmoject
Spasmolin
Spasmophen
Spasquid
Susano
tizanidine HCl
Transderm Scōp
Zanaflex

---

# Antituberculosis Agents
[*see also: Antibiotics*]
aminosalicylate sodium (*p*-aminosal-
icylate sodium)
aminosalicylic acid (4-aminosalicylic
acid)
aminosidine
BCG vaccine (bacillus Calmette-
Guérin)
Capastat Sulfate
capreomycin sulfate
clofazimine
cycloserine (L-cycloserine)
ethambutol HCl
ethionamide
Gabbromicina
isoniazid
Lamprene
Laniazid
Laniazid C.T.
Myambutol
Nydrazid
Paromomycin
Paser
Priftin
pyrazinamide (PZA)
Rifadin
Rifamate
rifampin
rifapentine
Rifater
Rimactane
Rimactane/INH
Seromycin
Sodium P.A.S.
streptomycin sulfate
Tice BCG
Trecator-SC

# Antitussives
## Antitussives, Narcotic
Actagen-C Cough
Actifed with Codeine Cough
Allerfrin with Codeine
Ambenyl Cough
Amgenal Cough
Anaplex HD
Aprodine with Codeine
Atuss EX
Atuss G
Atuss HD
Bromanate DC Cough
Bromanyl
Bromotuss with Codeine
Bromphen DC with Codeine Cough
Brompheniramine DC Cough
Brontex
Calcidrine
Calmylin Codeine ⒸⒶⓃ
Cheracol Cough
Chlorgest-HD
Co-Tuss V
Codamine
Codegest Expectorant
Codehist DH
codeine phosphate
codeine sulfate
Codiclear DH
Codimal DH
Conex with Codeine
Cophene XP
Cotridin ⒸⒶⓃ
Cotridin Expectorant ⒸⒶⓃ
Cyclofed Pediatric
Cycofed Pediatric
Decohistine DH
Deconamine CX
Decongestant Expectorant
Deconsal Pediatric
Deproist Expectorant with Codeine
Detussin
Detussin Expectorant
Dihistine Expectorant
Dilaudid Cough
Dimetane-DC Cough
Donatussin DC
Duratuss HD
ED-TLC; ED Tuss HC
Endagen-HD

## Antitussives, Narcotic (cont.)

Endal Expectorant
Endal-HD; Endal-HD Plus
Entuss-D
Entuss-D Jr.
Entuss Expectorant
Guiatuss AC
Guiatuss DAC
Guiatussin DAC
Guiatussin with Codeine Expectorant
H-Tuss-D
Histinex HC
Histinex PV
Histussin D
Histussin HC
HycoClear Tuss
Hycodan
Hycomine
Hycomine Compound
Hycotuss Expectorant
hydrocodone bitartrate
hydrocodone polistirex
Hydrocodone Compound
Hydrocodone CP; Hydrocodone HD
Hydrocodone GF
Hydrocodone PA
Hydromet
Hyphed
Iodal HD
Iophen-C
Iotussin HC
Isoclor Expectorant
Kwelcof
Marcof Expectorant
Myphetane DC Cough
Mytussin AC Cough
Mytussin DAC
Naldecon CX Adult
Novagest Expectorant with Codeine
Novahistine DH
Novahistine Expectorant
Nucofed
Nucofed Expectorant; Nucofed
    Pediatric Expectorant
Nucotuss Expectorant; Nucotuss
    Pediatric Expectorant
Oncet
P-V-Tussin
Pancof-HC
Para-Hist HD

## Antitussives, Narcotic (cont.)

Pediacof
Pedituss Cough
Pentazine VC with Codeine
Phenergan VC with Codeine
Phenergan with Codeine
Phenhist DH with Codeine
Phenhist Expectorant
Pherazine VC with Codeine
Pherazine with Codeine
Pneumotussin HC
Poly-Histine CS
Prometh VC with Codeine
Prometh with Codeine
Promethazine VC with Codeine
Promethist with Codeine
Protuss
Protuss-D
Robafen AC Cough
Robafen DAC
Robitussin A-C
Robitussin-DAC
Rolatuss Expectorant
Rolatuss with Hydrocodone
Ru-Tuss with Hydrocodone
Ryna-C
Ryna-CX
S-T Forte 2
SRC Expectorant
Statuss Expectorant
Statuss Green
T-Koff
Triacin-C Cough
Triafed with Codeine
Triaminic Expectorant DH
Triaminic Expectorant with Codeine
Tricodene Cough and Cold
Trifed-C Cough
Tussafed HC
Tussafin Expectorant
Tussanil DH
Tussar SF; Tussar-2
Tussend
Tussgen
Tussi-Organidin NR; Tussi-Organi-
    din-S NR
Tussigon
Tussionex Pennkinetic
Tussirex
Tyrodone

**Indications**

**Antitussives, Narcotic (cont.)**
　Unituss HC
　Vanex Expectorant
　Vanex-HD
　Vetuss HC
　Vicodin Tuss
**Antitussives, Non-narcotic**
　Anatuss
　Atuss DM
　benzonatate
　Bromadine-DM
　Bromadine-DX
　Bromarest DX Cough
　Bromatane DX Cough
　Bromfed-DM Cough
　Bromphen DX Cough
　Brotane DX Cough
　caramiphen edisylate
　carbetapentane citrate
　carbetapentane tannate
　Carbinoxamine Compound
　Carbodec DM
　Cardec-DM
　Cophene-X
　dextromethorphan
　dextromethorphan hydrobromide
　dextromethorphan polistirex
　Dimetane-DX Cough
　Donatussin
　Fenesin DM
　Guaifenex DM
　Histine DM
　Humibid DM
　Humibid DM Sprinkle
　Iobid DM
　Iohist DM
　Iophen-DM
　Liqui-Histine DM
　MED-Rx DM
　Monafed DM
　MorphiDex
　Muco-Fen-DM
　Myphetane DX Cough
　Ordrine AT
　Phenameth DM
　Phenergan with Dextromethorphan
　Pherazine DM
　Poly-Histine DM
　Profen II DM
　Prometh with Dextromethorphan

**Antitussives, Non-narcotic (cont.)**
　Promethazine DM
　Protuss DM
　Pseudo-Car DM
　Rentamine Pediatric
　Rescaps-D S.R.
　Respa-DM
　Rondamine-DM
　Rondec-DM
　Rynatuss
　Sildec-DM
　Siltapp with Dextromethorphan
　　HBr Cold & Cough
　Tessalon
　Tri-Tannate Plus Pediatric
　Tusquelin
　Tuss-Allergine Modified T.D.
　Tuss-Genade Modified
　Tuss-Ornade
　Tussafed
　Tussi-Organidin DM NR; Tussi-
　　Organidin DM-S NR
　Tussi-12
　Tusso-DM
　Tussogest
**Antivenin** [*see: Immunizing Agents,*
*Immune Extracts*]

# Antivirals
[*see also: HIV Infections, Viral*]
**Antivirals, Systemic**
　acyclovir
　acyclovir sodium
　adefovir dipivoxil
　amantadine HCl
　Apo-Acyclovir ⒸⒶⓃ
　Aztec
　Combivir
　Crixivan
　Cytovene
　didanosine
　Epivir
　Epivir-HBV
　famciclovir
　Famvir
　Flumadine
　Fortovase
　ganciclovir
　ganciclovir sodium

**Antivirals, Systemic (cont.)**
Genvir
Heptovir ⒸⒶⓃ
Hivid
indinavir sulfate
interferon alfa-n1
Invirase
lamivudine
lysine (L-lysine)
Norvir
Ostavir
Papirine
Preveon
Rebetol
Rebetron
Relenza
Retrovir
ribavirin
rimantadine HCl
ritonavir
saquinavir
saquinavir mesylate
Scriptene
stavudine
Symadine
Symmetrel
tuvirumab
valacyclovir HCl
Valtrex
vidarabine
Videx
Vira-A
Virazole
Wellferon
zalcitabine
zanamivir
Zeffix
Zerit
zidovudine
Zovirax
**Antivirals, Topical**
[see also: Ophthalmologicals, Antibiotics]
acyclovir
acyclovir sodium
Denavir
n-docosanol
Herplex
idoxuridine (IDU)
Lidakol
penciclovir

**Antivirals, Topical (cont.)**
trifluridine
Viroptic
Zovirax

---

# Asthma Agents
[see also: Corticosteroids, Systemic;
  Respiratory System Agents]
**Asthma Agents, Inhalants**
Adrenalin Chloride
Advair
AeroBid; AeroBid-M
Airet
albuterol
albuterol sulfate
Alupent
Apo-Cromolyn ⒸⒶⓃ
Apo-Ipravent ⒸⒶⓃ
Atrovent
Azmacort
Becloforte Inhaler ⒸⒶⓃ
beclomethasone dipropionate
Beclovent
Beclovent Inhaler ⒸⒶⓃ
Beta-2
bitolterol mesylate
Brethaire
Bronalide ⒸⒶⓃ
Bronkometer
Bronkosol
budesonide
Combivent
cromolyn sodium
Dexacort Phosphate
dexamethasone sodium phosphate
Duo-Medihaler
epinephrine
epinephrine bitartrate
epinephrine HCl
Flovent
flunisolide
fluticasone propionate
Foradil ⒸⒶⓃ
formoterol fumarate
Intal
ipratropium bromide
isoetharine
isoetharine HCl
isoetharine mesylate

**Indications**

**Asthma Agents, Inhalants (cont.)**
isoproterenol HCl
isoproterenol sulfate
Isuprel
levalbuterol HCl
Maxair
Medihaler-Iso
Metaprel
metaproterenol sulfate
mometasone furoate
nedocromil sodium
Norisodrine
Oxeze (CAN)
phenylephrine bitartrate
pirbuterol acetate
Proventil
Proventil HFA
Pulmicort
racepinephrine HCl
salmeterol xinafoate
Serevent
terbutaline sulfate
Tilade
Tornalate
triamcinolone acetonide
Vanceril; Vanceril Double Strength
Ventolin
Xopenex

**Asthma Agents, Systemic**
A-Methapred
A-Hydrocort
Accolate
Accurbron
Adlone
Adrenalin Chloride
Aerolate Sr.; Aerolate Jr.; Aerolate III
albuterol sulfate
Alupent
Amcort
aminophylline
Ana-Guard
Ana-Kit
Aquaphyllin
Aristocort
Aristocort Forte
Articulose L.A.
Asbron-G
Asmalix
Atolone
Berotec

**Asthma Agents, Systemic (cont.)**
Brethine
Bricanyl
Bronchial
Brondelate
Bronkephrine
Bronkodyl
Choledyl
Choledyl SA
Contramid
Cordox
Cortef
dehydroepiandrosterone sulfate
   (DHEAS)
Deltasone
depMedalone 40; depMedalone 80
Depo-Medrol
Depoject
Depopred-40; Depopred-80
Dilor
Dilor 400
Dilor-G
Duralone-40; Duralone-80
Dy-G
Dyflex-200
Dyflex-G
Dyline-GG
dyphylline
Elixomin
Elixophyllin
Elixophyllin GG
Elixophyllin-KI
epinephrine
epinephrine HCl
Epinephrine Pediatric
ethylnorepinephrine HCl
fenoterol
fructose-1,6-diphosphate (FDP)
Glyceryl-T
hydrocortisone (HC)
hydrocortisone acetate (HCA)
hydrocortisone sodium phosphate
hydrocortisone sodium succinate
Hydrocortone
Hydrocortone Acetate
Hydrocortone Phosphate
Hydrophed
Iophylline
isoproterenol HCl
isoproterenol sulfate

**Asthma Agents, Systemic (cont.)**
  Isuprel
  Kenacort
  Kenaject-40
  Kenalog-10; Kenalog-40
  Lanophyllin
  levalbuterol
  Liquid Pred
  Lufyllin
  Lufyllin 400
  Lufyllin-EPG
  Lufyllin-GG
  M-Prednisol-40; M-Prednisol-80
  Marax
  Marax-DF
  Medralone 40; Medralone 80
  Medrol
  Metaprel
  metaproterenol sulfate
  methylprednisolone
  methylprednisolone acetate
  methylprednisolone sodium succinate
  Meticorten
  montelukast sodium
  Mudrane
  Mudrane-2
  Mudrane GG
  Mudrane GG-2
  Neothylline
  Neothylline-GG
  Norisodrine with Calcium Iodide
  Orasone
  oxtriphylline
  Panasol-S
  Phyllocontin
  Prednicen-M
  prednisone
  Prometa
  Proventil
  Quadrinal
  Quibron; Quibron-300
  Quibron-T
  Quibron-T/SR
  Respbid
  Singulair
  Slo-bid
  Slo-phyllin
  Slo-phyllin GG
  Solu-Cortef
  Solu-Medrol

**Asthma Agents, Systemic (cont.)**
  Sterapred
  Sterapred DS
  Sus-Phrine
  Sustaire
  Synophylate-GG
  T-Phyl
  Tac-3
  Tac-40
  terbutaline sulfate
  Theo-24
  Theo-Dur
  Theo-Dur Sprinkle
  Theo-Organidin
  Theo-Sav
  Theo-X
  Theobid
  Theobid Jr.
  Theochron
  Theoclear-80
  Theoclear L.A.
  Theolair
  Theolair-SR
  Theolate
  Theomax DF
  Theophyllin KI
  theophylline (TH)
  Theospan-SR
  Theostat 80
  Theovent
  Thylline-GG
  Tri-Kort
  Triam-A
  Triam Forte
  triamcinolone
  triamcinolone acetonide
  Triamolone 40
  Triamonide 40
  Trilog
  Trilone
  Tristoject
  Truphylline
  Uni-Dur
  Uniphyl
  Volmax
  Zaditen
  zafirlukast
  zileuton
  Zyflo

Indications

**Anxiolytics** [see: Psychotherapeutics, Anxiolytics]

**Arrhythmias** [see: Cardiac Agents, Antiarrhythmics]

**Attention Deficit Hyperactivity Disorder (ADHD)** [see: Central Nervous System Stimulants]

**Benign Prostatic Hypertrophy (BPH)** [see: Prostatic Hyperplasia Agents]

## Biliary Tract Agents

Actigall
Bilezyme
Chenix
chenodiol
CholestaGel
colesevelam HCl
dehydrocholic acid
desoxycholic acid
Digestozyme
flumecinol
Moctanin
monoctanoin
Urso
ursodiol
Zixoryn

**Bipolar Disorder** [see: Psychotherapeutics, Antidepressants; Psychotherapeutics, Antimanic]

## Blood Expanders and Substitutes

albumin, human
Albuminar-5; Albuminar-25
Albutein 5%; Albutein 25%
Buminate 5%; Buminate 25%
dextran 40
dextran 70
dextran 75
Fluosol
Gendex 75
Gentran 40
Gentran 70
Gentran 75
hemoglobin, recombinant human (rHb1.1)

**Blood Expanders and Substitutes (cont.)**
Hemolink
Hemopure
Hespan
hetastarch
Hextend
intravascular perfluorochemical emulsion
LiquiVent
10% LMD
Macrodex
Oxygent
Pentaspan
pentastarch
perflubron
Plasbumin-5; Plasbumin-25
plasma protein fraction
Plasma-Plex
Plasmanate
Plasmatein
PolyHeme
Protenate
Rheomacrodex

**Bronchodilators** [see: Asthma agents; Respiratory System Agents]

**Burns** [see: Wound Treatment]

**Cancer** [see: Antineoplastics]

## Cardiac Agents
[see also: Antihypertensives; Diuretics]

**Cardiac Agents, Antianginals**
acebutolol HCl
Adalat
Adalat CC; Adalat Oros
amlodipine
amlodipine besylate
atenolol
bepridil HCl
Betachron E-R
Blocadren
Calan
Calan SR
Cardene
Cardilate
Cardizem
Cardizem SR; Cardizem CD
celiprolol HCl
Corgard

**Cardiac Agents, Antianginals (cont.)**
  Covera-HS
  Deponit
  Dilacor XR
  Dilatrate-SR
  diltiazem HCl
  diltiazem malate
  Duotrate; Duotrate 45
  erythrityl tetranitrate
  Imdur
  Inderal
  Inderal LA
  Ipran
  Ismo
  Iso-Bid
  Isoptin
  Isoptin SR
  Isordil
  isosorbide dinitrate
  isosorbide mononitrate
  Isotrate
  Isotrate ER
  Lopressor
  metoprolol succinate
  metoprolol tartrate
  mibefradil dihydrochloride
  Minitran
  Monoket
  nadolol
  nicardipine HCl
  nifedipine
  Nitrek
  Nitro-Bid
  Nitro-Bid IV
  Nitro-Derm
  Nitro-Dur
  Nitro-Time
  Nitrocine
  Nitrodisc
  Nitrogard
  nitroglycerin
  Nitroglyn
  Nitrol
  Nitrolingual Pumpspray ⒸⒶⓃ
  Nitrong
  NitroQuick
  Nitrostat
  Norvasc
  NTS
  pentaerythritol tetranitrate (PETN)

**Cardiac Agents, Antianginals (cont.)**
  Pentylan
  Peritrate
  Peritrate SA
  pindolol
  Posicor
  Procardia
  Procardia XL
  propranolol HCl
  ranolazine HCl
  Sectral
  Selecor
  Sorbitrate
  Sorbitrate SA
  Tenormin
  Tiamate
  Tiazac
  timolol maleate
  Toprol XL
  Transderm-Nitro
  Tridil
  Trinipatch ⒸⒶⓃ
  Vascor
  verapamil HCl
  Verelan
  Visken

**Cardiac Agents, Antiarrhythmics**
  Adenocard
  adenosine
  Amio-Aqueous
  amiodarone HCl
  Betachron E-R
  Betapace
  bretylium tosylate
  Bretylol
  Brevibloc
  Calan
  Calan SR
  Cardioquin
  Cardizem
  Cardizem SR; Cardizem CD
  cifenline succinate
  Cipralan
  Cordarone
  Corvert
  Covera-HS
  Crystodigin
  digitoxin
  digoxin
  Dilacor XR

Indications

**Cardiac Agents, Antiarrhythmics (cont.)**
diltiazem HCl
diltiazem malate
disopyramide phosphate
esmolol HCl
Ethmozine
flecainide acetate
ibutilide fumarate
Inderal
Inderal LA
Ipran
Isoptin
Isoptin SR
Lanoxicaps
Lanoxin
lidocaine HCl
LidoPen
mexiletine HCl
Mexitil
moricizine HCl
Napamide
Norpace
Norpace CR
Pacerone
procainamide HCl
Procan SR
Procanbid
Promine
Pronestyl
Pronestyl-SR
propafenone HCl
propranolol HCl
Quin-Release
Quinaglute
Quinalan
Quinidex
quinidine gluconate
quinidine polygalacturonate
quinidine sulfate
Quinora
Rhythmin
RSD-921
Rythmol
sotalol HCl
Tambocor
Tiamate
Tiazac
tocainide HCl
Tonocard

**Cardiac Agents, Antiarrhythmics (cont.)**
verapamil HCl
Verelan
Xylocaine HCl IV for Cardiac Arrhythmias
**Cardiac Agents, Congestive Heart Failure Agents**
Accupril
Accuretic (CAN)
Aldactazide
Aldactone
amiloride HCl
amrinone lactate
Aquatensen
Arkin Z
bumetanide
Bumex
Capoten
Capozide 25/15; Capozide 25/25; Capozide 50/15; Capozide 50/25
captopril
carvedilol
chlorthalidone
cilazapril
Combipres 0.1; Combipres 0.2; Combipres 0.3
Coreg
Crystodigin
Demadex
Demi-Regroton
digitoxin
digoxin
dobutamine HCl
Dobutrex
dopamine HCl
Dyazide
Dyrenium
Edecrin
Edecrin Sodium
enalapril maleate
enalaprilat
Enbrel
Enduron
Esidrix
etanercept
ethacrynate sodium
ethacrynic acid
Ezide
furosemide

**Cardiac Agents, Congestive Heart Failure Agents (cont.)**
Hydro-Par
hydrochlorothiazide (HCT; HCTZ)
HydroDIURIL
Hygroton
Inhibace
Inocor
Intropin
Lanoxicaps
Lanoxin
Lasix
levosimendan
lisinopril
Maxzide
methyclothiazide
metolazone
Microzide
Midamor
milrinone lactate
Moduretic
Mykrox
Natrecor
nesiritide
Oretic
Primacor
Primacor in 5% Dextrose
Prinivil
Prinzide
Prinzide 12.5; Prinzide 25
quinapril HCl
Simdax
spironolactone
Thalitone
torsemide
triamterene
Vaseretic 5-12.5; Vaseretic 10-25
Vasotec
Vasotec I.V.
vesnarinone
Zaroxolyn
Zestoretic
Zestril
**Cardiac Agents, Vasopressors**
Adrenalin Chloride
Ana-Guard
Aramine
dobutamine HCl
Dobutrex
dopamine HCl

**Cardiac Agents, Vasopressors (cont.)**
dopamine HCl in 5% dextrose
ephedrine sulfate
epinephrine
epinephrine HCl
Epinephrine Pediatric
EpiPen; EpiPen Jr.
Intropin
isoproterenol HCl
Isuprel
Levophed
mephentermine sulfate
metaraminol bitartrate
methoxamine HCl
midodrine HCl
Neo-Synephrine
norepinephrine bitartrate
phenylephrine HCl
ProAmatine
Sus-Phrine
Vasoxyl
Wyamine Sulfate
**Cardiac Agents, Other**
5G1.1-SC
alprostadil
Berinert-P
C1-esterase-inhibitor, human
Indocin I.V.
indomethacin sodium trihydrate
Pravachol
pravastatin sodium
Prostin VR Pediatric
simvastatin
TNK-tPA
Vasoprost
Zocor

# Central Nervous System Stimulants
Adderall
Alertec ⒸⒶⓃ
amphetamine aspartate
amphetamine sulfate
caffeine
caffeine, citrated
Cylert
d-methylphenidate HCl (d-MPH)
Desoxyn

Indications

**Central Nervous System Stimulants (cont.)**
Dexedrine
dextroamphetamine saccharate
dextroamphetamine sulfate
Dextrostat
Dopram
doxapram HCl
methamphetamine HCl
Methylin
methylphenidate
methylphenidate HCl (MPH)
modafinil
Neocaf
Oxydess II
pemoline
Provigil
Ritalin
Ritalin-SR
Spancap No. 1
**Chelating Agents** [see: Antidotes, Chelating Agents]
**Chemonucleolytic Agents** [see: Enzymes, Proteolytic]
**Chemotherapy Protocols** [see: Antineoplastics, Chemotherapy Protocols]
**Cholelithics** [see: Biliary Tract Agents]
**Cholesterol-lowering Agents** [see: Lipid-lowering Agents]
**Chronic Obstructive Pulmonary Disease (COPD)** [see: Respiratory System Agents]
**Cold Sores and Fever Blisters** [see: Mouth and Throat Preparations]
**Congestive Heart Failure** [see: Cardiac Agents, Congestive Heart Failure Agents]
**Contraceptives** [see: Sex Hormones, Oral Contraceptives; Sex Hormones, Parenteral Contraceptives; Vaginal Preparations, Contraceptives]

# Contrast Media
**Contrast Media, Paramagnetic**
AngioMark
Combidex
Dynospheres M-035
Feridex
ferristene

**Contrast Media, Paramagnetic (cont.)**
ferucarbotran
ferumoxides
ferumoxsil
ferumoxtran-10
gadodiamide
gadopentetate dimeglumine
gadoteridol
GastroMARK
Imagent GI
Magnevist
mangafodipir trisodium
mangofodipir trisodium
MS-325
Omniscan
Optimark
perflubron
ProHance
Resovist
Teslascan
**Contrast Media, Radiopaque**
Amipaque
Anatrast
Angio-Conray
Angiovist 282
Angiovist 292; Angiovist 370
arcitumomab
Baricon
barium sulfate
Baro-cat
Barobag
Baroflave
Barosperse
Barosperse, Liquid
Bear-E-Bag Pediatric
Bear-E-Yum CT
Bear-E-Yum GI
Bilivist
Bilopaque
CEA-Scan
Cholebrine
Cholografin Meglumine
Conray 325
Conray 400
Conray; Conray 30; Conray 43
Cysto-Conray; Cysto-Conray II
Cystografin; Cystografin Dilute
diatrizoate meglumine
diatrizoate sodium

## Contrast Media, Radiopaque (cont.)

Dionosil Oily
Enecat
Enhancer
Entrobar
Epi-C
ethiodized oil
Ethiodol
Flo-Coat
Gastrografin
HD 200 Plus
HD 85
Hexabrix
Hypaque-76
Hypaque-Cysto
Hypaque-M 75; Hypaque-M 90
Hypaque Meglumine 30%; Hypaque
    Meglumine 60%
Hypaque Sodium
Hypaque Sodium 20%
Hypaque Sodium 25%; Hypaque
    Sodium 50%
Imager ac
Intropaste
iocetamic acid
iodamide meglumine
iodipamide meglumine
iodixanol
iohexol
iopamidol
iopanoic acid
iopromide
iosulfan blue
iothalamate meglumine
iothalamate sodium
iotrolan
ioversol
ioxaglate meglumine
ioxaglate sodium
ipodate calcium
ipodate sodium
Isovue-M 200; Isovue-M 300
Isovue-128; Isovue-200; Isovue-250;
    Isovue-300; Isovue-370
Liqui-Coat HD
Liquipake
Lymphazurin 1%
MD-60; MD-76
MD-76 R
MD-Gastroview

## Contrast Media, Radiopaque (cont.)

Medebar Plus
Medescan
metrizamide
Novopaque
OctreoScan
Omnipaque
Optiray 160; Optiray 240; Optiray
    300; Optiray 320; Optiray 350
Oragrafin Calcium
Oragrafin Sodium
Osmovist
oxidronate sodium
polyvinyl chloride, radiopaque
Prepcat
propyliodone
Quick AC Enema Kit
Reno-30
Reno-Dip; Reno-60
RenoCal-76
Renografin-60
Renografin-76
Renovist; Renovist II
Renovue-Dip; Renovue-65
Sinografin
Sitzmarks
Telepaque
Tomocat
Tonopaque
tyropanoate sodium
Ultravist
Urovist Cysto
Urovist Meglumine DIU/CT
Urovist Sodium 300
Vascoray
Visipaque

## Contrast Media, Ultrasound

albumin, human (sonicated with
    chlorofluorocarbons)
Albunex
Definity
EchoGen
Echovist ⒸⒶⓃ
Filmix
galactose
Imagent US
Levovist ⒸⒶⓃ
microbubble contrast agent
Optison
perflenapent

## Contrast Media, Ultrasound (cont.)
perflisopent
perflutren

---

## Corticosteroids, Systemic
[see also: Asthma Agents; Gout
   Agents; Immunosuppressants;
   Rheumatic Disease Agents]
A-Methapred
A-Hydrocort
ACTH
ACTH-80
Acthar
Adlone
Amcort
Aristocort
Aristocort Forte
Aristospan Intra-articular
Articulose-50
Articulose L.A.
Atolone
betamethasone
betamethasone acetate
betamethasone sodium phosphate
Cel-U-Jec
Celestone
Celestone Phosphate
Celestone Soluspan
Cortef
corticotropin
cortisone acetate
Cortone Acetate
Dalalone
Dalalone D.P.
Dalalone L.A.
Decadron
Decadron-LA
Decadron Phosphate
Decadron with Xylocaine
Decaject
Decaject-L.A.
Delta-Cortef
Deltasone
depMedalone 40; depMedalone 80
Depo-Medrol
Depoject
Depopred-40; Depopred-80
Dexameth
dexamethasone

## Corticosteroids, Systemic (cont.)
dexamethasone acetate
dexamethasone sodium phosphate
Dexasone
Dexasone L.A.
Dexone
Dexone LA
Duralone-40; Duralone-80
Florinef Acetate
fludrocortisone acetate
H.P. Acthar Gel
Hexadrol
Hexadrol Phosphate
Hydeltra-T.B.A.
Hydeltrasol
hydrocortisone (HC)
hydrocortisone acetate (HCA)
hydrocortisone sodium phosphate
hydrocortisone sodium succinate
Hydrocortone
Hydrocortone Acetate
Hydrocortone Phosphate
Kenacort
Kenaject-40
Kenalog-10; Kenalog-40
Key-Pred 25; Key-Pred 50
Key-Pred-SP
Liquid Pred
M-Prednisol-40; M-Prednisol-80
Medralone 40; Medralone 80
Medrol
methylprednisolone
methylprednisolone acetate
methylprednisolone sodium phosphate
methylprednisolone sodium succinate
Meticorten
Orasone
Panasol-S
Pediapred
Predaject-50
Predalone 50
Predcor-50
Prednicen-M
Prednisol TBA
prednisolone
prednisolone acetate
prednisolone sodium phosphate
prednisolone tebutate
prednisone
Prelone

**Corticosteroids, Systemic (cont.)**
Selestoject
Solu-Cortef
Solu-Medrol
Solurex
Solurex LA
Sterapred
Sterapred DS
Tac-3
Tac-40
Tri-Kort
Triam-A
Triam Forte
triamcinolone
triamcinolone acetonide
triamcinolone diacetate
triamcinolone hexacetonide
Triamolone 40
Triamonide 40
Trilog
Trilone
Tristoject
**Cough** [see: Antitussives]
**Crohn's Disease:** [see: Inflammatory Bowel Disease Agents]
**Debriding Agents** [see: Wound Treatment, Debriding Agents]

---

# Decongestants, Systemic
Aclophen
Actagen-C Cough
Actifed with Codeine Cough
AH-chew
AH-chew D
Alersule
Allegra-D
Allent
Allerfrin with Codeine
Alumadrine
Ami-Drix
Ami-Tex LA
Anamine
Anamine T.D.
Anaplex
Anaplex HD
Anaplex SR
Anatuss
Anatuss LA
Aprodine with Codeine

**Decongestants, Systemic (cont.)**
Atrohist Pediatric
Atrohist Plus
Atuss DM
Atuss G
Atuss HD
Banex
Biohist-LA
Brexin-L.A.
Brofed
Bromadine-DM
Bromadine-DX
Bromanate DC Cough
Bromarest DX Cough
Bromatane DX Cough
Bromfed
Bromfed-DM Cough
Bromfed-PD
Bromfenex
Bromfenex PD
Bromophen T.D.
Bromphen DC with Codeine Cough
Bromphen DX Cough
Brompheniramine DC Cough
Broncholate
Bronkotuss Expectorant
Brotane DX Cough
Calmylin Codeine ⓒⓐⓝ
Carbinoxamine Compound
Carbiset
Carbiset-TR
Carbodec
Carbodec DM
Carbodec TR
Cardec-DM
Cardec-S
Chlorafed; Chlorafed HS
Chlordrine S.R.
Chlorgest-HD
Chlorphedrine SR
Claritin-D; Claritin-D 12 Hour; Claritin-D 24 Hour
Codamine
Codegest Expectorant
Codehist DH
Codimal DH
Codimal-L.A.; Codimal-L.A. Half
Coldloc
Coldloc-LA
Colfed-A

Indications

**Decongestants, Systemic (cont.)**
  Comhist
  Comhist LA
  Condrin-LA
  Conex with Codeine
  Congess JR
  Congess SR
  Contuss
  Cophene No. 2
  Cophene-X
  Cophene XP
  Cotridin ⒸⒶⓃ
  Cotridin Expectorant ⒸⒶⓃ
  Cyclofed Pediatric
  Cycofed Pediatric
  D.A.
  D.A. II
  Dallergy
  Dallergy-JR
  Decohistine DH
  Deconamine
  Deconamine CX
  Deconamine SR
  Decongestabs
  Decongestant
  Decongestant Expectorant
  Decongestant S.R.
  Deconhist L.A.
  Deconomed SR
  Deconsal II
  Deconsal Pediatric
  Deconsal Sprinkle
  Defen-LA
  Deproist Expectorant with Codeine
  Despec
  Detussin
  Detussin Expectorant
  Dexaphen S.A.
  Dihistine Expectorant
  Dimetane-DC Cough
  Dimetane-DX Cough
  Disobrom
  Donatussin
  Donatussin DC
  Drixomed
  Drize
  Dura-Gest
  Dura-Vent
  Dura-Vent/A
  Dura-Vent/DA

**Decongestants, Systemic (cont.)**
  Dura-Tap/PD
  Duralex
  Duratuss
  Duratuss HD
  E.N.T.
  Ed A-Hist
  ED-TLC; ED Tuss HC
  Endafed
  Endagen-HD
  Endal
  Endal Expectorant
  Endal-HD; Endal-HD Plus
  Enomine
  Entex
  Entex LA
  Entex PSE
  Entuss-D
  Entuss-D Jr.
  ephedrine HCl
  ephedrine sulfate
  ephedrine tannate
  Eudal-SR
  Ex-Histine
  Exgest LA
  Extendryl
  Extendryl JR
  Extendryl SR
  Fedahist
  GP-500
  Guai-Vent/PSE
  Guaifed
  Guaifed-PD
  Guaifenex
  Guaifenex PPA 75
  Guaifenex PSE 60; Guaifenex PSE
    120; Guaifenex Rx DM
  Guaifenex Rx
  GuaiMAX-D
  Guaipax
  Guaitex
  Guaitex LA
  Guaitex PSE
  Guaivent
  Guaivent PD
  Guiatex LA
  Guiatex PSE
  Guiatuss DAC
  Guiatussin DAC
  Guipax

**Decongestants, Systemic (cont.)**

H-Tuss-D
Hista-Vadrin
Histalet
Histalet Forte
Histalet X
Histamic
Histine DM
Histinex HC
Histinex PV
Histor-D
Histussin D
Histussin HC
Hycomine
Hycomine Compound
Hydrocodone CP; Hydrocodone HD
Hydrocodone PA
Hydrophed
Hyphed
Iodal HD
Iofed
Iofed PD
Iohist D
Iohist DM
Iosal II
Iotussin HC
Isoclor Expectorant
KIE
Klerist-D
Kronofed-A
Kronofed-A Jr.
Liqui-Histine-D
Liqui-Histine DM
Liquibid-D
Lodrane LD
Lufyllin-EPG
Marax
Marax-DF
MED-Rx
MED-Rx DM
Mescolor
methscopolamine nitrate
Mudrane
Mudrane GG
Myphetane DC Cough
Myphetane DX Cough
Mytussin DAC
Naldec Pediatric
Naldecon
Naldecon CX Adult

**Decongestants, Systemic (cont.)**

Naldelate
Nalgest
Nasabid
Nasabid SR
Nasatab LA
ND Clear
No-Hist
Nolamine
Norel
Norel Plus
Novafed
Novafed A
Novagest Expectorant with Codeine
Novahistine DH
Novahistine Expectorant
Nucofed
Nucofed Expectorant; Nucofed
    Pediatric Expectorant
Nucotuss Expectorant; Nucotuss
    Pediatric Expectorant
OMNIhist L.A.
Ordrine AT
Ordrine S.R.
Ornade
P-V-Tussin
Pancof-HC
Panmist JR
Pannaz
Para-Hist HD
Parhist SR
Partapp TD
Partuss LA
Pediacof
Pedituss Cough
Phenahist-TR
Phenate
Phenchlor S.H.A.
Phenergan VC
Phenergan VC with Codeine
Phenhist DH with Codeine
Phenhist Expectorant
phenylephrine HCl
phenylephrine tannate
Phenylfenesin L.A.
phenylpropanolamine HCl
Pherazine VC with Codeine
Polaramine Expectorant
Poly-Histine CS
Poly-Histine-D

Indications

**Decongestants, Systemic (cont.)**
Poly-Histine-D Ped Caps
Poly-Histine DM
Prehist
Prehist D
Profen II DM
Profen II; Profen LA
Prometh VC Plain
Prometh VC with Codeine
Promethazine VC
Promethazine VC Plain
Promethazine VC with Codeine
Promethist with Codeine
Protuss-D
Protuss DM
Pseudo-Car DM
Pseudo-Chlor
pseudoephedrine HCl
pseudoephedrine sulfate
pseudoephedrine tannate
Quadra-Hist
Quadra-Hist Pediatric
Quadrinal
R-Tannamine
R-Tannate
Rentamine Pediatric
Resaid
Rescaps-D S.R.
Rescon
Rescon-ED
Rescon JR
Respa-1st
Respahist
Respaire-60; Respaire-120
Rhinatate
Rhinolar
Rhinolar-EX; Rhinolar-EX 12
Rinade B.I.D.
Robafen DAC
Robitussin-DAC
Rolatuss Expectorant
Rolatuss with Hydrocodone
Rondamine-DM
Rondec
Rondec-DM
Rondec-TR
Ru-Tuss
Ru-Tuss DE
Ru-Tuss II
Ru-Tuss with Hydrocodone

**Decongestants, Systemic (cont.)**
Rymed
Rymed-TR
Ryna-C
Ryna-CX
Rynatan
Rynatan-S
Rynatuss
Seldane-D
Semprex-D
Sil-Tex
Sildec-DM
Siltapp with Dextromethorphan
    HBr Cold & Cough
Sinufed
Sinupan
SinuVent
SRC Expectorant
Stahist
Stamoist E
Stamoist LA
Statuss Expectorant
Statuss Green
Sudal 120/600
Sudal 60/500
Sudex
Syn-Rx
T-Koff
Tamine S.R.
Tanafed
Tanoral
Theomax DF
Time-Hist
Touro A & H
Touro LA
Tri-P
Tri-Phen-Chlor
Tri-Phen-Chlor T.R.
Tri-Phen-Mine
Tri-Phen-Mine S.R.
Tri-Tannate
Tri-Tannate Plus Pediatric
Triacin-C Cough
Triafed with Codeine
Triaminic
Triaminic Expectorant DH
Triaminic Expectorant with Codeine
Trifed
Trifed-C Cough
Trinalin

**Decongestants, Systemic (cont.)**
Triotann
Tritan
Tritan Pediatric
Tusquelin
Tuss-Allergine Modified T.D.
Tuss-Genade Modified
Tuss-LA
Tuss-Ornade
Tussafed
Tussafed HC
Tussafin Expectorant
Tussanil DH
Tussanil Plain
Tussar SF; Tussar-2
Tussend
Tussgen
Tussi-12
Tussirex
Tussogest
Tyrodone
ULR-LA
UltraBrom
UltraBrom PD
Uni-Decon
Unituss HC
V-Dec-M
Vanex Expectorant
Vanex Forte
Vanex Forte-R
Vanex-HD
Vanex-LA
Versacaps
Vetuss HC
Zephrex
Zephrex LA
**Dementia** [see: Alzheimer's Disease Agents]
**Depigmenting Agents** [see: Dermatological Preparations, Depigmenting Agents]

---

# Dermatological Preparations
**Dermatological Preparations, Acne Products, Systemic**
[see also: Antibiotics; Corticosteroids, Systemic]
Accutane
Achromycin V

**Dermatological Preparations, Acne Products, Systemic (cont.)**
cyproterone acetate
Diane-35 (CAN)
Dynacin
E-Base
E-Mycin
Ery-Tab
ERYC
erythromycin
erythromycin estolate
Ilosone
isotretinoin
Minocin
minocycline HCl
Nor-Tet
Ortho Tri-Cyclen
Panmycin
PCE
Robimycin
Robitet
Sumycin
Sumycin '250'; Sumycin '500'
Teline; Teline-500
Tetracap
tetracycline HCl
Tetracyn; Tetracyn 500
Tetralan
Tetralan "250"; Tetralan-500
Tetram
Vectrin
**Dermatological Preparations, Acne Products, Topical**
[see also: Antibiotics, Topical; Antiseptics; Dermatological Preparations, Keratolytics]
A/T/S
adapalene
Akne-mycin
Avita
azelaic acid
Azelex
Benzac AC 2½; Benzac W 2½; Benzac 5; Benzac AC 5; Benzac W 5; Benzac 10; Benzac AC 10; Benzac W 10
Benzac AC Wash 2½; Benzac AC Wash 5; Benzac W Wash 5; Benzac AC Wash 10; Benzac W Wash 10
5 Benzagel; 10 Benzagel

**Indications**

## Dermatological Preparations, Acne Products, Topical (cont.)

Benzamycin
Benzashave
Benzox-10
benzoyl peroxide
Brevoxyl
C/T/S
Cleocin T
Clinda-Derm
clindamycin
clindamycin phosphate
Clindets
Dalacin T ⓒⒶⓝ
Del Aqua-5; Del Aqua-10
Del-Mycin
Desquam-E; Desquam-E 5; Desquam-E 10
Desquam-X 2.5
Desquam-X 5 Wash; Desquam-X 10 Wash
Desquam-X 5; Desquam-X 10
Differin
Emgel
Ery-Sol
Erycette
EryDerm 2%
Erygel
Erymax
Erythra-Derm
erythromycin
Hyacne
Klaron
Meclan
meclocycline sulfosalicylate
Novacet
Panoxyl
Panoxyl AQ 2½; Panoxyl 5; Panoxyl AQ 5; Panoxyl 10; Panoxyl AQ 10
Peroxin A 5; Peroxin A 10
Persa-Gel; Persa-Gel W 5%; Persa-Gel W 10%
PROPApH Foaming Face Wash
pyrithione zinc
Rejuva-A ⓒⒶⓝ
Renova
Retin-A
Retin-A Micro
Romycin
salicylic acid (SA)

## Dermatological Preparations, Acne Products, Topical (cont.)

Septi-Soft
Septisol
Staticin
Sulfacet-R
sulfacetamide sodium
Sulfoxyl Regular; Sulfoxyl Strong
sulfur, precipitated
sulfur, sublimed
T-Stat
tazarotene
Tazorac
tetracycline HCl
Theramycin Z
Topicycline
tretinoin
Triaz
triclosan
Vanoxide-HC
Vitinoin ⓒⒶⓝ

## Dermatological Preparations, Anti-hyperhidrotics

aluminum chloride
aluminum chlorohydrate
aluminum sulfate
Drysol
formaldehyde solution
Formalyde-10
Lazer Formalyde

## Dermatological Preparations, Anti-inflammatory Agents

Aclovate
Acticort 100
Aeroseb-Dex
Aeroseb-HC
Ala-Cort
Ala-Quin
alclometasone dipropionate
Alphatrex
amcinonide
Aristocort
Aristocort A
Aristocort Intralesional
Aristospan Intralesional
Beta-Val
betamethasone benzoate
betamethasone dipropionate
betamethasone dipropionate, augmented

## Dermatological Preparations, Anti-inflammatory Agents (cont.)

betamethasone sodium phosphate
betamethasone valerate
Betatrex
Carmol HC
Celestone Soluspan
Cetacort
clobetasol propionate
clocortolone pivalate
Cloderm
Cordran
Cordran SP
Cormax
Corque
Cort-Dome
Cortin
cortisone acetate
Cortisporin
Cortone Acetate
Cutivate
Cyclocort
Dalalone
Dalalone L.A.
Decadron-LA
Decadron Phosphate
Decaject
Decaject-L.A.
Decaspray
Delta-Tritex
depMedalone 40; depMedalone 80
Depo-Medrol
Depoject
Depopred-40; Depopred-80
Derma Comb
Derma-Smoothe/FS
Dermabet
Dermacort
Dermatop
desonide
DesOwen
desoximetasone
dexamethasone
dexamethasone acetate
dexamethasone sodium phosphate
Dexasone
Dexasone L.A.
Dexone
Dexone LA
diclofenac potassium

## Dermatological Preparations, Anti-inflammatory Agents (cont.)

diflorasone diacetate
Diprolene
Diprolene AF
Diprosone
Duralone-40; Duralone-80
Eldecort
Elocon
Enzone
Epifoam
1+1-F Creme
Florone
Florone E
fluocinolone acetonide
fluocinonide
Fluonex
Fluonid
flurandrenolide
Flurosyn
Flutex
fluticasone propionate
FS Shampoo
Fungoid-HC
halcinonide
halobetasol propionate
Halog
Halog-E
1% HC
Hexadrol Phosphate
Hi-Cor 1.0; Hi-Cor 2.5
Hyanalgese-D
Hycort
Hydeltra-T.B.A.
HydroTex
Hydrocort
hydrocortisone (HC)
hydrocortisone acetate (HCA)
hydrocortisone buteprate
hydrocortisone butyrate
hydrocortisone probutate
hydrocortisone valerate
Hydrocortone Acetate
Hytone
Hytone 1%
Kenaject-40
Kenalog
Kenalog-H
Kenalog-10; Kenalog-40
Kenonel

## Dermatological Preparations, Anti-inflammatory Agents (cont.)

Kutapressin
LactiCare-HC
Lida-Mantle-HC
Lidex
Lidex-E
liver derivative complex
Locoid
Lotrisone
Luxiq
M-Prednisol-40; M-Prednisol-80
Mantadil
Maxiflor
Maxivate
Medralone 40; Medralone 80
methylprednisolone acetate
mometasone furoate
Myco-Biotic II
Myco-Triacet II
Mycogen II
Mycolog-II
Myconel
Mytrex
N.G.T.
Nasonex
Neo-Cortef
Neo-Synalar
NeoDecadron
Nutracort
Olux
orgotein
OxSODrol
Pandel
Pedi-Cort V Creme
Penecort
Pramosone
prednicarbate
Prednisol TBA
prednisolone tebutate
Psorcon
Psorion
S-T Cort
Solurex
Solurex LA
Synacort
Synalar
Synalar-HP
Synemol
Tac-3

## Dermatological Preparations, Anti-inflammatory Agents (cont.)

Teladar
Temovate
Temovate Emollient
Texacort
Topicort
Topicort LP
Tri-Kort
Tri-Statin II
Triacet
Triam-A
triamcinolone acetonide
triamcinolone diacetate
triamcinolone hexacetonide
Triamonide 40
Triderm
Tridesilon
Trilog
U-Cort
UAD
Ultravate
Uticort
Valisone
Valisone Reduced Strength
Vanoxide-HC
Vasoderm; Vasoderm-E
ViaFoam
Vytone
Westcort
Zemaphyte
Zone-A Forte

## Dermatological Preparations, Depigmenting Agents

hydroquinone
Lustra
Melanex
Melpaque HP
Melquin HP
Nuquin HP
Solaquin Forte
Viquin Forte

## Dermatological Preparations, Emollients and Protectants

[see also: Wound Treatment, Vulneraries]
Accuzyme
allantoin
aloe
aluminum acetate

**Dermatological Preparations, Emollients and Protectants (cont.)**
ammonium lactate (lactic acid neutralized with ammonium hydroxide)
bismuth subnitrate
Carmol HC
cocoa butter
cod liver oil
colloidal oatmeal
Derma-Smoothe/FS
dimethicone
glycerin
glycolic acid
Gordon's Urea 40%
Lac-Hydrin
lactic acid
Lactinol
Lactinol-E
lanolin
Lustra
mineral oil
Panafil
Panafil White
Peruvian balsam
petrolatum
propylene glycol
shark liver oil
silicone
urea
Ureacin-40
vitamin A
vitamin A palmitate
vitamin E
zinc oxide

**Dermatological Preparations, Hair and Scalp Agents**
Ala-Scalp
betamethasone valerate
Capitrol
chloroxine
coal tar
Drithocreme; Drithocreme HP 1%; Dritho-Scalp
finasteride
ketoconazole
Luxiq
minoxidil
Nizoral
Olux

**Dermatological Preparations, Hair and Scalp Agents (cont.)**
phenol
povidone-iodine
Propecia
pyrithione zinc
Sal-Oil-T
salicylic acid (SA)
sulfur, precipitated

**Dermatological Preparations, Keratolytic Agents**
[see also: Dermatological Preparations, Acne Products, Topical; Dermatological Products, Wart and Corn Removers]
Bensal HP
Castellani Paint Modified
Emersal
glycolic acid
Lustra
Mono-Chlor
Monocete
monochloroacetic acid
resorcinol
salicylic acid (SA)
silver nitrate
Tinver
Tri-Chlor
trichloroacetic acid
Versiclear

**Dermatological Preparations, Photodamaged Skin Agents**
Actinex
ALA Photodynamic Therapy
5-aminolevulinic acid HCl (5-ALA HCl)
Avita
diclofenac potassium
Levulan
masoprocol
Rejuva-A ⒸⒶⓃ
Renova
Retin-A
Retin-A Micro
Solarase
tretinoin
Vitinoin ⒸⒶⓃ

**Dermatological Preparations, Psoriasis Agents, Systemic**
Abitrexate

**Dermatological Preparations, Psoriasis Agents, Systemic (cont.)**
acitretin
etretinate
Folex PFS
methotrexate (MTX)
methotrexate sodium
Methotrexate LPF Sodium
methoxsalen (8-methoxsalen)
Oxsoralen-Ultra
P-53
Rheumatrex
Soriatane
Tegison

**Dermatological Preparations, Psoriasis Agents, Topical**
[see also: Dermatological Preparations, Hair and Scalp Agents]
ALA Photodynamic Therapy
Anthra-Derm
anthralin
calcipotriene
coal tar
Dovonex
Drithocreme; Drithocreme HP 1%; Dritho-Scalp
Lasan
Lasan HP-1
mercury, ammoniated
methenamine sulfosalicylate
methoxsalen (8-methoxsalen)
Miconal
Sal-Oil-T
salicylic acid (SA)
Unguentum Bossi
Zetar Emulsion

**Dermatological Preparations, Rosacea Agents**
MetroCream
MetroGel; MetroLotion
metronidazole
Noritate

**Dermatological Preparations, Vitiligo Agents**
Benoquin
methoxsalen (8-methoxsalen)
monobenzone
8-MOP
Oxsoralen
trioxsalen

**Dermatological Preparations, Vitiligo Agents (cont.)**
Trisoralen

**Dermatological Preparations, Wart and Corn Removers**
[see also: Dermatological Preparations, Keratolytics]
Bichloracetic Acid
cantharidin
Condylox
dichloroacetic acid
DuoPlant
Gordofilm
Paplex Ultra
Podocon-25
podofilox
Podofin
podophyllum
podophyllum resin
salicylic acid (SA)
Verr-Canth
Verrex
Verrusol
Wartec ⒸⒶⓃ

**Dermatological Preparations, Other**
aminobenzoate potassium
Glylorin
monolaurin
Potaba

---

# Diabetes Agents
**Diabetes Agents, Insulin**
Humalog
insulin
insulin aspart
insulin lispro
NovoPen 1.5
NovoRapid
Oralgen; Oralin ⒸⒶⓃ
Regular Iletin II U-500 (concentrated)

**Diabetes Agents, Oral Agents**
acetohexamide
Actos
Amaryl
Avandia
bromocriptine mesylate
chlorpropamide
Diab II

**Diabetes Agents, Oral Agents (cont.)**
  Diabinese
  Diapid
  Diaβeta (or DiaBeta)
  Dymelor
  Ergoset
  Euglucon ⒸⒶ⒩
  glimepiride
  glipizide
  Glucophage
  Glucotrol
  Glucotrol XL
  glyburide
  Glynase
  Glyset
  INS-1
  lypressin
  metformin HCl
  Micronase
  Micronized Glyburide
  miglitol
  Oralgen; Oralin ⒸⒶ⒩
  Oramide
  Orinase
  pioglitazone HCl
  pramlintide
  Prandase ⒸⒶ⒩
  Prandin
  Precose
  repaglinide
  Rezulin
  rosiglitazone maleate
  Symlin
  tolazamide
  tolbutamide
  Tolinase
  troglitazone
**Diabetes Agents, Related Disorders**
  alprostadil, liposomal
  Alredase
  Apligraf
  Apo-Domperidone ⒸⒶ⒩
  Axokine
  becaplermin
  Cytolex
  Dermagraft; Dermagraft-TC
  domperidone
  epalrestat
  graftskin
  memantine

**Diabetes Agents, Related Disorders (cont.)**
  Motilium ⒸⒶ⒩
  Novo-Domperidone ⒸⒶ⒩
  pexiganan acetate
  pimagedine HCl
  Regranex
  tolrestat

# Diagnostic Agents
  [see also: Ophthalmologicals, Diagnostic Agents; Radiopharmaceuticals]
  AcuTect
  Acthrel
  AD7C
  Adenoscan
  adenosine
  AlaSTAT
  Albay
  allergenic extracts (aqueous, glycerinated, or alum-precipitated)
  Allpyral
  Altropane
  aminohippurate sodium
  Aplisol
  Aplitest
  arbutamine
  arginine (L-arginine)
  Bactigen B Streptococcus-CS
  Bactigen N meningitidis
  Baros
  bentiromide
  benzylpenicillin
  benzylpenicilloyl polylysine
  BioCox
  BTA Rapid Urine Test
  BTA Stat Test
  Calypte
  Candida albicans skin test antigen
  Candin
  capromab pendetide
  carbon C 14 urea
  Cardiac T
  Cardio-Green (CG)
  Cardiolite
  Center-Al
  Chymex
  coccidioidin
  Color Allergy Screening Test (CAST)

Indications

## Diagnostic Agents (cont.)

corticorelin ovine triflutate
Cortrosyn
cosyntropin
depreotide
Dermatophytin
Dermatophytin "O"
DiaScreen
dipyridamole
Evans blue
Flu OIA
Gadolite
GenESA
Geref
GlucaGen Diagnostic Kit
glucagon
Glucagon Diagnostic Kit
glucose, liquid
gonadorelin acetate
HercepTest
histamine phosphate
Histolyn-CYL
histoplasmin
Hyskon
imciromab pentetate
ImmuRAID-AFP
ImmuRAID-hCG
indium In 111 IGIV pentetate
indium In 111 pentetreotide
indium In 111 satumomab pendetide
indocyanine green
inulin
iodine I 123 murine MAb to human
    chorionic gonadotropin (hCG)
iodine I 131 6B-iodomethyl-19-nor-
    cholesterol
Kinevac
latex agglutination test
LeuTech
LeukoScan
LymphoScan
Macroscint
mespiperone C 11
methacholine chloride
methylene blue (MB)
Metopirone
metyrapone
Miraluma
Mono-Vacc Test (O.T.)
MSTA (Mumps Skin Test Antigen)

## Diagnostic Agents (cont.)

Multitest CMI
mumps skin test antigen (MSTA)
Myoscint
NeoTect
Neurolite
NG-29
NicCheck I
NicCheck II
NMP-22
nofetumomab merpentan
OctreoScan 111
OncoTrac
OncoScint CR/OV
OraSure HIV-1
Orinase Diagnostic
Osteomark
P-748
Parathar
pentagastrin
Peptavlon
Perchloracap
Persantine IV
Pharmalgen
phentolamine mesylate
potassium perchlorate
Pre-Pen
Pre-Pen/MDM
ProstaScint
protirelin
Provocholine
Pylori-Check
PYtest
R-gene 10
Riba 3.0 SIA
RIGScan
rose bengal
Sclavo PPD Solution
Sclavo Test-PPD
secretin
Secretin Ferring
Sentinel
sermorelin acetate
simethicone
sincalide
sodium iodide I 123
Somatrel
SonoRx
Spherulin
T.R.U.E. Test

**Diagnostic Agents (cont.)**

technetium ($^{99m}$Tc) dimercaptosuccinic acid

technetium ($^{99m}$Tc) methylenediphosphonate

technetium Tc 99m albumin aggregated

technetium Tc 99m antimelanoma
murine MAb

technetium Tc 99m apcitide

technetium Tc 99m arcitumomab

technetium Tc 99m bectumomab

technetium Tc 99m biciromab

technetium Tc 99m bicisate

technetium Tc 99m disofenin

technetium Tc 99m furifosmin

technetium Tc 99m medronate

technetium Tc 99m mertiatide

technetium Tc 99m murine MAb to
human alpha-fetoprotein (AFP)

technetium Tc 99m murine MAb to
human chorionic gonadotropin
(hCG)

technetium Tc 99m oxidronate

technetium Tc 99m sestamibi

technetium Tc 99m siboroxime

technetium Tc 99m succimer

technetium Tc 99m sulesomab

technetium Tc 99m teboroxime

technetium Tc 99m tetrofosmin

teriparatide

Thypinone

Thyrel-TRH

Thyrogen

thyrotropin

thyrotropin alfa

Thytropar

Tine Test PPD

tolbutamide sodium

tolonium chloride

toluidine blue O

Trichophyton extract

tuberculin

Tuberculin Tine Test, Old

Tubersol

Venomil

Verluma

xylose (D-xylose)

**Diet Aids** [see: Weight Reduction Agents]

**Digestive Enzymes** [see: Enzymes,
Digestive]

# Diuretics

[see also: Antihypertensives, Diuretics;
Cardiac Agents, Congestive Heart
Failure Agents]

acetazolamide

acetazolamide sodium

ammonium chloride

caffeine

caffeine, citrated

chlorothiazide

Daranide

Dazamide

Diamox

dichlorphenamide

Diurese

Diurigen

Diuril

Ismotic

isosorbide

Metahydrin

Naqua

Sodium Diuril

urea

Ureaphil

**Dressings** [see: Hemostatics; Wound
Treatment, Medicated Dressings]

# Electrolytes

Aminosyn 3.5% M; Aminosyn II
3.5% M

Aminosyn 7% (8.5%) with Electrolytes; Aminosyn II 7% (8.5%,
10%) with Electrolytes

Aminosyn-HBC 7%

Aminosyn II 3.5% M in 5% Dextrose; Aminosyn II 4.25% M in
10% Dextrose

betaine HCl

calcium carbonate

calcium chloride

calcium citrate

calcium gluconate (calcium D-gluco-
nate)

calcium glycerophosphate

**Electrolytes (cont.)**
   calcium lactate
   calcium lactobionate
   Cena-K
   Cystadane
   5% Dextrose and Electrolyte #48;
      5% Dextrose and Electrolyte #75;
      10% Dextrose and Electrolyte #48
   50% Dextrose with Electrolyte Pat-
      tern A (or N)
   Dialyte Pattern LM
   Effer-K
   Effervescent Potassium
   FreAmine HBC 6.9%
   FreAmine III 3% (8.5%) with Elec-
      trolytes
   Gen-K
   HepatAmine
   Hyperlyte; Hyperlyte CR; Hyperlyte R
   Inpersol; Inpersol-LM
   Isolyte E (G; H; M; P; R; S) with
      5% Dextrose
   Isolyte E; Isolyte S; Isolyte S pH 7.4
   Isolyte S pH 7.4
   K-vescent
   K+ 8; K+ 10
   K+ Care
   K+ Care ET
   K-Lyte; K-Lyte DS
   K-Tab
   K-Dur 10; K-Dur 20
   K-G Elixir
   K-Lease
   K-Lor
   K-Lyte/Cl
   K-Lyte/Cl; K-Lyte/Cl 50
   K-Norm
   Kaochlor 10%; Kaochlor S-F
   Kaon
   Kaon-Cl 20%
   Kaon-Cl; Kaon-Cl 10
   Kato
   Kay Ciel
   Kaylixir
   Klor-Con 8; Klor-Con 10
   Klor-Con; Klor-Con/25
   Klor-Con/EF
   Klorvess
   Klotrix
   Kolyum

**Electrolytes (cont.)**
   Lypholyte; Lypholyte II
   magnesium chloride
   magnesium gluconate
   magnesium sulfate
   Micro-K LS
   Micro-K; Micro-K 10
   Multilyte-20; Multilyte-40
   NephrAmine 5.4%
   Normosol-M and 5% Dextrose; Nor-
      mosol-R and 5% Dextrose
   Normosol-R; Normosol-R pH 7.4
   Nutrilyte; Nutrilyte II
   Plasma-Lyte A pH 7.4; Plasma-Lyte
      R; Plasma-Lyte 56; Plasma-Lyte 148
   Plasma-Lyte M (R; 56; 148) and 5%
      Dextrose
   Plegisol
   Potasalan
   potassium acetate
   potassium bicarbonate
   potassium chloride (KCl)
   potassium citrate
   potassium gluconate
   potassium phosphate, dibasic
   potassium phosphate, monobasic
   ProcalAmine
   RenAmin
   Rum-K
   Slow-K
   sodium acetate
   sodium bicarbonate
   sodium chloride (NaCl)
   sodium lactate (SL)
   sodium phosphate, dibasic
   Ten-K
   TPN Electrolytes; TPN Electrolytes
      II; TPN Electrolytes III
   Tracelyte; Tracelyte II; Tracelyte
      with Double Electrolytes; Trace-
      lyte II with Double Electrolytes
   Travasol 3.5% (5.5%, 8.5%) with
      Electrolytes
   5% Travert and Electrolyte No. 2;
      10% Travert and Electrolyte No. 2
   Tri-K
   Twin-K
   Uro-KP-Neutral
**Emphysema** [*see: Respiratory System
   Agents*]

**Endometriosis** [see: Gynecological Agents, Endometriosis Agents]

**Enuresis** [see: Urinary Tract Agents, Enuresis Agents]

---

# Enzymes
## Enzymes, Digestive
amylase
Arco-Lase Plus
bile salts
Bilezyme
cellulase
Cotazym
Cotazym-S
Creon
Creon 10; Creon 20
Digepepsin
Digestozyme
Donnazyme
Gustase Plus
Ilozyme
Ku-Zyme
Ku-Zyme HP
Kutrase
lactase enzyme
lipase
Pancrease; Pancrease MT 4; Pancrease MT 10; Pancrease MT 16; Pancrease MT 20
pancreatin
Pancrecarb MS-8
pancrelipase
pepsin
protease
Protilase
Ultrase MT 12; Ultrase MT 20
Viokase
Zymase
## Enzymes, Proteolytic
[see also: Wound Treatment, Debriding Agents]
Accuzyme
ananain
bromelains
Chymodiactin
chymopapain
collagenase
comosain
Dermuspray

## Enzymes, Proteolytic (cont.)
Elase
Elase-Chloromycetin
fibrinolysin, human
Granulderm
Granulex
GranuMed
Panafil
Panafil White
papain
Santyl
sutilains
Travase
trypsin, crystallized
Vianain
## Enzymes, Thrombolytic
[see also: Thrombolytic Agents]
Abbokinase
Abbokinase Open-Cath
anistreplase
Eminase
Kabikinase
r-ProUK
Retavase
reteplase
saruplase
Streptase
streptokinase (SK)
urokinase
## Enzymes, Other
Adagen
alglucerase
alpha-galactosidase A
CC-Galactosidase
Ceredase
Cerezyme
FABRase
imiglucerase
Lysodase
PEG-glucocerebrosidase
pegademase bovine
sacrosidase
Sucraid

**Epilepsy** [see: Anticonvulsants]

**Erectile Dysfunction** [see: Sexual Dysfunction Agents, Male]

**Estrogens** [see: Sex Hormones, Estrogens]

Indications

# Expectorants

Ami-Tex LA
ammonium chloride
Anatuss
Anatuss LA
Asbron-G
Atuss EX
Atuss G
Banex
Bronchial
Broncholate
Brondelate
Bronkotuss Expectorant
Brontex
Calcidrine
calcium iodide
Calmylin Codeine (CAN)
Cheracol Cough
Co-Tuss V
Codegest Expectorant
Codiclear DH
Coldloc
Coldloc-LA
Conex with Codeine
Congess JR
Congess SR
Contuss
Cophene-X
Cophene XP
Cotridin Expectorant (CAN)
Cyclofed Pediatric
Cycofed Pediatric
Deconamine CX
Decongestant Expectorant
Deconsal II
Deconsal Pediatric
Deconsal Sprinkle
Defen-LA
Deproist Expectorant with Codeine
Despec
Detussin Expectorant
Dihistine Expectorant
Dilaudid Cough
Dilor-G
Donatussin
Donatussin DC
Dura-Gest
Dura-Vent
Duratuss
Duratuss-G

# Expectorants (cont.)

Duratuss HD
Dy-G
Dyflex-G
Dyline-GG
Elixophyllin GG
Elixophyllin-KI
Endal
Endal Expectorant
Enomine
Entex
Entex LA
Entex PSE
Entuss-D
Entuss-D Jr.
Entuss Expectorant
Eudal-SR
Exgest LA
Fenesin
Fenesin DM
glycerol, iodinated
Glyceryl-T
GP-500
Guai-Vent/PSE
Guaifed
Guaifed-PD
guaifenesin
Guaifenex
Guaifenex DM
Guaifenex LA
Guaifenex PPA 75
Guaifenex PSE 60; Guaifenex PSE
    120; Guaifenex Rx DM
Guaifenex Rx
GuaiMAX-D
Guaipax
Guaitex
Guaitex LA
Guaitex PSE
Guaivent
Guaivent PD
Guiatex LA
Guiatex PSE
Guiatuss AC
Guiatuss DAC
Guiatussin DAC
Guiatussin with Codeine Expectorant
Guipax
Histalet X
Humibid DM

**Expectorants (cont.)**
  Humibid DM Sprinkle
  Humibid L.A.
  Humibid Sprinkle
  HycoClear Tuss
  Hycotuss Expectorant
  Hydrocodone GF
  Iobid DM
  Iophen
  Iophen-C
  Iophen-DM
  Iophylline
  Iosal II
  Isoclor Expectorant
  KIE
  Kwelcof
  Liquibid-D
  Liquibid; Liquibid-1200
  Lufyllin-EPG
  Lufyllin-GG
  Marcof Expectorant
  MED-Rx
  MED-Rx DM
  Monafed
  Monafed DM
  Muco-Fen-DM
  Muco-Fen-LA
  Mudrane
  Mudrane-2
  Mudrane GG
  Mudrane GG-2
  Mytussin AC Cough
  Mytussin DAC
  Naldecon CX Adult
  Nasabid
  Nasabid SR
  Nasatab LA
  Neothylline-GG
  Norel
  Norisodrine with Calcium Iodide
  Novagest Expectorant with Codeine
  Novahistine Expectorant
  Nucofed Expectorant; Nucofed
    Pediatric Expectorant
  Nucotuss Expectorant; Nucotuss
    Pediatric Expectorant
  Organidin NR
  P-V-Tussin
  Panmist JR
  Par Glycerol

**Expectorants (cont.)**
  Partuss LA
  Pediacof
  Pedituss Cough
  Phenhist Expectorant
  Phenylfenesin L.A.
  Pima
  Pneumomist
  Pneumotussin HC
  Polaramine Expectorant
  potassium guaiacolsulfonate
  potassium iodide
  Profen II DM
  Profen II; Profen LA
  Protuss
  Protuss-D
  Protuss DM
  Quadrinal
  Quibron; Quibron-300
  R-Gen
  Respa-DM
  Respa-GF
  Respa-1st
  Respaire-60; Respaire-120
  Robafen AC Cough
  Robafen DAC
  Robitussin A-C
  Robitussin-DAC
  Rolatuss Expectorant
  Ru-Tuss DE
  Rymed
  Rymed-TR
  Ryna-CX
  Sil-Tex
  Sinufed
  Sinumist-SR
  Sinupan
  SinuVent
  Slo-phyllin GG
  SRC Expectorant
  SSKI
  Stamoist E
  Stamoist LA
  Statuss Expectorant
  Sudal 120/600
  Sudal 60/500
  Sudex
  Syn-Rx
  Synophylate-GG
  terpin hydrate

**Indications**

**Expectorants (cont.)**
Theo-Organidin
Theolate
Theophyllin KI
Thylline-GG
Touro Ex
Touro LA
Triaminic Expectorant DH
Triaminic Expectorant with Codeine
Tuss-LA
Tussafed HC
Tussafin Expectorant
Tussanil DH
Tussar SF; Tussar-2
Tussi-Organidin DM NR; Tussi-Organidin DM-S NR
Tussi-Organidin NR; Tussi-Organidin-S NR
Tusso-DM
ULR-LA
V-Dec-M
Vanex Expectorant
Vanex-LA
Versacaps
Vicodin Tuss
Zephrex
Zephrex LA
**Fertility Agents** [see: Sex Hormones, Fertility Stimulants]
**Gallbladder Disease and Gallstones** [see: Biliary Tract Agents]
**Gastroesophageal Reflux Disease (GERD)** [see: Peptic Ulcer and Gastric Reflux Agents]
**Glucocorticoids** [see: Corticosteroids, Systemic; Dermatological Preparations, Anti-inflammatory Agents; Ophthalmologicals, Anti-inflammatory]

---

# Gout Agents
[see also: Analgesics, Nonsteroidal; Corticosteroids, Systemic]
allopurinol
Anturane
Aprazone
Benemid ⒸⒶⓃ
Benuryl ⒸⒶⓃ
Col-Probenecid
Colabid

**Gout Agents (cont.)**
ColBenemid
colchicine
Probalan
Proben-C
probenecid
Purinol ⒸⒶⓃ
sulfinpyrazone
Zurinol
Zyloprim

---

# Gynecological Agents
[see also: Sex Hormones; Vaginal Preparations]
**Gynecological Agents, Endometriosis Agents**
Amen
Aygestin
Curretab
Cycrin
danazol
Danocrine
leuprolide acetate
Lupron Depot
medroxyprogesterone acetate
nafarelin acetate
norethindrone
norethindrone acetate
Norlutate
Norlutin
Provera
Synarel
**Gynecological Agents, Labor Suppressants**
ritodrine HCl
Yutopar
**Gynecological Agents, Labor Stimulants**
carboprost tromethamine
Cervidil
dinoprostone
ergonovine maleate
Ergotrate Maleate
Hemabate
Methergine
methylergonovine maleate
Mifegyne
mifepristone
oxytocin

## Gynecological Agents, Labor Stimulants (cont.)
Pitocin
Prepidil
Prostin E2
Syntocinon

## Gynecological Agents, Lactation Suppressants
bromocriptine mesylate
cabergoline
Dostinex
Parlodel

## Gynecological Agents, Menopause Agents
[see also: Mineral Replacement, Calcium]
Activelle
alendronate sodium
Allelix
Calcimar
calcitonin (salmon)
Evista
Fortical
Fosamax
Macritonin
Miacalcin
Osteo-F
Osteocalcin
parathyroid hormone (1-84), recombinant human
raloxifene HCl
Salmonine
Slow Fluoride
sodium fluoride

## Hemorrhoidal Agents
[see also: Analgesics, Topical; Antihistamines, Topical; Dermatological Preparations, Anti-inflammatory]
Analpram-HC
Anogesic
Anucort HC
Anumed HC
Anuprep HC
Anusol-HC
Anusol-HC 1
Cort-Dome High Potency
Dermol HC
Hemorrhoidal HC

## Hemorrhoidal Agents (cont.)
Hemril-HC
hydrocortisone (HC)
hydrocortisone acetate (HCA)
phenol
Pramoxine HC
Proctocort
ProctoCream-HC
Proctofoam-HC
Rectacort

## Hemostatics
[see also: Wound Treatment, Medicated Dressings]
Alphanate
AlphaNine
AlphaNine SD
Amicar
aminocaproic acid
anti-inhibitor coagulant complex
antihemophilic factor (AHF)
Antihemophilic Factor (Porcine) Hyate:C
aprotinin
AquaMEPHYTON
argatroban
Autoplex T
Avitene Hemostat
Benefix
Bioclate
calcium alginate fiber
cellulose, oxidized
collagen sponge, absorbable
Cyklokapron
DDAVP
desmopressin acetate
Ethamolin
ethanolamine oleate
factor IX complex
factor VIIa, recombinant
factor VIII SQ, recombinant
factor XIII, plasma-derived
Feiba VH Immuno
Fibrogammin P
gelatin film, absorbable
gelatin powder, absorbable
gelatin sponge, absorbable
Gelfilm; Gelfilm Ophthalmic
Gelfoam

**Hemostatics (cont.)**
Helistat
Helixate
Hemaseel HMN
Hemofil M
Hemonyne
Hemopad
Hemotene
Humate-P
Koāte-DVI
Koāte-HP
KoGENate
KoGENate SF
Konakion
Konyne 80
Mephyton
microfibrillar collagen hemostat
  (MCH)
Monoclate
Monoclate P
Mononine
Novastan
NovoSeven
Oxycel
phytonadione
Profilate HP
Profilate OSD
Profilnine Heat-Treated
Profilnine SD
Proplex T
Recombinate
ReFacto
Sorbsan
Stimate
Surgicel
thrombin
Thrombin-JMI
Thrombinar
Thrombogen
Thrombostat
tranexamic acid
Trasylol
**Herpes Simplex** [see: Mouth and
  Throat Preparations]

---

# HIV Infections

[see also: Antibiotics; Antifungals; Anti-
  diarrheal Agents, Intestinal Antibac-
  terials; Antiemetics and Antinause-
ants; Antiprotozoals; Antituberculosis
  Agents; Antivirals; Immunizing
  Agents; Immunostimulants]
**HIV Infections, Bacterial**
aminosidine
azithromycin
Biaxin
clarithromycin
ethambutol HCl
Gabbromicina
gentamicin sulfate
isoniazid
Laniazid
Laniazid C.T.
Maitec
Myambutol
Mycobutin
Nydrazid
Paromomycin
Priftin
rifabutin
Rifadin
Rifamate
rifampin
rifapentine
Rifater
Rimactane
Rimactane/INH
Zithromax
Zithromax ⒸⒶⓃ
**HIV Infections, Fungal**
Abelcet
AmBisome
Amphotec
amphotericin B cholesteryl sulfate
amphotericin B deoxycholate
amphotericin B lipid complex
  (ABLC)
Apo-Ketoconazole ⒸⒶⓃ
Diflucan
fluconazole
Fungizone
itraconazole
ketoconazole
Nizoral
Sporanox
TLC ABLC
**HIV Infections, Parasitic**
albendazole
atovaquone

**HIV Infections, Parasitic (cont.)**
azithromycin
Bactrim IV
Bactrim Pediatric
Bactrim; Bactrim DS
Biaxin
clarithromycin
Cotrim Pediatric
Cotrim; Cotrim D.S.
Daraprim
Mepron
NeuTrexin
NebuPent
Pentacarinat
Pentam 300
pentamidine isethionate
Pneumopent
pyrimethamine
Septra
Septra DS
Septra IV
sulfadiazine
sulfamethoxazole (SMX; SMZ)
Sulfatrim
trimethoprim (TMP)
trimetrexate glucuronate
Zithromax
Zithromax ⓒⒶⓃ
**HIV Infections, Viral**
abacavir sulfate
acemannan
adefovir dipivoxil
Agenerase
AIDS vaccine
AIDSVax
Ampligen
amprenavir
AR-177
Aztec
Bravavir
Bucast
Carrisyn
CD4, human truncated 369 AA
    polypeptide
CD4, recombinant soluble human
    (rCD4)
celgosivir HCl
cidofovir
Combivir
Coviracil

**HIV Infections, Viral (cont.)**
Crixivan
Cytovene
delavirdine mesylate
dextran sulfate
didanosine
efavirenz
emtricitabine
Epivir
fomivirsen sodium
Fortovase
foscarnet sodium
Foscavir
ganciclovir
ganciclovir sodium
Genevax-HIV-Px
gp160 (glycoprotein 160) antigens
HIV immunotherapeutic (HIV-IT);
    HIV therapeutic
HIV-1 peptide vaccine
Hivid
hypericin
indinavir sulfate
inosine pranobex
Invirase
Isoprinosine
lamivudine
lopinavir
nelfinavir mesylate
nevirapine
Norvir
Novapren
Panavir
poly I: poly C12U
Preveon
probucol
Protovir
Receptin
Remune
Rescriptor
Retrovector
Retrovir
ritonavir
saquinavir
saquinavir mesylate
Scriptenc
sevirumab
Soluble T4
sorivudine
stavudine

**HIV Infections, Viral (cont.)**
Sustiva
tetrachlorodecaoxide
Uendex
VaxSyn HIV-1
vidarabine
Videx
VIMRxyn
Vira-A
Viracept
Viramune
Virend
Vistide
Vitrasert
Vitravene
zalcitabine
Zerit
Ziagen
zidovudine
Zintevir

**HIV Infections, Other Related Disorders**
Alferon LDO
Alferon N
alitretinoin
Androgel
Androgel-DHT
Avonex
BACI
Betaseron
bexarotene
Cachexon
Cryptaz
*Cryptosporidium parvum* bovine
    colostrum IgG concentrate
DaunoXome
daunorubicin citrate, liposomal
dihydrotestosterone (DHT)
dronabinol
epoetin alfa (EPO)
Epogen
Geref
L-glutathione, reduced
Hepandrin
Immuno-C
interferon alfa
interferon alfa-2a (IFN-αA)
interferon alfa-2b (IFN-α2)
interferon alfa-n3
interferon beta (IFN-B)

**HIV Infections, Other Related Disorders (cont.)**
interferon beta-1a
interferon beta-1b
Intron A
Marinol
Megace
megestrol acetate
memantine
nitazoxanide (NTZ)
Omniferon
Oxandrin
oxandrolone
Panretin
PEG-Intron A
poloxamer 331
Procrit
Protox
Provir
r-IFN-beta
R-Frone
Roferon-A
sermorelin acetate
SP-303
Sporidin-G
SU-5416
Targretin
testosterone
TheraDerm
Veldona

# Hormones
[see also: Sex Hormones]
**Hormones, Anterior Pituitary**
Cortrosyn
cosyntropin
Genotropin
Geref
Humatrope
Norditropin
Nutropin
Nutropin AQ
Nutropin Depot
Protropin
Protropin II
Saizen
sermorelin acetate
Serostim
somatrem

**Hormones, Anterior Pituitary (cont.)**
somatropin
**Hormones, Hypothalamic**
buserelin acetate
deslorelin
DUROS
Factrel
gonadorelin acetate
gonadorelin HCl
goserelin acetate
histrelin
leuprolide acetate
Lupron Depot
Lupron Depot-Ped
Lupron Depot–3 month; Lupron Depot–4 month
Lupron; Lupron Pediatric
Lutrepulse
nafarelin acetate
octreotide acetate
ProMaxx-100
Reducin
Sandostatin
Sandostatin LAR Depot
Somagard
somatostatin (SS)
Supprelin
Suprefact ⒸⒶⓃ
Suprefact; Suprefact Depot ⒸⒶⓃ
Synarel
Zecnil
Zoladex
**Hormones, Pancreatic**
GlucaGen Emergency Kit
glucagon
Glucagon Emergency Kit
**Hormones, Posterior Pituitary**
DDAVP
desmopressin acetate
Diapid
lypressin
oxytocin
Pitocin
Pitressin Synthetic
Stimate
Syntocinon
vasopressin (VP)

# Hypercalcemia Agents
Actonel
alendronate sodium
Aredia
Bondronat
Bonefos
Bonviva
Calcimar
calcitonin (human)
calcitonin (salmon)
Cibacalcin
clodronate disodium
Didronel
disodium clodronate tetrahydrate
doxercalciferol
etidronate disodium
Fortical
Fosamax
gallium nitrate
Ganite
Hectorol
ibandronate sodium
Miacalcin
Ostac ⒸⒶⓃ
Osteo-D
Osteocalcin
risedronate sodium
Salmonine
secalciferol
Skelid
tiludronate disodium
**Hyperhidrosis** [see: Dermatological Preparations, Antihyperhidrotics]

# Hyperkalemia Agents
Kayexalate
sodium polystyrene sulfonate
SPS
**Hyperlipidemia** [see: Lipid-lowering Agents]

# Hyperphosphatemia Agents
calcium acetate
calcium carbonate
PhosLo
R & D Calcium Carbonate/600
Renagel

**Indications**

**Hyperphosphatemia Agents (cont.)**
sevelamer HCl
**Hyperuricemia** [*see: Gout Agents*]
**Hypoglycemics** [*see: Diabetes Agents*]

---

# Immunizing Agents
[*see also: Immunostimulants*]
**Immunizing Agents, Bacterial Vaccines**
Acel-Imune
Acel-P ⓒⒶⓃ
ActHIB
ActHIB/Tripedia
BCG vaccine (bacillus Calmette-Guérin)
Certiva
cholera vaccine
Comvax
diphtheria & tetanus toxoids & acellular pertussis vaccine (DTaP)
diphtheria & tetanus toxoids & whole-cell pertussis vaccine (DTwP)
diphtheria & tetanus toxoids, adsorbed (DT; Td)
diphtheria toxoid, adsorbed
Hemophilus b conjugate vaccine
HibTITER
ImmuCyst ⓒⒶⓃ
Infanrix
lipoprotein OspA, recombinant
LYMErix
meningococcal polysaccharide vaccine, group A
meningococcal polysaccharide vaccine, group C
meningococcal polysaccharide vaccine, group W-135
meningococcal polysaccharide vaccine, group Y
Menomune-A/C/Y/W-135
mixed respiratory vaccine (MRV)
MRV
OmniHIB
OncoTICE ⓒⒶⓃ
Pacis ⓒⒶⓃ
PedvaxHIB
pertussis vaccine adsorbed
plague vaccine

**Immunizing Agents, Bacterial Vaccines (cont.)**
Pneumo 23 ⓒⒶⓃ
pneumococcal polysaccharide vaccine
pneumococcal vaccine, polyvalent
Pneumovax 23
Pnu-Imune 23
ProHIBiT
Quilimmune-P
SPL-Serologic types I and III
staphage lysate (SPL)
StaphVAX
tetanus toxoid
Tetramune
TheraCys
Tice BCG
Tri-Immunol
TriHIBit
Tripedia
Typherex
Typhim Vi
typhoid vaccine
typhoid Vi capsular polysaccharide vaccine
Typhoid Vaccine (AKD)
Typhoid Vaccine (H-P)
Vivotif Berna
**Immunizing Agents, Immune Extracts**
antivenin (Crotalidae) polyvalent (ovine) Fab
antivenin (*Latrodectus mactans*)
CroTab
diphtheria antitoxin
**Immunizing Agents, Immunoglobulins**
Atgam
CytoGam
cytomegalovirus immune globulin, human
Gamastan
Gamimune N
Gammagard S/D
Gammar
Gammar-IV
Gammar-P IV
Gamulin Rh
globulin, immune
H-BIG
Hep-B-Gammagee

**Immunizing Agents, Immunoglob-
ulins (cont.)**
hepatitis B immune globulin (HBIG)
HIV immune globulin (HIVIG)
HIV-IG
Hyper-Tet
Hyperab
HyperHep
Hypermune RSV
HypRho-D; HypRho-D Mini-Dose
Imogam
Iveegam
lymphocyte immune globulin, anti-
thymocyte
MICRhoGAM
Mini-Gamulin Rh
Nabi-HB
Nashville Rabbit Antithymocyte
Serum
Polygam
Polygam S/D
rabies immune globulin (RIG)
RespiGam
respiratory syncytial virus immune
globulin (RSV-IG)
$Rh_0(D)$ immune globulin
Rhesonativ
RhoGAM
Sandoglobulin
tetanus immune globulin
varicella-zoster immune globulin
(VZIG)
Venoglobulin-I
Venoglobulin-S
WinRho SD; WinRho SDF
**Immunizing Agents, Viral Vaccines**
[see also: HIV Infections, Viral]
AIDS vaccine
AIDSVax
ALVAC-HIV 1
Attenuvax
Biavax II
ChimeriVax
Comvax
Engerix-B
FluMist
Fluogen
FluShield
Fluvirin
Fluzone

**Immunizing Agents, Viral Vaccines
(cont.)**
Genevax-HIV-Px
Havrix
Hepagene
hepatitis A vaccine, inactivated
hepatitis B virus vaccine, inactivated
HIV-1 peptide vaccine
Imovax
influenza virus vaccine
IPOL
Japanese encephalitis (JE) virus vac-
cine
JE-VAX
M-M-R II
M-R-Vax II
measles & rubella virus vaccine, live
measles, mumps & rubella virus vac-
cine, live
measles virus vaccine, live
Meruvax II
mumps virus vaccine, live
Mumpsvax
Orimune
poliovirus vaccine, inactivated (IPV)
poliovirus vaccine, live oral (OPV)
Priorix
RabAvert
rabies vaccine
Recombivax HB
Rotamune
RotaShield
rotavirus vaccine
rubella & mumps virus vaccine, live
rubella virus vaccine, live
thymalfasin
Vaqta
varicella virus vaccine
Varivax
Vaxigrip ⒸⒶⓃ
yellow fever vaccine
YF-Vax
Zadaxin
**Immunizing Agents, Immunostim-
ulating Adjuncts**
aldesleukin
Alferon LDO
Alferon N
ancestim
Avonex

**Indications**

## Immunizing Agents, Immunostimulating Adjuncts (cont.)

Betaseron
diethyldithiocarbamate
filgrastim
Infergen
interferon alfa
interferon alfa-2a (IFN-αA)
interferon alfa-2b (IFN-α2)
interferon alfa-n1
interferon alfa-n3
interferon alfacon-1
interferon beta (IFN-B)
interferon beta-1a
interferon beta-1b
interferon gamma-1b
Intron A
levamisole HCl
Maxamine
Neupogen
Omniferon
PEG-Intron A
Proleukin
r-IFN-beta
R-Frone
Rebetron
Rebif (CAN)
Roferon-A
Stemgen
tetrachlorodecaoxide
Veldona
Wellferon
Wellferon (CAN)

## Immunostimulants

[see also: HIV Infections; Immunizing Agents]
acetylcysteine (N-acetylcysteine)
Actimmune
Aldara
Aliminase
Ampligen
Betafectin
cilmostim
Copaxone
disaccharide tripeptide glycerol dipalmitoyl
Ergamisol
Fluimucil

## Immunostimulants (cont.)

glatiramer acetate
Iamin
ImmTher
imiquimod
Imreg-1
Imuthiol
interleukin-4 receptor (IL-4R)
Leucomax
Leucotropin
Leukine
Linomide
lisofylline (LSF)
Macstim
Megagen
megakaryocyte growth and development factor, pegylated, recombinant human
milodistim
molgramostim
Neumega
Nuvance
oprelvekin
oxothiazolidine carboxylate (L-2-oxothiazolidine-4-carboxylic acid)
PGG glucan
Pixykine
poly I: poly C12U
prezatide copper acetate
Procysteine
ProTec
regramostim
Remune
roquinimex
sargramostim
Stimulon
Sulfasim
T-cell gene therapy
thalidomide
Thalomid
thymopentin
Timunox
Vendona

## Immunosuppressants

[see also: Antineoplastics; Corticosteroids, Systemic; Rheumatic Disease Agents]

**Immunosuppressants (cont.)**
anti-human thymocyte immuno-
globulin, rabbit
Atgam
azathioprine
azathioprine sodium
Campath 1H
CellCept
Centara
cyclosporine
dacliximab
Imuran
LJP-394
lymphocyte immune globulin, anti-
thymocyte
muromonab-CD3
mycophenolate mofetil
mycophenolate mofetil HCl
Nashville Rabbit Antithymocyte
Serum
Neoral
Orthoclone OKT3
priliximab
Prograf
Rapamune
Sandimmune
Sandimmune Neoral (CAN)
SangCya
sirolimus
tacrolimus
Thymoglobulin
Zenapax
**Impotence** [see: Sexual Dysfunction
Agents, Male]

## Inflammatory Bowel Disease
## Agents
[see also: Dermatological Preparations,
Anti-inflammatory; Hemorrhoidal
Agents]
Aliminase
aminosalicylic acid (4-aminosalicylic
acid)
anakinra
Antril
Asacol
Azulfidine
Azulfidine EN-tabs

**Inflammatory Bowel Disease
Agents (cont.)**
balsalazide disodium
budesonide
Colazide
Colomed
Cortenema
Cortifoam
Dipentum
Entocort (CAN)
infliximab
mesalamine
olsalazine sodium
Pamisyl
Pentasa
Remicade
Rezipas
Rowasa
Salofalk (CAN)
short chain fatty acids
sulfasalazine
**Intestinal Parasites** [see: Anthelmin-
tics; Antiprotozoals]
**Keratolytics** [see: Dermatological
Preparations, Keratolytic Agents]
**Kidney Stones** [see: Urinary Tract
Agents, Antiurolithic]
**Labor Stimulants and Suppressants**
[see: Gynecological Agents, Labor
Stimulants; Gynecological Agents,
Labor Suppressants]
**Lactation Suppressants** [see: Gyneco-
logical Agents, Lactation Suppressants]

## Laxatives
bisacodyl
carboxymethylcellulose sodium
casanthranol
cascara sagrada
Chronulac
Constilac
Constulose
Duphalac
Evalose
glycerin
Heptalac
lactulose
magnesium citrate
magnesium sulfate

**Indications**

**Laxatives (cont.)**
mineral oil
MiraLax
Osmoglyn
phenolphthalein
phenolphthalein, yellow
psyllium hydrophilic mucilloid
senna
sennosides
sodium phosphate, dibasic
sodium phosphate, monobasic
**Laxatives, Pre-procedure Bowel
Evacuants**
bisacodyl
bisacodyl tannex
Clysodrast
Co-Lav
Colovage
Colyte
Go-Evac
GoLYTELY
NuLytely
OCL
polyethylene glycol-electrolyte solution (PEG-ES)
senna
**Laxatives, Stool Softeners**
docusate calcium
docusate potassium
docusate sodium
**Leukemia** [see: Antineoplastics]
**Lice** [see: Pediculicides and Scabicides]

---

**Lipid-lowering Agents**
Apo-Gemfibrozil Ⓒ
atorvastatin calcium
Atromid-S
Baycol
cerivastatin sodium
CholestaGel
cholestyramine resin
Choloxin
clofibrate
colesevelam HCl
Colestid
colestipol HCl
dextrothyroxine sodium
fenofibrate
fluvastatin sodium

**Lipid-lowering Agents (cont.)**
Gemcor
gemfibrozil
lecithin
Lescol
Lipitor
Lipo-Nicin/100
Lipo-Nicin/300
LoCholest; LoCholest Light
Lopid
Lorelco
lovastatin
Mevacor
niacin
Niacor
Niaspan
Nicolar
Novo-Gemfibrozil Ⓒ
Pravachol
pravastatin sodium
Prevalite
probucol
Questran; Questran Light
simvastatin
Tricor
ZD 4522
Zocor
**Manic-Depressive Disorder** [see:
Psychotherapeutics, Antidepressants;
Psychotherapeutics, Antimanic]
**Menopause Agents** [see: Gynecologi-
cal Agents, Menopause Agents]

---

**Mineral Replacement**
**Mineral Replacement, Calcium**
[see also: Gynecological Agents,
Menopause Agents]
Adeflor M
calcium
calcium carbonate
calcium gluceptate
calcium glycerophosphate
calcium lactate
Calphosan
Filibon F.A.; Filibon Forte
Lactocal-F
Marnatal-F
Materna
Mission Prenatal Rx

## Mineral Replacement, Calcium (cont.)
Mynatal
Mynatal FC
Mynatal P.N.
Mynatal P.N. Forte
Mynatal Rx
Mynate 90 Plus
Natabec Rx
Natafort
NatalCare Plus
Natalins Rx
Natarex Prenatal
Nestabs FA
Niferex-PN Forte
Norlac Rx
O-Cal f.a.
Par-F
Par-Natal Plus 1 Improved
Pramet FA
Pramilet FA
Pre-H Cal
Prenatal H.P.
Prenatal Maternal
Prenatal MR 90
Prenatal One
Prenatal Plus Iron
Prenatal Plus with Betacarotene
Prenatal Plus; Prenatal Plus Improved
Prenatal Rx
Prenatal Rx with Betacarotene
Prenatal Z
Prenatal-1 + Iron
Prenate 90; Prenate Ultra
Secran Prenatal
Stuartnatal Plus

## Mineral Replacement, Fluoride
ADC with Fluoride
Adeflor M
Apatate with Fluoride
Chewable Multivitamins with Fluoride
Chewable Triple Vitamins with Fluoride
Florvite
Florvite + Iron
Florvite + Iron; Half Strength Florvite + Iron
Florvite; Florvite Half Strength

## Mineral Replacement, Fluoride (cont.)
Fluoritab
Flura
Flura-Drops
Karidium
Luride
Multivitamin with Fluoride
Mulvidren-F
O-Cal f.a.
Pediaflor
Pharmaflor; Pharmaflur df; Pharmaflur 1.1
Poly-Vi-Flor
Poly-Vi-Flor with Iron
Polytabs-F
Polyvitamin Fluoride
Polyvitamin Fluoride with Iron
Polyvitamin with Iron and Fluoride
Polyvitamins with Fluoride and Iron
sodium fluoride
Soluvite C.T.
Soluvite-f
Tri-A-Vite F
Tri-Flor-Vite with Fluoride
Tri-Vi-Flor
Tri-Vi-Flor with Iron
Tri Vit with Fluoride
Tri-Vitamin with Fluoride
Triple Vitamin ADC with Fluoride
Triple Vitamins with Fluoride
Trivitamin Fluoride
Vi-Daylin/F ADC
Vi-Daylin/F ADC + Iron
Vi-Daylin/F Multivitamin
Vi-Daylin/F Multivitamin + Iron

## Mineral Replacement, Iron
[see also: Anemia Agents, Iron]
Adeflor M
B-C with Folic Acid Plus
Bacmin
Berocca Plus
Berplex Plus
Estrostep Fe
ferrous fumarate
ferrous gluconate
ferrous sulfate
ferrous sulfate, dried
Filibon F.A.; Filibon Forte
Florvite + Iron

Indications

**Mineral Replacement, Iron (cont.)**
Florvite + Iron; Half Strength
    Florvite + Iron
Formula B Plus
iron
Lactocal-F
Loestrin Fe 1/20; Loestrin Fe 1.5/30
Marnatal-F
Materna
Mission Prenatal Rx
Mynatal
Mynatal FC
Mynatal P.N.
Mynatal P.N. Forte
Mynatal Rx
Mynate 90 Plus
Natabec Rx
Natafort
NatalCare Plus
Natalins Rx
Natarex Prenatal
Nestabs FA
Niferex-PN
Niferex-PN Forte
Norlac Rx
Nu-Iron V
O-Cal f.a.
Par-F
Par-Natal Plus 1 Improved
Poly-Vi-Flor with Iron
Polyvitamin Fluoride with Iron
Polyvitamin with Iron and Fluoride
Polyvitamins with Fluoride and Iron
Pramet FA
Pramilet FA
Pre-H Cal
Prenatal H.P.
Prenatal Maternal
Prenatal MR 90
Prenatal One
Prenatal Plus Iron
Prenatal Plus with Betacarotene
Prenatal Plus; Prenatal Plus
    Improved
Prenatal Rx
Prenatal Rx with Betacarotene
Prenatal Z
Prenatal-1 + Iron
Prenate 90; Prenate Ultra
Secran Prenatal

**Mineral Replacement, Iron (cont.)**
Senilezol
Stuartnatal Plus
Theragran Hematinic
Tri-Vi-Flor with Iron
Vi-Daylin/F ADC + Iron
Vi-Daylin/F Multivitamin + Iron
Vitafōl; Vitafōl-PN
Zenate, Advanced Formula
Zodeac-100
**Mineral Replacement, Magnesium**
magnesium amino acid chelate
magnesium carbonate
magnesium gluconate
magnesium oxide
**Mineral Replacement, Zinc**
zinc gluconate
zinc sulfate
Zinca-Pak
Zincate
**Mineral Replacement, Trace Elements**
ammonium molybdate
Chroma-Pak
chromic chloride
Chromium Chloride
ConTE-Pak-4
cupric sulfate
M.T.E.-4; M.T.E.-5; M.T.E.-6;
    M.T.E.-7; M.T.E.-4 Concentrated
    M.T.E.-5 Concentrated; M.T.E.-6
    Concentrated
manganese chloride
manganese sulfate
Molypen
MulTE-Pak-4; MulTE-Pak-5
Multiple Trace Element with Selenium; Multiple Trace Element
    with Selenium Concentrated
Multiple Trace Element; Multiple
    Trace Element Concentrated;
    Multiple Trace Element Neonatal
    Multiple Trace Element Pediatric
Multitrace-5 Concentrate
Neotrace-4
P.T.E.-4; P.T.E.-5
PedTE-Pak-4
Pedtrace-4
Sele-Pak
selenious acid

**Mineral Replacement, Trace Elements (cont.)**
Selepen
Trace Metals Additive in 0.9% NaCl
Tracelyte; Tracelyte II; Tracelyte with Double Electrolytes; Tracelyte II with Double Electrolytes
**Mineral Replacement, Multiple (not listed)**
B-C with Folic Acid Plus
Bacmin
Berocca Plus
Berplex Plus
Cezin-S
Eldercaps
Florvite + Iron
Florvite + Iron; Half Strength Florvite + Iron
Formula B Plus
Hemocyte Plus
Heptuna Plus
Lactocal-F
Marnatal-F
Materna
Megaton
Mynatal
Mynatal FC
Mynatal P.N. Forte
Mynatal Rx
NatalCare Plus
Niferex-PN
Niferex-PN Forte
Norlac Rx
O-Cal f.a.
Par-F
Poly-Vi-Flor with Iron
Polyvitamin Fluoride with Iron
Pramilet FA
Prenatal Maternal
Strovite Plus; Strovite Forte
Theragran Hematinic
Vicon Forte
Zincvit
Zodeac-100

---

# Mouth and Throat Preparations
[see also: Antiseptics]
acidulated phosphate fluoride (sodium fluoride & hydrofluoric acid)

**Mouth and Throat Preparations (cont.)**
Actisite
Americaine Anesthetic Lubricant
amlexanox
Anestacon
Aphthasol
Astracaine; Astracaine Forte (CAN)
Atrisorb FreeFlow GTR Barrier
benzocaine
benzydamine HCl
carbamide peroxide
chlorhexidine gluconate
chlorobutanol
chlorophyllin
choline salicylate
Citanest Forte
Dey-Pak Sodium Chloride 3% & 10%
n-docosanol
Duo-Trach Kit
Fluoride Loz
Fluorinse
Flura-Loz
Gel-Kam
itraconazole
Karigel; Karigel-N
Kenalog in Orabase
Lidakol
lidocaine HCl
Luride SF
Minute-Gel
Mycostatin
Nilstat
nystatin
Nystex
Orabase HCA
Oralease
Oralone Dental
Peridex
PerioChip
PerioGard
phenol
Phos-Flur
pilocarpine HCl
Point-Two
Pontocaine HCl
povidone-iodine
PreviDent
PreviDent Rinse

**Indications**

## Mouth and Throat Preparations (cont.)

Ravocaine & Novocaine with Levophed
Salagen
sodium chloride (NaCl)
sodium fluoride
Sporanox
stannous fluoride
Stop
Tantrum
tetracaine HCl
tetracycline
Thera-Flur; Thera-Flur-N
triamcinolone acetonide
Trilisate
Xylocaine
Xylocaine 10% Oral
Xylocaine Viscous

## MRI Contrast Media [see: Contrast Media, Paramagnetic]

## Multiple Sclerosis Agents

Antegren
bovine myelin
Myloral

## Muscle Relaxants

[see also: Psychotherapeutics, Anxiolytics; Sedatives and Hypnotics]

## Muscle Relaxants, Skeletal

Anectine
Arduan
atracurium besylate
baclofen (L-baclofen)
Banflex
carisoprodol
chlorphenesin carbamate
chlorzoxazone
cisatracurium besylate
cyclobenzaprine HCl
Dantrium
dantrolene sodium
Diazemuls ⓒⒶⓃ
diazepam
Dizac
doxacurium chloride

## Muscle Relaxants, Skeletal (cont.)

Flaxedil
Flexaphen
Flexeril
Flexoject
Flexon
gallamine triethiodide
Lioresal
Maolate
metaxalone
methocarbamol
metocurine iodide
Metubine Iodide
Mivacron
mivacurium chloride
Mus-Lax
Myolin
Nimbex
Norcuron
Norflex
Norgesic; Norgesic Forte
Nuromax
orphenadrine citrate
Orphengesic; Orphengesic Forte
pancuronium bromide
Paraflex
Parafon Forte DSC
Pavulon
pipecuronium bromide
Quelicin
Remular-S
Robaxin
Robaxisal
rocuronium bromide
Skelaxin
Sodol
Sodol Compound
Soma
Soma Compound
Soma Compound with Codeine
succinylcholine chloride
Sucostrin
Tracrium
tubocurarine chloride
Valium
Valium Roche Oral ⓒⒶⓃ
Valrelease
vecuronium bromide
Zemuron
Zetran

**Muscle Relaxants, Smooth**
Cerespan
Cyclan
cyclandelate
Cyclospasmol
Cyclospasmol (CAN)
flavoxate HCl
Genabid
papaverine HCl
Pavabid
Pavabid HP
Pavagen TD
Pavarine
Pavased
Pavatine
Paverolan
Urispas

# Muscle Stimulants
ambenonium chloride
carbachol
edrophonium chloride
Enlon
Enlon Plus
guanidine HCl
IGF-BP3 complex
Mestinon
Mytelase
neostigmine bromide
neostigmine methylsulfate
Prostigmin
pyridostigmine bromide
Regonol
Reversol
SomatoKine
Tensilon
**Narcolepsy** [see: Central Nervous System Stimulants]

# Nasal Preparations
**Nasal Preparations, Antiallergic**
[see also: Allergy and Anaphylaxis Agents; Antihistamines, Topical]
Apo-Cromolyn (CAN)
Astelin
Atrovent
azelastine HCl

**Nasal Preparations, Antiallergic (cont.)**
cromolyn sodium
ipratropium bromide
levocabastine HCl
Livostin (CAN)
pheniramine maleate
**Nasal Preparations, Anti-inflammatory**
beclomethasone dipropionate
Beconase
Beconase AQ
budesonide
Dexacort Phosphate
dexamethasone sodium phosphate
Flonase
flunisolide
fluticasone propionate
Nasacort
Nasacort AQ
Nasalide
Nasarel
Rhinocort
Rhinocort Aqua (CAN)
Rhinocort Turbuhaler (CAN)
triamcinolone acetonide
Vancenase
Vancenase AQ
**Nasal Preparations, Decongestants**
Adrenalin Chloride
Benzedrex
ephedrine sulfate
epinephrine HCl
naphazoline HCl
oxymetazoline HCl
phenylephrine HCl
propylhexedrine
tetrahydrozoline HCl
Tyzine
**Nasal Preparations, Moisturizers**
sodium chloride (NaCl)
**Nausea** [see: Antiemetics and Antinauseants]

# Nutritional Agents
5% Alcohol and 5% Dextrose in Water; 10% Alcohol and 5% Dextrose in Water
Aminess 5.2%

**Indications**

## Nutritional Agents (cont.)

Aminosyn 3.5% (5%, 7%, 8.5%, 10%); Aminosyn (pH6) 10%; Aminosyn II 3.5% (5%, 7%, 8.5%, 10%, 15%); Aminosyn-PF 7% (10%)

Aminosyn 3.5% M; Aminosyn II 3.5% M

Aminosyn 7% (8.5%) with Electrolytes; Aminosyn II 7% (8.5%, 10%) with Electrolytes

Aminosyn-HBC 7%

Aminosyn II 3.5% in 5% (25%) Dextrose; Aminosyn II 4.25% in 10% (20%, 25%) Dextrose; Aminosyn II 5% in 25% Dextrose

Aminosyn II 3.5% M in 5% Dextrose; Aminosyn II 4.25% M in 10% Dextrose

Aminosyn-RF 5.2%

BranchAmin 4%

Carnitor

Cernevit-12

choline

choline chloride

cysteine HCl (L-cysteine HCl)

D-2.5-W; D-5-W; D-10-W; D-20-W; D-25-W; D-30-W; D-40-W; D-50-W; D-60-W; D-70-W

dextrose

5% Dextrose and Electrolyte #48; 5% Dextrose and Electrolyte #75; 10% Dextrose and Electrolyte #48

50% Dextrose with Electrolyte Pattern A (or N)

Dialyte Pattern LM

Dianeal Peritoneal Dialysis Solution with 1.1% Amino Acids

Extraneal Peritoneal Dialysis Solution

fat emulsion, intravenous

FreAmine HBC 6.9%

FreAmine III 3% (8.5%) with Electrolytes

FreAmine III 8.5%; FreAmine III 10%

glutamic acid (L-glutamic acid)

glycine

HepatAmine

icodextrin

inositol

## Nutritional Agents (cont.)

Inpersol; Inpersol-LM

Intrachol

Intralipid 10%; Intralipid 20%

Iodo-Pak

Iodopen

Isolyte E (G; H; M; P; R; S) with 5% Dextrose

levocarnitine

Liposyn II 10%; Liposyn III 10%

Liposyn II 20%; Liposyn III 20%

lysine (L-lysine)

NephrAmine 5.4%

Normosol-M and 5% Dextrose; Normosol-R and 5% Dextrose

Novamine; Novamine 15%

Nutrineal Peritoneal Dialysis Solution with 1.1% Amino Acid

Plasma-Lyte M (R; 56; 148) and 5% Dextrose

ProcalAmine

ProSol 20%

RenAmin

sodium iodide

sugar, invert (50% dextrose & 50% fructose)

threonine (L-threonine)

Travasol 2.75% in 5% (10%, 25%) Dextrose; Travasol 4.25% in 5% (10%, 25%) Dextrose

Travasol 3.5% (5.5%, 8.5%) with Electrolytes

Travasol 5.5% (8.5%, 10%)

Travert

5% Travert and Electrolyte No. 2; 10% Travert and Electrolyte No. 2

TrophAmine 6%; TrophAmine 10%

VitaCarn

## Obsessive-Compulsive Disorder (OCD) [see: Psychotherapeutics, Antiobsessional]

# Ophthalmologicals
## Ophthalmologicals, Antiallergic

[see also: Antihistamines, Topical]

AK-Con-A

Alomide

antazoline phosphate

Antazoline-V

**Nutritional Agents (cont.)**
ciprofloxacin HCl
Crolom
cromolyn sodium
Emadine
emedastine difumarate
ketotifen fumarate
levocabastine HCl
Livostin
lodoxamide tromethamine
Mireze ⒸⒶⓃ
Nafazair A
Naphazole-A
Naphoptic-A
nedocromil sodium
olopatadine HCl
Opticrom 4%
Patanol
pheniramine maleate
Vasocon-A
Zaditor

**Ophthalmologicals, Antibiotics**
[see also: Antibiotics, Topical]
Achromycin
AK-Chlor
AK-Mycin
AK-Poly-Bac
AK-Spore
AK-Spore H.C.
AK-Sulf
AK-Trol
AKTob
Argyrol S.S. 20%
Aureomycin
bacitracin zinc
Bacticort
Bleph-10
Blephamide
Cetamide
Cetapred
Chibroxin
chloramphenicol
chlorobutanol
Chloromycetin
Chloromycetin Hydrocortisone
Chloroptic
Chloroptic S.O.P.
chlortetracycline HCl
Ciloxan
Coracin

**Ophthalmologicals, Antibiotics (cont.)**
Cortisporin
Defy
Dexacidin
Dexasporin
erythromycin
FML-S
Gantrisin
Garamycin
Genoptic
Genoptic S.O.P.
Gentacidin
Gentak
gentamicin sulfate
gramicidin
Herplex
idoxuridine (IDU)
Ilotycin
Isopto Cetamide
Isopto Cetapred
Maxitrol
Metimyd
Natacyn
natamycin
neomycin sulfate
Neosporin
Neotal
Neotricin HC
norfloxacin
Ocuflox
Ocusulf-10
Ocutricin
ofloxacin
Ophthocort
Optimyd
oxytetracycline HCl
Poly-Pred
polymyxin B sulfate
Polytrim
Pred-G
Pred-G S.O.P.
silver nitrate
silver protein, mild
Sodium Sulamyd
Storz-N-P-D
Storz-Sulf
Sulf-10
Sulf-15
sulfacetamide sodium

**Indications**

## Ophthalmologicals, Antibiotics (cont.)

sulfisoxazole diolamine
Sulpred
Sulster
Terak
Terra-Cortril
Terramycin with Polymyxin B
tetracycline HCl
TobraDex
tobramycin
Tobrex
trifluridine
Triple Antibiotic
Vasocidin
Vasocine
Vasosulf
vidarabine
Vira-A
Viroptic

## Ophthalmologicals, Antiglaucoma

acetazolamide
acetazolamide sodium
Adrenalin Chloride
Adsorbocarpine
Akarpine
AKBeta
AKPro
Alphagan
apraclonidine HCl
Azopt
Beta-Tim ⒸⒶⓃ
Betagan Liquifilm
betaxolol HCl
Betimol
Betoptic; Betoptic S
brimonidine tartrate
brinzolamide
carbachol
Carboptic
carteolol HCl
Cosopt
demecarium bromide
Diamox
dipivefrin HCl
dorzolamide HCl
E-Pilo-3
E-Pilo-1; E-Pilo-2; E-Pilo-4; E-Pilo-6
echothiophate iodide
Epifrin

## Ophthalmologicals, Antiglaucoma (cont.)

Epinal
epinephrine bitartrate
epinephrine borate
epinephrine HCl
epinephryl borate
Eppy/N 1%; Eppy/N 2%
Eserine Salicylate
Eserine Sulfate
Floropryl
Glaucon
GlaucTabs
Humorsol
Iopidine
isoflurophate
isopropyl unoprostone
Isopto Carbachol
Isopto Carpine
latanoprost
levobunolol HCl
Med Timolol ⒸⒶⓃ
methazolamide
metipranolol HCl
MZM
Neptazane
Novo-Timol ⒸⒶⓃ
Nu-Timolol ⒸⒶⓃ
Ocu-Carpine
Ocupress
Ocusert Pilo-20; Ocusert Pilo-40
OptiPranolol
$P_1E_1$; $P_2E_1$; $P_4E_1$; $P_6E_1$
$P_3E_1$
Phospholine Iodide
physostigmine
physostigmine salicylate
physostigmine sulfate
Pilagan
Pilocar
pilocarpine
pilocarpine HCl
pilocarpine nitrate
Pilopine HS
Piloptic-½; Piloptic-1; Piloptic-2; Piloptic-3; Piloptic-4; Piloptic-6
Pilopto-Carpine
Pilostat
Propine
Rescula

**Ophthalmologicals, Antiglaucoma (cont.)**
Storzine 2
Timodal (CAN)
timolol hemihydrate
timolol maleate
Timoptic
Timoptic-XE
Trusopt
Xalatan

**Ophthalmologicals, Anti-inflammatory**
Acular; Acular PF
AK-Dex
AK-Neo-Dex
AK-Pred
AK-Spore H.C.
AK-Trol
Alrex
Bacticort
Blephamide
Cetapred
Chloromycetin Hydrocortisone
Coracin
Cortisporin
Decadron Phosphate
Dexacidin
dexamethasone
dexamethasone sodium phosphate
Dexasporin
diclofenac sodium
Diodex (CAN)
Econopred; Econopred Plus
Eflone
Flarex
Fluor-Op
fluorometholone
fluorometholone acetate
flurbiprofen sodium
FML-S
FML S.O.P.
FML; FML Forte
HMS
hydrocortisone (HC)
hydrocortisone acetate (HCA)
Inflamase Mild; Inflamase Forte
Isopto Cetapred
Lotemax
loteprednol etabonate
Maxidex

**Ophthalmologicals, Anti-inflammatory (cont.)**
Maxitrol
medrysone
Metimyd
Neo-Dexair
Neo-Dexameth
NeoDecadron
Neotricin HC
Ocufen
Ophthocort
Optimyd
Poly-Pred
Pred-G
Pred-G S.O.P.
Pred Mild; Pred Forte
prednisolone acetate
prednisolone sodium phosphate
Profenal
R.O.-Dexsone (CAN)
Spersadex (CAN)
Storz-N-D
Storz-N-P-D
Sulpred
Sulster
suprofen
Surodex
Terra-Cortril
TobraDex
Vasocidin
Vasocine
Vexol
Voltaren

**Ophthalmologicals, Contact Lens Preparations**
[see also: Antiseptics]
hydrogen peroxide
sodium chloride (NaCl)

**Ophthalmologicals, Decongestants**
AK-Con
AK-Con-A
AK-Dilate
Albalon
Antazoline-V
Muro's Opcon
Mydfrin 2.5%
Nafazair
Nafazair A
Naphazole-A
naphazoline HCl

**Ophthalmologicals, Decongestants (cont.)**
Naphcon Forte
Naphoptic-A
Neo-Synephrine
oxymetazoline HCl
Phenoptic
phenylephrine HCl
Storzfen
tetrahydrozoline HCl
Vasocon-A
Vasocon Regular
Vasosulf

**Ophthalmologicals, Diagnostic Agents**
AK-Fluor
Flu-Oxinate
Fluor-I-Strip; Fluor-I-Strip A.T.
Fluoracaine
fluorescein
fluorescein sodium
Fluorescite
Fluoresoft
fluorexon
Flurate
Fluress
Ful-Glo
Funduscein-10; Funduscein-25
Healon Yellow
Ophthifluor

**Ophthalmologicals, Local Anesthetics**
[see also: Anesthetics, Local]
AK-Taine
Alcaine
benoxinate HCl
Flu-Oxinate
Fluoracaine
Flurate
Fluress
Ophthaine
Ophthetic
Pontocaine HCl
proparacaine HCl
tetracaine HCl

**Ophthalmologicals, Miotics**
acetylcholine chloride
Adsorbocarpine
Akarpine
carbachol

**Ophthalmologicals, Miotics (cont.)**
Carbastat
Carboptic
dapiprazole HCl
demecarium bromide
echothiophate iodide
Eserine Salicylate
Eserine Sulfate
Floropryl
Humorsol
isoflurophate
Isopto Carbachol
Isopto Carpine
Miochol
Miochol-E
Miostat
Ocu-Carpine
Ocusert Pilo-20; Ocusert Pilo-40
Phospholine Iodide
physostigmine
physostigmine salicylate
physostigmine sulfate
Pilagan
Pilocar
pilocarpine
pilocarpine HCl
pilocarpine nitrate
Pilopine HS
Piloptic-½; Piloptic-1; Piloptic-2; Piloptic-3; Piloptic-4; Piloptic-6
Pilopto-Carpine
Pilostat
Rēv-Eyes
Storzine 2

**Ophthalmologicals, Moisturizers, Lubricants, and Emollients**
Albalon
boric acid
carboxymethylcellulose sodium
collagen
glycerin
Herrick Lacrimal Plug
hydroxypropyl cellulose
hydroxypropyl methylcellulose
methylcellulose
polyethylene glycol (PEG)
polyvinyl alcohol (PVA)
Punctum Plug
silicone
vitamin A

**Ophthalmologicals, Mydriatics and Cycloplegics**
AK-Dilate
AK-Homatropine
AK-Pentolate
atropine sulfate
Atropine Care
Atropine-1
Atropisol
Cyclogyl
Cyclomydril
cyclopentolate HCl
homatropine hydrobromide
hydroxyamphetamine hydrobromide
Isopto Atropine
Isopto Homatropine
Isopto Hyoscine
Murocoll-2
Mydfrin 2.5%
Mydriacyl
Neo-Synephrine
Opticyl
Paredrine
Paremyd
Pentolair
Phenoptic
phenylephrine HCl
scopolamine hydrobromide
Storzfen
Tropi-Storz
Tropicacyl
tropicamide

**Ophthalmologicals, Surgical Preparations**
AdatoSil 5000
AMO Vitrax
Amvisc; Amvisc Plus
Argyrol S.S. 20%
Betadine 5% Sterile Ophthalmic Prep
Catarase 1:5000
chymotrypsin
gelatin film, absorbable
gelatin powder, absorbable
gelatin sponge, absorbable
Gelfilm; Gelfilm Ophthalmic
Gelfoam
glycerin
Healon Yellow
Healon; Healon GV
hyaluronate sodium

**Ophthalmologicals, Surgical Preparations (cont.)**
hydroxypropyl methylcellulose
Occucoat
Ophthalgan
polydimethylsiloxane
povidone-iodine
Profenal
silver protein, mild
Staarvisc
suprofen
Viscoat

**Ophthalmologicals, Other**
aminocaproic acid
AMO Endosol; AMO Endosol Extra
B-Salt Forte
Botox
botulinum toxin, type A
BSS; BSS Plus
Caprogel
cyclosporine
Dysport
fomivirsen sodium
Galardin
glucose, liquid
Glucose-40
ilomastat
Lu-Tex
lutetium texaphyrin
matrix metalloproteinase (MMP) inhibitors
Optimmune
PhotoPoint
Salagen
Sandimmune
sodium chloride (NaCl)
Succus Cineraria Maritima
tin etiopurpurin dichloride
tyloxapol
verteporfin
Visudyne
Vitrase
Vitravene

**Organ Transplant Rejection** [see: Immunosuppressive Agents]
**Osteoarthritis** [see: Antiarthritics; Analgesics, Nonsteroidal]
**Osteoporosis** [see: Gynecological Agents, Menopause Agents; Mineral Replacement, Calcium; Sex Hormones]

**Indications**

# Otologicals

[see also: Anesthetics, Local; Antibiotics,
   Topical; Antiseptics; Dermatological
   Preparations, Anti-inflammatory]
AA-HC Otic
Acetasol
Acetasol HC
acetic acid
AK-Spore H.C.
Allergen Ear Drops
Americaine Otic
AntibiŌtic
Antibiotic Ear Solution
Antibiotic Ear Suspension
antipyrine
Auralgan Otic
Auroto Otic
benzocaine
boric acid
Borofair Otic
carbamide peroxide
Cerumenex
chloramphenicol
chlorobutanol
Chloromycetin Otic
chloroxylenol
Cipro HC Otic
colistin sulfate
Coly-Mycin S Otic
Cortatrigen Modified
Cortic
Cortisporin Otic
Cortisporin-TC
Cresylate
Drotic
Ear-Eze
hydrocortisone (HC)
hydrocortisone acetate (HCA)
LazerSporin-C
neomycin sulfate
Octicare
Oti-Med
Otic-Care
Otic Domeboro
Otic Tridesilon
OtiTricin
Otobiotic Otic
Otocain
Otocalm
Otocort

# Otologicals (cont.)

Otomar-HC
Otomycet-HC
Otomycin-HPN Otic
Otosporin
Pediotic
Pedotic
polymyxin B sulfate
Tri-Otic
trolamine polypeptide oleate-con-
   densate
Tympagesic
UAD Otic
VōSol HC Otic
VōSol Otic
Vasotate HC
Zoto-HC

**Paget's Disease** [see: Hypercalcemia
   Agents]
**Panic Disorder** [see: Psychotherapeu-
   tics, Antipanic]
**Parasites, Intestinal** [see: Anthelmin-
   tics; Antiprotozoals]
**Parkinson's Disease** [see: Antiparkin-
   sonian Agents]

# Pediculicides and Scabicides

Acticin
crotamiton
Elimite
Eurax
G-Well
Kwell
Kwildane
lindane
malathion
Ovide
permethrin
piperonyl butoxide
pyrethrins
Scabene

# Peptic Ulcer and Gastric Reflux Agents

[see also: Antacids]
Aciphex
anisotropine methylbromide

**Peptic Ulcer and Gastric Reflux Agents (cont.)**
Arthrotec
Axid
Banthīne
Cantil
Carafate
cimetidine
cimetidine HCl
cisapride
Cytotec
Daricon
enprostil
famotidine
Gardrin
Gastrozepine
Iamin
lansoprazole
Losec Ⓒ
mepenzolate bromide
methantheline bromide
misoprostol
nizatidine
omeprazole
oxyphencyclimine HCl
pantoprazole
Pantozol
Pathilon
Pepcid
Pepcid RPD
pirenzepine HCl
Prepulsid Ⓒ
Prevacid
Prevpac
Prilosec
Propulsid
Pylorid Ⓒ
rabeprazole sodium
ranitidine
ranitidine bismuth citrate
ranitidine HCl
roxatidine acetate HCl
Roxin
sucralfate
Tagamet
tridihexethyl chloride
Tritec
Zantac
Zantac EFFERdose
Zantac GELdose

**Peripheral Vasodilators**
Cerespan
cilostazol
Cyclan
cyclandelate
Cyclo-Prostin
Cyclospasmol
Cyclospasmol Ⓒ
epoprostenol
Ethaquin
Ethatab
ethaverine HCl
Ethavex-100
Flolan
flunarizine HCl
Genabid
Isovex
isoxsuprine HCl
Lipo-Nicin/100
Lipo-Nicin/300
niacin
Niacor
Niaspan
papaverine HCl
Pavabid
Pavabid HP
Pavagen TD
Pavarine
Pavased
Pavatine
Paverolan
pentoxifylline
Pletal
Priscoline HCl
Sibelium
tolazoline HCl
Trental
Vasodilan
Voxsuprine
**Plasma Expanders** [see: Blood Expanders and Substitutes]

**Platelet Aggregation Inhibitors**
[see also: Cardiac Agents]
abciximab
Aggrastat
Aggrenox
Apo-Ticlopidine Ⓒ
aspirin

Indications

**Platelet Aggregation Inhibitors (cont.)**
cilostazol
clopidogrel bisulfate
dipyridamole
Easprin
eptifibatide
Integrilin
Persantine
Plavix
Pletal
ReoPro
Ticlid
ticlopidine HCl
tirofiban HCl
ZORprin

**Progestins** [*see: Sex Hormones, Progestins*]

---

# Prostatic Hyperplasia Agents
Apo-Terazosin ⒸⒶⓃ
Cardura
doxazosin mesylate
finasteride
Flomax
HP-4
Hytrin
Hytrin ⒸⒶⓃ
Novo-Terazosin ⒸⒶⓃ
PPRT-321
Proscar
tamsulosin HCl
terazosin HCl

**Psoriasis** [*see: Dermatological Preparations, Psoriasis Agents*]

---

# Psychotherapeutics
**Psychotherapeutics, Antidepressants**
Adapin
amitriptyline HCl
amoxapine
Anafranil
Apo-Moclobemide ⒸⒶⓃ
Asendin
Aventyl HCl
benactyzine HCl
bupropion HCl

**Psychotherapeutics, Antidepressants (cont.)**
Catatrol
Celexa
citalopram hydrobromide
clomipramine HCl
Deprol
desipramine HCl
Desyrel
dothiepin HCl
doxepin HCl
Edronax
Effexor
Effexor XR
Elavil
Endep
Enovil
Etrafon; Etrafon 2–10; Etrafon-A; Etrafon-Forte
fluoxetine HCl
fluvoxamine maleate
imipramine HCl
imipramine pamoate
isocarboxazid
Janimine
Limbitrol DS 10-25
Ludiomil
Luvox
Manerex ⒸⒶⓃ
maprotiline HCl
Marplan
mirtazapine
moclobemide
Nardil
nefazodone HCl
Norpramin
nortriptyline HCl
Pamelor
Parnate
paroxetine HCl
Paxil
Paxil CR
Pertofrane
phenelzine sulfate
Prothiaden
protriptyline HCl
Prozac
reboxetine
Remeron
sertraline HCl

Psychotherapeutics, Antipsychotics 195

**Psychotherapeutics, Antidepressants (cont.)**
Serzone
Sinequan
Surmontil
Tofranil
Tofranil-PM
tranylcypromine sulfate
trazodone HCl
Triavil 2-10; Triavil 2-25; Triavil 4-10; Triavil 4-25; Triavil 4-50
trimipramine maleate
venlafaxine HCl
viloxazine
Vivactil
Wellbutrin
Wellbutrin SR
Zoloft
Zoloft ⒸⒶⓃ

**Psychotherapeutics, Antimanic**
Atretol
carbamazepine
Carbatrol
Carbolith ⒸⒶⓃ
Depitol
Duralith ⒸⒶⓃ
Epitol
Eskalith
Eskalith CR
Lithane ⒸⒶⓃ
lithium carbonate
lithium citrate
Lithobid
Lithonate
Lithotabs
PMS-Lithium Carbonate ⒸⒶⓃ
PMS-Lithium Citrate ⒸⒶⓃ
Tegretol
Tegretol-XR

**Psychotherapeutics, Antiobsessional**
Anafranil
clomipramine HCl
fluoxetine HCl
fluvoxamine maleate
Luvox
paroxetine HCl
Paxil
Paxil CR
Prozac
sertraline HCl

**Psychotherapeutics, Antiobsessional (cont.)**
Zoloft
Zoloft ⒸⒶⓃ

**Psychotherapeutics, Antipanic**
alprazolam
Pagoclone
paroxetine HCl
Paxil
Paxil CR
sertraline HCl
Xanax
Zoloft
Zoloft ⒸⒶⓃ

**Psychotherapeutics, Antipsychotics**
acetophenazine maleate
Apo-Fluphenazine ⒸⒶⓃ
Apo-Loxapine ⒸⒶⓃ
Apo-Perphenazine ⒸⒶⓃ
Apo-Thioridazine ⒸⒶⓃ
Apo-Trifluoperazine ⒸⒶⓃ
chlorpromazine
chlorpromazine HCl
clozapine
Clozaril
Compazine
Etrafon; Etrafon 2-10; Etrafon-A; Etrafon-Forte
fluphenazine decanoate
fluphenazine enanthate
fluphenazine HCl
Haldol
Haldol Decanoate 50; Haldol Decanoate 100
haloperidol
haloperidol decanoate
haloperidol lactate
Haloperidol LA ⒸⒶⓃ
iloperidone
Loxapac ⒸⒶⓃ
loxapine
loxapine HCl
loxapine succinate
Loxitane
Loxitane C
Loxitane IM
Mellaril
Mellaril-S
mesoridazine besylate
Moban

**Indications**

## Psychotherapeutics, Antipsychotics (cont.)

Modecate (CAN)
Moditen Enanthate (CAN)
Moditen HCl (CAN)
molindone HCl
Navane
Nu-Prochlor (CAN)
olanzapine
Orap
Ormazine
Permitil
perphenazine
pimozide
PMS-Fluphenazine (CAN)
PMS-Haloperidol; PMS-Haloperidol LA (CAN)
prochlorperazine
prochlorperazine bimaleate
prochlorperazine edisylate
prochlorperazine maleate
prochlorperazine mesylate
Prolixin
Prolixin Decanoate
Prolixin Enanthate
promazine HCl
Prozine-50
quetiapine fumarate
Raudixin
Rauverid
rauwolfia serpentina
reserpine
Rho-Fluphenazine (CAN)
Risperdal
risperidone
Serentil
Seroquel
Serpalan
Sparine
Stelazine
Stemetil (CAN)
thioridazine HCl
thiothixene
thiothixene HCl
Thorazine
Tindal
Triavil 2-10; Triavil 2-25; Triavil 4-10; Triavil 4-25; Triavil 4-50
trifluoperazine HCl
triflupromazine HCl

## Psychotherapeutics, Antipsychotics (cont.)

Trilafon
Vesprin
Zeldox
ziprasidone
Zomaril
Zyprexa

## Psychotherapeutics, Anxiolytics

[see also: Sedatives and Hypnotics]
acecarbromal
alprazolam
Anxanil
Apo-Trifluoperazine (CAN)
Atarax
Atarax 100
Ativan
BuSpar
buspirone HCl
Centrax
chlordiazepoxide
chlordiazepoxide HCl
chlormezanone
Clindex
Clinoxide
Clipoxide
clobazam
clorazepate dipotassium
Deprol
Diazemuls (CAN)
diazepam
Dizac
E-Vista
Epromate
Equagesic
Equanil
Equazine M
Frisium
Gen-Xene
halazepam
hydroxyzine HCl
hydroxyzine pamoate
Hyzine-50
Librax
Libritabs
Librium
Lidox
Limbitrol DS 10-25
lorazepam

**Psychotherapeutics, Anxiolytics (cont.)**
Menrium 5-2; Menrium 5-4; Menrium 10-4
meprobamate
Meprogesic Q
Meprospan
Micrainin
Miltown; Miltown-600
Mitran
Neuramate
· oxazepam
Paxarel
Paxipam
PMB 200; PMB 400
prazepam
Quiess
Reposans-10
Rezine
Serax
Stelazine
Trancopal
Tranxene
Tranxene-SD
trifluoperazine HCl
Valium
Valium Roche Oral ⒸⒶⓃ
Valrelease
Vistacon
Vistaject-25; Vistaject-50
Vistaquel 50
Vistaril
Vistazine 50
Xanax
Zetran

**Psychotherapeutics, Other**
ritanserin

**Radiopaque Contrast Media** [see: Contrast Media, Radiopaque]

# Radiopharmaceuticals

[see also: Diagnostic Agents]
AcuTect
Bexxar
Cardiolite
chromic phosphate P 32
depreotide
ImmuRAID-AFP
ImmuRAID-hCG

**Radiopharmaceuticals (cont.)**
ImmuRAIT-LL2
indium In 111 IGIV pentetate
indium In 111 pentetreotide
indium In 111 satumomab pendetide
iodine I 123 murine MAb to alpha-fetoprotein (AFP)
iodine I 123 murine MAb to human chorionic gonadotropin (hCG)
iodine I 131 6B-iodomethyl-19-norcholesterol
iodine I 131 Lym-1 MAb
iodine I 131 murine MAb $IgG_2a$ to B cell
iodine I 131 murine MAb to alpha-fetoprotein (AFP)
iodine I 131 murine MAb to human chorionic gonadotropin (hCG)
iodine I 131 radiolabeled B1 MAb
iodine I 131 tositumomab
Iodotope
LeuTech
LeukoScan
LymphoScan
Macroscint
mespiperone C 11
Metastron
Miraluma
NeoTect
Neurolite
nofetumomab merpentan
OctreoScan 111
OncoTrac
Oncolym
OncoScint CR/OV
Phosphocol P 32
Quadramet
samarium Sm 153 lexidronam
sodium iodide ($^{131}$I)
sodium iodide I 123
sodium iodide I 131
sodium phosphate P 32
strontium chloride Sr 89
technetium ($^{99m}$Tc) dimercaptosuccinic acid
technetium ($^{99m}$Tc) methylenediphosphonate
technetium Tc 99m albumin aggregated

Indications

**Radiopharmaceuticals (cont.)**
technetium Tc 99m antimelanoma murine MAb
technetium Tc 99m apcitide
technetium Tc 99m arcitumomab
technetium Tc 99m bectumomab
technetium Tc 99m biciromab
technetium Tc 99m bicisate
technetium Tc 99m disofenin
technetium Tc 99m furifosmin
technetium Tc 99m medronate
technetium Tc 99m mertiatide
technetium Tc 99m murine MAb to human alpha-fetoprotein (AFP)
technetium Tc 99m murine MAb to human chorionic gonadotropin (hCG)
technetium Tc 99m oxidronate
technetium Tc 99m sestamibi
technetium Tc 99m siboroxime
technetium Tc 99m succimer
technetium Tc 99m sulesomab
technetium Tc 99m teboroxime
technetium Tc 99m tetrofosmin
Verluma

**Respiratory System Agents**
[see also: Allergy and Anaphylaxis Agents; Antituberculosis Agents; Asthma Agents; Expectorants]
acetylcysteine (N-acetylcysteine)
acetylcysteine sodium
Aeropin
Alec
alpha$_1$-proteinase inhibitor (alpha$_1$ PI)
beractant
calfactant
colfosceril palmitate
Curosurf
Delaprem
dextran sulfate
dornase alfa
Exosurf
Exosurf Neonatal
heparin, 2-0-desulfated
hexoprenaline sulfate
HP-3
Infasurf
KL4 surfactant

**Respiratory System Agents (cont.)**
LiquiVent
Mucomyst
Mucomyst 10
Mucosil-10; Mucosil-20
Neuprex
nitric oxide
orgotein
OxSODrol
palivizumab
perflubron
phosphatidylglycerol
Prolastin
protirelin
Pseudostat
pulmonary surfactant replacement, porcine
Pulmozyme
Sclerosol
Surfaxin
Survanta
Synagis
talc, sterile aerosol
Thymone
Uendex

**Rheumatic Disease Agents**
[see also: Analgesics; Corticosteroids, Systemic]
5G1.1-SC
Abitrexate
AE-941
amiprilose HCl
anakinra
Antril
Arava
auranofin
Aurolate
aurothioglucose
azathioprine
azathioprine sodium
Azulfidine
Azulfidine EN-tabs
Bispan
Cuprimine
Depen
Enbrel
etanercept
Folex PFS

**Rheumatic Disease Agents (cont.)**
 gold sodium thiomalate
 hydroxychloroquine sulfate
 Imuran
 infliximab
 IPL-423
 leflunomide
 methotrexate (MTX)
 methotrexate sodium
 Methotrexate LPF Sodium
 Myochrysine
 orgotein
 OxSODrol
 penicillamine
 Plaquenil Sulfate
 Prosorba Column
 protein A
 Remicade
 Rheumatrex
 Ridaura
 Solganal
 sulfasalazine
 T-cell receptor (TCR) peptide
 Therafectin
**Rosacea** [see: Dermatological Preparations, Rosacea Agents]
**Sarcoma** [see: Antineoplastics]
**Schizophrenia** [see: Psychotherapeutics, Antipsychotics]

# Sedatives and Hypnotics
 [see also: Psychotherapeutics, Anxiolytics]
**Sedatives and Hypnotics, Barbiturates**
 Alurate
 amobarbital sodium
 Amytal Sodium
 Antispasmodic
 Antrocol
 aprobarbital
 Arco-Lase Plus
 Barbidonna
 Barbidonna; Barbidonna No. 2
 Barophen
 Bel-Phen-Ergot SR
 Bellacane
 Bellacane SR
 Bellatal

**Sedatives and Hypnotics, Barbiturates (cont.)**
 Bellergal-S
 butabarbital
 butabarbital sodium
 Butibel
 Butisol Sodium
 Cafatine-PB
 Chardonna-2
 Dilantin with Phenobarbital
 Donna-Sed
 Donnamor
 Donnapine
 Donnatal
 Donnatal No. 2
 Folergot-DF
 Gustase Plus
 Hyosophen
 Kinesed
 Levsin PB
 Levsin-PB
 Levsin with Phenobarbital
 Lufyllin-EPG
 Luminal Sodium
 Malatal
 Mebaral
 mephobarbital
 Mudrane
 Mudrane GG
 Nembutal
 Nembutal Sodium
 pentobarbital
 pentobarbital sodium
 Phenerbel-S
 phenobarbital
 phenobarbital sodium
 Pyridium Plus
 Quadrinal
 Relaxadon
 secobarbital sodium
 Seconal Sodium
 Solfoton
 Spasmolin
 Spasmophen
 Spasquid
 Susano
 Tuinal
**Sedatives and Hypnotics, Benzodiazepines**
 alprazolam

Indications

**Sedatives and Hypnotics, Benzodiazepines (cont.)**
Ativan
Centrax
clobazam
clorazepate dipotassium
Dalmane
Diazemuls (CAN)
diazepam
Dizac
Doral
flurazepam HCl
Frisium
Gen-Xene
halazepam
Halcion
lorazepam
midazolam HCl
Mogadon
nitrazepam
oxazepam
Paxipam
prazepam
quazepam
Restoril
Serax
temazepam
Tranxene
Tranxene-SD
triazolam
Valium
Valium Roche Oral (CAN)
Valrelease
Versed
Xanax
Zetran
**Sedatives and Hypnotics, Nonprescription Sleep Aids**
diphenhydramine HCl
pyrilamine maleate
**Sedatives and Hypnotics, Other**
acecarbromal
Ambien
Aquachloral
chloral hydrate
dichloralphenazone (chloral hydrate & phenazone)
Diprivan
estazolam
ethchlorvynol

**Sedatives and Hypnotics, Other (cont.)**
glutethimide
Imovane (CAN)
Isocom
Isopap
Largon
Levoprome
methotrimeprazine
Midchlor
Midrin
Migratine
Paral
paraldehyde
Paxarel
Placidyl
propiomazine HCl
propofol
ProSom
Sonata
zaleplon
zolpidem tartrate
zopiclone
**Senile Dementia** [see: Alzheimer's Disease Agents]

---

# Sex Hormones
[see also: Gynecological Preparations; Vaginal Preparations]
**Sex Hormones, Androgenic/Anabolic Steroids**
Anadrol-50
Andro L.A. 200
Andro/Fem
Androderm
Androgel
Androgel-DHT
Android-10; Android-25
Androlone-D 200
Andropository-200
Androtest-SL
Deca-Durabolin
Deladumone
Delatestryl
depAndro 100; depAndro 200
depAndrogyn
Depo-Testadiol
Depo-Testosterone
Depotest 100; Depotest 200

## Sex Hormones, Androgenic/Anabolic Steroids (cont.)
Depotestogen
dihydrotestosterone (DHT)
Duo-Cyp
Durabolin
Duratest 100; Duratest 200
Duratestrin
Durathate-200
Estra-Testrin
Estratest; Estratest H.S.
Everone 200
fluoxymesterone
Halotestin
Hepandrin
Histerone 100
Hybolin Decanoate-50; Hybolin Decanoate-100
Hybolin Improved
Menogen; Menogen H.S.
methyltestosterone
nandrolone decanoate
nandrolone phenpropionate
Neo-Durabolic
Oreton Methyl
Oxandrin
oxandrolone
oxymetholone
Premarin with Methyltestosterone
stanozolol
Tesamone
Teslac
Test-Estro Cypionates
Testandro
Testoderm TTS
Testoderm; Testoderm with Adhesive
testolactone
Testopel
testosterone
testosterone cypionate
testosterone enanthate
testosterone propionate
Testosterone Aqueous
Testred
TheraDerm
TheraDerm-MTX
Valertest No. 1
Virilon
Winstrol

## Sex Hormones, Estrogens
Alora
Andro/Fem
Aquest
Cenestin
chlorotrianisene
Climara
CombiPatch
Deladiol-40
Deladumone
Delestrogen
depAndrogyn
depGynogen
Depo-Estradiol Cypionate
Depo-Testadiol
DepoGen
Depotestogen
dienestrol
Dioval XX; Dioval 40
Duo-Cyp
Dura-Estrin
Duragen-20; Duragen-40
Duratestrin
DV
E2III
Enovid
Esclim
Estinyl
Estra-D
Estra-L 20
Estra-L 40
Estra-Testrin
Estrace
Estraderm
estradiol
estradiol cypionate
estradiol hemihydrate
estradiol valerate
Estrasorb
Estratab
Estratest; Estratest H.S.
Estring
Estro-Cyp
Estrogenic Substance Aqueous
estrogens, conjugated
estrogens, esterified
Estroject-L.A.
estrone
Estrone 5
Estrone Aqueous

**Sex Hormones, Estrogens (cont.)**
estropipate
Estrovis
ethinyl estradiol
FemPatch
Gynogen L.A. 20
Gynogen L.A. 40
Kestrone 5
Menest
Menogen; Menogen H.S.
Menorest
Menrium 5-2; Menrium 5-4; Menrium 10-4
mestranol
Ogen
Ortho Dienestrol
Ortho-Est
PMB 200; PMB 400
Premarin
Premarin Intravenous
Premarin with Methyltestosterone
Premphase
Prempro
quinestrol
sodium estrone sulfate
Tace
Test-Estro Cypionates
Theelin Aqueous
TheraDerm-MTX
Vagifem
Valergen 10
Valergen 20; Valergen 40
Valertest No. 1
Vivelle; Vivelle-Dot
Wehgen

**Sex Hormones, Fertility Stimulants**
A.P.L.
Chorex-5; Chorex-10
Chorigon
Choron-10
Clomid
clomiphene citrate
Factrel
Fertinex
Follistim
follitropin alfa
follitropin beta
Follutein
Glukor
gonadorelin acetate

**Sex Hormones, Fertility Stimulants (cont.)**
gonadorelin HCl
gonadotropin, chorionic
Gonal-F
Gonic
Humegon
Lutrepulse
menotropins
Metrodin
Milophene
Pergonal
Pregnyl
Profasi
Puregon ⒸⒶⓃ
Repronex
Serophene
urofollitropin

**Sex Hormones, Oral Contraceptives**
Alesse
Brevicon
Demulen 1/35; Demulen 1/50
Desogen
Estrostep 21
Estrostep Fe
Genora 0.5/35; Genora 1/35
Genora 1/50
Jenest-28
Levlen
Levlite 21; Levlite 28
Levora
Lo/Ovral
Loestrin 21 1/20; Loestrin 21 1.5/30
Loestrin Fe 1/20; Loestrin Fe 1.5/30
Micronor
Minesse
Mircette
Modicon
N.E.E. 1/35
Necon 0.5/35-21; Necon 0.5/35-28
Necon 1/35-21; Necon 1/35-28
Necon 1/50-21; Necon 1/50-28
Necon 10/11-21; Necon 10/11-28
Nelova 1/35E; Nelova 0.5/35E
Nelova 1/50M
Nelova 10/11
Nor-Q.D.
Nordette
Norethin 1/35E
Norethin 1/50M

**Sex Hormones, Oral Contraceptives (cont.)**
norethindrone
Norinyl 1 + 35
Norinyl 1 + 50
Ortho-Cept
Ortho-Cyclen
Ortho-Novum 1/35
Ortho-Novum 1/50
Ortho-Novum 10/11
Ortho-Novum 7/7/7
Ortho Tri-Cyclen
Ovcon-35; Ovcon-50
Ovral
Ovrette
Plan B
Preven
Tri-Levlen
Tri-Norinyl
Triphasil
Trivora-28
Zovia
**Sex Hormones, Parenteral Contraceptives**
Depo-Provera
levonorgestrel
Norplant
**Sex Hormones, Progestins**
Amen
Aygestin
CombiPatch
Crinone
Curretab
Cycrin
Depo-Provera
desogestrel
Duralutin
Enovid
ethynodiol diacetate
gestodene
hydroxyprogesterone caproate
Hylutin
Hyprogest 250
levonorgestrel
medroxyprogesterone acetate
Megace
megestrol acetate
norethindrone
norethindrone acetate
norethynodrel

**Sex Hormones, Progestins (cont.)**
norgestimate
norgestrel
Norlutate
Norlutin
Premphase
Prempro
Progestasert
progesterone
Prometrium
Provera

# Sexual Dysfunction Agents, Male
alprostadil
Alprox-TD
aminobenzoate potassium
Aphrodyne
Caverject
Dayto Himbin
Edex
Invicorp
Muse
Plaquase
Potaba
sildenafil citrate
Topiglan
vasoactive intestinal polypeptide (VIP)
Vasomax
Viagra
Yocon
yohimbe (*Corynanthe johimbe; Pausinystalia johimbe*)
yohimbine HCl
Yohimex
**Shampoos** [*see: Dermatological Preparations, Hair and Scalp Agents*]

# Smoking Cessation Aids
benzocaine
bupropion HCl
Habitrol
lobeline sulfate
NicErase-SL
Nicoderm
Nicorette DS

Indications

**Smoking Cessation Aids (cont.)**
nicotine
nicotine polacrilex
Nicotrol
Nicotrol NS
ProStep
Zyban
**Steroids** [see: Corticosteroids, Systemic; Dermatological Preparations, Anti-inflammatory Agents; Ophthalmologicals, Anti-inflammatory; Sex Hormones, Androgenic/Anabolic Steroids]
**Surfactants, Lung** [see: Respiratory System Agents]

---

# Thrombolytic Agents
[see also: Enzymes, Thrombolytic]
Abbokinase
Abbokinase Open-Cath
Activase
Agrylin
alteplase
Eminase
Kabikinase
lanoteplase
r-ProUK
saruplase
Streptase
urokinase
xemilofiban HCl
**Thrush** [see: Mouth and Throat Preparations]

---

# Thyroid Agents
Armour Thyroid
Cytomel
Eltroxin
Levo-T
Levothroid
Levothroid (CAN)
levothyroxine sodium (T$_4$)
Levoxyl
liothyronine sodium (T$_3$)
liotrix
Lugol
methimazole
potassium iodide

**Thyroid Agents (cont.)**
S-P-T
Strong Iodine
Synthroid
Tapazole
Thyrar
Thyro-Block
thyroid
Thyroid Strong
Thyrolar-0.25; -0.5; -1; -2; -3
thyrotropin
Thytropar
Triacana
Triostat
**Total Parenteral Nutrition (TPN)** [see: Nutritional Agents]
**Tuberculosis** [see: Antituberculosis Agents]
**Ulcerative Colitis** [see: Inflammatory Bowel Disease Agents]
**Ulcers, Decubitus** [see: Diabetes Agents, Related Disorders; Wound Treatment]
**Ulcers, Gastric** [see: Peptic Ulcer and Gastric Reflux Agents]
**Ultrasound Contrast Media** [see: Contrast Media, Ultrasound]

---

# Urinary Tract Agents
**Urinary Tract Agents, Analgesics**
Atrosept
Azo Gantanol
Azo Gantrisin
Azo-Sulfisoxazole
Baridium
Cystex
Dolsed
Eridium
Geridium
Phenazo (CAN)
Phenazodine
phenazopyridine HCl
phenyl salicylate
Prosed/DS
Pyridiate; Pyridate No. 2
Pyridium
Pyridium Plus
salicylamide
sodium salicylate (SS)

**Urinary Tract Agents, Analgesics (cont.)**
Trac Tabs 2X
UAA
Uridon Modified
Urimar-T
Urinary Antiseptic No. 2
Urised
Uristat
Uritin
Urobiotic-250
Urodine
Urogesic
Urogesic Blue
**Urinary Tract Agents, Antineoplastics**
[see also: Antineoplastics]
BCG vaccine (bacillus Calmette-Guérin)
doxorubicin HCl
eflornithine HCl
ImmuCyst ⓒ
OncoTICE ⓒ
Pacis ⓒ
Photofrin
Platinol-AQ
Regressin
TheraCys
Tice BCG
Valstar
Vumon
**Urinary Tract Agents, Antibacterials**
[see also: Antibiotics]
Atrosept
Azo Gantanol
Azo Gantrisin
Azo-Sulfisoxazole
Cinobac
cinoxacin
Cystex
Dolsed
fosfomycin tromethamine
Furadantin
Furalan
Hiprex
Macrobid
Macrodantin
Mandameth
Mandelamine
Methblue 65

**Urinary Tract Agents, Antibacterials (cont.)**
methenamine
methenamine hippurate
methenamine mandelate
methylene blue (MB)
Monurol
nalidixic acid
NegGram
nitrofurantoin
Prosed/DS
sulfamethizole
sulfamethoxazole (SMX; SMZ)
sulfisoxazole
Trac Tabs 2X
UAA
Urex
Uridon Modified
Urimar-T
Urinary Antiseptic No. 2
Urised
Urisedamine
Uritin
Uro-Phosphate
Urobak
Urobiotic-250
Urogesic Blue
Urolene Blue
Uroqid-Acid No. 2
**Urinary Tract Agents, Antispasmodics**
[see also: Antispasmodics]
Atrosept
belladonna extract
Ditropan
Ditropan XL
Dolsed
flavoxate HCl
hyoscyamine (L-hyoscyamine)
hyoscyamine sulfate
oxybutynin chloride
Prosed/DS
Pyridium Plus
Trac Tabs 2X
UAA
Uridon Modified
Urimar-T
Urinary Antiseptic No. 2
Urised
Urisedamine

**Urinary Tract Agents, Antispasmodics (cont.)**
Urispas
Uritin
Urogesic Blue
**Urinary Tract Agents, Antiurolithic**
Calcibind
cellulose sodium phosphate (CSP)
Cystagon
cysteamine bitartrate
magnesium hydroxycarbonate
Renacidin
Renacidin Irrigation
Thiola
tiopronin
**Urinary Tract Agents, Cystitis Agents**
dimethyl sulfoxide (DMSO)
Elmiron
Kemsol ⓒ
pentosan polysulfate sodium
Rimso-50
**Urinary Tract Agents, Enuresis Agents**
collagen
Contigen
DDAVP
desmopressin acetate
Detrol
Hylagel Uro
imipramine HCl
Janimine
Tofranil
tolterodine tartrate
**Urinary Tract Agents, pH Modifiers**
ammonium chloride
Bicitra
Citrolith
Cytra-2
Cytra-3
Cytra-K
Cytra-LC
K-Lyte ⓒ
K-Phos M.F.
K-Phos Neutral
K-Phos No. 2
K-Phos Original
M-Caps
methionine (DL-methionine)

**Urinary Tract Agents, pH Modifiers (cont.)**
Neut
Oracit
Pedameth
PMS-Dicitrate ⓒ
Polycitra
Polycitra-K
Polycitra-LC
potassium acid phosphate
potassium citrate
racemethionine
sodium acid phosphate
sodium bicarbonate
sodium biphosphate
sodium citrate
Uracid
Urimar-T
Uro-Phosphate
Urocit-K
Urogesic Blue
**Urinary Tract Agents, Urinary Retention Agents**
bethanechol chloride
Duvoid
Myotonachol
neostigmine methylsulfate
PMS-Bethanechol Chloride ⓒ
Prostigmin
Urecholine
**Urinary Tract Agents, Other**
acetohydroxamic acid (AHA)
Lithostat
Resectisol
sorbitol
**Vaccines** [see: Immunizing Agents]

# Vaginal Preparations
**Vaginal Preparations, Antibacterial**
[see also: Antibiotics, Topical]
Alasulf
aminacrine HCl
AVC
Cleocin
clindamycin phosphate
D.I.T.I.-2
Dalacin ⓒ
Dayto Sulf
Deltavac

**Vaginal Preparations, Antibacterial (cont.)**
Gyne-Sulf
MetroGel Vaginal
metronidazole
Nidagel ⓒⒶⓃ
sulfabenzamide
sulfacetamide
sulfanilamide
sulfathiazole
sulfisoxazole
Sultrin Triple Sulfa
Triple Sulfa
Trysul
V.V.S.
Vagisec Plus
**Vaginal Preparations, Antifungal**
[see also: Antifungals, Topical]
Amino-Cerv pH 5.5
butoconazole nitrate
clotrimazole (CLT)
Femstat
miconazole nitrate
Monistat Dual-Pak
Mycelex-G
Mycelex Twin Pack
Mycostatin
nystatin
sodium propionate
Terazol 3
Terazol 7
terconazole
tioconazole
**Vaginal Preparations, Antiseptic Cleansers**
[see also: Antiseptics]
povidone-iodine
Vagisec Douche
**Vaginal Preparations, Contraceptives**
nonoxynol 9
octoxynol 9
Progestasert
progesterone
**Vaginal Preparations, Other**
PRO-2000

## Varicose Vein Agents
adenosine phosphate
Kaysine

**Varicose Vein Agents (cont.)**
morrhuate sodium
Scleromate
sodium tetradecyl (STD) sulfate
Sotradecol
**Verruca** [see: Dermatological Preparations, Wart and Corn Removers]

## Vitamin Replacement
**Vitamin Replacement, Vitamin A**
ADC with Fluoride
Aquasol A
beta carotene
Chewable Triple Vitamins with Fluoride
Del-Vi-A
Solatene
Soluvite-f
Tri-A-Vite F
Tri-Flor-Vite with Fluoride
Tri-Vi-Flor
Tri-Vi-Flor with Iron
Tri Vit with Fluoride
Tri-Vitamin with Fluoride
Triple Vitamin ADC with Fluoride
Triple Vitamins with Fluoride
Trivitamin Fluoride
Vi-Daylin/F ADC
Vi-Daylin/F ADC + Iron
vitamin A
vitamin A palmitate
**Vitamin Replacement, B Vitamins**
[see also: Anemia Agents, B Vitamins]
Apatate with Fluoride
B-C with Folic Acid
B-Plex
Berocca
calcium pantothenate (calcium D-pantothenate)
cyanocobalamin
folic acid
Formula B
hydroxocobalamin
Lipo-Nicin/100
Lipo-Nicin/300
liver, desiccated; liver extracts
niacin
niacinamide
Niacor

**Indications**

**Vitamin Replacement, B Vitamins (cont.)**
Niaspan
Nicolar
pyridoxine HCl
riboflavin
thiamine HCl

**Vitamin Replacement, Vitamin C**
ADC with Fluoride
ascorbic acid (L-ascorbic acid)
B Complex with C and B-12
B-C with Folic Acid
B-Plex
Berocca
calcium ascorbate
Cenolate
Cevalin
Cevi-Fer
Chewable Triple Vitamins with Fluoride
Chromagen
Contrin
Fergon Plus
Fero-Folic-500
Ferotrinsic
Foltrin
Formula B *
Fumatinic
Hem Fe
Hemocyte Plus
Iberet-Folic-500
Key-Plex
Livitamin with Intrinsic Factor
Livitrinsic-f
Lypholized Vitamin B Complex & Vitamin C with $B_{12}$
Multibret-500 Hematinic
Multibret-Folic-500
Nephlex Rx
Nephro-Vite Rx
Nephro-Vite Rx + Fe
Nephrocaps
Nephron FA
Neurodep
Pronemia Hematinic
sodium ascorbate
Soluvite-f
Strovite
Tabron
Tri-A-Vite F

**Vitamin Replacement, Vitamin C (cont.)**
Tri-Flor-Vite with Fluoride
Tri-Vi-Flor
Tri-Vi-Flor with Iron
Tri Vit with Fluoride
Tri-Vitamin with Fluoride
Tri-Tinic
TriHemic 600
Trinsicon
Triple Vitamin ADC with Fluoride
Triple Vitamins with Fluoride
Trivitamin Fluoride
Vi-Daylin/F ADC
Vi-Daylin/F ADC + Iron
Vicam

**Vitamin Replacement, Vitamin D**
ADC with Fluoride
calcifediol
Calciferol
Calcijex
calcitriol
Calderol
Chewable Triple Vitamins with Fluoride
cholecalciferol
dihydrotachysterol (DHT)
Drisdol
ergocalciferol
Hytakerol
paricalcitol
Rocaltrol
Soluvite-f
Tri-A-Vite F
Tri-Flor-Vite with Fluoride
Tri-Vi-Flor
Tri-Vi-Flor with Iron
Tri Vit with Fluoride
Tri-Vitamin with Fluoride
Triple Vitamin ADC with Fluoride
Triple Vitamins with Fluoride
Trivitamin Fluoride
Vi-Daylin/F ADC
Vi-Daylin/F ADC + Iron
Zemplar

**Vitamin Replacement, Vitamin E**
Aquavit-E
Tabron
TriHemic 600
vitamin E

**Vitamin Replacement, Other**
AquaMEPHYTON
Konakion
Mephyton
phytonadione
**Vitamin Replacement, Multiple
(not listed)**
Adeflor M
B-C with Folic Acid Plus
Bacmin
Berocca Parenteral Nutrition
Berocca Plus
Berplex Plus
Cefol
Cezin-S
Chewable Multivitamins with Fluoride
Eldercaps
Filibon F.A.; Filibon Forte
Florvite
Florvite + Iron
Florvite + Iron; Half Strength
    Florvite + Iron
Florvite; Florvite Half Strength
Formula B Plus
Heptuna Plus
Lactocal-F
Lipo-Nicin/100
Lipo-Nicin/300
M.V.C. 9+3
M.V.C. 9+4 Pediatric
M.V.I. Neonatal
M.V.I. Pediatric
M.V.I.-12
Marnatal-F
Materna
Mission Prenatal Rx
Multi Vitamin Concentrate
Multivitamin with Fluoride
Mulvidren-F
Mynatal
Mynatal FC
Mynatal P.N.
Mynatal P.N. Forte
Mynatal Rx
Mynate 90 Plus
Natabec Rx
Natafort
NatalCare Plus
Natalins Rx

**Vitamin Replacement, Multiple
(not listed) (cont.)**
Natarex Prenatal
Nestabs FA
Niferex-PN
Niferex-PN Forte
Norlac Rx
Nu-Iron V
O-Cal f.a.
Par-F
Par-Natal Plus 1 Improved
Poly-Vi-Flor
Poly-Vi-Flor with Iron
Polytabs-F
Polyvitamin Fluoride
Polyvitamin Fluoride with Iron
Polyvitamin with Iron and Fluoride
Polyvitamins with Fluoride and Iron
Pramet FA
Pramilet FA
Pre-H Cal
Prenatal H.P.
Prenatal Maternal
Prenatal MR 90
Prenatal One
Prenatal Plus Iron
Prenatal Plus with Betacarotene
Prenatal Plus; Prenatal Plus
    Improved
Prenatal Rx
Prenatal Rx with Betacarotene
Prenatal Z
Prenatal-1 + Iron
Prenate 90; Prenate Ultra
Secran Prenatal
Soluvite C.T.
Strovite Plus; Strovite Forte
Stuartnatal Plus
Theragran Hematinic
Vi-Daylin/F Multivitamin
Vi-Daylin/F Multivitamin + Iron
Vicon Forte
Vitafōl; Vitafōl-PN
Zenate, Advanced Formula
Zincvit
Zodeac-100
**Vitiligo** [see: Dermatological Preparations, Vitiligo Agents]

# Weight Reduction Agents
## Weight Reduction Agents, CNS Modifiers
[see also: Central Nervous System Stimulants]
Adipex-P
Adipost
Anorex
benzphetamine HCl
Bontril
Bontril PDM
dexfenfluramine HCl
Didrex
diethylpropion
diethylpropion HCl
Dital
Dyrexan-OD
Fastin
fenfluramine HCl
Ionamin
Mazanor
mazindol
Melfiat-105
Meridia
Obalan
Obenix
Obephen
Oby-Cap
phendimetrazine tartrate
phentermine HCl
Phentrol
Phentrol 2; Phentrol 4; Phentrol 5
Plegine
Pondimin
Prelu-2
Redux
Rexigen Forte
Sanorex
sibutramine HCl
Tenuate
Tepanil
Trimstat
Wehless
Weightrol
Zantryl
## Weight Reduction Agents, Digestion Modifiers
bromocriptine mesylate
Ergoset
orlistat

## Weight Reduction Agents, Digestion Modifiers (cont.)
Xenical
## Weight Reduction Agents, Nonprescription Diet Aids
benzocaine
phenylpropanolamine HCl

---

# Wound Treatment
## Wound Treatment, Debriding Agents
Accuzyme
ananain
collagenase
comosain
Debrisan
Dermuspray
desoxyribonuclease
dextranomer
Elase
Elase-Chloromycetin
fibrinolysin, human
Granulderm
Granulex
GranuMed
Panafil
Panafil White
papain
Santyl
sutilains
Travase
trypsin, crystallized
Vianain
## Wound Treatment, Medicated Dressings
[see also: Antibiotics, Topical; Hemostatics]
Adcon-L
Adcon-P Adhesion Control Barrier
Apligraf
carbohydrate polymer gel
DuraGen
Furacin Soluble Dressing
Iamin
mafenide
mafenide acetate
nitrofurazone
povidone-iodine
prezatide copper acetate

Indications

# Xref: Investigational Code Names to Generic Names

A code name is a temporary identification assigned to a product by the manufacturer. The number or letter-number combination is used while the substance is undergoing testing, before a generic name is given. Code names appearing in this list cross-reference to the assigned generic name (3737 entries) or are designated "generic not yet assigned" (177 entries), which indicates that testing is ongoing or has been discontinued within the past five years. Both generic names and code names appearing here without generic names are listed alphabetically in *Saunders Pharmaceutical Word Book*. Additional information may be obtained there.

**10275-S** epitiostanol
**106223** cefamandole nafate
**10 80 07** omoconazole nitrate
**10-EDAM** edatrexate
**110264** cefaparole
**125 I NM-113** iomethin I 125
**129Y83** colfosceril palmitate
**12C** velaresol
**1314 TH** ethionamide
**131 I NM-113** iomethin I 131
**1380U** baquiloprim
**141W94** amprenavir
**1589 RB** pefloxacin
**1592U89** abacavir succinate
**1592U89** abacavir sulfate
**15AU81** generic not yet assigned
**16726** symetine HCl
**16842** bitoscanate
**1709 CERM** niaprazine
**177 J.D.** aminocaproic acid
**1875 CERM** fepromide
**18894** nifungin
**194-B** zolamine HCl
**20025** clorprenaline HCl
**205 E** calcium dobesilate
**21401-Ba** tribenoside
**21679-CH** malethamer
**22-708** endralazine mesylate
**24281** mitocarcin
**249-16** deditonium bromide
**2-5410-3A** iodixanol

**256U87 HCl** valacyclovir HCl
**26383** thiphencillin potassium
**26P** aliflurane
**27165** temefos
**27-400** cyclosporine
**28002** epipropidine
**29060-LE** vinblastine sulfate
**2936** proscillaridin
**29866** levopropoxyphene napsylate
**30038CB** minaprine HCl
**3-01003** guanoxan sulfate
**3-01029** guanoclor sulfate
**30109** noracymethadol HCl
**30639** polyethadene
**311C90** zolmitriptan
**3123L** puromycin
**31518** pyrroliphene HCl
**31595C** mitosper
**31814** heteronium bromide
**32-046** edetate dipotassium
**32379** dromostanolone propionate
**32645** vinleurosine sulfate
**33006** acetohexamide
**33355** mestranol
**33379** flurandrenolide
**33876** anthelmycin
**34977** capreomycin sulfate
**349 C59** moxipraquine
**35483** cyclothiazide
**36781** vinrosidine sulfate
**36-801** etifoxine

**37 162 R.P.** suproclone
**37231** vincristine sulfate
**38000** clometherone
**38253** cephalothin sodium
**38389** levopropylcillin potassium
**38489** nortriptyline HCl
**38851** bolmantalate
**39435** cephaloglycin
**3 MS** hydroxytoluic acid
**3TC** lamivudine
**40 045** articaine
**40045** trimetazidine
**40602** cephaloridine
**4091 C.B.** benfurodil hemisuccinate
**41071** cefalonium
**41-123** clazolam
**41 982 RP** pefloxacin mesylate
**42-348** lifibrate
**42406** metoquizine
**42-548** mazindol
**4306 CB** clorazepate dipotassium
**4311 CB** clorazepate monopotassium
**43-663** guanoxabenz
**43-715** proquazone
**43853** clobenoside
**44089** valproic acid
**44106** toquizine
**44328** dexproxibutene
**46083** cefazolin sodium
**46236** dobutamine HCl
**46-790** fluproquazone
**46 R.P.** benzylsulfamide
**47-210 (as sodium)** tetriprofen
**47599** pyrazofurin
**47657** apramycin
**47663** tobramycin
**48-674** furacrinic acid
**49040** vinglycinate sulfate
**4909 RP** chlorproethazine HCl
**49825** nylestriol
**4A65** imidocarb HCl
**4-C-32** ticlopidine HCl
**5048** dimethisterone
**5052** acetylcysteine
**5054** prodilidine HCl
**5058** oxybutynin chloride
**506U** nelzarabine
**5071** megestrol acetate
**5107** chloral betaine
**516 MD** cinnarizine

**5190** amidephrine mesylate
**51W89** cisatracurium besylate
**520C9x22** generic not yet assigned
**52230** pyrrolnitrin
**524W91** emtricitabine
**53183** aranotin
**53-32C** ticlopidine HCl
**5373** melengestrol acetate
**53858** fenoprofen
**566C** atovaquone
**566C80** atovaquone
**57C65** cloguanamil
**589C** tucaresol
**59156** enpromate
**5A8** generic not yet assigned
**5G1.1-SC** generic not yet assigned
**5IUDR** idoxuridine
**60284** cyclophenazine HCl
**611 C 65** thenium closylate
**640/1** cefuracetime
**640/359** cefuroxime
**64716** cinoxacin
**65-318** bidimazium iodide
**66-269** pretamazium iodide
**66873** cephalexin
**673-082** nexeridine HCl
**67314** monensin
**68618** mycophenolic acid
**69323** fenoprofen calcium
**711 SE** pipratecol
**7162 RP** trimipramine
**7432-S** ceftibuten
**776C85** eniluracil
**786-723** anilopam HCl
**79907** lergotrile
**79 T61** lucanthone HCl
**7-OMEN** menogaril
**80066** bufilcon A
**8088 C.B.** benfotiamine
**8102 CB** bamifylline HCl
**83636** lergotrile mesylate
**8599 R.P. mesylate** fonazine mesylate
**882C** generic not yet assigned
**88BV59** votumumab
**935U83** raluridine
**[99mTc]-P246** technetium Tc 99m apcitide
**A-118** sultroponium
**A-12253A** nebramycin
**A-157378.0** lopinivir

A-16612 teroxalene HCl
A-16686 ramoplanin
A-17624 ditolamide
A-19120 paragyline HCl
A-19757 encyprate
A-1981-12 prodilidine HCl
A-20968 piposulfan
A-2205 profadol HCl
A-2371 plicamycin
A-2655 dioxamate
A-27053 chromonar HCl
A-272 rutamycin
A-3217 ocfentanil HCl
A-32686 proscillaridin
A-3331 brifentanil HCl
A-33547 remoxipride
A-33547.HCl·H$_2$O remoxipride HCl
A-3508.HCl mirfentanil HCl
A-35957 altrenogest
A-3665.HCl trefentanil HCl
A-4020 Linz midodrine HCl
A 40664 (as tartrate) raclopride
A-41-304 desoximetasone
A-4180 isometamidium chloride
A-4492 pentamorphone
A 46 745 gestrinone
A-4696 actaplanin
A-4828 trofosfamide
A-53986 fostedil
A-5610 azelastine HCl
A 5MP adenosine phosphate
A-60386X beractant
A-61589 docebenone
A-65006 lansoprazole
A-7283 guanoctine HCl
A-73001 seratrodast
A-75200 mesylate napitane mesylate
A-77000 pazinaclone
A-8103 pipobroman
A-82 nitroxoline
A-85761.0 atreleuton
A-8999 aspartocin
AA-2414 seratrodast
AA-673 amlexanox
AA-861 docebenone
AAFC flurocitabine
AB08 doxycycline fosfatex
AB-100 uredepa
AB-103 benzodepa
AB-132 meturedepa

AB-A 663 cimaterol
Abbott-16900 teflurane
Abbott-19957 lorbamate
Abbott-22370 trimetozine
Abbott-24091 berythromycin
Abbott-34842 butamben picrate
Abbott-35616 clorazepate dipotassium
Abbott-36581 butamirate citrate
Abbott-38579 protirelin
Abbott-38642 fosfonet sodium
Abbott-39083 clorazepate
  monopotassium
Abbott-40728 cetocycline HCl
Abbott-41070 gonadorelin acetate
Abbott-43326 carteolol HCl
Abbott-43818 leuprolide acetate
Abbott 44090 valproate sodium
Abbott-44747 astromicin sulfate
Abbott-45975 terazosin HCl
Abbott-46811 cefsulodin sodium
Abbott-47631 estazolam
Abbott-48999 cefotiam HCl
Abbott-50192 (HCl) cefmenoxime
  HCl
Abbott-50711 divalproex sodium
Abbott-56268 clarithromycin
Abbott-56619 difloxacin HCl
Abbott-56620 sarafloxacin HCl
Abbott-57135 sarafloxacin HCl
Abbott-61827 tosufloxacin
Abbott-62254 temafloxacin HCl
Abbott-64077 zileuton
Abbott-64662 enalkiren
Abbott 70569.1 tiagabine HCl
Abbott 70569 HCl tiagabine HCl
Abbott-72517 zankiren HCl
Abbott-73001 seratrodast
Abbott-76120 urokinase alfa
Abbott-76745 fenleuton
Abbott-84538 ritonavir
Abbott-85761 atreleuton
ABC 12/3 doxofylline
ABOB moroxydine
ABS-205 generic not yet assigned
ABT-001 seratrodast
ABT-120 urokinase alfa
ABT-378 lopinavir
ABT-538 ritonavir
ABT-569 tiagabine HCl
ABT-719 generic not yet assigned

**ABT-761** atreleuton
**ABX-CBL** generic not yet assigned
**AC001** amlintide
**AC0137** pramlintide
**AC 1198** dimethadione
**AC 1370** cefpimizole
**AC 263,780** cimaterol
**AC 3810** bamifylline HCl
**AC4464** torsemide
**AC-528** dioxation
**AC-601** buramate
**ACC-9089** flestolol sulfate
**ACC-9653-010** fosphenytoin sodium
**ACEA 1021** licostinel
**AD 106** cicrotoic acid
**AD-439** generic not yet assigned
**AD-519** generic not yet assigned
**AD-810** zonisamide
**ADD-3878** ciglitazone
**ADR-033** tripamide
**ADR-529** dexrazoxane
**AE-705W** neutramycin
**AE-9** feclobuzone
**AE-941** generic not yet assigned
**AF102B** cevimeline HCl
**AF-1161** trazodone HCl
**AF 1934 (lysine)** bendazac
**AF-2139** dapiprazole HCl
**AF 2838** bindarit
**AF-438 (as citrate)** oxolamine
**AF-634** proxazole citrate
**AF-864** benzydamine HCl
**AG-1343** nelfinavir mesylate
**AG-1749** lansoprazole
**AG-3** chromonar HCl
**AG331** metesind glucuronate
**AG-3340** generic not yet assigned
**AG 58107** ioxitalamic acid
**Agent M-01** sucrosofate potassium
**AGN 190168** tazarotene
**AGN 190342-LF** brimonidine tartrate
**AGN 192013** alitretinoin
**AGN 20** metamfazone
**AGN 511 (as HCl)** prazitone
**AGN 616** fantridone HCl
**AGR-1240** minaprine
**AH 19065** ranitidine HCl
**AH 22216** lamtidine
**AH 23844** lavoltidine succinate
**AH 23844A** lavoltidine succinate

**AH 25352X** sufotidine
**AH 3923** salmefamol
**AH 5158A** labetalol HCl
**AH 8165D** fazadinium bromide
**AHR-10282B** bromfenac sodium
**AHR-10718** suricainide maleate
**AHR-1118** pridefine HCl
**AHR-11190-B** zacopride HCl
**AHR-11325-D** rocastine HCl
**AHR-11748** dezinamide
**AHR-1680** fenpipalone
**AHR-224** pyroxamine maleate
**AHR-2277 (as HCl)** lenperone
**AHR-2438B** polignate sodium
**AHR-3000** butaperazine
**AHR-3002** fenfluramine HCl
**AHR-3015** cintazone
**AHR-3018** apazone
**AHR-3053** carbocysteine
**AHR-3070-C** metoclopramide HCl
**AHR-438** metaxalone
**AHR-4698** isosorbide mononitrat
**AHR-504** glycopyrrolate
**AHR-5531C** dazopride fumarate
**AHR-5850D** amfenac sodium
**AHR-6134** cloroperone HCl
**AHR-619** doxapram HCl
**AHR 6646** duoperone fumarate
**AHR-8559** fluzinamide
**AHR-857** sulfameter
**AHR-9377** tampramine fumarate
**AHR-9434** nepafenac
**AI-27,303** cetamolol HCl
**AICA** orazamide
**AIT-082** leteprinim potassium
**A IX** demecycline
**AJ-2615** monatepil maleate
**AL02145** apraclonidine HCl
**AL02725** pyrithione sodium
**Al-0361** hydroxyphenamate
**AL 0559** fenamole
**AL-1021** carperone
**AL1577A** levobetaxolol HCl
**AL 20 (as HCl)** clemizole
**AL-3432A** emedastine difumarate
**AL-3789** anecortave acetate
**AL-4862** brinzolamide
**AL-6515** nepafenac
**AL-721** generic not yet assigned
**AL 842** deterenol HCl

**ALCA** alcloxa
**ALDA** aldioxa
**Allergan 211** idoxuridine
**ALO 1401-02** betaxolol HCl
**ALO 2184** resocortol butyrate
**ALO4943A** olopatadine HCl
**ALRT 1057** alitretinoin
**AL-T150** oxyfilcon A
**AL-T30** vinafocon A
**ALVAC-120TMG** generic not yet assigned
**ALVAC-HIV 1** generic not yet assigned
**ALX1-11** parathyroid hormone (1-84), recombinamt human
**AM-1155** gatifloxacin
**AM-684-Beta** relomycin
**AMA 1080(2Na)** carumonam sodium
**AMI-121** ferumoxsil
**AMI-25** ferumoxides
**AMR-69** pirfenidone
**AN021** tizanidine HCl
**AN-051** dezinamide
**AN 1317** perimetazine
**AN 1324** glybuzole
**anesthetic compound no. 347** enflurane
**ANP 246** clofexamide
**ANP 3260** clofezone
**antibiotic 241a** biniramycin
**antibiotic 273a₁** paldimycin
**antibiotic A-5283** natamycin
**antifoam A** simethicone
**antifoam AF** simethicone
**AO-407** hydrofilcon A
**AOD-9604** generic not yet assigned
**AOMA** surfomer
**AO-PLUTO** mesifilcon A
**AP 67** chlorthenoxazine
**APC-366** generic not yet assigned
**APL 400-020** generic not yet assigned
**APM** aspartame
**APSAC** anistreplase
**AQ-110** tretoquinol
**AR 12008** trapidil
**AR-121** nystatin liposomal
**AR-177** generic not yet assigned
**ARC I-K-1** methopholine
**ARDF 26** gliquidone

**AS-013** generic not yet assigned
**AS 101** arsanilic acid
**AS-17665** nifurthiazole
**ASA 158/5 (as phosphate)** benproperine
**ASL-279** dopamine HCl
**ASL-601** acecainide HCl
**ASL-603** bretylium tosylate
**ASL-607** pentastarch
**ASL-8052** esmolol HCl
**Asta 3746** ciclonium bromide
**Astra 1512** prilocaine HCl
**Astra 1572** iron sorbitex
**AT-101** isosorbide
**AT-125** acivicin
**AT-2266** enoxacin
**AT 327** tipepidine
**AT-4140** sparfloxacin
**ATI 01** sinapultide
**ATM-027** generic not yet assigned
**AW 10** sitogluside
**AW 105-843** naftifine HCl
**AW 14′2333** perlapine
**AW-14′2446** clodazon HCl
**AY-11,440** clogestone acetate
**AY-11,483** estrofurate
**AY-15,613** citenamide
**AY-20,385** nequinate
**AY-20,694** dexpropranolol HCl
**AY-21,011** practolol
**AY-21,367** furobufen
**AY-21,554** talopram HCl
**AY-22,124** intriptyline HCl
**AY-22,214** taclamine HCl
**AY-22,241** actodigin
**AY-22,284A** alrestatin sodium
**AY-22,469** deprostil
**AY-22989** sirolimus
**AY-23,028** butaclamol HCl
**AY-23,289** prodolic acid
**AY-23,713** pirandamine HCl
**AY-23,946** tandamine HCl
**AY-24,031** gonadorelin HCl
**AY-24,169** dexclamol HCl
**AY-24,236** etodolac
**AY-24,269** proroxan HCl
**AY-24,559** doxaprost
**AY-24,856** pareptide sulfate
**AY-25,329** azaclorzine HCl
**AY-25,712** acifran

**Code Names**

**AY-27,110** ciladopa HCl
**AY-27,255** vinpocetine
**AY-27,773** tolrestat
**AY-28,228** atiprosin maleate
**AY-28,768** pelrinone HCl
**AY-30,715** pemedolac
**AY-5312** chlorhexidine HCl
**AY-5710** magaldrate
**AY-6108** ampicillin
**AY-61122** methallibure
**AY-61123** clofibrate
**AY-62014** butriptyline HCl
**AY-62021** clopenthixol
**AY-62022** medrogestone
**AY 6204 (as HCl)** pronetalol
**AY-64043** propranolol HCl
**AY-6608** pentagastrin
**AY-8682** cyheptamide
**AZQ** diaziquone
**AZT-P-ddI** zidovudine + didanosine
**B 10610** iodoxamic acid
**B 11420** iopronic acid
**B 1312 (as HCl)** bupranolol
**B 1464** guanacline sulfate
**B1 61.012** sargramostim
**B19036/7** gagobenate dimeglumine
**B1Q 16** hedaquinium chloride
**B2036-PEG** generic not yet assigned
**B-2311** morinamide
**B28-Asp-Insulin** insulin aspart
**B-35251** mitocromin
**B-360** paroxypropione
**B-4130** iodamide
**B-436** prenylamine
**Ba 13155 (as tartrate)** meladrazine
**Ba-20684** etonitazene
**Ba-29038** boldenone undecylenate
**Ba-29837** deferoxamine HCl
**Ba-30803** benzoctamine HCl
**BA 32644** niridazole
**Ba-32968** delfantrine
**Ba-33112** deferoxamine mesylate
**Ba-34,276 (as HCl)** maprotiline
**Ba-34,647** baclofen
**BA 36278A** cephacetrile sodium
**Ba-39,089** oxprenolol HCl
**Ba-40088** proxibutene
**Ba 41166/E** rifampin
**BA 4164-8** diflumidone sodium
**Ba-41795** codactide

**BA 4197** flucrylate
**BA 4223** triflumidate
**BA 7602-06** talniflumate
**BA 7604-02** talosalate
**BA 7605-06** talmetacin
**BAQD 10** dequalinium chloride
**BASF 43915** pelretin
**BASF 47011** doretinel
**BASF 52404** linarotene
**BAX 1400Z** dimethadione
**BAX 1515** sutilains
**BAX 1526** chymopapain
**BAX 2739Z** bamifylline HCl
**BAX 422Z** albutoin
**BAY 12-8039** moxifloxacin HCl
**BAY 1500** mefruside
**BAY 1521** noxiptiline
**BAY 2353** niclosamide
**BAY 4059 Va** brotianide
**BAY 4503** propiram fumarate
**BAY 5097** clotrimazole
**BAY 9002** naftalofos
**Bay a 1040** nifedipine
**BAY B 4231** glisoxepide
**Bay d 1107** etofenamate
**BAY d 8815 (HCl)** amidantel
**Bay e 5009** nitrendipine
**BAY e 9736** nimodipine
**Bayer 1362** butaperazine
**Bayer 1420** propanidid
**Bayer 205** suramin sodium
**Bayer 21199** coumaphos
**Bayer 2502** nifurtimox
**Bayer 3231** triaziquone
**Bayer 5360** metronidazole
**Bayer 9015** niclofolan
**Bayer 9037** quintiofos
**Bayer 9053** phoxim
**Bayer A 128** aprotinin
**Bayer L 1359** metrifonate
**BAY g 2821** muzolimine
**Bay g 5421** acarbose
**Bay g 6575** nafazatrom
**BAY h 2049** daniquidone
**Bay h 4502** bifonazole
**Bay h 5757** febantel
**BAY i 3930** isomalt
**BAY i 7433** copovithane
**Bay k 5552** nisoldipine
**BAY m 1099** miglitol

**BAYNAC** fenfluthrin
**BAY o 1248** emiglitate
**Bay o 9867 monohydrate** ciprofloxacin HCl
**Bay q 3939** ciprofloxacin
**Bay q 4218** butaprost
**BAY q 7821** ipsapirone HCl
**BAY V1 4718** etisomicin
**BAY V1 6045** flumethrin
**BAY Va 1470** xylazine HCl
**Bay VA 9387** etisazole
**BAY Va 9391** olaquindox
**BAY Vh 5757** febantel
**Bay Vi 9142** toltrazuril
**BAY Vk 4999** fuzlocillin
**Bay Vl 1704** cyfluthrin
**Bay Vn 6528** fenfluthrin
**Bay Vp 2674** enrofloxacin
**BAY w 6228** cerivastatin sodium
**BAY w 6240** factor VIII (rDNA)
**BAY X 1352** nerelimomab
**BAY y 7432** ecadotril
**BB-10010** nagrestipen
**BB-2516** marimastat
**BB-2893** generic not yet assigned
**BB-882** lexipafant
**BB-94** batimastat
**BB-K8** amikacin sulfate
**BBM-2478A** elsamitrucin
**BC-105** pizotyline
**BCM** mannomustine
**BCX-1470** generic not yet assigned
**BCX 2600** stiripentol
**BCX-34** peldesine
**BD 40A** formoterol fumarate
**BDH 1298** megestrol acetate
**BDH 1921** melengestrol acetate
**Be-100** ibuprofen piconol
**Be-1293** xipamide
**BE 419** ioglycamic acid
**BEC-2** generic not yet assigned
**BG 8301** teceleukin
**BG8967** bivalirudin
**BIBR 277 SE** telmisartan
**BIIP 20 XX** apaxifylline
**BI-L-239** enofelast
**BILA 2011 BS** palinavir
**BIM-23014C** lanreotide acetate
**BIMT 17** flibanserin
**BIMT 17 BS** flibanserin

**BIRG 0587** nevirapine
**BIRM-270** ontazolast
**BI-RR-0001** enlimomab
**BL 191** pentoxifylline
**BL-3912A** dimoxamine HCl
**BL-4162a** anagrelide HCl
**BL-5111** tiodazosin
**BL-5572M** proxorphan tartrate
**BL-5641A** etintidine HCl
**BL-P 1322** cephapirin sodium
**BL-P 1462** suncillin sodium
**BL-P 1761** sarpicillin
**BL-P 1780** sarmoxicillin
**BLP-25** generic not yet assigned
**BL-P 804** hetacillin
**BL-R 743** intrazole
**BL-S578** cefadroxil
**BL-S640** cefatrizine
**BL-S786** ceforanide
**BM01.004** metipranolol
**BM02.015** torsemide
**BM 06.019** epoetin beta
**BM 06.022** reteplase
**BM 13.177** sulotroban
**BM 13.505** daltroban
**BM 14.190** carvedilol
**BM 15.075** bezafibrate
**BM 21.0955·Na·H$_2$O** ibandronate sodium
**BM 22.145** isosorbide mononitrate
**BM 41.332** ciamexon
**BM 41.440** ilmofosine
**BM 51052** carazolol
**BMS 180048** avitriptan fumarate
**BMS 180048-02** avitriptan fumarate
**BMS-180194** lobucavir
**BMS-180291** ifetroban
**BMS-180291-02** ifetroban sodium
**BMS 180549** ferumoxtran-10
**BMS-181173** gusperimus trihydrochloride
**BMS-181339-01** paclitaxel
**BMS-186091** ammonium lactate
**BMS-186295** irbesartan
**BMS 200980** lanoteplase
**BMS-205603-01** uracil
**BMS-206584-01** gatifloxacin
**BMS-234475** generic not yet assigned
**BMY-05763-1-D** dexsotalol HCl
**BMY 13754** nefazodone HCl

Code Names

**BMY 13805-1** gepirone HCl
**BMY 13859-1** tiospirone HCl
**BMY-21891** belfosdil
**BMY-25182** cefbuperazone
**BMY-25801-01** batanopride HCl
**BMY-26517** pemirolast potassium
**BMY-27857** stavudine
**BMY-28090** elsamitrucin
**BMY-28100-03-800** cefprozil
**BMY-28142** cefepime
**BMY-28142 2HCl·H₂O** cefepime HCl
**BMY-30056** halobetasol propionate
**BMY-30120** chlorhexidine phosphanilate
**BMY-40327** modecainide
**BMY 40481** etoposide phosphate
**BMY-40900** didanosine
**BMY-41606** vapreotide
**BMY-42215-1** gusperimus trihydrochloride
**BN-1270** cicletanine
**BOF-A2** emitefur
**BP 1.02; S.049** ecadotril
**BP-1184** guanoctine HCl
**BP 400** pimethixene
**BRL-1241** methicillin sodium
**BRL 12594** ticarcillin cresyl sodium
**BRL-1288** benapryzine HCl
**BRL-1341** ampicillin
**BRL 13856** clopirac
**BRL 14151** clavulanic acid
**BRL 14151K** clavulanate potassium
**BRL 14777** nabumetone
**BRL-1621** cloxacillin sodium
**BRL-1702** dicloxacillin
**BRL 17421 (as sodium)** temocillin
**BRL-2039** floxacillin
**BRL-2064** carbenicillin disodium
**BRL 2288** ticarcillin disodium
**BRL 2333** amoxicillin
**BRL 2333AB-B** amoxicillin sodium
**BRL 2534** azidocillin
**BRL 26921** anistreplase
**BRL-284** levopropylcillin potassium
**BRL 29060** paroxetine
**BRL 30892** denbufylline
**BRL-3475** carbenicillin phenyl sodium
**BRL 34915** cromakalim
**BRL-38227** levcromakalim
**BRL 38705** epsiprantel

**BRL-39123** penciclovir
**BRL 40015** diproteverine
**BRL-42810** famciclovir
**BRL 43694** granisetron
**BRL 43694A** granisetron HCl
**BRL 4664** nonabine
**BRL 4910A** mupirocin
**BRL 4910F** mupirocin calcium
**BRL-49653-C** rosiglitazone maleate
**BRL 61063** cipamfylline
**BRL-804** hetacillin
**BRL 8988 HCl** talampicillin HCl
**BS 100-141** guanfacine HCl
**B.S. 6534** bufenadrine
**BS 6748** xyloxemine
**BS 6987** deptropine citrate
**BS 7161D (as HCl)** pytamine
**B.S. 7173-D** xylocoumarol
**BS 749** metacetamol
**B.S. 7561 (as HCl)** tixadil
**B.S. 7573-a** acridorex
**BS 7723 (as maleate)** tropirine
**BS 7977 D (as dihydrochloride)** xipranolol
**BSH** borocaptate sodium B 10
**BSSG** sitogluside
**BT 621 (as HCl)** todralazine
**BTI-322** generic not yet assigned
**BTPABA, PFT** bentiromide
**BTS 13622** hexaprofen
**BTS 17345** fluprofen
**BTS 18,322** flurbiprofen
**BTS 24332** esflurbiprofen
**BTS 49 465** flosequinan
**BTS 54524** sibutramine HCl
**BTS 7706** debropol
**BU-2231A** talisomycin
**BW 12C** generic not yet assigned
**BW 207U** xenalipin
**BW 234U dihydrochloride** rimcazole HCl
**BW 248U sodium** acyclovir sodium
**BW256U** valacyclovir
**BW 301U isethionate** piritrexim isethionate
**BW 325U** trifenagrel
**BW 33A** atracurium besylate
**BW 33-T-57** methisazone
**BW 356-C-61** gloxazone
**BW 430C** lamotrigine

**BW-467-C-60** bethanidine sulfate
**BW 49-210** diaveridine
**BW-524W91** emtricitabine
**BW 532U** cinflumide
**BW 56-158** allopurinol
**BW 56-72** trimethoprim
**BW-57-322** azathioprine
**BW 57-323** thiamiprine
**BW 58-271** rolodine
**BW-61-32** stilbazium iodide
**BW 63-90** butacetin
**BW 647U HCl** bipenamol HCl
**BW 64-9** butoxamine HCl
**BW 72U** trimethoprim sulfate
**BW 759U** ganciclovir
**BW 825C** acrivastine
**BW A256C** palatrigine
**BW A509U** zidovudine
**BW A515U** desciclovir
**BW A770U mesylate** crisnatol mesylate
**BW A938U dichloride** doxacurium chloride
**BW B1O9OU** mivacurium chloride
**Bx 311** cinoxolone
**BX 341** bifluranol
**BX 363A (as disodium salt)** cicloxolone
**BX 591** acefluranol
**BX 650A** ipsalazide
**BX 661A** balsalazide; balsalazide disodium
**BY 1023** pantoprazole
**BZ 55** carbutamide
**C-1** edrecolomab
**C-11925** phanquone
**C-12669** demecolcine
**C-1428** cyclarbamate
**C 1656** clometacin
**C-225** generic not yet assigned
**C-238** pridinol
**C242-DM1** generic not yet assigned
**C-3** capobenate sodium
**C-3** capobenic acid
**C-4** imciromab pentetate
**C-434** trimedoxime bromide
**C-49802B-Ba** oxaprotiline HCl
**c7E3** abciximab
**Ca 1022** carbutamide
**CA-7** brinolase

**CAB-2001** trafermin
**CAM-807** bialamicol HCl
**CARN 750** acemannan
**CAS 276** molsidomine
**CAS 936** pirsidomine
**CB 1048** chlornaphazine
**CB 10615** nifurmazole
**CB 11380** nifurizone
**CB 11 (as HCl)** phenadoxone
**CB 12592** subendazole
**CB-154** bromocriptine
**CB-154 mesylate** bromocriptine mesylate
**CB 1664** aceprometazine
**CB 1678** propiomazine
**CB 2201** amfepentorex
**CB-30038** minaprine
**CB 302** ferric fructose
**CB 3025** melphalan
**CB 304** azaribine
**CB 309** fenabutene
**CB-311** somatropin
**CB 313** mitotane
**CB-337** meglutol
**CB 3697** racefemine
**CB 4260** nortetrazepam
**CB 4261** tetrazepam
**CB 4857** menitrazepam
**CB 4985** acequinoline
**CB 7432** idoxifene
**CB 804** bucloxic acid
**CBP-1011** generic not yet assigned
**CCA** lobenzarit sodium
**CCD 1042** ganaxolone
**C.C.I. 12923** minaxolone
**CCI 15641** cefuroxime axetil
**CCI 18773** cloticasone propionate
**CCI 18781** fluticasone propionate
**CCI 23628** cefuroxime pivoxetil
**CCI 4725** clobetasol propionate
**CCI 5537** clobetasone butyrate
**CD 271** adapalene
**CDDD 1815** alprenoxime HCl
**CDDD 2803** adaprolol maleate
**CDDD 3602** tematropium methylsulfate
**CDDD 5604** loteprednol etabonate
**CDP571** generic not yet assigned
**CEN 000029** priliximab
**CEP 1538** modafinil

**CEPH (as HCl)** todralazine
**CERM 1978** bepridil HCl
**CERM 730** amoproxan
**CG 201** bevonium metilsulfate
**CG-315E** tramadol HCl
**GCA 18809** azamethiphos
**CGA-23654** nitroscanate
**CGA 72662** cyromazine
**CGP-14221/E** cefotiam HCl
**CGP 14,458** halobetasol propionate
**CGP 21690E** oxiracetam
**CGP 2175C** metoprolol fumarate
**CGP-2175E** metoprolol tartrate
**CGP 23339AE** pamidronate disodium
**CGP 25827A** formoterol fumarate
**CGP 30694** edatrexate
**CGP 32349** formestane
**CGP 39393** desirudin
**CGP 42446** zoledronic acid
**CGP 42446A** zoledronate disodium
**CGP 42446B** zoledronate trisodium
**CGP 45840B** diclofenac potassium
**CGP 48933** valsartan
**CGP-64128A** ggeneric not yet assigned
**CGP-69846A** generic not yet assigned
**CGP-7174/E** cefsulodin sodium
**CGP 7760B** prenalterol HCl
**CGP 9000** cefroxadine
**CGS 10078B** bendacalol mesylate
**CGS 10746B** pentiapine maleate
**CGS 10787D** prinomide tromethamine
**CGS 13080** pirmagrel
**CGS 13429A** batelapine maleate
**CGS 13945** pentopril
**CGS 14824A HCl** benazepril HCl
**CGS 14831** benazeprilat
**CGS 15040A** serazapine HCl
**CGS 16617** libenzapril
**CGS 16949A** fadrozole HCl
**CGS 18416A** zoniclezole HCl
**CGS 19755** selfotel
**CGS 20267** letrozole
**CGS 25019C** moxilubant maleate
**CGS 5391B (anhydrous)** enolicam sodium
**CGS 7135A** azaloxan fumarate
**CGS 7525A** aptazapine maleate
**CH 3565** triclosan

**CHX-100** masoprocol
**CHX-3673** amlexanox
**CI-100** acetosulfone sodium
**CI-1003** suramin hexasodium
**CI-1004** darbufelone mesylate
**CI-1006** diethylnorspermine
**CI-1008** pregabalin
**CI-1011** avasimibe
**CI-1012** generic not yet assigned
**CI-1019** igmesine HCl
**CI-1020** generic not yet assigned
**CI-107** argipressin tannate
**CI-301** bialamicol HCl
**CI-336** carbocloral
**CI-366** ethosuximide
**CI-379** benzilonium bromide
**CI-395** phencyclidine HCl
**CI 403A** pararosaniline pamoate
**CI-406** oxymetholone
**CI-416** triclofenol piperazine
**CI-419** fenimide
**CI 427** prodilidine HCl
**CI-433** clamoxyquin HCl
**CI 440** flufenamic acid
**CI-456** diapamide
**CI-473** mefenamic acid
**CI-501** cycloguanil pamoate
**CI-515** guanoxyfen sulfate
**CI-546** alipamide
**CI 556** acedapsone
**CI-572** profadol HCl
**CI-581** ketamine HCl
**CI-583** meclofenamic acid
**CI-633** clioxanide
**CI-634** tiletamine HCl
**CI-636** sulfacytine
**CI-642** butirosin sulfate
**CI 673** vidarabine
**CI-686 HCl** trebenzomine HCl
**CI-705** methaqualone
**CI-716** zolazepam HCl
**CI-718** bentazepam
**CI-719** gemfibrozil
**CI-720** gemcadiol
**CI-781** zometapine
**CI 787** tioperidone HCl
**CI-825** pentostatin
**CI-874** indeloxazine HCl
**CI-879** pramiracetam HCl
**CI-879 (sulfate)** pramiracetam sulfate

CI-880 amsacrine
CI-881 ametantrone acetate
CI-882 sparfosate sodium
CI-888 procaterol HCl
CI-897 tebuquine
CI-898 trimetrexate
CI-904 diaziquone
CI-906 quinapril HCl
CI-907 indolapril HCl
CI-908 dezaguanine
CI-908 **mesylate** dezaguanine mesylate
CI-909 tiazofurin
CI-911 rolziracetam
CI-912 zonisamide
CI-914 imazodan HCl
CI-9148 cysteamine HCl
CI-919 enoxacin
CI-920 fostriecin sodium
CI 925 moexipril HCl
CI-928 quinaprilat
CI-942 piroxantrone HCl
CI-945 gabapentin
CI-946 ralitoline
CI-958 ledoxantrone trihydrochloride
CI-960 **HCl** clinafloxacin HCl
CI-970 tacrine HCl
CI-977 enadoline HCl
CI-978 sparfloxacin
CI-979 milameline HCl
CI-980 mivobulin isethionate
CI-981 atorvastatin calcium
CI-982 fosphenytion sodium
CI-983 cefdinir
CI-991 troglitazone
CIBA 1906 thiambutosine
CJ 91B olsalazine sodium
CK-0383 verofylline
CK-0569 **(as the base)** ipexidine
  mesylate
CK-1752A sematilide HCl
CL09 icomethasone enbutate
CL 10304 aminocaproic acid
CL 106359 triamcinolone acetonide
  sodium phosphate
CL 108,756 brocresine
CL 112,302 buprenorphine HCl
CL 115,347 viprostol
CL 118,532 triptorelin
CL 12,625 natamycin
CL-1388R guanadrel sulfate

CL 13,900 puromycin
CL 14377 methotrexate
CL 16,536 puromycin HCl
CL 184,116 porfimer sodium
CL 184,824 alovudine
CL-1848C etoxadrol HCl
CL 186,815 biapenem
CL 203,821 cetaben sodium
CL 205925 iprocinodine HCl
CL 206,214 butamisole HCl
CL 206,576 sulbenox
CL 206,797 cypothrin
CL 216,942 bisantrene HCl
CL 217,658 imcarbofos
CL 220,075 bicifadine HCl
CL 22415 demecycline
CL 227,193 piperacillin sodium
CL 232,315 mitoxantrone HCl
CL 2422 guancydine
CL 25477 azetepa
CL 26193 simtrazene
CL 27,071 descinolone acetonide
CL 273,547 ocinaplon
CL 273,703 maduramicin
CL 274,471 colestolone
CL 284,635 cefixime
CL 284,846 zaleplon
CL 286,558 zeniplatin
CL 287,088 nemadectin
CL 287,110 enloplatin
CL 287,389 nilvadipine
CL 291,894 somagrebove
CL 297,939 bisoprolol
CL 297,939 bisoprolol fumarate
CL 298,741 tazobactam
CL 301,423 moxidectin
CL 307,579 tazobactam sodium
CL 307,782 levoleucovorin calcium
CL 318,952 verteporfin
Cl 337 azaserine
CL 34433 triamcinolone hexacetonide
CL 34699 amcinonide
CL 36467 methotrimeprazine
CL 369 ketamine HCl
CL 39743 methotrimeprazine
CL 39808 thozalinone
CL 399 tiletamine HCl
CL 40881 ethambutol HCl
CL 48156 imidoline HCl
CL 5,279 nithiamide

CL 53415 cyproximide
CL 54131 piperamide maleate
CL 54998 brocresine
Cl-583.Na salt meclofenamate sodium
CL 59112 roletamide
CL 61965 triamcinolone acetonide sodium phosphate
CL 62,362 loxapine
CL-639C dioxadrol HCl
Cl-64,976 zilantel
CL 65205 boxidine
CL 65336 tranexamic acid
CL 65,562 triflocin
Cl-661 oxiramide
CL 67,772 amoxapine
Cl-683 ripazepam
CL 71563 loxapine succinate
Cl-775 bevantolol HCl
Cl-808 vidarabine phosphate
Cl-808 sodium vidarabine sodium phosphate
CL 81,587 avoparcin
CL 82,204 fenbufen
CL 83,544 felbinac
Cl-845 pirmenol HCl
CL 84,633 nimidane
CL-867 piridicillin sodium
Cl-871 piracetam
CL 88,893 clazolimine
CL 90,748 azolimine
CL-911C dexoxadrol HCl
CL-912C levoxadrol HCl
CL 98984 cinodine HCl
CLY-503 simfibrate
CM 31-916 ceftiofur sodium
CN-10,395 ethosuximide
CN-14,329-23A cycloguanil pamoate
CN-15,573-23A pararosaniline pamoate
CN-15,757 azaserine
CN-16146 carbocloral
CN-17,900-2B clamoxyquin HCl
CN-1883 acedapsone
CN-20,172-3 benzilonium bromide
CN-25,253-2 phencyclidine HCl
CN-27,554 flufenamic acid
CN-34,799-5A guanoxyfen sulfate
CN-35355 mefenamic acid
CN-36,337 diapamide
CN-38,474 alipamide

CN 38703 methaqualone
CN-52,372-2 ketamine HCl
CN-54521-2 tiletamine HCl
CN-5834-5931B triclofenol piperazine
CN 59,567 clioxanide
CNS 1102 aptiganel HCl
CNS-5161 generic not yet assigned
CO 405 butidrine
Code 7277 ferumoxtran-10
compound 109168 nifluridide
compound 112531 vindesine
compound 113878 ciprefadol succinate
compound 113935 pentomone
compound 122587 drobuline
compound 133314 trioxifene mesylate
compound 24266 pentetate calcium trisodium Yb 169
compound 42339 acronine
compound 469 isoflurane
compound 497 dieldrin
compound 53616 frentizole
compound 56063 melizame
compound 57926 sinefungin
compound 68-198 diamfenetide
compound 79891 narasin
compound 81929 dobutamine
compound 83405 cefamandole
compound 83846 aprindine HCl
compound 85287 nibroxane
compound 89218 nisoxetine
compound 904 alexidine
compound 90459 benoxaprofen
compound 90606 isamoxole
compound 93819 fluretofen
compound 99170 aprindine
compound 99638 cefaclor
compound LY 131126 butopamine
compound S zidovudine
COP-1 glatiramer acetate
CP-0127 deltibant
CP-10,188 fenclonine
CP-10,303-8 quinterenol sulfate
CP-10,423-16 pyrantel pamoate
CP-10,423-18 pyrantel tartrate
CP 1044 J3 bufexamac
CP-11,332-1 quinazosin HCl
CP-116,517-27 alatrofloxacin mesylate
CP-118,954-11 icopezil maleate
CP-12,009-18 morantel tartrate

**CP-12,252-1** thiothixene HCl
**CP-12,299-1** prazosin HCl
**CP-12,521-1** piquizil HCl
**CP-12,574** tinidazole
**CP-13,608** tesicam
**CP-14,185-1** hoquizil HCl
**CP-14,368-1** lometraline HCl
**CP-14,445-16** oxantel pamoate
**CP-148,623** pamaqueside
**CP-15,464-2** carbenicillin indanyl sodium
**CP-15,467-61** lithium carbonate
**CP 1552 S** milacemide HCl
**CP-15-639-2** carbenicillin disodium
**CP-15,973** sudoxicam
**CP-16,171** piroxicam
**CP-16,171-85** piroxicam olamine
**CP-16,533-1** verapamil
**CP 172 AP** clopirac
**CP-18,524** tibric acid
**CP-19,106-1** trimazosin HCl
**CP-20,961** avridine
**CP-22,341** temodox
**CP-22,665** flumizole
**CP-24,314-1** pirbuterol HCl
**CP-24,314-14** pirbuterol acetate
**CP-24,441-1** tametraline HCl
**CP-24,877** drinidene
**CP-25,673** tiazuril
**CP-26,154** tolimidone
**CP-27,634** gliamilide
**CP-28,720** glipizide
**CP-31,081** polydextrose
**CP-32,387** pirolate
**CP-33,994-2** pirbenicillin sodium
**CP-34,089** sulprostone
**CP-36,584** flutroline
**CP-38,754** plauracin
**CP-44,001-1** nantradol HCl
**CP-45,634** sorbinil
**CP-45,899-2** sulbactam sodium
**CP-45,899-99** sulbactam benzathine
**CP-47,904** sulbactam pivoxil
**CP-48,810-27** fanetizole mesylate
**CP-48,867-9** ristianol phosphate
**CP-49,952** sultamicillin
**CP-50,556-1** levonantradol HCl
**Cp-51,974-1** sertraline HCl
**CP-52,640-2** cefoperazone sodium
**CP-54,802** alitame

**CP-556S** suloctidil
**CP-57,361-01** zaltidine HCl
**CP-62,993** azithromycin
**CP-65703** ampiroxicam
**CP-66,248** tenidap
**CP-66,248-2** tenidap sodium
**CP-70,429** sulopenem
**CP-70,490-09** enazadrem phosphate
**CP-72,133** ilonidap
**CP-72,467-2** englitazone sodium
**CP-73,049** binfloxacin
**CP-73,850** zopolrestat
**CP-76,136-27** danofloxacin mesylate
**CP-80,794** terlakiren
**CP-86,325-2** darglitazone sodium
**CP-88,059** ziprasidone
**CP-88,059-1** ziprasidone HCl
**CP-88,818** tiqueside
**CP-93,393-1** sunepitron HCl
**CP-99,219-27** trovafloxacin mesylate
**CPC-111** generic not yet assigned
**CPC-211** generic not yet assigned
**Cpd 109514** nabilone
**Cpd. 5411** iopentol
**CPT-11** irinotecan
**CR/662** tipepidine
**CRL 40476** modafinil
**CS-045** troglitazone
**CS-151** crofilcon A
**CS-514** pravastatin sodium
**CS-622** temocapril HCl
**CS-807** cefpodoxime proxetil
**CSAG-144** mebeverine HCl
**CT 1501R** lisofylline
**CTLA4-Ig** generic not yet assigned
**CTP-37** generic not yet assigned
**CTR 6110** nitrodan
**CTX** lornoxicam
**CV-11974** candesartan
**CV 57533** xenyhexenic acid
**CV 58903** xenazoic acid
**CVT-124** generic not yet assigned
**CVT-313** generic not yet assigned
**CVT-510** generic not yet assigned
**CY-116** aminocaproic acid
**CY-1503** generic not yet assigned
**CY 153** acexamic acid
**CY-1899** generic not yet assigned
**CY 216** nadroparin calcium
**CY2301** generic not yet assigned

**CY 39** psilocybine
**CYT-103** [111]In indium In 111 satu-
momab pendetide
**CYT-103-Y-90** generic not yet
assigned
**CYT-356** capromab pendetide
**CYT-424** samarium Sm 153 lex-
idronam pentasodium
**D 00079** anoxomer
**D-1262** cloxypendyl
**D-1593** diapamide
**D-1721** alipamide
**D-1959 HCl** reproterol HCl
**D2083** desonide
**D-2163** generic not yet assigned
**D 237** cloforex
**D-254** pipazethate
**D-365** verapamil
**D 4028** enprofylline
**D 47** sulbentine
**d4T** stavudine
**D 7093** mesna
**D-775** homofenazine
**D-9998** flupirtine maleate
**DA 1773** sodium picosulfate
**DA 2370** feprazone
**DA-398** epirizole
**DA 688** gefarnate
**DA-708** teflurane
**DA-808** nafcaproic acid
**DA-893** roflurane
**DA-914** nafiverine
**DA-992** naftypramide
**DAB-389** generic not yet assigned
**DAC** decitabine
**D.A.T.** acetiamine
**DATC** tiocarlide
**DAU6215CL** itasetron
**DBV** buformin
**DCH 21 (as sodium salt)** exiproben
**DCL Hb** hemoglobin crosfumaril
**DETF** trichlorfon
**DF 118** dihydrocodeine bitartrate
**DH-524** fenmetozole HCl
**DH-581** probucol
**DIM-SA** succimer
**DK-7419** argatroban
**DL 152** bietaserpine
**DL-164** tiodonium chloride
**DL-588** napactadine HCl

**DL-8280** ofloxacin
**dl HM-PAO** exametazime
**dl HM-PAO** hexametazime
**DMI** desipramine HCl
**DMP-115** generic not yet assigned
**DMP 266** efavirenz
**DMP 450** generic not yet assigned
**DMP 504** generic not yet assigned
**DMP 754** roxifiban acetate
**DMP 777** generic not yet assigned
**DMP 840** bisnafide dimesylate
**DMSC** doxycycline fosfatex
**DN-2327** pazinaclone
**DO6** lexipafant
**DPDP** fodipir
**DR-3355** levofloxacin
**DS 103-282** tizanidine HCl
**DS-4152** tecogalan sodium
**DT-3** detrothyronine
**DT-327** clopamide
**DTPA-SMS** pentetreotide
**D-Trp LHRH-PEA** deslorelin
**DU-21220** ritodrine
**DU-21445** tiprenolol HCl
**DU 22550 (as sulfate)** caproxamine
**DU23000** fluvoxamine maleate
**DU-23187** quincarbate
**DuP 128** lecimibide
**DuP 753** losartan potassium
**Dup 785** brequinar sodium
**DuP 921** sibopirdine
**DUP 937** teloxantrone HCl
**DUP 941** losoxantrone
**DuP 996** linopirdine
**DV-1006** cetraxate HCl
**DW-61** flavoxate HCl
**DW-62** dimefline HCl
**DW 75** norleusactide
**DyDTPA-BMA** sprodiamide
**E-0659** azelastine HCl
**E-106-E (as cyclamate)** furfenorex
**E 141** ethamsylate
**E-2020** donepezil HCl
**E25** generic not yet assigned
**E-2663** bentiromide
**E-3810** rabeprazole sodium
**E 39** inproquone
**E-52** pentafilcon A
**E-614** tripamide
**E 9002** naftalofos

EA-166 guanoxyfen sulfate
EDU edoxudine
EE₃ME mestranol
EF-27 generic not yet assigned
EF9 temoporfin
EGTA egtazic acid
EGYT 201 bencyclane fumarate
EHB 776 foscarnet sodium
EL10 dehydroepiandrosterone
EL349 somidobove
EL737 ractopamine HCl
EL-857 apramycin
EL870 tilmicosin
EL-970 fampridine
EL-974 ticarbodine
ELD 950 eledoisin
EMBAY 8440 praziquantel
EMD 15 700 nitrefazole
EMD 19698 (as hydrogen maleate) peratizole
EMD 33 512 bisoprolol
EMD 9806 pramiverine
EN-1010 pyrrocaine
EN-141 josamycin
EN-15304 naloxone HCl
EN-1620A nalmexone HCl
EN-1639A (as HCl) naltrexone
EN-1661L bisobrin lactate
EN-1733A molindone HCl
EN-2234A nalbuphine HCl
EN-313 moricizine
EN-970 fluquazone
ENT-20852 butonate
ENT-23969 carbaril
ENT-25567 naftalofos
ENT 29,106 nimidane
EPI-2010 generic not yet assigned
EPOCH epoetin beta
ES 304 nicofuranose
ET-394 tribromsalan
ET-495 piribedil
ETTN propatyl nitrate
EU-1063 proquinolate
EU-1085 leniquinsin
EU-1093 buquinolate
EU-1806 nafronyl oxalate
EU-2826 benurestat
EU-2972 nolinium bromide
EU-3120 acodazole HCl
EU-3325 triafungin

EU-3421 oxifungin HCl
EU-4093 azumolene sodium
EU-4200 piribedil
EU-4534 flurofamide
EU-4584 tolfamide
EU-4891 diacetolol HCl
EU-4906 sitogluside
EU-5306 pefloxacin
EUDR edoxudine
EV2-7 sevirumab
EX 10-029-C elantrine
EX 10-781 metizoline HCl
EX 12-095 eterobarb
EX 4355 desipramine HCl
EX 4810 ambuside
Ex 4883 rolicyprine
EXP-105-1 amantadine HCl
EXP 126 rimantadine HCl
EXP 338 midaflur
EXP 999 metopimazine
F 1500 succisulfone
F 1983 pyrovalerone HCl
F28249α nemadectin
F-368 dantrolene
F-413 clodanolene
F-440 dantrolene sodium
F-605 (as the sodium) clodanolene
F 6066 cyclofenil
F-691 furodazole
F-776 orpanoxin
F-853 nitrafudam HCl
Fa 402 fentonium bromide
FBA 1420 propanidid
FBA 4059 brotianide
FBB 4231 glisoxepide
FBB 6896 clenpirin
FC-1157a toremifene citrate
FC 41-12 perflenapent + perflisopent
FCE 21336 cabergoline
FCF 89 roquinimex
FER-1443 ticlatone
FG-10571 panadiplon
FG 5111 melperone
FGN-1 exisulind
FI 5852 oxabolone cipionate
F.I. 6146 buzepide metiodide
FI 6337 metergoline
FI 6339 (as the base) daunorubicin HCl
F.I. 6426 stallimycin HCl

**F.I. 6654** caroxazone
**F.I. 6820** brofoxine
**FK 027** cefixime
**FK-201** quinotolast
**FK 235** nilvadipine
**FK 482** cefdinir
**FK-506** tacrolimus
**FK-565** generic not yet assigned
**FK 749** ceftizoxime sodium
**FKS-508** cevimeline HCl
**FLA 731** remoxipride
**FLA 731(–)** remoxipride HCl
**FPL 12924AA** remacemide HCl
**FPL 58668KC** probicromil calcium
**FPL 59002** nedocromil
**FPL 59002KC** nedocromil calcium
**FPL 59002KP** nedocromil sodium
**FPL 59360** minocromil
**FPL 60278** dopexamine
**FPL 60278AR** dopexamine HCl
**FPL.670** cromolyn sodium
**FR 13749** ceftizoxime sodium
**FR 17027** cefixime
**(–)-FTC** emtricitabine
**FTC-(–)**
**FU-02** fumoxicillin
**FUT-175** nafamostat mesylate
**FWH 399** troxonium tosilate
**G-101** erythromycin salnacedin
**G-201** salnacedin
**G-203** fluocinonide
**G-24480** dimpylate
**G-25178** prodeconium bromide
**G-25766** clorindione
**G 26,872** phenbutazone sodium glycerate
**G 30320** clofazimine
**G-32883** carbamazepine
**G-33040** opipramol HCl
**G-33182** chlorthalidone
**G 34586** clomipramine HCl
**G-35020** desipramine HCl
**G 35259** ketipramine fumarate
**G-4** dichlorophen
**G-704,650** alendronate sodium
**GEA 654** alaproclate
**GEM-231** generic not yet assigned
**GEM-91** trecovirsen sodium
**GER-11** pimagedine HCl
**GF 120918A** elacridar

**GG-167** zanamivir
**GG-745** dutasteride
**GI147211C** lurtotecan dihydrochloride
**GI 198745** dutasteride
**GI 87084B** remifentanil HCl
**GL-701** dehydroepiandrosterone
**GLQ 223** trichosanthin
**GMC 89-107** regramostim
**GN1600** argatroban
**Go 1213** atolide
**Go 1733** suloxifen oxalate
**Go 2782** iproxamine HCl
**Go 3026A** ciclafrine HCl
**Go-560** febarbamate
**Go 919** piprozolin
**GOE 3450** gabapentin
**Goedecke 3282** ozolinone
**GP-1-110** acadesine
**gp120** generic not yet assigned
**GP-121** phencyclidine HCl
**gp 160** generic not yet assigned
**GP-2-121-3** arbutamine HCl
**GP 31406** depramine
**GP 45840** diclofenac sodium
**GP 51084** glibutimine
**GPA-878** metazamide
**GPI-1046** generic not yet assigned
**GPI-200** iometopane I 123
**GPI-5000** generic not yet assigned
**GR109714X** lamivudine
**GR 114297A** picumeterol fumarate
**GR 114297X (picumeterol)** picumeterol fumarate
**GR 116526X** isotretinoin anisatil
**GR 121167X** zanamivir
**GR 122311X** ranitidine bismuth citrate
**GR 138950C** saprisartan potassium
**GR 20263** ceftazidime
**GR 2/1214** clobetasone butyrate
**GR 2/1574** alfadolone
**GR 2/234** alfaxalone
**GR 2/443 (as propionate)** doxibetasol
**GR 2/925** clobetasol propionate
**Gr 30921** mitoquidone
**GR 32191** vapiprost HCl
**GR 32191B** vapiprost HCl
**GR 33207** ovandrotone albumin
**GR 33343 G** salmeterol xinafoate
**GR 33343 X** salmeterol
**GR 38032F** ondansetron HCl

**GR 412** dodeclonium bromide
**GR 43175C** sumatriptan succinate
**GR 43659X** lacidipine
**GR50360A** fluparoxan HCl
**GR 50692** cefempidone
**GR 53992B (GX 1296B)** teludipine HCl
**GR 63178K** fosquidone
**GR 68755C** alosetron HCl
**GR 81225C** galdansetron HCl
**GR 85548A** naratriptan HCl
**GR 87442 N** luroseron mesylate
**GR92132** troglitazone
**GR 69153X** cefetecol
**GRF1-44** generic not yet assigned
**GS-0504** cidofovir
**GS-0840** adefovir dipivoxil
**GS-1339** dymanthine HCl
**GS 2147** sancycline
**GS-2876** methacycline
**GS-2989** meclocycline
**GS-3065** doxycycline
**GS-3159** carbenicillin potassium
**GS 393** generic not yet assigned
**GS-4104** generic not yet assigned
**GS-6244** carbadox
**GS-6742** sulfomyxin
**GS-7443** mequidox
**GS 840** adefovir dipivoxil
**GS-95** thiethylperazine maleate
**GT16-026A** sevelamer HCl
**GT31-104HB** colesevelam HCl
**GV 104326B** sanfetrinem sodium
**GV 118819X** sanfetrinem cilexetil
**GV 150526X** gavestinel
**GW-80126** seprilose
**H 102/09 HCl** zimeldine HCl
**H 104/08** pamatolol sulfate
**H 133/22** prenalterol HCl
**H 154/82** felodipine
**H 168/68** omeprazole
**H 168/68 sodium** omeprazole sodium
**H 365** paroxypropione
**H 3774** alibendol
**II 4132** dotefonium bromide
**H 4170** tolpiprazole
**H 4723** clobazam
**H 56/28** alprenolol HCl
**H65-RTA** zolimomab aritox

**H 93/26 succinate** metoprolol succinate
**HA-1A** nebacumab
**HB 115** nifurprazine
**HB 419** glyburide
**H.B.F. 386** cactinomycin
**HBY097** generic not yet assigned
**HC 1528** decoquinate
**HC 20,511 fumarate** ketotifen fumarate
**HCP-30** generic not yet assigned
**HF 1854** clozapine
**HF 1927** dibenzepin HCl
**HF-2159** clothiapine
**HF 241** bufeniode
**HGP-1** loteprednol etabonate
**HGP-2** adaprolol maleate
**HGP-30W** generic not yet assigned
**HGP-5** alprenoxime HCl
**HGP-6** tematropium methylsulfate
**HH105** butetamate
**HH 197** butamirate citrate
**HL 267** dipenine bromide
**HL 362** colforsin
**HL 523 (as HCl)** tiformin
**HMD** oxymetholone
**HMR-3480** generic not yet assigned
**HNK-20** generic not yet assigned
**Hoe 045** articaine
**HOE 062** roxatidine acetate HCl
**HOE 077** lufironil
**Hoe 105** citenazone
**HOE 118** piretanide
**HOE 140** icatibant acetate
**HOE 18 680** embutramide
**HOE 216V** luxabendazole
**HOE 280** ofloxacin
**HOE 296** ciclopirox olamine
**HOE 296b** ciclopirox
**Hoe 296 V** resorantel
**HOE 304** desoximetasone
**HOE 36801** etifoxine
**HOE 39-893d** penbutolol sulfate
**HOE 42-440** tiamenidine HCl
**HOE440** tiamenidine
**Hoe 473** aclantate
**HOE 490** glimepiride
**HOE 498** ramipril
**HOE 760** roxatidine acetate HCl
**HOE 766** buserelin acetate

**HOE 777** prednicarbate
**Hoe 881V** fenbendazole
**HOE 893d** penbutolol sulfate
**HOE 984** nomifensine maleate
**Hoechst 10495** norpipanone
**Hoechst 10582** normethadone
**HP 029** velnacrine maleate
**HP 128** suronacrine maleate
**HP 1598** guanoxyfen sulfate
**HP 290** quilostigmine
**HP-3** generic not yet assigned
**HP 3522** brocrinat
**HP-4** generic not yet assigned
**HP 494** fluradoline HCl
**HP 522** brocrinat
**HP 549** isoxepac
**HP 749** besipirdine HCl
**HP 873** iloperidone
**HPEK-1** tetroquinone
**hPTH 1-34 (acetate salt)** teriparatide acetate
**HR111V-sulfate** cefquinome sulfate
**HR 221 (as sodium)** cefodizime
**HR 376** clobazam
**HR 756** cefotaxime sodium
**HR 810 sulfate** cefpirome sulfate
**HR 930** fosazepam
**HRP 543** dazepinil HCl
**HRP 913** neflumozide HCl
**HS-592** clemastine
**HSP 2986** pramiverine
**HT-11** cloperastine
**HTO** tritiated water
**HU-1124** generic not yet assigned
**HU-211** dexanabinol
**Hu23F2G** generic not yet assigned
**HUF-2446** clodazon HCl
**HWA 285** propentofylline
**HY-185** carbocloral
**¹²³I labeled IMP** iofetamine HCl I 123
**¹²³I-M123** iofetamine HCl I 123
**I-2105** afovirsen sodium
**I-653** desflurane
**IA-307** acetosulfone sodium
**IB-367** generic not yet assigned
**IBT-9302** heparinase III
**IC-351** generic not yet assigned
**ICI 118,587** xamoterol
**ICI 118,630** goserelin
**ICI 125,211** tiotidine

**ICI 128,436** ponalrestat
**ICI 136,753** tracazolate
**ICI 139603** tetronasin
**ICI 141,292** epanolol
**ICI 156,834** cefotetan
**ICI 176,334** bicalutamide
**ICI 194,660** meropenem
**ICI 204,219** zafirlukast
**ICI 204,636** quetiapine fumarate
**ICI 28257** clofibrate
**ICI 29661** pyrimitate
**ICI 32865** etoglucid
**ICI-33,828** methallibure
**ICI 35,868** propofol
**ICI 38174 (as HCl)** pronetalol
**ICI 45520** propranolol HCl
**ICI 45763 (as HCl)** toliprolol
**ICI 46,474** tamoxifen citrate
**ICI 46683** oxyclozanide
**I.C.I. 47,319** dexpropranolol HCl
**ICI 48213** cyclofenil
**ICI 50,123** pentagastrin
**I.C.I. 50,172** practolol
**I.C.I. 54,450** fenclozic acid
**ICI 54,594 (as sodium salt)** brofezil
**ICI 55,052** nequinate
**ICI 55,897** clobuzarit
**ICI 58,834** viloxazine HCl
**ICI 59118** razoxane
**ICI 66,082** atenolol
**ICI 80,008 (as sodium salt)** fluprostenol sodium
**ICI 80,996** cloprostenol sodium
**ICI 81,008** fluprostenol sodium
**ICI 8173** quindoxin
**ICI D1033** anastrozole
**ICI-U.S. 457** octazamide
**ICN-542** ribaminol
**ICRF 159** razoxane
**ICRF-187** dexrazoxane
**IDEC-102** rituximab
**IDEC-131** generic not yet assigned
**IDEC-151** clenoliximab
**IDEC-C2B8** rituximab
**IDEC-CE9.1** generic not yet assigned
**IDEC-Y2B8** generic not yet assigned
**IL-17803A (as HCl)** acebutolol
**IL-19552** pipotiazine palmitate
**IL 22811 HCl** meptazinol HCl
**IL 5902** spiramycin

**IL 6001** trimipramine
**IL-6302 mesylate** fonazine mesylate
**IMI-28** epirubicin HCl
**IMI 30** idarubicin HCl
**IMI 58** esorubicin HCl
**IMMU-4** arcitumomab
**IMMU-LL2** bectumomab
**IMMU-MN3** sulesomab
**IN 1060** cyprolidol HCl
**IN 29-5931B** triclofenol piperazine
**IN 379** pimetine HCl
**IN 461** benzindopyrine HCl
**IN 511** phenyramidol HCl
**IN 836** fenyripol HCl
**INA-X14** insulin aspart
**INF-1837** flufenamic acid
**INF-3355** mefenamic acid
**INF 4668** meclofenamic acid
**INGN-201** generic not yet assigned
**INS-1** generic not yet assigned
**insulin X14** insulin aspart
**IP-2105** afovirsen sodium
**IP 302 sodium** citicoline sodium
**IP 456** pagoclone
**IPA** riboprine
**IPL-576** generic not yet assigned
**IR-501** generic not yet assigned
**IR-502** generic not yet assigned
**IS 2596** domoxin
**I.S. 499** poldine methylsulfate
**ISIS-13312** generic not yet assigned
**ISIS 2105** afovirsen sodium
**ISIS-2302** generic not yet assigned
**ISIS 2503** generic not yet assigned
**ISIS 2922** generic not yet assigned
**ISIS 3521** generic not yet assigned
**ISIS-5132** generic not yet assigned
**isomer A** zuclomiphene
**isomer B** enclomiphene
**ISV-205** generic not yet assigned
**ISV-208** generic not yet assigned
**Janssen R 4929** benzetimide HCl
**JAV 852** benfosformin
**JB-8181** desipramine HCl
**JD-96** vinylbital
**JF-1** nalmefene
**JL-1078** dihexyverine HCl
**JL 512** fenadiazole
**JM-8** carboplatin
**JM-83** oxaliplatin

**JM-9** iproplatin
**JO-1784** igmesine HCl
**JTT-501** generic not yet assigned
**K 11941** alfaprostol
**K 12148** lifibrol
**K-17** thalidomide
**K-1900** nimorazole
**K-38** glycyclamide
**K-386** glycyclamide
**K 4024** glipizide
**K 4277** indoprofen
**K 9147** tolciclate
**Kabi 2234** tolterodine
**KABI 925** emylcamate
**KAT 256 (as HCl)** clobutinol
**KB-944** fostedil
**KB 95** benzpiperylon
**K-F 224** naftoxate
**KL-255 (as HCl)** bupranolol
**KNI-272** generic not yet assigned
**Ko 1173 Cl** mexiletine HCl
**KO 1366** bunitrolol
**Ko 592 (as HCl)** toliprolol
**KP-363** butenafine HCl
**KRM-1648** rifalazil
**KS 33** oxyridazine
**KVX-478** amprenavir
**KW-110** aceglutamide aluminum
**KW4679** olopatadine HCl
**KWD 2019** terbutaline sulfate
**L1** deferiprone
**L-1573** cysteamine
**L-1633** sodium dibunate
**L-1718** osalmid
**L-1777** medazomide
**L 2197** benzarone
**L-2214** benzbromarone
**L 2329** benziodarone
**L 2642** etabenzarone
**L-3428** amiodarone
**L-364,718** devazepide
**L-4269** pyridarone
**L-5103 Lepetit** rifampin
**L-5418** diftalone
**L 542** mercurobutol
**L-554** tritoqualine
**L 566** dibemethine
**L 5818 (as HCl)** coumazoline
**L-6257** oxetorone fumarate
**L-627** biapenem

Code Names

L-637,510 nelezaprine maleate
L-6400 fluazacort
L-647,339 naxagolide HCl
L-668,019 verlukast
L-669,455 dexibuprofen lysine
L-67 prilocaine HCl
L-735,524 indinavir sulfate
L-749 salacetamide
L 75 1362B colforsin
L-8 lypressin
L 8027 nictindole
L-9394 butoprozine HCl
LA-012 (as HCl) quatacaine
LA 1221 (as HCl) butalamine
LA III diazepam
LA 391 sodium picosulfate
La 6023 metformin
LAC-43 bupivacaine HCl
LAS 30451 pancopride
LAS 31025 arofylline
LAS 31416 almotriptan
LAS 3876 almagate
LAS 9273 clebopride
LAS W-090 ebastine
LB 125 cyprodenate
LB-46 pindolol
LB-502 furosemide
LC 44 flupentixol
LD 2351 (as hydrobromide)
  butopiprine
LD 2480 piprocurarium iodide
LD 2630 difencloxazine HCl
LD 2988 folescutol
LD 3055 oxypyrronium bromide
LD 335 propyromazine bromide
LD 3394 fenozolone
LD 3612 paraflutizide
LD 4644 pipebuzone
LD 935 dipiproverine HCl
LDI-200 generic not yet assigned
LDP-02 generic not yet assigned
Leo 1031 prednimustine
Leo 114 polyestradiol phosphate
levo-BC-2605 oxilorphan
levo-BC-2627 butorphanol
levo-BC-2627 tartrate butorphanol
  tartrate
levo-BL-4566 moxazocine
LEX-032 generic not yet assigned
LG100057 alitretinoin

LG100069 bexarotene
LGD1057 alitretinoin
LGD 1069 bexarotene
LJ 206 carbocysteine
LJC 10,141 felbinac
LJ C10,627 biapenem
LJP-394 generic not yet assigned
LL 1530 nadoxolol
LL-705W neutramycin
LM-1404 lortalamine
LM 176 cobamamide
LM 192 viquidil
LM 2717 clobazam
LM-427 rifabutin
LM-94 hymecromone
L.N. 107 broparestrol
l-OHP oxaliplatin
LP-2307 generic not yet assigned
LS-121 nafronyl oxalate
LS 2616 roquinimex
LS 519 C12 pirenzepine HCl
Lu 23-174 sertindole
LU3-010 talopram HCl
LVD dextran 40
LY031537 ractopamine HCl
LY 048 740 avilamycin
LY061188 cephalexin HCl
LY097964 cefetamet
LY099094 vindesine sulfate
LY104208 vinzolidine sulfate
LY 108380 doxpicomine HCl
LY110140 fluoxetine HCl
LY 119863 vinepidine sulfate
LY120363 flumezapine
LY121019 cilofungin
LY 122512 anitrazafen
LY 12271-72 viroxime
LY 122772 enviroxime
LY 123508 lorzafone
LY 127123 enviradene
LY 127623 metkephamid acetate
LY 127809 pergolide mesylate
LY 127935 moxalactam disodium
LY 135837 indecainide HCl
LY137998 somatropin
LY 139037 nizatidine
LY 139381 ceftazidime
LY 139603 tomoxetine HCl
LY 141894 amflutizole
LY 146032 daptomycin

LY 150378 clofilium phosphate
LY 150720 picenadol HCl ·
LY156758 raloxifene HCl
LY163502 quinelorane HCl
LY163892 **monohydrate** loracarbef
LY167005 proinsulin human
LY170053 olanzapine
LY170680 sulukast
LY171555 quinpirole HCl
LY171883 tomelukast
LY 174008 dobutamine tartrate
LY 175326 isomazole HCl
LY177370 tilmicosin
LY177370 **phosphate** tilmicosin
   phosphate
LY177837 somidobove
LY186641 sulofenur
LY 186655 tibenelast sodium
LY188011 gemcitabine
LY188011 **HCl** gemcitabine HCl
LY 195115 indolidan
LY 201116 ameltolide
LY206243 **lactobionate** levdobuta-
   mine lactobionate
LY207506 dobutamine lactobionate
LY210448 **HCl** dapoxetine HCl
LY 213829 tazofelone
LY215229 **HCl** seproxetine HCl
LY231514 pemetrexed disodium
LY 237216 dirithromycin
LY237733 amesergide
LY246708 xanomeline
LY246708 **tartrate** xanomeline tartrate
LY248686 **HCl** duloxetine HCl
LY253351 tamsulosin HCl
LY264618 lometrexol sodium
LY275585 insulin lyspro
LY277359 zatosetron maleate
LY281067 sergolexole maleate
LY287041 tazomeline citrate
LY293404 rismorelin porcine
LY294468 **sulfate** efegatran sulfate
LY295337 basifungin
LY307640 **sodium** rabeprazole sodium
LY-315535 generic not yet assigned
LY 333334 teriparatide
LY335348 denileukin diftitox
LY353381·HCl arzoxifene HCl
LYO31537 ractopamine HCl
M-1028 (Meiji) haloprogin

M-14 rifamycin
M-141 spectinomycin HCl
M 285 cyprenorphine HCl
M. 5050 diprenorphine
M-811 salverine
M. 99 (as HCl) etorphine
MA 1277 zolertine HCl
MA 1291 quipazine maleate
MA 1337 cloperidone HCl
MA-1443 letimide HCl
MA-540 quinuclium bromide
MA-593 salethamide maleate
MAB35 indium In 111 altumomab
   pentetate
MAK 195 F generic not yet assigned
MAS-1 polyglyconate
Material A pentetate calcium triso-
   dium Yb 169
MAY nelzarabine
M&B 15497 decoquinate
M&B 16942A diacetolol HCl
M&B 17803A (as HCl) acebutolol
M&B 22948 zaprinast
M&B 33153 oxoprostol
M&B 39831 temozolomide
M&B 5062 A amicarbalide
M&B 782 (as isethionate) propami-
   dine
MB 800 (as isethionate) pentamidine
M&B 9302 clorgiline
MBR-4164-8 diflumidone sodium
MBR-4197 flucrylate
MBR 4223 triflumidate
MC 903 calcipotriene
MCE metergoline
MCI-9038 argatroban
McN-1075 fenmetramide
McN-1107 clominorex
McN-1210 pyrinoline
McN-1231 fluminorex
McN-1546 flumetramide
McN-1589 mixidine
McN-2378 mefenidil
McN-2378-46 mefenidil fumarate
McN-2453 azepindole
McN-2559 tolmetin
McN-2559-21-98 tolmetin sodium
McN-2783-21-98 zomepirac sodium
McN-3113 xilobam
McN-3377-98 fenobam

Code Names

McN-3495 pirogliride tartrate
McN-3716 methyl palmoxirate
McN-3802-21-98 palmoxirate sodium
McN-3802 (anhydrous free acid) palmoxirate sodium
McN 3935 linogliride
McN-3935 linogliride fumarate
McN-4097-12-98 fenoctimine sulfate
McN-4853 topiramate
McN-742 aminorex
McN-A-2673-11 etoperidone HCl
McN-A-2833 perindopril
McN-A-2833-109 perindopril erbumine
McN-JR-13,558-11 fetoxylate HCl
McN-JR-15,403-11 difenoxin
McN-JR-1625 haloperidol
McN-JR-16,341 penfluridol
McN-JR-2498 trifluperidol
McN-JR-4263-49 fentanyl citrate
McN-JR-4584 benperidol
McN-JR-4749 droperidol
McN-JR-4929-11 benzetimide HCl
McN-JR-6218 fluspirilene
McN-JR-6238 pimozide
McN-JR-7242-11 difluanine HCl
McN-JR-7904 lidoflazine
McN-JR-8299-11 tetramisole HCl
McN-R-1162-22 potassium glucaldrate
McN-R-1967 fenretinide
McN-R-726-47 poldine methylsulfate
McN-R-73-Z rotoxamine
McN-X-181 valnoctamide
McN-X-94 capuride
MD 141 ethamsylate
MD 2028 fluanisone
MD 67350 (as maleate) cinepazide
MD-805 argatroban
mda-7 generic not yet assigned
MDL 11,939 glemanserin
MDL 14,042 lofexidine HCl
MDL 16,455A fexofenadine HCl
MDL 17,043 enoximone
MDL 18,962 plomestane
MDL 19,205 piroximone
MDL 19,744 tipentosin HCl
MDL-201129 beraprost sodium
MDL-201229 beraprost
MDL 257 zindotrine
MDL 26,024G0 tetrazolast meglumine

MDL 26,479 suritozole
MDL 28,574A celgosivir HCl
MDL 458 deflazacort
MDL 473 rifapentine
MDL 507 teicoplanin
MDL 62,198 ramoplanin
MDL 62,769 rifamexil
MDL 71,754 vigabatrin
MDL 71,782 A eflornithine HCl
MDL 72,222 bemesetron
MDL 72,422 tropanserin HCl
MDL 72,974A mofegiline HCl
MDL 73,005EF binospirone mesylate
MDL 73,147EF dolasetron mesylate
MDL 73,745 zifrosilone
MDL 73,945 camiglibose
MDX-210 generic not yet assigned
MDX-240 generic not yet assigned
MDX-RA generic not yet assigned
MEDI 493 palivizumab
MER-29 triparanol
MER-41 clomiphene citrate
MF 934 rufloxacin
M.G. 13054 fenquizone
M.G. 13608 domiodol
M.G. 143 sulmarin
M.G. 1559 xenbucin
Mg 4833 fencibutirol
M.G. 5454 guaiapate
MG 559 metamfepramone
M.G. 5771 butixirate
M.G. 624 stilonium iodide
M.G. 652 oxamarin HCl
M.G. 8823 exaprolol HCl
M.G. 8926 (as HCl) droprenilamine
MGI-114 generic not yet assigned
MH-532 phenprobamate
MI-216 iothalamic acid
Mi-85 apazone
MIM D2A21 generic not yet assigned
MJ 10061 benzbromarone
MJ 12,175-170 tiprinast meglumine
MJ 12,880-1 tipropidil HCl
MJ 13,105-1 bucindolol HCl
MJ 13401-1-3 fenprinast HCl
MJ 13,754-1 nefazodone HCl
MJ 1986 indriline HCl
MJ 1987 mesuprine HCl
MJ 1988 quazodine
MJ 1992 soterenol HCl

**MJ 1998** metalol HCl
**MJ 1999** sotalol HCl
**MJ 4309-1** oxybutynin chloride
**MJ 505** phenyramidol HCl
**MJ 9022-1** buspirone HCl
**MJ 9067-1** encainide HCl
**MJ 9184-1** zinterol HCl
**MJF 10,938** xipamide
**MJF 11567-3** cefadroxil
**MJF-12264** tegafur
**MJF 12637** suloctidil
**MJF 9325** ifosfamide
**MK-0462** rizatriptan benzoate
**MK-0677** ibutamoren mesylate
**MK-0681** trientine HCl
**MK-0699** rofecoxib
**MK-0787** imipenem
**MK-0936** abamectin
**MK-0991** caspofungin acetate
**MK-130 (as the base)** cyclobenza-
    prine HCl
**MK-188** zeranol
**MK-196** indacrinone
**MK-208** famotidine
**MK-217** alendronate sodium
**MK-233** dexibuprofen lysine
**MK-240** protriptyline HCl
**MK-250** emylcamate
**MK-329** devazepide
**MK-341** tranilast
**MK-351** methyldopa
**MK-360** thiabendazole
**MK-366** norfloxacin
**MK-383** tirofiban HCl
**MK-397** eprinomectin
**MK-401** clorsulon
**MK-417** sezolamide HCl
**MK-422** enalaprilat
**MK-458** naxagolide HCl
**MK-462** rizatriptan benzoate
**MK-476** montelukast sodium
**MK-507** dorzolamide HCl
**MK-521** lisinopril
**MK 57** methyldesorphine
**MK-591** quiflapon sodium
**MK-595** ethacrynic acid
**MK-621** efrotomycin
**MK-639** indinavir sulfate
**MK-678** seglitide acetate
**MK-733** simvastatin

**MK790** levomethadyl acetate HCl
**MK-791** cilastatin sodium
**MK-793** diltiazem maleate
**MK-801** dizocilpine maleate
**MK-803** lovastatin
**MK-869** generic not yet assigned
**MK-906** finasteride
**MK-966** rofecoxib
**MK-A462** rizatriptan sulfate
**MKC-442** generic not yet assigned
**ML-1024** theofibrate
**ML 1034** celucloral
**ML-1129** beraprost sodium
**ML-1229** beraprost
**MO-1255** encyprate
**MO-911** pargyline HCl
**MP-10013** iogulamide
**MP-1051** silodrate
**MP-1177** gadoversetamide
**MP-1196** versetamide
**MP-1554** technetium Tc 99m furifos-
    min
**MP-1727** indium In 111 pentetreotide
**MP 2032** iocarmic acid
**MP 2032-meglumine** iocarmate
    meglumine
**MP-271** iosefamic acid
**MP 302 (with ioxaglate sodium)**
    ioxaglate meglumine
**MP 328** ioversol
**MP-351** generic not yet assigned
**MP 4006** albumin, aggregated
**MP 4018** stannous pyrophosphate
**MP-537** iomethin I 125
**MP-537** iomethin I 131
**MP-600** betiatide
**MP-6026** ioglucol
**MP-620** iocetamic acid
**MP 7010** stannous sulfur colloid
**MP-8000** ioglucomide
**MPV-1248** atipamezole
**MPV-1440** dexmedetomidine
**MPV-253 AII** detomidine HCl
**MPV-785** medetomidine HCl
**MR6S4** sevoflurane
**MRL 38** hexadiline
**MRL-41** clomiphene citrate
**MRP-10** pentetate calcium trisodium
    Yb 169
**MS-325** generic not yet assigned

**MSI-78** pexiganan acetate
**MSL-109** sevirumab
**MTS 263** tropenziline bromide
**MUC-1** generic not yet assigned
**MX-6** generic not yet assigned
**MY-25 (as bitartrate)** metergotamine
**MY-33-7 (as HCl)** lotucaine
**MY-5116** repirinast
**MYC 8003** mocimycin
**MZ-144** rimazolium metilsulfate
**N-0252** laurocapram
**N-0923** generic not yet assigned
**N-137** carbetimer
**N-3** methetoin
**N-399** xenytropium bromide
**N-553 (as HCl)** tolperisone
**N-7009** flupentixol
**N-7020** meprotixol
**N-714** chlorprothixene
**N-746** clopenthixol
**NA-119** bromamid
**NA 274** bromhexine HCl
**NA-66** pimeclone
**NAB 365** clenbuterol
**NASH** borocaptate sodium B 10
**NAT-327** trimoxamine HCl
**NAT-333** fenspiride HCl
**NB 68** dacuronium bromide
**NC-123** mesoridazine
**NC 1264** thonzonium bromide
**NC 150** phenazopyridine HCl
**NC-1968** fungimycin
**NC-7197** esproquin HCl
**NCNU** pentamustine
**ND 50** octopamine
**NDC 0082-4155** daunorubicin HCl
**NDR 263** propenzolate HCl
**NDR 304** ethyl dibunate
**NDR-5061A** aletamine HCl
**NDR-5523A** trimoxamine HCl
**NDR-5998A** fenspiride HCl
**NE-10064** azimilide dihydrochloride
**NE 11740** tebufelone
**NE-1530** generic not yet assigned
**NE-19550** olvanil
**NE-58095** risedronate sodium
**NE 97221** piridronate sodium
**NF-1010** nifurdazil
**NF-1088** nifurquinazol
**NF-1120** nifurimide

**NF-1425** furazolium tartrate
**NF-161** nifursemizone
**NF-246** nifuradene
**NF-602** levofuraltadone
**NF-71** nifurmerone
**NF-84** nifuraldezone
**NF-902 (as HCl)** levofuraltadone
**NF-963** furazolium chloride
**NG-29** generic not yet assigned
**NIB** nabitan HCl
**NIH 2933** dimepheptanol
**NIH 7574** benzethidine
**NIH 7607** etonitazene
**NIH 7667** noracymethadol HCl
**NIH 7672** methopholine
**NIH 8805** buprenorphine HCl
**NK 1006** bekanamycin
**NK 204** basifungin
**NK-631** peplomycin sulfate
**NKK-105** malotilate
**NKT-01** gusperimus trihydrochloride
**NMP-22** generic not yet assigned
**NNC-05-0328** tiagabine HCl
**NO-05-0328** tiagabine HCl
**NPAP** prajmalium bitartrate
**NPT 15392** nosantine
**NS-2710** generic not yet assigned
**NSC-266046** oxaliplatin
**NSC 613792** lodenosine
**NSC 659772** alitretinoin
**NSD 1055** brocresine
**Nu-1779** betaprodine
**Nu-1932** betameprodine
**NU-2121** nicotinyl alcohol
**NU-445** sulfisoxazole diolamine
**NXX-066** quilostigmine
**NY-198** lomefloxacin HCl
**ODA 914** demoxytocin
**OGT-918** generic not yet assigned
**l-OHP** oxaliplatin
**OK-B7** generic not yet assigned
**OM 401** generic not yet assigned
**OM-977** etaminile
**OMDS** dipyrithione
**OMS No 1825** azamethiphos
**ONYX-015** generic not yet assigned
**OP 21-23** parnaparin sodium
**OPC-1085** carteolol HCl
**OPC-13013** cilostazol
**OPC-14117** generic not yet assigned

OPC-14597 aripiprazole
OPC-17116 grepafloxacin HCl
OPC-18790 toborinone
OPC-21 cilostazol
OPC-31 aripiprazole
OPC-8212 vesnarinone
(−)-OR-1259 levosimendan
OR-611 entacapone
ORF 10131 norgestimate
ORF 11676 nalmefene
ORF 15244 thymopentin
ORF 15817 edoxudine
ORF 15927 rioprostil
ORF 16600 bemarinone HCl
ORF 17070 histrelin
ORF 18704 pelretin
ORF 20257 doretinel
ORF 20485 tepoxalin
ORF 22164 atosiban
ORF 22867 bemoradan
ORF-8063 triflubazam
ORF 9326 nisterime acetate
ORG 10172 danaparoid sodium
ORG 2969 desogestrel
ORG 3236 etonogestrel
ORG 3770 mirtazapine
Org 4428 beloxepin
Org 6216 rimexolone
ORG7417 resocortol butyrate
Org 817 epimestrol
ORG 9426 rocuronium bromide
Org 9487 rapacuronium bromide
Org GB 94 mianserin HCl
Org NA 97 pancuronium bromide
ORG NC 45 vecuronium bromide
Org OD 14 tibolone
OST-577 generic not yet assigned
P 071 cetirizine HCl
P-1011 dicloxacillin sodium
P-113 saralasin acetate
P-12 oxacillin sodium
P-1306 glyparamide
P-1496 zeranol
P-1560 taleranol
P-165 azaserine
P-1742 fluperolone acetate
P-1779 althiazide
P-1888 isosulfan blue
P-2105 epithiazide
P-248 levopropylcillin potassium

P-25 cloxacillin sodium
P-2525 polythiazide
P-2530 methalthiazide
P-2647 benzquinamide
P-280 bibapcitide
P-286 ioxaglic acid
P-301 hydroxyphenamate
P-3232 somfasepor
P-3693A doxepin HCl
P-3895 somfasepor
P-3896 guanisoquin sulfate
P-4125 isosulfan blue
P-414 generic not yet assigned
P-4385B clothixamide maleate
P-4599 cidoxepin HCl
P-463 fenamole
P-4657 B thiothixene
P-50 ampicillin
P-5227 pinoxepin HCl
P53 tetrofosmin
P-54 generic not yet assigned
P-5604 loteprednol etabonate
P-638 puromycin
P 7 lauroguadine
P-71 lycetamine
P 71-0129 fendosal
P-7138 nifurpirinol
P 720549 isoxepac
P-748 generic not yet assigned
P 76 2494A fluradoline HCl
P 76 2543 dazepinil HCl
P 78 3522 brocrinat
P79 3913 neflumozide HCl
P829 depreotide
P83 6029A velnacrine maleate
PA-144 plicamycin
PA-1648 rifalazil
PAA-3854 clamoxyquin HCl
PAA-701 bialamicol HCl
PAM-MR-1165 acedapsone
PAM-MR-807-23a cycloguanil pamoate
PAMN (as methonitrate) prampine
PASIT glyprothiazol
PAT fenamole
PB-005 dehydroepiandrosterone sulfate
PB 89 (as HCl) fominoben
p-BIDA butilfenin
PC1020 acetate prezatide copper acetate

Code Names

**PC-1421** piperacetazine
**PC-603** iproclozide
**PD 107779** enoxacin
**PD-110843** zonisamide
**PD 81565** pentostatin
**PD 90,695-73** dezaguanine mesylate
**PD-93** piromidic acid
**PDB** prifinium bromide
**PE1-1** tuvirumab
**pentapeptide DSDPR** pentigetide
**PF-26** mepramidil
**PFA-186** salicylate meglumine
**PG 430** febuverine
**PG-501** mazaticol
**PH 218** edogestrone
**pierrel-TQ 86** azipramine HCl
**PIXY321** milodistim
**PK 10169** enoxaparin
**PM 1807** fenimide
**PM-185184** secnidazole
**PM-1952** fenacetinol
**PM-3944** flucetorex
**PM-671** ethosuximide
**PMD-387** crilvastatin
**PN 200-110** isradipine
**PNU-140690E** tipranavir disodium
**PNU-180638E** almotriptan malate
**POLI 67** tetrydamine
**POR 8** ornipressin
**PP 563** cyhalothrin
**PPI-002** generic not yet assigned
**PPI-149** abarelix
**PPRT-321** generic not yet assigned
**PR-0818-156A** verilopam HCl
**PR-122** redox phenytoin
**PR-225** redox acyclovir
**PR-239** redox penicillin G
**PR-320** molecusol & carbamazepine
**PR-3847** teroxalene HCl
**PR-741-976A** somantadine HCl
**PR-870-714A** veradoline HCl
**PR-877-530L** flavodilol maleate
**PR 879-317A** oxamisole HCl
**PR 934-423A** remacemide HCl
**PR-G 138-CL (as HCl)**
   ciclosidomine
**PRO-542** generic not yet assigned
**protease 1** brinolase
**PS-1286** pararosaniline pamoate

**PS 2383** trimetozine
**PSC-833** generic not yet assigned
**PT-14** generic not yet assigned
**PT-9** betahistine HCl
**PU-239** benzilonium bromide
**PY 108-068** darodipine
**PZ 1511** carpipramine dihydrochloride
**PZ68** pentosan polysulfate sodium
**Q-12** technetium Tc 99m furifosmin
**QB-1** cloquinozine
**QS-21** generic not yet assigned
**QZ-2** methaqualone
**R 10.100** ethonam nitrate
**R106-1** basifungin
**R 10,948** diamocaine cyclamate
**R 11,333** bromperidol
**R-121919** generic not yet assigned
**R 12,563 (as HCl)** dexamisole
**R 12,564** levamisole HCl
**R 1303** carbofenotion
**R-13423** dicloxacillin
**R 13,558** fetoxylate HCl
**R-13,672** haloperidol decanoate
**R 1406** phenoperidine
**R-148** methaqualone
**R 14,827** econazole nitrate
**R 14,889** miconazole nitrate
**R 14,950** flunarizine HCl
**R 15,403 (as HCl)** difenoxin
**R-15,454 (as nitrate salt)** isoconazole
**R 15,556** orconazole nitrate
**R 1575** cinnarizine
**R 15,889** lorcainide HCl
**R-1625** haloperidol
**R 16,341** penfluridol
**R 16,470 (as HCl)** dexetimide
**R 1658** moperone
**R 1707** glafenine
**R 17,147** cyclobendazole
**R 17,635** mebendazole
**R 17,889** flubendazole
**R 17,934** nocodazole
**R 18,553** loperamide HCl
**R 1881** metribolone
**R 18,910** fluperamide
**R 1929** azaperone
**R 19,317** rodocaine
**R 2028** fluanisone
**R 2113** desoximetasone
**R 2159** anisopirol

**R 2167** fluanisone
**R 22,700 (as HCl)** rodocaine
**R 23,050** salantel
**R 2323** gestrinone
**R 23,633** fludazonium chloride
**R 23,979** enilconazole
**R 2453** demegestone
**R-2498** trifluperidol
**R-25,061** suprofen
**R-25,160** cliprofen
**R 25,540** imafen HCl
**R 25,831 (as the free base)** carnidazole
**R 26,412** sulnidazole
**R 27,500** sepazonium chloride
**R 28,096 (as HCl)** carnidazole
**R 2858** moxestrol
**R-28,644** azaconazole
**R 28,930** fluspiperone
**R 2962** amiperone
**R 29,764** clopimozide
**R 29,860** nitramisole HCl
**R 30,730** sufentanil
**R 31,520** closantel
**R 3248** aceperone
**R 33,204** declenperone
**R 3345** pipamperone
**R 3365** piritramide
**R 33,799** carfentanil citrate
**R 33800** sufentanil citrate
**R 33,812** domperidone
**R 34,000** doconazole
**R 34,009** milenperone
**R 34,301** halopemide
**R-34,803** etibendazole
**R 34,995** lofentanil oxalate
**R 35,443** oxatomide
**R 38,198** buterizine
**R3827** abarelix
**R 39,209** alfentanil HCl
**R 39,500** parconazole HCl
**R 3959** clometacin
**R 4082** propyperone
**R 41,400** ketoconazole
**R-41,468** ketanserin
**R-42,470** terconazole
**R-4263** fentanyl citrate
**R 4318** floctafenine
**R 43,512** astemizole
**R 4444** duometacin

**R-45,486** flumeridone
**R-4584** benperidol
**R-46,541** bromperidol decanoate
**R 46,846** tubulozole HCl
**R 4714** oxiperomide
**R-47,465** pirenperone
**R-4749** droperidol
**R 48** chlornaphazine
**R 4845** bezitramide
**R 5046** cinperene
**R 50,547** levocabastine HCl
**R 50 970** metrenperone
**R 51 163** tameridone
**R 51,211** itraconazole
**R-51,469** mioflazine HCl
**R 5147** spiperone
**R 516** cinnarizine
**R-51,619** cisapride
**R 5188** spiroxatrine
**R-52** mannosulfan
**R 52,245** setoperone
**R-53,200** altanserin tartrate
**R 5385** acoxatrine
**R 54,718** transcainide
**R-548** tricetamide
**R 55104** erbulozole
**R 55,667** ritanserin
**R 5808** spiramide
**R58425** loperamide oxide
**R 58735** sabeluzole
**R 60844** irtemazole
**R 610** racemoramide
**R 6109** spirilene
**R 6218** fluspirilene
**R 6238** pimozide
**R62,690** clazuril
**R 62 818** lorcinadol
**R 6438** antazonite
**R64,433** diclazuril
**R 64 766** risperidone
**R 64947** noberastine
**R65,824** nebivolol
**R 661** buzepide metiodide
**R 66905** saperconazole
**R 67408** fenclofenac
**R 68070** ridogrel
**R 72063** loreclezole
**R 7242** difluanine HCl
**R 7464** propoxate
**R 75231** draflazine

**R 75251** liarozole HCl
**R 77975** pirodavir
**R 7904** lidoflazine
**R 79598** ocaperidone
**R 798** rimiterol hydrobromide
**R 8025** antienite
**R-803** furaprofen
**R 805** nimesulide
**R 8141** antienite
**R-8193** antafenite
**R 8284** proclonol
**R 8299** tetramisole HCl
**R-830** prifelone
**R-830T** prifelone
**R-835** ibafloxacin
**R-837** imiquimod
**R 83842** vorozole
**R 85246** liarozole fumarate
**R-87926** lubeluzole
**R-89439** loviride
**R 91,274** alniditan dihydrochloride
**R 9298** seperidol HCl
**RA-8** dipyridamole
**RA-C-384** iodocetylic acid I 123
**RBC-CD4** generic not yet assigned
**RC-160** vapreotide
**RC-167** niceverine
**RC-172** aldioxa
**RC-173** alcloxa
**RC-27109** nifuroxazide
**RC 61-91** ifenprodil
**RCH 314** benhepazone
**RCM 258** fepentolic acid
**RD 11654** ibufenac
**RD 17345** fluprofen
**RD 2801** pyritidium bromide
**Rd 292** fenpentadiol
**RD 328** pasiniazid
**RD 406** cyprodenate
**RD 9338 (as HCl)** norbudrine
**Rec 15 0122** nifurpipone
**Rec 15/1476** fenticonazole nitrate
**Rec 7/0267** dimefline HCl
**REV 3659-(S)** pivopril
**REV 6000A** delapril HCl
**RFS-2000** 9-nitrocamptothecin
**RG 12561** dalvastatin
**RG 201** generic not yet assigned
**RG 270** iomeglamic acid
**RG 83606** diltiazem HCl

**RGG0853,E1A** generic not yet assigned
**RGH 1106** pipecuronium bromide
**rgp160** generic not yet assigned
**rgp160 MN** generic not yet assigned
**RGW-2938** prinoxodan
**RH-32,565** uredofos
**RH-565** uredofos
**RHC 2871** eclazolast
**RHC 2906** flordipine
**RHC 3659-(S)** pivopril
**RHC 3988** quazolast
**rhuTNFR:Fc** etanercept
**RI-64** pifexole
**Riker 52G** aprotinin
**Riker 594** sulthiame
**Riker 595** butaperazine
**Riker 601** triaziquone
**RIT 1140** apicycline
**RJW 49004** cedelizumab
**RJW 60235** becaplermin
**r-metHuG-CSF** filgrastim
**RMI 10,482A** metizoline HCl
**RMI 16,238** eterobarb
**RMI 16,289** enclomiphene
**RMI 16,312** zuclomiphene
**RMI 80,029** elantrine
**RMI 8090DJ** quindecamine acetate
**RMI 81,182EF** cilobamine mesylate
**RMI 81,968** medroxalol
**RMI 81,968 A** medroxalol HCl
**RMI 83,027** rolicyprine
**RMI 83,047** ambuside
**RMI 9,384A** desipramine HCl
**RMI 9918** terfenadine
**RMP-7** generic not yet assigned
**Ro 01-6794/706** dextrorphan HCl
**Ro 03-7355/000** avizafone
**Ro 03-8799** pimonidazole
**Ro 09-1978/000** capecitabine
**Ro 10-1670/000** acitretin
**Ro 10-6338** bumetanide
**Ro107-9070/194** valganciclovir HCl
**Ro 10-9070** amdinocillin
**Ro 10-9071** amdinocillin pivoxil
**Ro 10-9359** etretinate
**Ro 11-1163/000** moclobemide
**Ro 11-1430** motretinide
**Ro 11-1781/023** tiapamil HCl
**Ro 12-0068/000** tenoxicam

Ro 13-5057 aniracetam
Ro 13-6438/006 quazinone
RO 13-8996 oxiconazole nitrate
Ro-13-9297 lornoxicam
Ro 13-9904 ceftriaxone sodium
Ro 14-4767/000 amorolfine
Ro 14-9706/000 sumarotene
RO 1-5155 nicotinyl alcohol
Ro 15-1570/000 etarotene
Ro 15-1788/000 flumazenil
Ro 16-6028/000 bretazenil
Ro 1-6794 dextrorphan
Ro 17-2301/006 carumonam sodium
Ro 18-0647/002 orlistat
Ro 1-9334/19 dehydroemetine
Ro 1-9569 tetrabenazine
Ro 19-6327/000 lazabemide
Ro 20-5720/000 carprofen
Ro 21-0702 flurocitabine
Ro 21-3981/001 midazolam maleate
Ro 21-3981/003 midazolam HCl
Ro 21-5535 calcitriol
Ro 21-5998 mefloquine
Ro 21-5998/001 mefloquine HCl
Ro 21-6937/000 trimoprostil
Ro 21-8837/001 estramustine phosphate sodium
Ro 22-1319/003 piquindone HCl
Ro 22-2296/000 estramustine
Ro 22-3747/000 tiacrilast
Ro 22-3747/007 tiacrilast sodium
Ro 22-7796 cifenline
Ro 22-7796/001 cifenline succinate
Ro 22-8181 interferon alfa-2a
Ro 22-9000 alfaprostol
Ro 2-2985 lasalocid
Ro 23-0731/000 sedecamycin
Ro 23-3544/000 ablukast
Ro 23-3544/001 ablukast sodium
Ro 23-6019 teceleukin
Ro 23-6240/000 fleroxacin
Ro 2-3773 clidinium bromide
Ro 24-2027/000 zalcitabine
Ro 24-5913 cinalukast
Ro 24-7375 dacliximab
Ro 24-7472/000 cdodckin alfa
Ro 2-9757 fluorouracil
Ro 2-9915 flucytosine
Ro-31-2848/006 cilazapril
Ro 31-3113 cilazaprilat

Ro-31-3948/000 romazarit
Ro 31-8959 saquinavir
Ro 31-8959/003 saquinavir mesylate
Ro 4-0403 chlorprothixene
Ro 40-5967/001 mibefradil dihydrochloride
Ro 40-7592 tolcapone
Ro 4-1544-6 sodium stibocaptate
Ro 4-1778/1 methopholine
Ro 4-2130 sulfamethoxazole
Ro 42-1611 arteflene
Ro 4-3780 isotretinoin
RO 4-3816 alcuronium chloride
Ro 4-4393 sulfadoxine
Ro 4-4602 benserazide
Ro 44-9883/000 lamifiban
Ro 45-2081 lenercept
Ro 4-5282 mefenorex HCl
Ro 4-5360 nitrazepam
Ro 4-6467/1 procarbazine HCl
Ro 46-6240/000 napsagatran
Ro 47-0203/029 bosentan
Ro 48347 trengestone
Ro 48-3657/001 sibrafiban
Ro 5-0690 chlordiazepoxide HCl
Ro 5-2092 demoxepam
Ro 5-2807 diazepam
Ro 5-3059 nitrazepam
RO 5-3307/1 debrisoquin sulfate
Ro 5-3350 bromazepam
Ro 5-4023 clonazepam
Ro 5-4200 flunitrazepam
Ro 5-4556 medazepam HCl
Ro 5-4645/010 coumermycin sodium
Ro 5-6901 flurazepam HCl
Ro 5-9110/1 dorastine HCl
Ro 5-9754 ormetoprim
Ro 64-0796 generic not yet assigned
Ro 6-4563 glibornuride
Ro 7-0207 ornidazole
Ro 7-0582 misonidazole
Ro 7-1554 ipronidazole
Ro 7-4488/1 cuprimyxin
RP 12222 penmesterol
RP 13057 (as the base) daunorubicin HCl
RP 13607 clotioxone
RP 14539 secnidazole
RP 16091 metiazinic acid
RP 19552 pipotiazine palmitate

Code Names

**R.P. 19,583** ketoprofen
**R.P. 20 578** bamnidazole
**RP 22,050 HCl** zorubicin HCl
**RP 22410** glisoxepide
**RP 2254** glyprothiazol
**RP 2259** glybuthiazol
**rp24** generic not yet assigned
**RP 2512 (as isethionate)** pentamidine
**RP 27267** zopiclone
**RP 2921** aminothiazole
**RP 2987** diethazine HCl
**RP 31264** suriclone
**RP 3854** melarsoprol
**RP 4763 (as sodium salt)** difetarsone
**RP 5171** proadifen HCl
**RP 5337** spiramycin
**RP 54274** rulizole
**RP 54476** dalfopristin
**RP 54563** enoxaparin sodium
**RP-54780** oxaliplatin
**RP 56976** docetaxel
**RP 57669** quinupristin
**RP 60475** intoplicine
**RP 62203** fanserin
**RP 62955** pagoclone
**RP 64305** ebastine
**RP 6484** etymemazine HCl
**RP 6847** oxomemazine
**RP 6870** inproquone
**RP 7044** methotrimeprazine
**RP 7204** cyamemazine
**RP 7293** pristinamycin
**RP 73401** piclamilast
**RP 7891** glybuzole
**RP 8595** dimetridazole
**RP 8823** metronidazole
**RP 8909** periciazine
**RP 9159** perimetazine
**RP 9671** nosiheptide
**RP 9778** protionamide
**RP 9921** aprotinin
**RP 9955** melarsonyl potassium
**RPI-4610** generic not yet assigned
**RR No. 32705** rutamycin
**RS-079070/194** valganciclovir HCl
**RS-10085-197** moexipril HCl
**RS-11988** laidlomycin propionate
   potassium
**RS-1301** delmadinone acetate
**RS-1320** flunisolide acetate

**RS 15385** delequamine
**RS-15385-197** delequamine HCl
**RS-21361** imiloxan HCl
**RS-21592** ganciclovir
**RS-21592 sodium** ganciclovir sodium
**RS-21607-197** azalanstat dihydro-
   chloride
**R&S 218-M** alletorphine
**RS-2208** amadinone acetate
**RS-2252** flucloronide
**RS-2362** procinonide
**RS-2386** ciprocinonide
**RS 25259** palonosetron HCl
**RS-26306** ganirelix acetate
**RS-3268R** nandrolone cyclotate
**RS-3540** naproxen
**RS-35887** butoconazole nitrate
**RS-35887-00-10-3** butoconazole
   nitrate
**RS-35909-00-00-0** ticabesone propio-
   nate
**RS-3650** naproxen sodium
**RS-3694R** cormethasone acetate
**RS-37326** anirolac
**RS-37449** temurtide
**RS-3999** flunisolide
**RS-4034** naproxol
**RS-40584** flumoxonide
**RS-40974-00-00-0** tiopinac
**RS-43179** lonapalene
**RS-43285** ranolazine HCl
**RS-4464** triclonide
**RS-44872** sulconazole nitrate
**RS-44872-00-10-3** sulconazole nitrate
**RS-4691** cloprednol
**RS-49014** tazifylline HCl
**R&S 5205-M** homprenorphine
**RS-61443** mycophenolate mofetil
**RS-61443-190** mycophenolate
   mofetil HCl
**RS-6245** tazolol HCl
**RS-6818** xanoxate sodium
**RS-68439** detirelix acetate
**RS-69216** nicardipine HCl
**RS-69216-XX-07-0** nicardipine HCl
**RS-7337** tixanox
**RS-82856** lixazinone sulfate
**RS-82917-030** tifurac sodium
**RS-84043** fenprostalene
**RS-84135** enprostil

RS-85446-007 timobesone acetate
RS-87476-000 lifarizine
RS-8858 oxfendazole
RS-9390 prostalene
RS-94991-298 nafarelin acetate
RSR-13 generic not yet assigned
RU 15060 tiaprofenic acid
Ru 15750 floctafenine
RU-1697 trenbolon acetate
RU-19110 halofuginone hydrobromide
RU-2267 altrenogest
RU 2323 gestrinone
RU 23908 nilutamide
RU 24756 cefotaxime sodium
RU 27987 trimegestone
RU 28965 roxithromycin
RU35926 milameline HCl
RU 38486 mifepristone
RU 38882 inocoterone acetate
RU 44570 trandolapril
RU 486 mifepristone
RU 882 inocoterone acetate
RU 965 roxithromycin
RWJ 10131 norgestimate
RWJ 15817 edoxudine
RWJ 15927 rioprostil
RWJ 16600 bemarinone HCl
RWJ-17021 topiramate
RWJ 17070 histrelin
RWJ 18704 pelretin
RWJ 20257 doretinel
RWJ 20485 tepoxalin
RWJ 21757 loroxibine
RWJ 22164 atosiban
RWJ 24517 carsatrin succinate
RWJ 24834 linarotene
RWJ-25213 levofloxacin
RWJ 26251 cladribine
RWJ 28299 immune globulin intrave-
nous pentetate
RWJ 37796 mazapertine succinate
RX 6029-M HCl buprenorphine HCl
Rx 67408 fenclofenac
RX77989 pentamorphone
R-(–)-YM-12617 tamsulosin HCl
S-041 gadodiamide
S-043 sprodiamide
S 10036 fotemustine
S-1210 bietaserpine
S-1320 budesonide

S 1530 nimetazepam
S-16820 prifelone
S-210 morsuximide
S-222 ditazole
S-2395 tertatolol
S-2539F phenothrin
S-25930 ibafloxacin
S26308 imiquimod
S 314 fusafungine
S 4105 medibazine
S 5614 HCl dexfenfluramine HCl
S-62 chlorphentermine HCl
S 7 fenticlor
S 73 4118 piretanide
S 77 0777 prednicarbate
S-940 naftalofos
S-9490 perindopril
S-9490-3 perindopril erbumine
S-9780 perindoprilat
SA-267 dipenine bromide
SB-202026-A sabcomeline HCl
SB-209247 ticolubant
SB 209509-AX frovatriptan succinate
SB 209763 felvizumab
SB-210396 generic not yet assigned
SB-214857-A lotrafiban HCl
SB-217969 generic not yet assigned
SB-223030 idoxifene
SB 7505 ibopamine
SBW-22 ketorfanol
SC 10363 megestrol acetate
SC 11585 oxandrolone
SC 11800 ethynodiol diacetate
SC-12350 nitralamine HCl
SC-12937 azacosterol HCl
SC-13504 ropizine
SC-13957 disopyramide phosphate
SC-14207 metogest
SC-14266 canrenoate potassium
SC-16148 silandrone
SC 1749 (as sodium salt) menbutone
SC-18862 aspartame
SC-19198 methynodiol diacetate
SC-21009 norgestomet
SC-23992 prorenoate potassium
SC-25469 pinadoline
SC-26100 difenoximide HCl
SC-26304 dicirenone
SC-26438 pirolazamide
SC-26714 mexrenoate potassium

**SC-27123** octriptyline phosphate
**SC-27166** nufenoxole
**SC-27761** pranolium chloride
**SC-29333** misoprostol
**SC-31828** disobutamide
**SC-32642** metronidazole HCl
**SC-32840** oxagrelate
**SC-33643** bemitradine
**SC-33963** reclazepam
**SC-34301** enisoprost
**SC-35135** edifolone acetate
**SC-36602** actisomide
**SC-37681** gemeprost
**SC-38390** zinoconazole HCl
**SC-39026** lodelaben
**SC-40230** bidisomide
**SC-4642** norethynodrel
**SC-47111** lomefloxacin HCl
**SC-47111A** lomefloxacin
**SC-47111B** lomefloxacin mesylate
**SC-48834** remiprostol
**SC-49483** generic not yet assigned
**SC-52151** telinavir
**SC-52458** forasartan
**SC-54684A** xemilofiban HCl
**SC-55389A** droxinavir HCl
**SC-55494** daniplestim
**SC-57099B** orbofiban acetate
**SC-58635** celecoxib
**SC-59046** deracoxib
**SC-66110** eplerenone
**SC-7031** disopyramide
**SC-7294** propetandrol
**SC-7525** bolandiol dipropionate
**SC-9376** canrenone
**SC-9880** flurogestone acetate
**SCE-1365 (Takeda) (base)** cefmenoxime HCl
**Sch 1000-Br-monohydrate** ipratropium bromide
**Sch 10144** tolnaftate
**Sch 10159** triclofos sodium
**Sch 10304** clonixin
**Sch 10595** bupicomide
**Sch 10649** azatadine maleate
**Sch 11460** betamethasone dipropionate
**Sch 11572** meclorisone dibutyrate
**Sch 11973** tosifen
**Sch 12041** halazepam
**Sch 12149** pazoxide

**Sch 12169** closiramine aceturate
**Sch 12650** dazadrol maleate
**Sch 12679** trepipam maleate
**Sch 12707** clonixeril
**Sch 13166 D fumarate** domazoline fumarate
**Sch 13430.2KH$_2$PO$_4$** megalomicin potassium phosphate
**Sch 13475 sulfate** sisomicin sulfate
**Sch 13521** flutamide
**Sch 13949W Sulfate** albuterol sulfate
**Sch 14342** betamicin sulfate
**Sch 14714** flunixin
**Sch 14714 meglumine** flunixin meglumine
**Sch 14947** rosaramicin
**Sch 14947.NaH$_2$PO$_4$** rosaramicin sodium phosphate
**Sch 14947 stearate** rosaramicin stearate
**Sch 15280** azanator maleate
**Sch 15427** carmantadine
**Sch 15507** dopamantine
**Sch 15698** fletazepam
**Sch 15719W** labetalol HCl
**Sch 16134** quazepam
**Sch 16524** repromicin
**Sch 17894** rosaramicin propionate
**Sch 18020W** beclomethasone dipropionate
**Sch 18667** rosaramicin butyrate
**Sch 19741** picotrin diolamine
**Sch 19927** dilevalol HCl
**Sch 20569** netilmicin sulfate
**Sch 21420** isepamicin
**Sch 21480** tioxidazole
**Sch 22219** alclometasone dipropionate
**Sch 22591** pentisomicin
**Sch 25298** florfenicol
**Sch 2544** cycliramine maleate
**Sch 28316Z** indenolol
**Sch 29851** loratadine
**Sch 30500** interferon alfa-2b
**Sch 31353** dexamethasone acefurate
**Sch 32088** mometasone furoate
**Sch 32481** netobimin
**Sch 33844** spirapril HCl
**Sch 33861** spiraprilat
**SCH 34117** desloratadine
**Sch 3444** parapenzolate bromide

**Sch 35852** cisconazole
**SCH 39166** ecopipam HCl
**Sch 39300** molgramostim
**Sch 39720** ceftibuten
**SCH 40054 HCl** nemazoline HCl
**Sch 4358** meprednisone
**Sch 4831** betamethasone
**Sch 4855** pseudoephedrine sulfate
**Sch 6620** prednazate
**Sch 6673** acetophenazine maleate
**Sch 6783** diazoxide
**Sch 7056** acrisorcin
**Sch 9384** oxymetazoline HCl
**Sch 9724** gentamicin sulfate
**Scha-306** cintazone
**SCL-70** alofilcon A
**SCT 1** salcatonin
**SCTZ (as edisylate)** clomethiazole
**SCY-Er** erythromycin salnacedin
**SD 1223-01** trazitiline
**SD 1248-17 (as HCl)** tropatepine
**SD 14112** sulclamide
**SD 149-01** feneritrol
**SD 15803** vincofos
**SD 17102** meticrane
**SD 1750** dichlorvos
**SD 2102-18** acrocinonide
**SD 2124-01** procinolol
**SD 25** dicarfen
**SD 270-07 (as succinate)** oxaprazine
**SD 270-31 (as disuccinate)** oxaflumazine
**SD 271-12** clobenzorex
**SD 27115 (as cyclamate)** furfenorex
**SD 286-03** cimemoxin
**SD 7859** clofenvinfos
**SDZ 215-811** pentetreotide
**SDZ 215-811s** pentetreotide
**SDZ ILE 964** muplestim
**SDZ MSL 109** sevirumab
**SDZ OST 577** tuvirumab
**SE 1702** gliclazide
**SeHCAT** tauroselcholic acid
**SERM 3** arzoxifene HCl
**SF 86-327** terbinafine
**SF-R11** bovactant
**SG-75** nicorandil
**SGD 301-76** oxiconazole nitrate
**SGP 3** unifocon A
**SH 100** oxapium iodide

**SH 1040** gestaclone
**SH 1051** glicetanile sodium
**SH 2.1139/H 248 AB** ioxotrizoic acid
**SH 213 AB** iotroxic acid
**SH 240** moxnidazole
**SH 263** droxacin sodium
**SH 3.1168** gliflumide
**SH 567** methenolone acetate
**SH 582** gestonorone caproate
**SH 601** methenolone enanthate
**SH 714** cyproterone acetate
**SH 717** glymidine sodium
**SH 723** mesterolone
**SH 741** clomegestone acetate
**SH 742** fluocortolone
**SH 770** fluocortolone caproate
**SH 818** clocortolone acetate
**SH 863** clocortolone pivalate
**SH 926** iodamide
**SH 968** diflucortolone pivalate
**SH B 331** gestodene
**SH E 199** etoformin HCl
**SH G 318 AB** sermetacin
**SH H 200 AB** ioglicic acid
**SH H 239 AB** ioseric acid
**SH K 203** fluocortin butyl
**SH L 451 A** gadopentetate dimeglumine
**SIB-1508Y** generic not yet assigned
**SJ 1977** methixene HCl
**SK&F 101468-A** ropinirole HCl
**SK&F 102,362** nilvadipine
**SK&F 104353-Q** pobilukast edamine
**SKF 105657** episteride
**SK&F 106615-A2** atiprimod dihydrochloride
**SF&F 106615-I2** atiprimod dimaleate
**SK&F 108566** eprosartan
**SK&F 108566-J** eprosartan mesylate
**SK&F 110679** generic not yet assigned
**SK&F 12866** clorethate
**SKF 13338** ampyrimine
**SK&F 13364-A** thyromedan HCl
**SK&F 1340** dimefadane
**SK&F 14287** idoxuridine
**SK&F 14336** clomacran phosphate
**SK&F 15601A** toliodium chloride
**SKF 16046** anisacril
**SK&F 18,667** poloxalene

SK&F 1995 dicloralurea
SKF 20716 periciazine
SK&F 2208 hetaflur
SK&F 24529 lobendazole
SKF 2599 doxenitoin
SK&F 28175 fluotracen HCl
SK&F 29044 parbendazole
SK&F 30310 oxibendazole
SK&F 3050 cortodoxone
SKF 33134-A amiodarone
SK&F 38094 dectaflur
SK&F 38095 olaflur
SK&F 39162 auranofin
SK&F 39186 amicloral
SK&F 40383 carbuterol HCl
SK&F 41558 cefazolin sodium
SK&F 478 diphenidol
SK&F 478-A diphenidol HCl
SK&F 478-J diphenidol pamoate
SK&F 51 octodrine
SK&F 5116 methotrimeprazine
SK&F 525-A proadifen HCl
SK&F 53705-A sulfonterol HCl
SK&F 59962 cefazaflur sodium
SK&F 61636 bromoxanide
SK&F 62698 ticrynafen
SK&F 62979 albendazole
SK&F 63797 dribendazole
SK&F 6539 flurothyl
SK&F 69634 clopipazan mesylate
SK&F 70230-A pipazethate
SK&F 72517 elfazepam
SK&F 7690 benorterone
SK&F 7988 virginiamycin
SK&F 82526-J fenoldopam mesylate
SKF-8318 xenazoic acid
SK&F 8542 triamterene
SK&F 88373-Z ceftizoxime sodium
SKF 8898-A moroxydine
SK&F 92058 metiamide
SK&F 92657-$A_2$ prizidilol HCl
SK&F 92676-$A_3$ impromidine HCl
SK&F 92994-$A_2$ oxmetidine HCl
SK&F 92994-$J_2$ oxmetidine mesylate
SK&F 93319 icotidine
SK&F 93479 lupitidine HCl
SK&F 93574 donetidine
SK&F 93944 temelastine
SK&F 94836 siguazodan
SK&F 95587 sulotroban

SK&F 96022 pantoprazole
SK&F 96148 daltroban
SKF 9976 (as citrate) oxolamine
SK&F D-39304 cephradine
SK&F D-75073-Z cefonicid monosodium
SK&F D-75073-$Z_2$ cefonicid sodium
SK&F S-104846-A topotecan HCl
SL 501 chlophedianol HCl
SL 75 177-10 ciclprolol HCl
SL 75.212-10 betaxolol HCl
SL 76 002 progabide
SL 77 499-10 alfuzosin HCl
SL 79.229-00 fengabine
SL 80.0342-00 alpidem
SL 80.0750-23N zolpidem tartrate
SL 81.0142-00 tolgabide
SM-1213 (free base) amiprilose HCl
SM-3997 tandospirone citrate
SM-7338 meropenem
SMP 68-40 pyrabrom
SMP-78 Acid S ambruticin
SMS-201-995 octreotide
SMS-201-995 ac octreotide acetate
SMS-201-995 pa octreotide pamoate
Sms2PA strontium chloride Sr 89
SN-166 (as the sodium salt) glucosulfone
SN-263 sodium amylosulfate
S.N. 44 insulin, dalanated
SN 654 mepartricin
SND-5008 cevimeline HCl
SNI-2011 cevimeline HCl
SNK-508 cevimeline HCl
SNR 1804 clamidoxic acid
SNX-111 ziconotide
SNX-482 generic not yet assigned
SP-106 nabitan HCl
SP-119 tinabinol
SP-175 nabazenil
SP-204 menabitan HCl
SP-303 generic not yet assigned
SP-304 pirnabine
SP-325 naboctate HCl
SP54 pentosan polysulfate sodium
SP63 otilonium bromide
SPA-S-132 partricin
SPA-S-160 mepartricin
SPA-S-510 piroxicam cinnamate
SPA-S-565 rifametane

SPC-100270 safingol
SPC-100271 safingol HCl
SPC-101210 cedefingol
SPC 297 D azidocillin
SPI-77 mitopodozide
SPM 925 moexipril HCl
SQ 10,269 carbiphene HCl
SQ 10,496 thiazesim HCl
SQ 10,643 cinanserin HCl
SQ 1089 hydroxyurea
SQ 11,302 epicillin
SQ 11436 cephradine
SQ 11725 nadolol
SQ 13050 econazole nitrate
SQ 13,396 iopamidol
SQ 13847 pirquinozol
SQ 14055 tiamulin
SQ 14,225 captopril
SQ 1489 thiram
SQ 15,101 algestone acetophenide
SQ 15,102 amcinafal
SQ 15,112 amcinafide
SQ 15,659 rolitetracycline
SQ 15,860 glyhexamide
SQ 15,874 pipazethate
SQ 16,123 methicillin sodium
SQ 16,150 estradiol enanthate
SQ 16360 fusidate sodium
SQ 16374 methenolone enanthate
SQ 16,401 halquinols
SQ 16,423 oxacillin sodium
SQ 16496 methenolone acetate
SQ 16,603 fusidic acid
SQ 18566 halcinonide
SQ 19844 sincalide
SQ 20009 etazolate HCl
SQ 20824 cicloprofen
SQ 20881 teprotide
SQ 2128 ethoxazene HCl
SQ 21982 iodoxamic acid
SQ 21983 iopronic acid
SQ 22022 (dihydrate) cephradine
SQ 22947 tiamulin fumarate
SQ 26490 naflocort
SQ 26,703 zofenoprilat arginine
SQ 26776 aztreonam
SQ 26962 mebrofenin
SQ 26991 zofenopril calcium
SQ 27,239 tipredane
SQ 27,519 fosinoprilat

SQ 28555 fosinopril sodium
SQ 29,852 ceronapril
SQ 30217 technetium Tc 99m teboroxime
SQ 30836 tigemonam dicholine
SQ-31,000 pravastatin sodium
SQ 32,097 technetium Tc 99m siboroxime
SQ 32,692 gadoteridol
SQ 32,756 sorivudine
SQ 33,248 calteridol calcium
SQ 34,514 lobucavir
SQ-6201 uracil
SQ 65396 cartazolate
SQ-7726 uracil
SQ 82291 oximonam
SQ 82531 gloximonam
SQ 82629 oximonam sodium
SQ 83360 pirazmonam sodium
SQ-8493 uracil
SQ 9343 phytate sodium
SQ 9453 dimethyl sulfoxide
SQ 9538 testolactone
SQ 9993 estradiol undecylate
SR-202 mifobate
SR 2508 etanidazole
SR 25990 C clopidogrel
SR 25990 C clopidogrel bisulfate
SR 33557 fantofarone
SR 41319B tiludronate disodium
SR 47436 irbesartan
SR-7037 belfosdil
SR 720-22 metolazone
SR 96225 adenosine
SR-96669 oxaliplatin
SRG 95213 diazoxide
St 1085 (as the base) midodrine HCl
ST12 dexamethasone dipropionate
St 1411 dimepregnen
ST1512/SO4 hexoprenaline sulfate
ST-155 clonidine HCl
ST-155-BS clonidine
ST 375 tolonidine
St 567-BR (as hydrobromide) alinidine
ST 600 flutonidine
ST-813 oxiconazole nitrate
ST 9067 azintamide
STA-307 tiomesterone
St. Peter 224 midodrine HCl

**SU-101** leflunomide
**Su-10568** clortermine HCl
**Su-13437** nafenopin
**Su-18137** cyproquinate
**Su 21524** pirprofen
**Su-4885** metyrapone tartrate
**SU-5416** generic not yet assigned
**Su-5864** guanethidine sulfate
**Su-6518** dimethindene maleate
**Su-8341** cyclopenthiazide
**Su-9064** metoserpate HCl
**SUD919CL2Y** pramipexole
**SUM 3170** loxapine
**SUN 9216** lanoteplase
**SUR 2647** sumacetamol
**SYD-230** clioxanide
**synthetic TRH** protirelin
**T-1220** piperacillin sodium
**T-1551** cefoperazone sodium
**T-1982** cefbuperazone
**T-20** pentafuside
**T-2636** sedecamycin
**T-2636A** sedecamycin
**T2G1s** biciromab
**T30177** ggeneric not yet assigned
**TA-3090** clentiazem maleate
**TA 5901** cefempidone
**TAK-603** generic not yet assigned
**TAP031 (as the base)** fertirelin acetate
**TAP-144** leuprolide acetate
**TAT-3** picoperine
**TATBA** triamcinolone hexacetonide
**TBC-11251** generic not yet assigned
**TBC-1269** generic not yet assigned
**TBC-3B** generic not yet assigned
**Tc 924 (DPD)** butedronate tetrasodium
**Tc99m-MP 4006** technetium Tc 99m albumin aggregated
**Tc99m RP-30A** technetium Tc 99m sestamibi
**Tc-MAG₃** technetium Tc 99m mertiatide
**TCV-116** candesartan cilexetil
**TE-031** clarithromycin
**TE 114** tiemonium iodide
**tenite butyrate formula 264 H4** cabufocon B
**TH 1165a (as hydrobromide salt)** fenoterol
**TH-1321** protionamide

**Th-152** metaproterenol sulfate
**TH-2151** hydracarbazine
**TH-2180** propanidid
**Th 322** metrifudil
**TH-9506** generic not yet assigned
**THFES (HM)** zeranol
**THR 221 (as sodium)** cefodizime
**TI-23** generic not yet assigned
**TJ-9** generic not yet assigned
**TLC ABLC** generic not yet assigned
**TLC C-53** generic not yet assigned
**TLC D-99** generic not yet assigned
**TMB-4** trimedoxime bromide
**TNF MAb** nerelinomab
**TNO-6** spiroplatin
**TNP-470** generic not yet assigned
**TP-1** thymostimulin
**TP-10** generic not yet assigned
**TP-20** generic not yet assigned
**TP-21** thioridazine
**TP-5** thymopentin
**TPN-12** sulforidazine
**TPS-23** mesoridazine
**TR-2378** broperamole
**TR-2515** pelanserin HCl
**TR-2855** cromitrile sodium
**TR-2985** ropitoin HCl
**TR-3369** indorenate HCl
**TR-4698** rioprostil
**TR-495** methaqualone
**TR-4979** butaprost
**TR-5109** conorphone HCl
**TR-5379M** xorphanol mesylate
**TS 408** hydrocortisone probutate
**TSAA-291** oxendolone
**TTFD** fursultiamine
**TVP-1012** rasagiline mesylate
**TVX485** etofenamate
**TWSB; TWSb** sodium stibocaptate
**U-100,592** eperezolid
**U-100,766** linezolid
**U-10,136** alprostadil
**U-101.440E** irinotecan HCl
**U-10,149** lincomycin
**U-10,858** minoxidil
**U-10,974** flumethasone
**U-10,997** mibolerone
**U-11100A** nafoxidine HCl
**U-12,019E** methylprednisolone sodium phosphate

U-12,062 dinoprostone
U-12,241 cirolemycin
U-12898 bluensomycin
U-13,933 asperlin
U-14,583 dinoprost
U-14,583E dinoprost tromethamine
U-14,743 porfiromycin
U-15167 nogalamycin
U-15,614 trestolone acetate
U-15,965 lydimycin
U-17312E etryptamine acetate
U-17,323 fluorometholone acetate
U-17835 tolazamide
U-18,409AE spectinomycin HCl
U-18,496 azacitidine
U-18,573 ibuprofen
U-18,573G ibuprofen aluminum
U-19183 sparsomycin
U-19,646 chlorphenesin carbamate
U-19,718 kalafungin
U-19763 bolasterone
U-19,920 cytarabine
U-19920A cytarabine HCl
U-2032 kethoxal
U-20,661 steffimycin
U-21,251 clindamycin
U-22020 indoxole
U-22,550 calusterone
U-22,559A dexoxadrol HCl
U-24,729A mirincamycin HCl
U-24,792 lomofungin
U-24,973A melitracen HCl
U-25,179 E clindamycin palmitate HCl
U-25,873 ranimycin
U-26,225A tramadol HCl
U-26,452 glyburide
U-27,182 flurbiprofen
U-28,009 denofungin
U-28,288D guanadrel sulfate
U-28,508 clindamycin phosphate
U-28,774 ketazolam
U-29,479 scopafungin
U-30,604 zorbamycin
U-31,889 alprazolam
U-31,920 uldazepam
U-32,070E calcifediol
U-32,921 carboprost
U-32,921E carboprost tromethamine
U-33,030 triazolam
U-34,865 diflorasone diacetate

U-36,059 amitraz
U-36,384 carboprost methyl
U-41,123 adinazolam
U-41,123F adinazolam mesylate
U-42,126 acivicin
U-42,585E lodoxamide tromethamine
U-42,718 lodoxamide ethyl
U-42,842 arbaprostil
U-43,120 paulomycin
U-4527 cycloheximide
U-46,785 meteneprost
U-47,931E bromadoline maleate
U-48,753E eclanamine maleate
U-52,047 menogaril
U-53,059 itazigrel
U-53,217 epoprostenol
U-53,217A epoprostenol sodium
U-53,996H tazadolene succinate
U-54,461 bropirimine
U-54,555 metronidazole phosphate
U-54,669F losulazine HCl
U-56,321 timefurone
U-57,930E pirlimycin HCl
U-5956 filipin
U-6013 isoflupredone acetate
U-60,257 piriprost
U-60,257B piriprost potassium
U-61,431F ciprostene calcium
U-62066E spiradoline mesylate
U-63,196 cefpimizole
U-63,196E cefpimizole sodium
U-63287 ciglitazone
U-63,366F trospectomycin sulfate
U-63,557A furegrelate sodium
U-64279A ceftiofur HCl
U-64279E ceftiofur sodium
U-66858 bunaprolast
U-67,590A methylprednisolone
U-69689E fertirelin acetate
U-6987 carbutamide
U-70138 paldimycin
U-70226E ibutilide fumarate
U-71038 ditekiren
U-72107A pioglitazone HCl
U-72791 cefmetazole
U-72791A cefmetazole sodium
U-73,975 adozelesin
U-74006F tirilazad mesylate
U-75630 ibuprofen piconol
U-76252 cefpodoxime proxetil

U-77,233 ormaplatin
U-7743 mercufenol chloride
U-7750 streptovarycin
U-77779 bizelesin
U-7800 fluprednisolone
U-78875 panadiplon
U-78,938 dexormaplatin
U-80244 carzelesin
U-82127 alexomycin
U-8344 uracil mustard
U-8471 medrysone
U-85,855 alvircept sudotox
U-87201E atevirdine mesylate
U-88943E artilide fumarate
U89 generic not yet assigned
U-90152S delavirdine mesylate
U-935 amiquinsin HCl
U-95376 premafloxacin
U-98079A itasetron
U-98528E pramipexole
U-9889 streptozocin
UCB 1402 decloxizine
UCB 1474 chlorbenzoxamine HCl
UCB 1549 minepentate
UCB 1967 dropropizine
UCB 2073 etoxeridine
UCB 3928 fedrilate
UCB 4445 buclizine HCl
UDCG-115 pimobendan
UF-021 isopropyl unoprostone
UH-AC 62XX meloxicam
UK-109,496 generic not yet assigned
UK-11,443 primidolol
UK-14304-18 brimonidine tartrate
UK-18,892 butikacin
UK-20,349 tioconazole
UK-2054 famotine HCl
UK-2371 memotine HCl
UK-25,842 oxfenicine
UK-31,214 propikacin
UK-31,557 carbazeran
UK-33,274-27 doxazosin mesylate
UK-3540-1 amedalin HCl
UK-3557-15 daledalin tosylate
UK-37,248-01 dazoxiben HCl
UK-38,485 dazmegrel
UK-4271 oxamniquine
UK-48,340-11 amlodipine maleate
UK-48,340-26 amlodipine besylate
UK-49,858 fluconazole

UK-61260-27 nanterinone
UK-61,689 semduramicin
UK-61,689-2 semduramicin sodium
UK-67,994 doramectin
UK-68,798 dofetilide
UK-738 ethybenztropine
UK-73,967 candoxatrilat
UK-76654-2 (as fumarate) zamife-
nacin
UK-79,300 candoxatril
UK-80067 modipafant
UK-88060 espatropate
UK-92,480-10 sildenafil citrate
UM 952 buprenorphine HCl
UP 106 propizepine
UP 107 bepiastine
UP 164 morniflumate
UP 74 nixylic acid
UP 83 niflumic acid
USV 3659-(S) pivopril
VA-10367 generic not yet assigned
V-C 13 dichlofenthion
VCP 205 generic not yet assigned
VK-57 glyprothiazol
VM-26 teniposide
VML 251 frovatriptan succinate
VML-262 generic not yet assigned
VP-16-213 etoposide
VP 63843 pleconaril
VUAB6453 (SPOFA) metipranolol
VX-105 arginine butyrate
VX-478 amprenavir
VX-497 generic not yet assigned
VX-710-3 biricodar dicitrate
VX-740 generic not yet assigned
W-1015 nisobamate
W 10168 vifilcon A
W-1372 beloxamide
W 1655 phenazopyridine HCl
W 1760A namoxyrate
W-19053 (as HCl) etidocaine
W 1929 colistimethate sodium
W 2180 suxemerid sulfate
W 2197 pentrinitrol
W 2291A mimbane HCl
W-2354 seclazone
W 2394A pemerid nitrate
W-2395 meseclazone
W 2426 chlorphentermine HCl
W 2900A etozolin

W-2946M reproterol HCl
W-2964M flupirtine maleate
W 2965 A acetryptine
W-2979M azelastine HCl
W 3207B modaline sulfate
W 3366A quindonium bromide
W3395 algestone acetonide
W 3399 quingestrone
W 3566 quinestrol
W 3580B ampyzine sulfate
W-36095 tocainide
W 3623 cyprazepam
W 3676 sulazepam
W 3699 piprozolin
W 37 buformin
W 3746 cetophenicol
W 3976B triampyzine sulfate
W 4020 prazepam
W 42782 iproxamine HCl
W 43026A ciclafrine HCl
W 4425 almadrate sulfate
W 4454A estrazinol hydrobromide
W 4540 quingestanol acetate
W 4565 oxolinic acid
W 4600 algeldrate
W 4701 hexedine
W 4744 mecloqualone
W 4869 prednival
W-5219 proglumide
W 5494A naranol HCl
W-554 felbamate
W 5733 atolide
W 5759A tilidine HCl
W-583 mebutamate
W 5975 betamethasone benzoate
W 6309 difluprednate
W 6412A bunolol HCl
W 6439A suloxifen oxalate
W 6495 oxisuran
W 7000A levobunolol HCl
W 713 tybamate
W 7320 alclofenac
W7783 ambruticin
W 8495 isoxicam
WA 184 sitogluside
W-A 335 danitracen
WAL 2014 FU talsaclidine fumarate
WAY-ACA-147 eldacimibe
WAY-ANA-756 tasosartan
WAY-ARI-509 minalrestat

WAY-GPA-748 pralmorelin dihydro-
chloride
WAY-PDA-641 filaminast
WAY-PEM-420 dexpemedolac
WAY-SEC-579 mirisetron maleate
WE352 triflubazam
We 941 brotizolam
We 973-BS ciclotizolam
WEB 2086 BS apafant
WF-10 tetrachlorodecaoxide
WG-253 rimiterol hydrobromide
WG 537 (as acetate) flumedroxone
WH 5668 propanidid
WHR-1051B biclodil HCl
WHR-1142A lidamidine HCl
WHR-2908A lofepramine HCl
WHR-5020 etofenamate
WHR-539 fenclorac
Win 11,318 bupivacaine HCl
Win 11450 benorilate
Win 11,464 fludorex
Win 11,530 menoctone
Win 11831 lorajmine HCl
Win 13,146 teclozan
Win 1344 gamfexine
Win 13820 becanthone HCl
Win 14833 stanozolol
Win 17625 azastene
Win 17665 topterone
Win 17,757 danazol
Win 1783 isomethadone
Win 18,320 nalidixic acid
Win 18,320-3 nalidixate sodium
Win 18,413-2 solypertine tartrate
Win 18,501-2 oxypertine
Win 18,935 milipertine
Win 19356 clorindanic acid
Win 20,228 pentazocine
Win 20,740 cyclazocine
Win 21,904 alexidine
WIN 22118 pegorgotein
Win 23,200 volazocine
Win 24,540 trilostane
Win 24,933 hycanthone
Win 25,347 nimazone
Win 25,978 amfonelic acid
Win 27147-2 cyclindole
Win 27,914 nivazol
Win 29194-6 carbantel lauryl sulfate
Win 31,665 alpertine

Win 32,729 epostane
Win 32,784 bitolterol mesylate
Win 3406 isoetharine
Win 34,276 ketazocine
Win 34284 oxarbazole
Win 34886 nisbuterol mesylate
Win 35150 flucindole
Win 35,213 rosoxacin
Win 35833 ciprofibrate
Win 38020 arildone
Win 38770 azarole
Win 39103 metrizamide
Win 39424 iohexol
Win 40014 quinfamide
Win 40350 durapatite
Win 40680 amrinone
Win 40808-7 sulfinalol HCl
Win 41464-2 octenidine HCl
Win 41,464-6 octenidine saccharin
Win 41528-2 fezolamine fumarate
Win 42156-2 tonazocine mesylate
Win 42,202 fosarilate
Win 42964-4 zenazocine mesylate
Win 44,441-3 quadazocine mesylate
Win 47,203-2 milrinone
Win 48,049 ofornine
Win 48,098-6 pravadoline maleate
Win 49,016 medorinone
Win 49,375 amifloxacin
Win 49,375-3 amifloxacin mesylate
Win 49,596 zanoterone
Win 5063 racephenicol
Win 5063-2 thiamphenicol
Win 51,181-2 napamezole HCl
Win 51,711 disoxaril
Win 54,177-4 ipazilide fumarate
Win 5563-3 colterol mesylate
WIN 59010 mangafodipir trisodium
Win 59075 tirapazamine
WIN 63843 pleconaril
Win 771 hydroxypethidine
Win 8851-2 tyropanoate sodium
Win 90,000 cicletanine
Win 9154 inositol niacinate
Win 9317 propatyl nitrate
Wl 140 calcium polycarbophil
Wl 287 euprocin HCl
Wl 291 zolamine HCl
WP-973 chlorhexidine phosphanilate
WR 142,490 mefloquine

WR-171669 halofantrine HCl
WR 180,409 enpiroline phosphate
WR-228,258 tebuquine
WR-2721 amifostine
WV 569 (as HCl) norfenefrine
WX 14812 alofilcon A
WX 14822 hydrofilcon A
WX 2412 fungimycin
Wy-1359 propiomazine
WY-15,705 ciramadol
WY-15,705 HCl ciramadol HCl
WY-16,225 dezocine
WY-18,251 tilomisole
Wy-2039 etoxeridine
WY-20,788 penamecillin
WY-21,743 oxaprozin
WY-21,894 fentiazac
Wy 21901 indoramin
WY-21,901 HCl indoramin HCl
WY-22811 HCl meptazinol HCl
WY-23,409 ciclazindol
WY-24,081 HCl tiquinamide HCl
WY-24,377 isotiquimide
Wy-2445 carphenazine maleate
WY-25,021 rolgamidine
Wy-2837 potassium aspartate & magnesium aspartate
Wy-2838 potassium aspartate & magnesium aspartate
Wy-3263 iprindole
Wy-3277 nafcillin sodium
Wy-3467 diazepam
Wy-3475 norbolethone
Wy-3478 sodium oxybate
Wy-3498 oxazepam
Wy-3707 norgestrel
Wy-3917 temazepam
Wy-4036 lorazepam
WY-4082 lormetazepam
WY-40,972 lutrelin acetate
WY-42,362 HCl recainam HCl
WY-42,362 tosylate recainam tosylate
WY-44,417 sodium apalcillin sodium
WY-44,635 cefpiramide
WY-44,635 sodium cefpiramide sodium
WY-45,030 venlafaxine HCl
Wy-4508 cyclacillin
WY-460E thiazinamium chloride
WY-47384 gevotroline HCl

**WY-47,663 acetate** anaritide acetate
**WY-47791 HCl** carvotroline HCl
**WY-47846 HCl** zalospirone HCl
**WY-48252** ritolukast
**WY-48314** lexithromycin
**WY-48624** enciprazine HCl
**WY-48986** risotilide HCl
**WY-50324 HCl** adatanserin HCl
**WY-5104** levonorgestrel
**Wy-806** oxethazaine
**Wy-8138** bisoxatin acetate
**Wy-8678** guanabenz
**WY-8678 acetate** guanabenz acetate
**WY-90493 RD** ardeparin sodium
**X-1497** methicillin sodium
**XA41** latanoprost
**XLG** polyglactin 910
**XM-72** polybutester
**XU 62-320** fluvastatin sodium
**XZ-450** azithromycin
**Y 3642** tinoridine
**Y 4153 (as HCl)** clocapramine
**Y 6124 (as HCl)** bufetolol
**YC-93** nicardipine HCl
**YKP-10A** generic not yet assigned
**YM-08316** formoterol fumarate
**YM-09330** cefotetan disodium

**YM-12617-1** tamsulosin HCl
**YM617** tamsulosin HCl
**YN-72** sorivudine
**YTR-830H** tazobactam
**Z 1282** fosfomycin tromethamine
**Z 326** fentonium bromide
**Z 424** viminol
**Z-4828** trofosfamide
**Z4942** ifosfamide
**Z 6000** troxerutin
**ZCE025** indium In 111 altumomab
**ZD1033** anastrozole
**ZD 1694** raltitrexed
**ZD 4522** generic not yet assigned
**ZD5077** quetiapine fumarate
**ZK 10 720** ioprocemic acid
**ZK 132281** ferucarbotran
**ZK 30595** drospirenone
**ZK 35760** iopromide
**ZK 39 482** iotrolan
**ZK 57 671** sulprostone
**ZK 62498** azelaic acid
**ZK 62 711** rolipram
**ZK 71 630** iotetric acid
**ZK 76 604** pirazolac
**ZK 79 112** iotasul
**ZM 204,636** quetirapine fumarate

**Code Names**

# Xref: Street Drug Slang to Pharmaceutical Names

Below are 1517 slang terms for illegally abused drugs. These slang terms are cross-referenced to the actual names of drugs, legal or illegal, that appear in the *Saunders Pharmaceutical Word Book*.

**A** [see: LSD; amphetamines]

**A-bomb** *marijuana and heroin smoked together in a cigarette* [see: marijuana; heroin]

**Acapulco gold; Acapulco red** *marijuana from southwest Mexico* [see: marijuana]

**ace** [see: marijuana; PCP]

**acid** [see: LSD]

**AD** [see: PCP]

**Adam** [see: MDMA]

**Adam and Eve** *a combination of MDMA and MDEA* [see: MDMA; MDEA]

**African black; African bush; African woodbine** [see: marijuana]

**ah-pen-yen** [see: opium]

**aimies; amys** *amphetamines, amyl nitrite, or Amytal (amobarbital; discontinued 1991)* [see: amphetamine; amyl nitrite; Amytal Sodium; amobarbital; amobarbital sodium]

**AIP** *heroin from Afghanistan, Iran, and Pakistan* [see: heroin]

**airplane** [see: marijuana]

**Alice B. Toklas** *marijuana brownies* [see: marijuana]

**all-American drug** [see: cocaine]

**alpha-ET** [see: alpha-ethyltryptamine]

**amoeba** [see: PCP]

**amp** [see: amphetamines]

**amp joint** *a marijuana cigarette laced with a narcotic* [see: marijuana]

**amys; aimies** *amphetamines, amyl nitrite, or Amytal (amobarbital; discontinued 1991)* [see: amphetamines; amyl nitrite; Amytal Sodium; amobarbital; amobarbital sodium]

**angel; angel dust; angel hair; angel mist; angel poke** [see: PCP]

**Angola** [see: marijuana]

**animal** [see: LSD]

**animal trank; animal tranquilizer** [see: PCP]

**antifreeze** [see: heroin]

**Apache** [see: fentanyl (citrate)]

**apple jacks** [see: cocaine, crack]

**Aries** [see: heroin]

**aroma of men** [see: isobutyl nitrite]

**ashes** [see: marijuana]

**Assassin of Youth** *from a 1930s film of the same name* [see: marijuana]

**atom bomb** *a combination of marijuana and heroin* [see: marijuana; heroin]

**atshitshi** [see: marijuana]

**aunt Hazel** [see: heroin]

**aunt Mary** [see: marijuana]

**aunt Nora** [see: cocaine]

**auntie; auntie Emma** [see: opium]

**aurora borealis** [see: PCP]

**baby; baby bhang** [see: marijuana]

**baby T** [see: cocaine, crack]

**backbreakers** *a combination of LSD and strychnine* [see: LSD; strychnine]

**back-to-back** *smoking crack after injecting heroin or vice versa* [see: heroin; cocaine, crack]

**backwards** *various CNS depressants*

**bad** [see: cocaine, crack]

**bad pizza** [see: PCP]

**bad seed** [see: mescaline; heroin; marijuana]

**bag** *1 to 15 g of heroin; also known as a "deck"* [see: heroin]

**bah-say** [see: cocaine, crack; coca paste]

**bale** *1 pound of marijuana* [see: marijuana]

**ball** [see: cocaine, crack]

**ballot** [see: heroin]

**bam** *various CNS depressants or amphetamines* [see: amphetamines]

**bambalacha** [see: marijuana]

**bambs** *various CNS depressants*

**bammy** [see: marijuana]

**banano** *(Spanish for "banana tree") a marijuana or tobacco cigarette laced with cocaine* [see: marijuana; tobacco; cocaine]

**bank bandit pills** *various CNS depressants*

**bar** [see: marijuana]

**barb; barbie doll; barbies; barbs** *various CNS depressants, primarily barbiturates*

**barbs** [see: cocaine]

**barrels** [see: LSD]

**base; baseball** *from "freebase"* [see: cocaine, crack]

**bash** [see: marijuana]

**basuco** *coca paste or coca paste residue sprinkled on a marijuana or tobacco cigarette* [see: coca paste; marijuana; tobacco]

**bathtub speed** [see: methcathinone]

**battery acid** [see: LSD]

**batu** *smokable methamphetamine* [see: methamphetamine HCl]

**bazooka** *crack or a combination of coca paste and marijuana* [see: cocaine, crack; coca paste; marijuana]

**bazulco** [see: cocaine]

**B-bomb** *1940s slang for a Benzedrine inhaler (amphetamine sulfate; discontinued)*

**beam me up Scotty** *crack dipped in PCP* [see: cocaine, crack; PCP]

**beans** *amphetamines, various CNS depressants, or mescaline* [see: amphetamines; mescaline]

**beast** [see: LSD]

**beautiful boulders** [see: cocaine, crack]

**bebe** [see: cocaine, crack]

**beemers** [see: cocaine, crack]

**Belushi** *a combination of cocaine and heroin (from the actor John Belushi, who died of an overdose)* [see: cocaine; heroin]

**belyando spruce** [see: marijuana]

**bennie; bennies; Benny and the Jets** *Benzedrine (amphetamine sulfate; discontinued 1982) or any of the amphetamines* [see: amphetamine sulfate; amphetamines]

**benz** *Benzedrine (amphetamine sulfate; discontinued 1982) or any of the amphetamines* [see: amphetamine sulfate; amphetamines]

**Bernice; Bernie; Bernie's flakes; Bernie's gold dust** [see: cocaine]

**bhang** *an Indian term* [see: marijuana]

**big 8** *⅛ kg of crack (about 4½ ounces)* [see: cocaine, crack]

**big bag** [see: heroin]

**big C** [see: cocaine]

**big chief** [see: mescaline]

**big D** [see: LSD]

**big flake** [see: cocaine]

**big H; big Harry** [see: heroin]

**big O** [see: opium]

**big rush** [see: cocaine]

**Bill Blass** [see: cocaine, crack]

**Billie hoke** [see: cocaine]

**bings** [see: cocaine, crack]

**birdie powder** [see: heroin; cocaine]

**biscuit** *50 rocks of crack* [see: cocaine, crack]

**black** [see: opium; marijuana]

**black acid** *LSD or a combination of LSD and PCP* [see: LSD; PCP]

**black and white** [see: amphetamines]

**black Bart** [see: marijuana]

**black beauties** *amphetamines or various CNS depressants* [see: amphetamines]

**black beauties** *Biphetamine (amphetamine + dextroamphetamine; discontinued 1993)* [see: amphetamines; amphetamine sulfate; dextroamphetamine]

**black birds; black bombers** [see: amphetamines]

**black ganga** *marijuana resin* [see: marijuana]

**black gold** *a high-potency marijuana* [see: marijuana]

**black gungi** *marijuana from India* [see: marijuana]

**black gunion** [see: marijuana]

**black hash** *a combination of opium and hashish* [see: opium; hashish]

**black mo; black moat** *highly potent marijuana* [see: marijuana]

**black mollies** [see: amphetamines]

**black mote** *marijuana mixed with honey* [see: marijuana]

**black pearl** [see: heroin]

**black pill** *an opium pill* [see: opium]

**black rock** [see: cocaine, crack]

**black Russian** *very potent hashish or a combination of hashish and opium* [see: hashish; opium]

**black star** [see: LSD]

**black stuff** [see: heroin]

**black stuff; black tar opium** *a tar-like opium for smoking* [see: opium]

**black sunshine** [see: LSD]

**black tabs** [see: LSD]

**black tar** [see: heroin; opium]

**black tar heroin; black Tootsie Roll** *a potent form of heroin from Mexico* [see: heroin]

**black whack** [see: PCP]

**blacks** [see: amphetamines]

**blanco** (Spanish for "white") [see: heroin]

**blanket** *a marijuana cigarette* [see: marijuana]

**block** *marijuana or crude opium or a cube of morphine* [see: marijuana; opium; morphine]

**blockbusters** *Nembutal (pentobarbital; discontinued 1979) or various CNS depressants*

**blonde** [see: marijuana]

**blood madman** [see: PCP]

**blotter** [see: LSD; cocaine]

**blotter acid; blotter cube** [see: LSD]

**blow up** *crack cocaine cut (diluted) with lidocaine to increase size and weight* [see: cocaine, crack]

**blowcaine** *crack cocaine cut (diluted) with powdered cocaine* [see: cocaine, crack; cocaine]

**blowing smoke** [see: marijuana]

**blowout** [see: cocaine, crack]

**blue** *crack or various CNS depressants* [see: cocaine, crack]

**blue acid** [see: LSD]

**blue and clears** *Fastin (phentermine HCl), which is a blue and clear capsule filled with blue and white balls* [see: Fastin; phentermine]

**blue angels** *various CNS depressants*

**blue barrels** [see: LSD]

**blue boy** [see: amphetamines]

**blue bullets** *various CNS depressants*

**blue caps** [see: mescaline]

**blue chairs; blue cheers** [see: LSD]

**blue de hue** *marijuana from Vietnam* [see: marijuana]

**blue devil** *various CNS depressants*

**blue dolls** *various CNS depressants*

**blue heaven** [see: LSD]

**blue heavens; bluebirds** *Amytal (amobarbital; discontinued 1991), Amytal Sodium (amobarbital sodium), or other depressants* [see: Amytal Sodium; amobarbital; amobarbital sodium]

**blue microdot; blue mist; blue moons** [see: LSD]

**blue sage** [see: marijuana]

**blue sky bond** *high-potency marijuana from Colombia* [see: marijuana]

**blue star** *a type of blotter LSD* [see: LSD]

**blue tabs** [see: LSD]

**blue tips** *various CNS depressants*

**blue velvet** *a combination of paregoric and tripelennamine, used as a weak heroin substitute*

**blue velvet** *a combination of terpin hydrate, codeine, and tripelennamine, used as a weak heroin substitute*

**blue vials** [see: LSD]

**bluebirds; blue heavens** *Amytal (amobarbital; discontinued 1991), Amytal Sodium (amobarbital sodium), or other depressants* [see: Amytal Sodium; amobarbital; amobarbital sodium]

**blues** *Amytal (amobarbital; discontinued 1991), named for the blue-colored capsules* [see: Amytal Sodium; amobarbital; amobarbital sodium]

**blues and reds** *Amytal (amobarbital; discontinued 1991) and Seconal (secobarbital; discontinued 1990)* [see: Amytal Sodium; amobarbital; Seconal Sodium; secobarbital]

**blunt** *marijuana or a combination of marijuana and cocaine in a cigar* [see: marijuana; cocaine]

**boat** [see: PCP]

**bobo; boubou; bobo bush** (Spanish for "fool" or "idiot") [see: marijuana; cocaine, crack]

**bohd** [see: marijuana; PCP]

**Bolivian marching powder** [see: cocaine]

**bolo** (Spanish and Italian for "bolus") [see: cocaine, crack]

**bolt** [see: butyl nitrite; isobutyl nitrite]

**bomb** [see: cocaine, crack; heroin; marijuana]

**bomber** *a marijuana cigarette* [see: marijuana]

**bombido; bombita** *injectable amphetamines, heroin, or various CNS depressants* [see: amphetamines; heroin]

**bombita** (Spanish for "little bomb") *injectable Desoxyn (methamphetamine HCl; discontinued 1980)* [see: methamphetamine HCl; amphetamines]

**bombs away** [see: heroin]

**bone** *marijuana or a $50 piece of crack* [see: marijuana; cocaine, crack]

**bonecrusher; bones** [see: cocaine, crack]

**bonita** (Spanish for "beautiful") [see: heroin]

**boo** [see: marijuana]

**boom** [see: marijuana]

**boomers** [see: psilocybin; psilocin]

**booster** *inhaled (snorted) cocaine* [see: cocaine]

**boppers** [see: amyl nitrite]

**botray** [see: cocaine, crack]

**bottles** [see: amphetamines]

**boubou; bobo** [see: cocaine, crack]

**boulder** *a $20 piece of crack, or crack in general* [see: cocaine, crack]

**boulya** [see: cocaine, crack]

**boy** [see: heroin]

**bozo** [see: heroin]

**brain ticklers** [see: amphetamines]

**breakdown** *a $40 piece of crack sold for $20* [see: cocaine, crack]

**brick** *1 kilo (kg) of marijuana or crack in general* [see: marijuana; cocaine, crack]

**brick gum** [see: heroin]

**Britton** [see: mescaline]

**broccoli** [see: marijuana]

**brother** [see: heroin]

**brown** [see: heroin; marijuana]

**brown and clears** *Dexedrine (dextroamphetamine sulfate) Spansules (brown and clear capsules)* [see: Dexedrine; dextroamphetamine sulfate; amphetamines]

**brown bombers** [see: LSD]

**brown crystal** [see: heroin]

**brown dots** [see: LSD]

**brown rhine; brown sugar** [see: heroin]

**brownies; browns** *amphetamines, especially Dexedrine Spansules (dextroamphetamine sulfate in brown capsules)* [see: Dexedrine; dextroamphetamine sulfate; amphetamines]

**bubble gum** [see: cocaine; cocaine, crack]

**bud** [see: marijuana]

**buda; budda; buddha** *potent, highgrade marijuana mixed with opium or crack* [see: marijuana; opium; cocaine, crack]

**bullet** [see: isobutyl nitrite]

**bullet bolt** *various inhalants*

**bullia capital** [see: cocaine, crack]

**bullion; bullyon** [see: cocaine, crack; marijuana]

**bumblebees** [see: amphetamines]

**bump** *crack, fake crack, or a $20 dose of ketamine* [see: cocaine, crack; ketamine HCl]

**bundle** [see: heroin]

**bunk** *fake cocaine* [see: cocaine]

**Burese** [see: cocaine]

**burnie** [see: marijuana]

**burrito** [see: marijuana]

**bush** [see: cocaine; marijuana]

**businessman's LSD; businessman's special; businessman's trip** [see: dimethyltryptamine]

busters *various CNS depressants*
busy bee [see: PCP]
butt naked [see: PCP]
butter [see: marijuana; cocaine, crack]
butter flower [see: marijuana]
buttons [see: mescaline]
butu [see: heroin]
buzz bomb *nitrous oxide or a device for inhaling nitrous oxide from small canisters* [see: nitrous oxide]
caballo (Spanish for "horse") [see: heroin]
cabello (Spanish for "hair") [see: cocaine]
cactus; cactus buttons; cactus head [see: mescaline]
Cadillac [see: PCP]
Cadillac express [see: methcathinone]
'caine [see: cocaine; cocaine, crack]
cakes *round disks of crack* [see: cocaine, crack]
California cornflakes [see: cocaine]
California sunshine [see: LSD]
Cam red; Cam trip; Cambodian red *high-potency marijuana from Cambodia* [see: marijuana]
came [see: cocaine]
can *1 oz. of marijuana* [see: marijuana]
Canadian black [see: marijuana]
canamo (Spanish for "hemp") [see: marijuana]
canappa [see: marijuana]
cancelled stick *a marijuana cigarette* [see: marijuana]
candy *illegal drugs in general*
candy C; candy cane; candycaine [see: cocaine]
cannabis tea [see: marijuana]
cap; caps [see: cocaine, crack; LSD; heroin; psilocin; psilocybin]
capital H [see: heroin]
caps; cap [see: cocaine, crack; LSD; heroin; psilocin; psilocybin]
Captain Cody [see: codeine]
carga (Spanish for "weight" or "load") [see: heroin]
carne; carnie (Spanish for "meat") [see: heroin; cocaine]
Carrie; Carrie Nation [see: cocaine]

cartucho (Spanish for "cartridge") *a pack of marijuana cigarettes* [see: marijuana]
cartwheels [see: amphetamines]
Casper the ghost [see: cocaine, crack]
cat [see: methcathinone]
cat valium [see: ketamine HCl]
catnip *a marijuana cigarette* [see: marijuana]
caviar [see: cocaine, crack]
cavite all star [see: marijuana]
C-dust; C-game [see: cocaine]
Cecil [see: cocaine]
chalk [see: methamphetamine HCl; amphetamines]
champagne of drugs [see: cocaine HCl]
chandoo; chandu [see: opium]
charas *marijuana from India* [see: marijuana]
charge [see: marijuana]
Charley; Charlie [see: heroin; cocaine]
chasing the dragon *inhaling vapors of heroin or cocaine (powder or crack) heated on tinfoil* [see: heroin; cocaine; cocaine, crack]
chasing the tiger *smoking heroin* [see: heroin]
cheap basing [see: cocaine, crack]
cheeba; cheeo [see: marijuana]
chemical [see: cocaine, crack]
cheroot *a tobacco and/or marijuana cigar* [see: tobacco; marijuana]
cherry menth [see: GHB]
chewies [see: cocaine, crack]
chiba chiba *high-potency marijuana from Colombia* [see: marijuana]
Chicago black; Chicago green [see: marijuana]
chick [see: heroin]
chicken powder [see: amphetamines]
chicle [see: heroin]
chief [see: LSD; mescaline]
chieva [see: heroin]
China cat *high-potency heroin* [see: heroin]
China girl; China town [see: fentanyl (citrate)]

**China white** *very pure heroin, fentanyl, or a fentanyl analog used as a heroin substitute* [see: heroin; fentanyl (citrate)]

**Chinese molasses** [see: opium]

**Chinese red** [see: heroin]

**Chinese tobacco** [see: opium]

**chip** [see: heroin]

**chippy** [see: cocaine]

**chips** *tobacco or marijuana cigarettes laced with PCP* [see: tobacco; marijuana; PCP]

**chira** [see: marijuana]

**chocolate** [see: hashish; opium; amphetamines]

**chocolate chips** [see: LSD]

**chocolate ecstasy** *crack made brown by adding chocolate milk powder during production* [see: cocaine, crack]

**cholly** [see: cocaine]

**chorals** *various CNS depressants*

**Chris; cris; Christina; Cristina** [see: methamphetamine HCl]

**Christmas rolls** *various CNS depressants*

**Christmas tree** *marijuana, various CNS depressants, or amphetamines* [see: marijuana; amphetamines]

**Christmas trees** *Dexamyl (dextroamphetamine sulfate + amobarbital; discontinued 1980) in green and clear capsules* [see: dextroamphetamine sulfate; amobarbital; amphetamines]

**Christy; Cristy** *smokable methamphetamine* [see: methamphetamine HCl]

**chronic** *marijuana or marijuana mixed with crack* [see: marijuana; cocaine, crack]

**churus** [see: marijuana]

**CIBAs** *Doriden (glutethimide; discontinued 1990)* [see: glutethimide]

**cid** [see: LSD]

**cigarette paper** *a packet of heroin* [see: heroin]

**cigarrode cristal** [see: PCP]

**circles** *Rohypnol (flunitrazepam; not marketed in the U.S.)* [see: Rohypnol; flunitrazepam]

**citrol** *high-potency marijuana from Nepal* [see: marijuana]

**clarity** [see: MDMA]

**clicker** *a combination of crack and PCP* [see: cocaine, crack; PCP]

**cliffhanger** [see: PCP]

**climax** [see: butyl nitrite; isobutyl nitrite; cocaine, crack; heroin]

**climb** *a marijuana cigarette* [see: marijuana]

**clips** *rows of vials heat-sealed together*

**cloud; cloud nine** [see: cocaine, crack]

**coast-to-coast** *a reference to truckers' use of amphetamines for long-distance runs* [see: amphetamines]

**coca** [see: cocaine]

**coca paste; cocaine paste** *a barely refined cocaine with adulterants* [see: cocaine]

**cochornis** [see: marijuana]

**cocktail** *a cigarette laced with cocaine, crack, or marijuana* [see: cocaine; cocaine, crack; marijuana]

**coco rocks** *dark brown crack made by adding chocolate pudding during production* [see: cocaine, crack]

**coco snow** *benzocaine used as a cutting agent for crack* [see: cocaine, crack; benzocaine]

**coconut** [see: cocaine]

**Cody** [see: codeine]

**coffee** [see: LSD]

**coke** [see: cocaine; cocaine, crack]

**cola** [see: cocaine]

**colas** *(Spanish for "tails") a reference to the flowering tops of marijuana plants* [see: marijuana]

**coli** [see: marijuana]

**coliflor tostada** *(Spanish for "brown or toasted cauliflower")* [see: marijuana]

**Colombian** [see: marijuana]

**Colorado cocktail** [see: marijuana]

**Columbo** [see: PCP]

**Columbus black** [see: marijuana]

**comeback** *the benzocaine and mannitol used in the conversion of cocaine to crack* [see: cocaine; cocaine, crack]

**conductor** [see: LSD]

**contact lens** [see: LSD]

**cookies** [see: cocaine, crack]

**cooler** *a regular cigarette laced with a drug*

**coolie** *a regular cigarette laced with cocaine* [see: cocaine]

**co-pilot** [see: amphetamines]

**coral** *various CNS depressants*

**cork the air** *inhaling (snorting) powdered cocaine* [see: cocaine]

**Corrine** [see: cocaine]

**cosa** (Spanish and Italian for "thing") [see: marijuana]

**Cozmo's** [see: PCP]

**'cotics** *from "narcotics"* [see: heroin]

**cotton brothers** *a combination of cocaine, heroin, and morphine* [see: cocaine; heroin; morphine]

**cotton fever** *septicemia caused by injecting small amounts of cotton fiber with the drugs*

**courage pills** *heroin or various CNS depressants* [see: heroin]

**crack** [see: cocaine, crack]

**crack back** *a combination of crack and marijuana* [see: cocaine, crack; marijuana]

**crack cooler** *crack soaked in a wine cooler* [see: cocaine, crack]

**crackers** [see: cocaine, crack]

**crank** *various amphetamines, especially methamphetamine, or methcathinone* [see: amphetamines; methamphetamine HCl; methcathinone]

**crazy coke; crazy Eddie** [see: PCP]

**crazy weed** [see: marijuana]

**cream and crimson** *Dalmane (flurazepam HCl), named for the white and red capsules* [see: Dalmane; flurazepam HCl]

**crib** [see: cocaine, crack]

**crimmie** *a regular cigarette laced with crack* [see: cocaine, crack]

**crink** [see: methamphetamine HCl]

**cripple** *a marijuana cigarette* [see: marijuana]

**cris; Chris; Cristina; Christina** [see: methamphetamine HCl]

**crisscross** [see: amphetamines]

**Cristina; Christina; cris; Chris** [see: methamphetamine HCl]

**Cristy; Christy** *smokable methamphetamine* [see: methamphetamine HCl]

**croak** *a combination of crack and methamphetamine* [see: cocaine, crack; methamphetamine HCl]

**crop** *low-quality heroin* [see: heroin]

**cross tops** [see: amphetamines]

**crossroads** [see: amphetamines]

**crown crap** [see: heroin]

**crumbs** *tiny pieces of crack* [see: cocaine, crack]

**crunch and munch** [see: cocaine, crack]

**'cruz** *opium from Veracruz, Mexico* [see: opium]

**crying weed** [see: marijuana]

**crypto** [see: methamphetamine HCl]

**crystal** [see: methamphetamine HCl; Desoxyn; amphetamines; PCP; cocaine]

**crystal; krystal; crystal joint; krystal joint** [see: PCP]

**crystal joint** [see: PCP]

**crystal meth** [see: methamphetamine HCl]

**crystal tea; crystal T** [see: LSD; PCP]

**cube; cubes** *morphine, LSD, marijuana tablets, or 1 oz. of any drug* [see: morphine; LSD; marijuana]

**culican** *high-potency marijuana from Mexico* [see: marijuana]

**cupcakes** [see: LSD]

**cura** (Spanish for "cure"; Italian for "care") [see: heroin]

**cut-deck** *heroin mixed with powdered milk* [see: heroin]

**cycline; cyclones** [see: PCP]

**cyclones; cycline** [see: PCP]

**dagga** [see: marijuana]

**dama blanca** (Spanish for "white lady") [see: cocaine]

**dance fever** [see: fentanyl citrate]

**date rape drug** *Rohypnol (flunitrazepam; not marketed in the U.S.)* [see: Rohypnol; flunitrazepam]

**dawamesk** [see: marijuana]

**dead on arrival; DOA** [see: heroin; PCP; cocaine, crack]

**decadence** [see: MDMA]

**deck** *1 to 15 g of heroin; also known as a "bag"* [see: heroin]

**deeda** [see: LSD]

**demo** *a sample-size piece of crack* [see: cocaine, crack]

**demolish** [see: cocaine, crack]

**Detroit pink** [see: PCP]

**deuce** *heroin or $2 worth of drugs* [see: heroin]

**devil's dandruff; devilsmoke** [see: cocaine, crack]

**devil's dust** [see: PCP]

**dew; 'due** *marijuana or the residue of oils left in a pipe after smoking crack* [see: marijuana; cocaine, crack]

**dexies** *Dexedrine (dextroamphetamine sulfate) or various other amphetamines, especially dextroamphetamine* [see: Dexedrine; dextroamphetamine sulfate; amphetamines]

**diamba; djamba** [see: marijuana]

**diet pills** [see: amphetamines]

**dillys** [see: Dilaudid; hydromorphone HCl]

**dimba** *marijuana from West Africa* [see: marijuana]

**dime** *$10 worth of crack* [see: cocaine, crack]

**dime store high** *glue sniffing* [see: petroleum distillate inhalants]

**dime's worth** *the amount of heroin needed to cause death* [see: heroin]

**ding** [see: marijuana]

**dinkie dow** [see: marijuana]

**dip** [see: cocaine, crack]

**dipper** [see: PCP]

**dirt** [see: heroin]

**dirt grass** *inferior-quality marijuana* [see: marijuana]

**dirty basing** [see: cocaine, crack]

**disco biscuits** *Quaalude (methaqualone; discontinued 1983) or other CNS depressants* [see: methaqualone]

**ditch; ditch weed** *inferior-quality marijuana from Mexico or any low-potency marijuana that grows wild* [see: marijuana]

**djamba; diamba** [see: marijuana]

**do a joint** *smoking marijuana* [see: marijuana]

**do a line** *inhaling (snorting) powdered cocaine* [see: cocaine]

**DOA; dead on arrival** [see: heroin; PCP; cocaine, crack]

**doctor** [see: MDMA]

**dog food** [see: heroin]

**dogie; doojee** [see: heroin]

**dollies** *methadone (from the brand name Dolophine)* [see: Dolophine HCl; methadone HCl]

**dolls** *various CNS depressants*

**domes** [see: LSD]

**domestic** *locally grown marijuana* [see: marijuana]

**domex** *a combination of PCP and MDMA* [see: PCP; MDMA]

**dominoes** [see: amphetamines]

**don jem** [see: marijuana]

**Dona Juana; Dona Juanita** [see: marijuana]

**doobie** [see: marijuana]

**doojee; dogie** [see: heroin]

**dooley** [see: heroin]

**doors** *Doriden (glutethimide; discontinued 1990)* [see: glutethimide]

**doors and fours** *Doriden (glutethimide; discontinued 1990) and codeine* [see: glutethimide; codeine]

**dope** *heroin, marijuana, or any other street drug* [see: heroin; marijuana]

**dope smoke** [see: marijuana]

**dopium** [see: opium]

**doradilla** [see: marijuana]

**dots** [see: LSD]

**doub** *a $20 piece of crack* [see: cocaine, crack]

**double bubble** [see: cocaine]

**double cross** [see: amphetamines]

**double dome** [see: LSD]

**double rock** *crack diluted with procaine* [see: cocaine, crack; procaine]

**double trouble** *Dexamyl (dextroamphetamine sulfate + amobarbital; discontinued 1980)* [see: dextroamphetamine sulfate; amobarbital]

**double trouble** *Tuinal (amobarbital sodium + secobarbital sodium) or other CNS depressants* [see: Tuinal; amobarbital sodium; secobarbital sodium]

**double yoke** [see: cocaine, crack]

**dove** *a $35 piece of crack* [see: cocaine, crack]

**Dover's powder** [see: opium]

**down; downer; downies** *various CNS depressants*

**down and dirty** Quaalude (methaqualone; discontinued 1983) [see: methaqualone]

**draf weed; drag weed** [see: marijuana]

**dream** [see: cocaine]

**dream gum; dream stick; dreams** [see: opium]

**dreamer** [see: morphine]

**dreck** [see: heroin]

**drink** [see: PCP]

**drowsy high** various CNS depressants

**drug store dope** [see: morphine]

**dry high** [see: marijuana]

**duct** [see: cocaine]

**'due; dew** marijuana or the residue of oils left in a pipe after smoking crack [see: marijuana; cocaine, crack]

**duji** [see: heroin]

**dummy dust** [see: PCP]

**durog; duros** [see: marijuana]

**dust** heroin, cocaine, PCP, or marijuana mixed with various other substances [see: heroin; cocaine; PCP; marijuana]

**dust joint; dust of angels; dusted parsley** [see: PCP]

**dusting** a combination of marijuana and PCP, heroin, or other powdered street drug [see: marijuana; PCP; heroin]

**dusty roads** a combination of cocaine and PCP for smoking [see: cocaine; PCP]

**dynamite** a combination of heroin and cocaine [see: heroin; cocaine]

**dyno; dyno-pure** [see: heroin]

**earth** a marijuana cigarette [see: marijuana]

**easing powder** [see: opium]

**eastside player** [see: cocaine, crack]

**easy lay** [see: GHB]

**ecstasy; ex; X** [see: MDMA]

**egg** [see: cocaine, crack]

**eight ball** heroin or 1/8 oz. of any drug [see: heroin]

**eighth** [see: heroin]

**el diablillo** (Spanish for "the little devil") a combination of marijuana, cocaine, heroin, and PCP [see: marijuana; cocaine; heroin; PCP]

**el diablo** (Spanish for "the devil") a combination of marijuana, cocaine, and heroin [see: marijuana; cocaine; heroin]

**electric Kool Aid** [see: LSD]

**elephant; elephant tranquilizer** [see: PCP]

**embalming fluid** [see: PCP]

**emsel** a pronunciation of the brand name MS/L (morphine sulfate liquid) [see: MS/L; morphine sulfate]

**endo** [see: marijuana]

**energizer** [see: PCP]

**ephedrone** [see: methcathinone]

**esrar** (Turkish for "secret preparation") a mixture of marijuana and tobacco [see: marijuana; tobacco]

**essence** [see: MDMA]

**estufa** (Spanish for "stove") [see: heroin]

**ET** [see: alpha-ethyltryptamine]

**Eve** [see: MDMA]

**ex; X; extasy** from "ecstasy" [see: MDMA]

**eye opener** [see: cocaine, crack; amphetamines]

**fairy dust** [see: heroin]

**fake STP** [see: PCP]

**Fallbrook redhair** marijuana from Fallbrook, California [see: marijuana]

**famous dimes** [see: cocaine, crack]

**fantasia** [see: dimethyltryptamine]

**fat bags** [see: cocaine, crack]

**fatty** a marijuana cigarette [see: marijuana]

**feenies** [see: phenobarbital]

**fennies; phennies** [see: phenobarbital]

**feno's; pheno's** [see: phenobarbital]

**fields** [see: LSD]

**fifty-one; one-fifty-one** [see: cocaine, crack]

**fine stuff** [see: marijuana]

**finger** a marijuana cigarette or a stick-shaped piece of hashish [see: marijuana; hashish]

**fir** [see: marijuana]

**fire** a combination of crack and methamphetamine [see: cocaine, crack; methamphetamine HCl]

**first line** [see: morphine]

**fish scales** [see: cocaine, crack]

**fives** [see: amphetamine]

**fizzies** [see: methadone]

**flake; flakes** [see: cocaine; PCP]

**flamethrowers** *a cigarette laced with cocaine and heroin* [see: cocaine; heroin]

**flash** *glue (for sniffing) or LSD* [see: petroleum distillate inhalants; LSD]

**flat blues** [see: LSD]

**flat chunks** *crack cocaine cut (diluted) with benzocaine* [see: cocaine, crack]

**flea powder** *low-purity heroin* [see: heroin]

**Florida snow** *cocaine or a cocaine look-alike* [see: cocaine]

**flower; flower tops** [see: marijuana]

**fly agaric** [see: *Amanita muscaria* mushrooms]

**Flying Saucers** [see: morning glory seeds]

**fo-do-nie** [see: opium]

**foo foo dust; foo foo stuff** [see: cocaine; heroin]

**foolish powder** [see: cocaine; heroin]

**footballs** *Dilaudid (hydromorphone HCl) or Biphetamine (dextroamphetamine + amphetamine; discontinued 1979)* [see: Dilaudid; hydromorphone HCl; amphetamines]

**forwards** [see: amphetamines]

**four doors** *a combination of Doriden (glutethimide; discontinued 1990) and codeine* [see: glutethimide; codeine]

**four ways** *a combination of LSD, methamphetamine, strychnine, and STP* [see: LSD; methamphetamine HCl; strychnine; STP]

**fours** [see: Tylenol with Codeine No. 4; Empirin with Codeine No. 4; codeine]

**fraho; frajo** [see: marijuana]

**freeze** [see: cocaine]

**French blue** [see: amphetamine]

**French fries; fries; fry** [see: cocaine, crack]

**fresh** [see: PCP]

**friend** [see: fentanyl]

**fries; French fries; fry** [see: cocaine, crack]

**frio** (Spanish for "cold") *marijuana laced with PCP* [see: marijuana; PCP]

**Frisco special; Frisco speedball** *a combination of cocaine, heroin, and LSD* [see: cocaine; heroin; LSD]

**Friskie powder** [see: cocaine]

**fry; fries; French fries** [see: cocaine, crack]

**fry daddy** *a regular or marijuana cigarette laced with crack* [see: marijuana; cocaine, crack]

**Fu** [see: marijuana]

**fuel** *PCP or marijuana mixed with insecticides* [see: PCP; marijuana]

**fumo d'Angola** (Spanish for "Angola smoke") [see: marijuana]

**fungus** *a reference to the source (mushrooms)* [see: psilocybin]

**funk** [see: marijuana]

**funny stuff** [see: marijuana]

**G; gee** [see: paregoric; opium]

**gaffel** *fake cocaine* [see: cocaine]

**gagers; gaggers** [see: methcathinone]

**galloping horse** [see: heroin]

**gamot** [see: heroin]

**ganga; gange; ganja; Ghana; ghanja; gunga; gungeon** [see: marijuana]

**gangster** [see: marijuana]

**gank** *fake crack* [see: cocaine, crack]

**garbage rock** [see: cocaine, crack]

**gas** [see: nitrous oxide]

**gash** [see: marijuana]

**gasper; gasper stick** *a marijuana cigarette* [see: marijuana]

**gato** (Spanish for "cat") [see: heroin]

**gauge; gauge butt** [see: marijuana]

**gee; G** [see: paregoric; opium]

**geek** *a combination of crack and marijuana* [see: cocaine, crack; marijuana]

**George smack** [see: heroin]

**Georgia home boy** [see: GHB]

**get your own** [see: cocaine]

**Ghana; ghanja; ganga; gange; ganja; gunga; gungeon** [see: marijuana]

**ghost** [see: LSD]

**GI gin** *an elixir of terpin hydrate and codeine (disapproved in 1991)* [see: terpin hydrate; codeine]

**gift of the sun** [see: cocaine]

**giggle weed; giggle smoke** [see: marijuana]

**gimmie** *a combination of crack and marijuana* [see: cocaine, crack; marijuana]

**gin** [see: cocaine]

**girl** [see: cocaine; cocaine, crack; heroin]

**girlfriend** [see: cocaine]

**glad stuff** [see: cocaine]

**glass** [see: amphetamines]

**glassines** *from the type of translucent glazed paper in which heroin is sold* [see: heroin]

**glo** [see: cocaine, crack]

**God's drug** [see: morphine]

**God's flesh** [see: psilocybin; psilocin]

**God's medicine** [see: opium]

**go-fast** [see: methcathinone]

**gold** [see: marijuana; cocaine, crack]

**gold star** [see: marijuana]

**golden dragon** [see: LSD]

**golden girl** [see: heroin]

**golden leaf** *very high quality marijuana* [see: marijuana]

**golf ball** [see: cocaine, crack]

**golpe** [see: heroin]

**goma** (Spanish for "rubber") *morphine, opium, or black tar heroin* [see: morphine; opium; black tar heroin]

**gondola** [see: opium]

**gong** [see: marijuana; opium]

**goob** [see: methcathinone]

**good** [see: PCP]

**good and plenty** [see: heroin]

**good butt** *a marijuana cigarette* [see: marijuana]

**good giggles** [see: marijuana]

**good H** [see: heroin]

**goodfellas** [see: fentanyl]

**goof butt** *a marijuana cigarette* [see: marijuana]

**goofball** *barbiturates or a combination of cocaine and heroin* [see: barbiturates; cocaine; heroin]

**goofers** [see: barbiturates]

**goofies** [see: LSD]

**goon; goon dust** [see: PCP]

**gooney birds** [see: LSD]

**'goric** *from "paregoric"* [see: paregoric; opium]

**gorilla biscuits; gorilla tabs** [see: PCP]

**gorilla pills** *barbiturate sleeping pills* [see: barbiturates]

**gram** [see: hashish]

**grape parfait** [see: LSD]

**grass; grass brownies** [see: marijuana]

**grata** (Spanish for "pleasing") [see: marijuana]

**gravel** [see: cocaine, crack]

**gravy** [see: heroin]

**great bear** [see: fentanyl]

**great tobacco** [see: opium]

**green** *inferior-quality marijuana, PCP, or ketamine* [see: marijuana; PCP; ketamine HCl]

**green double domes; green single domes** [see: LSD]

**green goddess** [see: marijuana]

**green gold** [see: cocaine]

**green leaves; green tea** [see: PCP]

**green single domes; green double domes** [see: LSD]

**green wedge** [see: LSD]

**greens and clears** *Dexamyl (dextroamphetamine sulfate + amobarbital; discontinued 1980), named for the capsule color* [see: dextroamphetamine sulfate; amobarbital]

**greeter** [see: marijuana]

**grefa; grifa; griff; griffa; griffo** [see: marijuana]

**Greta** [see: marijuana]

**grey shields** [see: LSD]

**grievous bodily harm** [see: GHB]

**grifa; grefa; griff; griffa; griffo** [see: marijuana]

**G-riffic** [see: GHB]

**grit** [see: cocaine, crack]

**groceries** [see: cocaine, crack]

**grocery store high** [see: nitrous oxide]

**g-rock** *one gram of crack* [see: cocaine, crack]

**groovy lemon** *a yellow LSD tablet* [see: LSD]

**gum; guma** *opium refined for smoking* [see: opium]

**gunga; gungeon; ganga; gange; ganja; Ghana; ghanja** [see: marijuana]

**gungeon; gungun** *potent Jamaican marijuana* [see: marijuana]

**gunny; gunnysack** *a reference to sacks made with hemp fiber* [see: marijuana]

Street Slang

**gutter glitter** *cocaine or illegal drugs in general* [see: cocaine]

**gyve** *a marijuana cigarette* [see: marijuana]

**hache** [see: heroin]

**hail** [see: cocaine, crack]

**hairy** [see: heroin]

**half moon** [see: mescaline]

**half track** [see: cocaine, crack]

**hamburger helper** [see: cocaine, crack]

**hanhich** [see: marijuana]

**hanyak** *smokable speed* [see: amphetamines]

**happy cigarette** *a marijuana cigarette* [see: marijuana]

**happy dust; happy powder; happy trails** [see: cocaine]

**hard candy** [see: heroin]

**hard line; hard rock** [see: cocaine, crack]

**hard on; heart on** [see: amyl nitrite]

**hard stuff** [see: heroin; opium]

**hardware** [see: isobutyl nitrite]

**Harry; Harry Jones** [see: heroin]

**hash** [see: hashish; marijuana]

**hats** [see: LSD]

**have a dust; haven dust** [see: cocaine]

**Hawaiian** *very high potency marijuana* [see: marijuana]

**Hawaiian sunshine** [see: LSD]

**hawk** [see: LSD]

**hay** [see: marijuana]

**hay butt** *a marijuana cigarette* [see: marijuana]

**haze** [see: LSD]

**Hazel** [see: heroin]

**H-caps** [see: heroin]

**head drugs** [see: amphetamines]

**headlights** [see: LSD]

**heart on; hard on** [see: amyl nitrite]

**hearts** [see: amphetamines]

**heaven and hell** [see: PCP]

**heaven dust** [see: cocaine; heroin]

**Heavenly Blue** *LSD or a variety of psychedelic morning glory seeds* [see: LSD; morning glory seeds]

**heavy stuff** [see: cocaine; heroin]

**Helen** [see: heroin]

**hell dust** [see: heroin]

**He-man** [see: fentanyl; isobutyl nitrite]

**hemp** [see: marijuana]

**Henry** [see: heroin]

**Henry VIII** [see: cocaine]

**Her** [see: cocaine]

**herb; herba** ("herbaje" is Spanish for "grass") [see: marijuana]

**Herb and Al** *a combination of marijuana and alcohol* [see: alcohol; marijuana]

**herms** [see: PCP]

**hero; heroina; heroine; hero of the underworld** [see: heroin]

**hessle** [see: heroin]

**hi speeds; high speed** [see: amphetamines]

**hikori** [see: mescaline]

**hikuli** [see: mescaline]

**Him** [see: heroin]

**Hinkley** [see: PCP]

**hiropon** *smokable methamphetamine* [see: methamphetamine HCl]

**hit** *crack or a marijuana cigarette* [see: cocaine, crack; marijuana]

**hocus** [see: marijuana; opium]

**hog** [see: PCP]

**hombre** (Spanish for "man") [see: heroin]

**hombrecitos** (Spanish for "little men") [see: psilocybin]

**homegrown** [see: marijuana]

**homer** *freebase cocaine* [see: cocaine, crack]

**honey blunts** *marijuana cigars sealed with honey* [see: marijuana]

**honey oil** [see: ketamine HCl]

**hong-yen** *heroin in pill form* [see: heroin]

**hooch** [see: marijuana]

**hooter** [see: cocaine; marijuana]

**hop; hops** [see: opium]

**horning** *powdered cocaine or heroin* [see: cocaine; heroin]

**horse** [see: heroin]

**horse heads** [see: amphetamines]

**horse tracks; horse tranquilizer** [see: PCP]

**hot dope** [see: heroin]

**hot heroin** *poisoned heroin to give to a police informant* [see: heroin]

**hot ice** *smokable methamphetamine* [see: methamphetamine HCl]

**hot stick** *a marijuana cigarette* [see: marijuana]

**hotcakes** [see: cocaine, crack]

**How do you like me now?** [see: cocaine, crack]

**hows** [see: morphine]

**hubba; hubbas; Hubba, I am back** [see: cocaine, crack]

**hug drug; huggers** [see: MDMA]

**hunter** [see: cocaine]

**hyatari** [see: mescaline]

**I am back** [see: cocaine, crack]

**ice** [see: cocaine; amphetamines; MDMA; methamphetamine HCl; PCP]

**ice cube** [see: cocaine, crack]

**icing** [see: cocaine]

**idiot pills** [see: barbiturates]

**in-betweens** [see: amphetamines]

**Inca message** [see: cocaine]

**incentive** [see: cocaine]

**Indian boy; Indian hay; Indian hemp** [see: marijuana]

**Indiana** [see: mescaline]

**Indiana ditchweed** *low-potency wild marijuana that grows wild from seeds originally bred for hemp rope* [see: marijuana]

**Indiana hay** [see: marijuana]

**Indica** *a species of cannabis found in hot climates* [see: cannabis]

**Indo; Indonesian bud** [see: marijuana; opium]

**instant Zen** [see: LSD]

**Isda** [see: heroin]

**issues** [see: cocaine, crack]

**jackpot** [see: fentanyl]

**jam** [see: amphetamine; cocaine]

**Jam Cecil** [see: amphetamine]

**Jane** [see: marijuana]

**Jay; Jay smoke** *a marijuana cigarette* [see: marijuana]

**jee gee; jojoe** [see: heroin]

**Jeff** [see: methcathinone]

**jellies** [see: chloral hydrate]

**jelly** [see: cocaine]

**jelly baby** [see: amphetamines]

**jelly beans** [see: amphetamines; chloral hydrate; cocaine, crack]

**jet** [see: ketamine HCl]

**jet fuel** [see: PCP]

**Jim Jones** *marijuana laced with cocaine and PCP* [see: marijuana; cocaine; PCP]

**jive** [see: heroin; marijuana]

**jive doo jee** [see: heroin]

**jive stick** *a marijuana cigarette* [see: marijuana]

**Joe Friday** *Quaalude (methaqualone; discontinued 1983), the tablet ID# matches Sgt. Friday's badge number on Dragnet* [see: methaqualone]

**Johnson** [see: cocaine, crack]

**Johnson grass** *low-potency Texas marijuana (President Lyndon Johnson was from Texas)* [see: marijuana]

**joint** *a marijuana cigarette* [see: marijuana]

**jojee; jee gee** [see: heroin]

**jolly bean** [see: amphetamines]

**jolly green** [see: marijuana]

**Jones** [see: heroin]

**joy flakes** [see: heroin]

**joy juice** *chloral hydrate in an alcoholic beverage* [see: alcohol; chloral hydrate]

**joy plant** [see: opium]

**joy powder** [see: cocaine; heroin]

**joy smoke** [see: marijuana]

**joy stick** *a marijuana cigarette* [see: marijuana]

**Juan Valdez** [see: marijuana]

**Juanita** [see: marijuana]

**Judas** *a reference to Jesus' disciple ("the one who betrays")* [see: heroin]

**jugs** [see: amphetamines]

**juice** [see: PCP; anabolic steroids]

**juice joint** *a marijuana cigarette sprinkled with crack* [see: cocaine, crack; marijuana]

**ju-ju** *a marijuana cigarette* [see: marijuana]

**junk** [see: cocaine; heroin]

**Kabayo** [see: heroin]

**Kaksonjae** *smokable methamphetamine* [see: methamphetamine HCl]

**Kali** [see: marijuana]

**kangaroo** [see: cocaine, crack]

**kaps** [see: PCP]

**Karachi** *a reference to Karachi, Pakistan* [see: heroin]

**kat; khat; q'at** *leaves of the Catha edulis plant* [see: *Catha edulis*, cathinone]
**kaya** [see: marijuana]
**K-blast** [see: PCP]
**Kentucky blue** [see: marijuana]
**keys to the kingdom** [see: LSD]
**KGB** *"killer green bud"* [see: marijuana]
**khat; kat; q'at** *leaves of the Catha edulis plant* [see: *Catha edulis*, cathinone]
**Kibbles and Bits** *a combination of Talwin (pentazocine HCl) and Ritalin (methylphenidate HCl) or crumbs of crack* [see: Talwin; pentazocine HCl; Ritalin; methylphenidate HCl; cocaine, crack]
**kick stick** *a marijuana cigarette* [see: marijuana]
**kif; kiff** *potent Moroccan marijuana or hashish* [see: hashish; marijuana]
**killer** [see: marijuana; PCP]
**killer weed** *marijuana (1960s and 70s) or a combination of marijuana and PCP (1980s–)* [see: marijuana; PCP]
**kilter** [see: marijuana]
**kind** [see: marijuana]
**king ivory** [see: fentanyl]
**King Kong pills** *barbiturate sleeping pills or other CNS depressants* [see: barbiturates]
**king's habit** [see: cocaine]
**Kleenex** [see: MDMA]
**knockout drops** *chloral hydrate mixed in an alcoholic beverage* [see: alcohol; chloral hydrate]
**Kokomo** [see: cocaine, crack]
**Kools** [see: PCP]
**Krypt Tonight** *a brand-name sound-alike to "kryptonite," the substance that makes Superman weak* [see: isobutyl nitrite]
**kryptonite** [see: cocaine, crack]
**krystal; crystal; krystal joint; crystal joint** [see: PCP]
**kumbo** [see: marijuana]
**L.A.** *a long-acting amphetamine* [see: amphetamines]
**L.A. glass; L.A. ice** *smokable methamphetamine* [see: methamphetamine HCl]

**L.A. turnarounds** *a reference to truckers' use of amphetamines for long-distance runs* [see: amphetamines]
**lace** *a combination of cocaine and marijuana* [see: cocaine; marijuana]
**lady; lady caine; lady snow** [see: cocaine]
**Lakbay diva** [see: marijuana]
**lamb's bread** [see: marijuana]
**las mujercitas** (Spanish for "the little women") [see: psilocybin]
**lason sa daga** [see: LSD]
**laughing gas** [see: nitrous oxide]
**laughing grass; laughing weed** [see: marijuana]
**leaf** [see: marijuana; cocaine]
**leaky bolla; leaky leak** [see: PCP]
**leapers** [see: amphetamines]
**Lebanese** *hashish from Lebanon* [see: hashish]
**legal speed** *Mini Thin (ephedrine HCl), an over-the-counter asthma drug* [see: Mini Thin; ephedrine HCl]
**Lemmon 714; Lemmons** *Quaalude (methaqualone; discontinued 1983), refers to the manufacturer (Lemmon) and tablet ID# (714)* [see: methaqualone]
**lemonade** *heroin or poor-quality street drugs in general* [see: heroin]
**Lennons** *Quaalude (methaqualone; discontinued 1983), probably a reference to musician John Lennon* [see: methaqualone]
**lens** [see: LSD]
**lethal weapon** [see: PCP]
**Lib** [see: Librium; chlordiazepoxide HCl]
**lid poppers; lip poppers** [see: amphetamines]
**light stuff** [see: marijuana]
**lightning** [see: amphetamines]
**Lima** [see: marijuana]
**limbo** [see: marijuana]
**lime acid** [see: LSD]
**line** [see: cocaine]
**liquid ecstasy; liquid E; liquid ex; liquid X** [see: GHB]
**little bomb** [see: amphetamines; heroin]
**little ones** [see: PCP]

**little smoke** [see: marijuana; psilocybin; psilocin]

**live ones** [see: PCP]

**Llesca** [see: marijuana]

**loads** *a combination of Doriden (glutethimide; discontinued 1990) and codeine* [see: glutethimide; codeine]

**loaf** [see: marijuana]

**lobo** (Spanish for "wolf") [see: marijuana]

**locker room** [see: isobutyl nitrite]

**loco** (Spanish for "crazy" or "insane") [see: marijuana]

**locoweed** [see: marijuana; jimsonweed]

**log** *a marijuana cigarette or PCP* [see: marijuana; PCP]

**logor** [see: LSD]

**love** [see: cocaine, crack]

**love affair** [see: cocaine]

**love boat** *PCP or marijuana dipped in formaldehyde* [see: marijuana; PCP]

**love drug** *Quaalude (methaqualone; discontinued 1983)* [see: methaqualone]

**love drug of the '80s and '90s** [see: MDMA]

**love pearls; love pills** [see: alpha-ethyltryptamine]

**love trip** *a combination of mescaline and MDMA* [see: mescaline; MDMA]

**love weed** [see: marijuana]

**lovelies** *marijuana laced with PCP* [see: marijuana; PCP]

**lovely** [see: PCP]

**lovers** *Quaalude (methaqualone; discontinued 1983)* [see: methaqualone]

**lubage** [see: marijuana]

**Lucas** [see: marijuana]

**Lucy; Lucy in the sky with diamonds** [see: LSD]

**'ludes** *Quaalude (methaqualone; discontinued 1983)* [see: methaqualone]

**lumber** *marijuana stems and waste* [see: marijuana]

**machinery** [see: marijuana]

**Macon** [see: marijuana]

**mad dog** *PCP or Mogen David 20/20 fortified wine* [see: PCP; alcohol]

**madman** [see: PCP]

**magic; magic dust** [see: PCP]

**magic mushroom** [see: psilocybin; psilocin]

**magic smoke** [see: marijuana]

**Mama Coca** [see: cocaine]

**man** [see: heroin]

**Manhattan silver** [see: marijuana]

**marathons** [see: amphetamines]

**Marley** [see: marijuana]

**Mary; Mari** [see: marijuana]

**Mary and Johnny** [see: marijuana]

**Mary Ann; Mary Jane; Mary Warner** [see: marijuana]

**Matsakow** [see: heroin]

**Maui wowie; Maui waui** *marijuana from Hawaii* [see: marijuana]

**Max** *GHB dissolved in water and mixed with amphetamine* [see: GHB; amphetamines]

**Mayo** [see: cocaine; heroin]

**mean green** [see: PCP]

**Meg; Megg; Meggie** [see: marijuana]

**mellow drug of America** *MDA (methylenedioxyamphetamine), now called MDMA (methylenedioxymethamphetamine)* [see: MDMA]

**mellow yellow** *LSD or banana peels used for smoking* [see: LSD]

**Merck** *a reference to the manufacturer of pharmaceutical cocaine* [see: cocaine]

**mesc'; mez** [see: mescaline]

**mescal** *mescaline or an intoxicating distilled beverage from the same plant* [see: mescaline]

**meserole** *a marijuana cigarette* [see: marijuana]

**meth** [see: methamphetamine HCl]

**Mexican brown** [see: heroin; marijuana]

**Mexican horse; Mexican mud** [see: heroin]

**Mexican mushrooms** [see: psilocybin; psilocin]

**Mexican red** [see: marijuana]

**Mexican Valium** [see: Rohypnol; flunitrazepam]

**mez; mesc'** [see: mescaline]

**Mickey Finn** *chloral hydrate mixed in an alcoholic beverage* [see: chloral hydrate; alcohol]

**microdot** [see: LSD]

Street Slang

**mic's; mikes** *microdots of LSD* [see: LSD]

**midnight oil** [see: opium]

**mighty mezz** *a marijuana cigarette* [see: marijuana]

**Mighty Quinn** [see: LSD]

**mikes; mic's** *microdots of LSD* [see: LSD]

**mind detergent** [see: LSD]

**minibennie** [see: amphetamines]

**mint leaf; mint weed** [see: PCP]

**45-minute psychosis** [see: dimethyltryptamine]

**mira** (Spanish for "look" or "watch") [see: opium]

**Miss Emma** [see: morphine]

**missile basing** *a combination of crack liquid and PCP* [see: cocaine, crack; PCP]

**mist** *crack smoke or PCP* [see: cocaine, crack; PCP]

**Mister Blue** [see: morphine]

**Mister Brownstone** *hashish or brown heroin* [see: hashish; heroin]

**Mister Natural** [see: LSD]

**M.O.; M.U.** [see: marijuana]

**modams** [see: marijuana]

**Mohasky** [see: marijuana]

**mojo** [see: cocaine; heroin; morphine]

**monkey** *a cigarette made from cocaine paste and tobacco* [see: cocaine; tobacco]

**monkey dust; monkey tranquilizer** [see: PCP]

**monos** *cigarettes made from cocaine paste and tobacco* [see: cocaine; tobacco]

**monte** (Spanish for "mountain") *marijuana from South America* [see: marijuana]

**mooca; moocah** [see: marijuana]

**moon** [see: mescaline]

**moonrock** *a combination of crack and heroin* [see: cocaine, crack; heroin]

**mooster** [see: marijuana]

**moota; mooter; mootie; mooto; muta; mutah** *a marijuana cigarette* [see: marijuana]

**mor a grifa** [see: marijuana]

**more** [see: PCP]

**morfina** (Spanish for "morphine") [see: morphine]

**morotgara** [see: heroin]

**morph; morphy** [see: morphine]

**mortal combat** *high-potency heroin* [see: heroin]

**mosquitos** [see: cocaine]

**mota; moto** (Spanish for "speck") [see: marijuana]

**mother** [see: marijuana]

**mother's little helper** [see: Valium; diazepam]

**movie star drug** [see: cocaine]

**M.U.; M.O.** [see: marijuana]

**mud** [see: heroin; morphine; opium]

**muggie; muggies; muggles** *a marijuana cigarette* [see: marijuana]

**mujer** (Spanish for "woman" or "wife") [see: cocaine]

**mulka** [see: methcathinone]

**murder 8** [see: fentanyl]

**murder one** *a combination of heroin and cocaine* [see: cocaine; heroin]

**Murphy** [see: morphine]

**mushrooms** [see: psilocybin; psilocin]

**musk** [see: psilocybin; psilocin]

**muta; mutah; moota; mooter; mootie; mooto** *a marijuana cigarette* [see: marijuana]

**muzzle** [see: heroin]

**nail** *a marijuana cigarette* [see: marijuana]

**Nanoo** [see: heroin]

**nebbies** [see: Nembutal Sodium; pentobarbital sodium]

**nemish** [see: Nembutal Sodium; pentobarbital sodium]

**new acid** [see: PCP]

**New Jack Swing** *a combination of heroin and morphine* [see: heroin; morphine]

**new magic** [see: PCP]

**nice and easy** [see: heroin]

**nickel desk** [see: heroin]

**nie; nigh** [see: nitrous oxide]

**niebla** (Spanish for "fog" or "haze") [see: PCP]

**nimbies** [see: Nembutal Sodium; pentobarbital sodium]

**nitro; nitrogen** [see: nitrous oxide]

**Nixon** *low-potency heroin* [see: heroin]

**noise** [see: heroin]

**nose** [see: heroin]

**nose candy; nose powder; nose stuff** [see: cocaine]

**nose drops** *liquefied heroin* [see: heroin]

**nubs** [see: mescaline]

**nuggets** [see: amphetamines; cocaine, crack]

**number** *a marijuana cigarette* [see: marijuana]

**number 3** [see: cocaine; heroin]

**number 4; number 8** [see: heroin]

**O; O.P.** [see: opium]

**octane** *PCP laced with gasoline* [see: PCP; petroleum distillate inhalants]

**ogoy** [see: heroin]

**oil** *hashish oil, heroin, or PCP* [see: hashish; heroin; PCP]

**O.J.** [see: marijuana]

**Old Steve** [see: heroin]

**one way** [see: LSD]

**one-fifty-one; fifty-one** [see: cocaine, crack]

**ope** [see: opium]

**O.P.P.** [see: PCP]

**optical illusions** [see: LSD]

**orange** *Desoxyn (methamphetamine HCl), a reference to the capsule color* [see: Desoxyn; methamphetamine HCl]

**orange barrels; orange cubes; orange haze; orange micro; orange wedges** [see: LSD]

**orange crystal** [see: PCP]

**orange cupcakes** *a combination of LSD, methamphetamine, strychnine, and STP* [see: LSD; methamphetamine HCl; strychnine; STP]

**oranges** [see: amphetamines]

**organic Quaalude** [see: GHB]

**outer limits** *a combination of crack and LSD* [see: cocaine, crack; LSD]

**Owsley; Owsley's acid; white Owsley** [see: LSD]

**ozone** [see: PCP]

**Ozzie's stuff** *probably a reference to Ozzie Osborne* [see: LSD]

**paca lolo; pakalolo** *a Hawaiian term* [see: marijuana]

**pack** [see: heroin; marijuana]

**pack of rocks** *a marijuana cigarette* [see: marijuana]

**Pakistani black** [see: marijuana]

**Panama cut; Panama gold; Panama red** [see: marijuana]

**panatella** *a large cigar-shaped marijuana cigarette* [see: marijuana]

**pancakes and syrup** *a combination of glutethimide and codeine cough syrup* [see: glutethimide; codeine]

**pane** *a short form of "window pane," a reference to the glassine packaging* [see: LSD]

**pangonadalot** [see: heroin]

**paper acid** [see: LSD]

**paper blunts** *a marijuana cigarette rolled in cigarette paper rather than a tobacco leaf casing* [see: marijuana]

**parachute** *heroin or crack and PCP smoked together* [see: cocaine, crack; PCP; heroin]

**paradise; paradise white** [see: cocaine]

**parlay** [see: cocaine, crack]

**parsley** [see: marijuana; PCP]

**paste** [see: cocaine, crack]

**Pat** [see: marijuana]

**'patico** *from the Spanish "simpático," meaning "nice" or "pleasant"* [see: cocaine, crack]

**paz** [see: PCP]

**PCPA** [see: PCP]

**P-dope** *20-30% pure heroin* [see: heroin]

**peace** [see: LSD; PCP]

**peace pill** [see: PCP]

**peace tablets** [see: LSD]

**peace weed** *PCP or a combination of marijuana and PCP* [see: marijuana; PCP]

**peaches** *Benzedrine (amphetamine sulfate; discontinued 1982)* [see: amphetamine sulfate]

**peanut butter** *PCP mixed with peanut butter* [see: PCP]

**peanuts** *barbiturate sleeping pills* [see: barbiturates]

**pearl** [see: cocaine]

**pearls** [see: amyl nitrite]

**pearly gates** *LSD or a variety of psychedelic morning glory seeds* [see: LSD; morning glory seeds]

**pebbles** [see: cocaine, crack]

**Pee Wee** [see: cocaine, crack]

Street Slang

**peep** [see: PCP]

**Peg** [see: heroin]

**pellets** [see: LSD]

**pen yan** [see: opium]

**pep pills** [see: amphetamines]

**perc's; perks** [see: Percodan; oxycodone HCl]

**perfect high** [see: heroin]

**perico** (Spanish for "parakeet") [see: cocaine]

**perp** *fake crack made of candle wax and baking soda (to "perpetrate" a fraud)*

**Peruvian; Peruvian flake; Peruvian lady** [see: cocaine]

**Peter** [see: chloral hydrate]

**Peter Pan** [see: PCP]

**peth** *from "pethidine," the official British and International name for meperidine HCl* [see: Demerol HCl; meperidine HCl]

**petrol** *a British term for gasoline* [see: petroleum distillate inhalants]

**peyote** [see: mescaline]

**P-funk** *heroin or a combination of crack and PCP* [see: heroin; cocaine, crack; PCP]

**phennies; fennies** [see: phenobarbital]

**pheno's; feno's** [see: phenobarbital]

**Phillies blunt** *a cigar hollowed out and filled with marijuana* [see: marijuana]

**piece** [see: cocaine; cocaine, crack]

**piedras** (Spanish for "stones") [see: cocaine, crack]

**pig killer** [see: PCP]

**piles** [see: cocaine, crack]

**pimp** [see: cocaine]

**pin; pinhead** *a thinly rolled marijuana cigarette* [see: marijuana]

**pin gun; pin yen** [see: opium]

**pineapple** *a combination of heroin and Ritalin (methylphenidate HCl) or amphetamine* [see: heroin; Ritalin; methylphenidate HCl; amphetamines]

**pink blotters** [see: LSD]

**pink hearts** [see: amphetamines]

**Pink Panther; pink robots; pink wedge; pink witches** [see: LSD]

**pink spoons** [see: Percodan; oxycodone HCl]

**pinks** [see: Seconal Sodium; secobarbital sodium]

**pit** [see: PCP]

**pixies** [see: amphetamines]

**platters** [see: hashish]

**pocket rocket** [see: marijuana]

**pod** [see: marijuana]

**poison** [see: heroin; fentanyl]

**poke** [see: marijuana]

**polvo** (Spanish for "powder" or "dust") [see: heroin; PCP]

**polvo blanco** (Spanish for "white powder") [see: cocaine]

**polvo de angel; polvo de estrellas** (Spanish for "angel dust"; "star dust") [see: PCP]

**pony** [see: cocaine, crack]

**poor man's speedball** *a combination of heroin and methamphetamine* [see: heroin; methamphetamine HCl]

**poppers** [see: isobutyl nitrite; amyl nitrite]

**poppy** [see: heroin]

**pot** [see: marijuana]

**pot liquor; pot likker** *a tea brewed from marijuana waste* [see: marijuana]

**potato** [see: LSD]

**potato chips** *crack cocaine cut (diluted) with benzocaine* [see: cocaine, crack]

**potten bush** [see: marijuana]

**powder** [see: heroin; amphetamines]

**powder diamonds** [see: cocaine]

**pox** [see: opium]

**P.R. (Panama Red)** [see: marijuana]

**preludes** *Preludin (phenmetrazine HCl; discontinued 1992)* [see: phenmetrazine HCl]

**prescription** *a marijuana cigarette* [see: marijuana]

**press** [see: cocaine; cocaine, crack]

**pretendica; pretendo** (Spanish for "pretender") [see: marijuana]

**primo** (Spanish for "priority") *crack, marijuana and crack, or cigarettes with cocaine and heroin* [see: cocaine, crack; marijuana; cocaine; heroin]

**pseudocaine** *phenylpropanolamine, an adulterant for cutting crack*

**puffy** [see: PCP]

**pulborn** [see: heroin]

**pure** [see: heroin]
**pure love** [see: LSD]
**purple** [see: ketamine HCl]
**purple barrels; purple flats; purple haze; purple ozoline** [see: LSD]
**purple hearts** *Luminal Sodium (phenobarbital sodium), LSD, amphetamines, or various CNS depressants* [see: Luminal Sodium; phenobarbital sodium; LSD; amphetamines]
**purple rain** [see: PCP]
**q'at; kat; khat** *leaves of the Catha edulis plant* [see: *Catha edulis*, cathinone]
**qua; quaa; quack; quad; quas** *Quaalude (methaqualone; discontinued 1983)* [see: methaqualone]
**quarter moon** [see: hashish]
**quartz** *smokable speed* [see: amphetamines]
**Queen Anne's lace** [see: marijuana]
**quicksilver** [see: isobutyl nitrite]
**quill** [see: methamphetamine HCl; heroin; cocaine]
**R and R** *reds (Seconal Sodium; secobarbital sodium) and Ripple (wine)* [see: Seconal Sodium; secobarbital sodium; alcohol]
**racehorse Charlie** [see: cocaine; heroin]
**ragweed** *inferior-quality marijuana or heroin* [see: marijuana; heroin]
**railroad weed** [see: marijuana]
**rainbows** *Tuinal (amobarbital sodium + secobarbital sodium), which comes in multicolored striped capsules* [see: Tuinal; amobarbital sodium; secobarbital sodium]
**rainy day woman** *a marijuana cigarette* [see: marijuana]
**Rambo** [see: heroin]
**Rane** [see: cocaine; heroin]
**rangood** *marijuana grown wild* [see: marijuana]
**Rasta weed** [see: marijuana]
**raw** [see: cocaine, crack]
**ready rock** [see: cocaine; cocaine, crack; heroin]
**recycle** [see: LSD]
**red and blues** [see: Tuinal; amobarbital sodium; secobarbital sodium]

**red birds; red bullets** [see: secobarbital sodium]
**red caps** [see: cocaine, crack]
**red chicken** [see: heroin]
**red chicken** *Chinese heroin* [see: heroin]
**red cross** [see: marijuana]
**red devils** *PCP or Seconal Sodium (secobarbital sodium) capsules* [see: PCP; Seconal Sodium; secobarbital sodium]
**red dirt** [see: marijuana]
**red eagle** [see: heroin]
**red phosphorus** *smokable speed* [see: amphetamines]
**red rum** *"murder" spelled backward; a potent form of heroin* [see: heroin]
**reds** [see: Seconal Sodium; secobarbital sodium]
**reds and Ripple** *a combination of Seconal Sodium (secobarbital sodium) and Ripple wine* [see: Seconal Sodium; secobarbital sodium; alcohol]
**reefer** [see: marijuana]
**regular P** [see: cocaine, crack]
**reindeer dust** [see: heroin]
**Rhine** [see: heroin]
**rhythm** [see: amphetamines]
**rib** [see: Rohypnol; flunitrazepam]
**rippers** [see: amphetamines]
**roach** *the butt of a marijuana cigarette* [see: marijuana]
**roach 2; roaches** [see: Rohypnol; flunitrazepam]
**road dope** [see: amphetamines]
**roca** (Spanish for "rock") [see: cocaine, crack]
**Roche** [see: Rohypnol; flunitrazepam]
**rock(s)** [see: cocaine, crack]
**rocket** *a marijuana cigarette* [see: marijuana]
**rocket fuel** [see: PCP]
**rocks; rox; rocks of hell** [see: cocaine, crack]
**Rocky III** [see: cocaine, crack]
**rolling** [see: MDMA]
**roofie; roofies** [see: Rohypnol; flunitrazepam]
**'rooms** *Psilocybe mushrooms* [see: psilocybin]
**roopies** [see: Rohypnol; flunitrazepam]
**rooster** [see: cocaine, crack]

Street Slang

**root** *a marijuana cigarette* [see: marijuana]

**rope** [see: marijuana; Rohypnol; fluni-trazepam]

**rophy; ropies; roples** [see: Rohypnol; flunitrazepam]

**rosa** (Spanish for "rose" or "pink") [see: amphetamines]

**Rose Maria** [see: marijuana]

**roses** *Benzedrine (amphetamine sulfate; discontinued 1982) tablets* [see: amphetamine sulfate]

**rox; rocks; rocks of Hell** [see: cocaine, crack]

**Roxanne** [see: cocaine; cocaine, crack]

**royal blues** [see: LSD]

**Roz** [see: cocaine, crack]

**ruderalis** *a species of cannabis found in Russia* [see: cannabis]

**ruffies; ruffles** [see: Rohypnol; flunitrazepam]

**running** [see: MDMA]

**rush; rush snappers** [see: isobutyl nitrite]

**Russian sickles** [see: LSD]

**sack** [see: heroin]

**sacrament** [see: LSD]

**sacred mushrooms** [see: psilocybin]

**salt** [see: heroin]

**salt and pepper** [see: marijuana]

**salty water** [see: GHB]

**Sandoz** *a reference to the manufacturer* [see: LSD]

**sandwich** *two layers of cocaine with a layer of heroin* [see: cocaine; heroin]

**Santa Marta** (Spanish for "Saint Marta") [see: marijuana]

**sassafras** [see: marijuana]

**sativa** *a species of cannabis found in cool, damp climates* [see: cannabis]

**scaffle** [see: PCP]

**scag** [see: heroin]

**scat; scate** [see: heroin]

**schmack; smack; schmeck; shmeck** [see: heroin]

**schoolboy** [see: cocaine; codeine]

**schoolboy scotch** *Scotch whiskey with codeine added* [see: codeine; alcohol]

**Schoolcraft** [see: cocaine, crack]

**scissors** [see: marijuana]

**scoop** [see: GHB]

**scorpion** [see: cocaine]

**Scott** [see: heroin]

**Scottie; Scotty** [see: cocaine; cocaine, crack]

**scramble** [see: cocaine, crack]

**scrubwoman's kick** *inhaled cleaning fluid, especially naphtha* [see: petroleum distillate inhalants]

**scruples** [see: cocaine, crack]

**scuffle; skuffle** [see: PCP]

**seccy; seggy** [see: Seconal Sodium; secobarbital sodium]

**seeds** [see: marijuana]

**seggy; seccy** [see: Seconal Sodium; secobarbital sodium]

**sen** [see: marijuana]

**seni** *peyote* [see: mescaline]

**serenity; serenity, tranquility, and peace** [see: STP]

**Sernyl** [see: PCP]

**Serpico 21** [see: cocaine]

**Sess** [see: marijuana]

**sets** *a combination of Talwin (pentazocine HCl) and PBZ (pyribenzamine)* [see: Talwin; pentazocine HCl; tripelennamine]

**seven fourteens** *Quaalude (methaqualone; discontinued 1983), from ID# 714 on the tablets* [see: methaqualone]

**Seven-Up** [see: cocaine; cocaine, crack]

**sezz** [see: marijuana]

**shabu** [see: cocaine; methamphetamine HCl; amphetamines; MDMA; PCP]

**shake** [see: marijuana]

**She** [see: cocaine]

**sheet rocking** *a combination of crack and LSD* [see: cocaine, crack; LSD]

**sheets** [see: PCP]

**Sherm(s); Sherman(s)** *a tobacco cigarette laced with PCP* [see: PCP]

**shmeck; schmeck; schmack; smack** [see: heroin]

**shoot the breeze** [see: nitrous oxide]

**'shrooms** *from "mushrooms"* [see: psilocybin; psilocin]

**siddi** [see: marijuana]

**sightball** [see: cocaine, crack]

**Silly Putty** [see: psilocybin; psilocin]

**Simple Simon** [see: psilocybin; psilocin]

**sinse; sinsemilla** *a potent variety of marijuana* [see: marijuana]

**sixty-second trip** [see: amyl nitrite]

**skee** [see: opium]

**skid** [see: heroin]

**skunk** [see: marijuana]

**slab** [see: cocaine, crack]

**sleeper** [see: heroin]

**sleet** [see: cocaine, crack]

**slick superspeed** [see: methcathinone]

**slime** [see: heroin]

**smack; schmack; shmeck; schmeck** [see: heroin]

**smears** [see: LSD]

**smoke** *marijuana, crack, or a combination of heroin and crack* [see: marijuana; cocaine, crack; heroin]

**smoke Canada** [see: marijuana]

**smoking** [see: PCP]

**smoking gun** [see: heroin; cocaine]

**snap** [see: amphetamines]

**snappers** [see: amyl nitrite; isobutyl nitrite]

**sniff** *methcathinone, an inhalant, or to inhale cocaine* [see: methcathinone; petroleum distillate inhalants; cocaine]

**snop** [see: marijuana]

**snort** *cocaine or inhalants* [see: cocaine; petroleum distillate inhalants]

**snorts** [see: PCP]

**snot** *the residue produced from smoking amphetamine* [see: amphetamines]

**snot balls** *rubber cement rolled into balls and burned* [see: petroleum distillate inhalants]

**snow** [see: cocaine; heroin; amphetamines]

**snow bird** [see: cocaine]

**snow pallets** [see: amphetamines]

**snow seals** *a combination of cocaine and amphetamine* [see: cocaine; amphetamines]

**snow soke** [see: cocaine, crack]

**snow white** [see: cocaine]

**snowball** *a combination of cocaine and heroin* [see: cocaine; heroin]

**snowcones** [see: cocaine]

**soap** [see: GHB]

**soaper; Sopors** *Sopor (methaqualone; discontinued 1981)* [see: methaqualone]

**society high** [see: cocaine]

**soda** *injectable cocaine* [see: cocaine]

**soles** [see: hashish]

**soma** (Italian for "burden" or "load") [see: PCP]

**somatomax** [see: GHB]

**Sopors; soaper** *Sopor (methaqualone; discontinued 1981)* [see: methaqualone]

**space base** *crack dipped in PCP or a hollowed-out cigar refilled with PCP and crack* [see: cocaine, crack; PCP]

**space cadet; space dust** *crack dipped in PCP* [see: cocaine, crack; PCP]

**sparkle plenty** [see: amphetamines]

**sparklers** [see: amphetamines]

**Special K** [see: ketamine HCl]

**special la coke** [see: ketamine HCl]

**speckled birds; speckled eggs** [see: amphetamines]

**specks** [see: LSD]

**speed** [see: methamphetamine HCl; amphetamine; cocaine, crack; methcathinone]

**speed boat** *a combination of marijuana, PCP, and crack* [see: marijuana; PCP; cocaine, crack]

**speed for lovers** [see: MDMA]

**speedball** *amphetamine or a combination of heroin and cocaine* [see: amphetamines; heroin; cocaine]

**spider blue** [see: heroin]

**splash** [see: amphetamines]

**spliff** *a marijuana cigarette* [see: marijuana]

**splim** [see: marijuana]

**splivins** [see: amphetamines]

**spores** [see: PCP]

**square mackerel** *marijuana from Florida* [see: marijuana]

**square time Bob** [see: cocaine, crack]

**squirrel** *LSD or a combination of cocaine, marijuana, and PCP for smoking* [see: LSD; cocaine; marijuana; PCP]

**stack** [see: marijuana]

**Stanley's stuff** [see: LSD]

Street Slang

**star** *methcathinone or LSD blotter acid with star-shaped design* [see: methcathinone; LSD]

**stardust** [see: cocaine; PCP]

**star-spangled powder** [see: cocaine]

**stat** [see: methcathinone]

**stems** [see: marijuana]

**stick** [see: marijuana; PCP]

**sticks** *marijuana stems and waste* [see: marijuana]

**stink weed** [see: marijuana]

**stones** [see: cocaine, crack]

**STP** *the hallucinogen 2,5-dimethoxy-4-methylamphetamine (DOM), derived from amphetamine*

**straw** *a marijuana cigarette* [see: marijuana]

**strawberry fields** [see: LSD]

**stuff** [see: heroin]

**stumblers** [see: barbiturates]

**sugar** [see: cocaine; LSD; heroin]

**sugar block** [see: cocaine, crack]

**sugar cubes; sugar lumps** [see: LSD]

**sugar weed** [see: marijuana]

**sunrise; sunshine** *yellow LSD* [see: LSD]

**super** [see: PCP]

**super acid; super C** [see: ketamine HCl]

**super cools; super kools** *PCP-laced cigarettes* [see: PCP]

**super grass; super weed** *PCP or marijuana laced with PCP* [see: marijuana; PCP]

**super ice** *smokable methamphetamine* [see: methamphetamine HCl]

**super joint** [see: PCP]

**super Sopors** *Parest (methaqualone; discontinued 1983)* [see: methaqualone]

**supers** [see: methaqualone]

**supper** *Sopor (methaqualone; discontinued 1981)* [see: methaqualone]

**surfer** [see: PCP]

**sweet Jesus** [see: heroin]

**sweet Lucy** [see: marijuana]

**sweet stuff** [see: heroin; cocaine]

**sweets** [see: amphetamines]

**swell up** [see: cocaine, crack]

**synthetic cocaine** [see: PCP]

**synthetic THT** [see: PCP]

**syrup and beans** *a combination of Doriden (glutethimide; discontinued 1990) and codeine* [see: glutethimide; codeine]

**tabs** [see: LSD]

**tac** [see: PCP]

**tail lights** [see: LSD]

**taima** [see: marijuana]

**taking a cruise** [see: PCP]

**Takkouri** [see: marijuana]

**tall** [see: Talwin; pentazocine HCl]

**Tango & Cash** [see: fentanyl]

**tar** [see: opium; heroin]

**tardust** [see: cocaine]

**taste** *heroin or a small sample of drugs* [see: heroin]

**T-birds** [see: Tuinal; amobarbital sodium; secobarbital sodium]

**T-buzz** [see: PCP]

**tea** [see: marijuana; PCP]

**tease and bees; T's and B's; tees and bees** *a combination of Talwin (pentazocine HCl) and PBZ (pyribenzamine), used as a heroin substitute* [see: Talwin; pentazocine HCl; tripelennamine]

**tease and blues; T's and blues; tees and blues** *a combination of Talwin (pentazocine HCl) and PBZ (pyribenzamine), used as a heroin substitute* [see: Talwin; pentazocine HCl; tripelennamine]

**tease and peas; T's and P's; tees and pees** *a combination of Talwin (pentazocine HCl) and PBZ (pyribenzamine), used as a heroin substitute* [see: Talwin; pentazocine HCl; tripelennamine]

**tecata; Tecate** [see: heroin]

**Teddies and Bettys** *a combination of Talwin (pentazocine HCl) and PBZ (pyribenzamine), used as a heroin substitute* [see: Talwin; pentazocine HCl; tripelennamine]

**tees and bees; T's and B's; tease and bees** *a combination of Talwin (pentazocine HCl) and PBZ (pyribenzamine), used as a heroin substitute* [see: Talwin; pentazocine HCl; tripelennamine]

**tees and blues; T's and blues; tease and blues** *a combination of Talwin (pentazocine HCl) and PBZ* (pyribenzamine), used as a heroin substitute [see: Talwin; pentazocine HCl; tripelennamine]

**tees and pees; T's and P's; tease and peas** a combination of Talwin (pentazocine HCl) and PBZ (pyribenzamine), used as a heroin substitute [see: Talwin; pentazocine HCl; tripelennamine]

**teeth** [see: cocaine; cocaine, crack]

**temple balls** [see: hashish]

**ten-cent pistol** a heroin dose laced with poison [see: heroin]

**tens** 10 mg amphetamine tablets [see: amphetamines]

**tension** [see: cocaine, crack]

**Texas pot; Texas tea; Tex-mex** [see: marijuana]

**Thai sticks** bundles of marijuana soaked in hashish oil or marijuana buds bound on short sections of bamboo [see: marijuana; hashish]

**The Beast** [see: heroin]

**The C** [see: methcathinone]

**the devil** [see: cocaine, crack]

**the witch** [see: heroin]

**Thing** [see: heroin; cocaine]

**thirteen** [see: marijuana]

**three hundreds** Quaaludes (methaqualone; discontinued 1983), a reference to 300 mg tablets [see: methaqualone]

**threes** [see: Tylenol with Codeine No. 3; Empirin with Codeine No. 3]

**thrust** [see: isobutyl nitrite]

**thrusters** [see: amphetamines]

**thumb** a marijuana cigarette [see: marijuana]

**tic; tic tac** [see: PCP]

**ticket; ticket to ride** [see: LSD]

**Tijuana** a reference to a Mexican town on the U.S. border [see: marijuana]

**tish** [see: PCP]

**tissue** [see: cocaine, crack]

**titch** [see: PCP]

**toncho** an octane booster, which is inhaled [see: petroleum distillate inhalants]

**tooey; tuie; twoie** [see: Tuinal; amobarbital sodium; secobarbital sodium]

**tooly** toluene, which is inhaled [see: petroleum distillate inhalants]

**toot** [see: cocaine]

**Tootsie Roll** [see: heroin]

**top gun** [see: cocaine, crack]

**topi** peyote cactus [see: mescaline]

**tops** peyote [see: mescaline]

**tops and bottoms** a combination of Talwin (pentazocine HCl) and PBZ (pyribenzamine), used as a heroin substitute [see: Talwin; pentazocine HCl; tripelennamine]

**torch** [see: marijuana]

**torpedo** chloral hydrate in an alcoholic beverage or a combination of crack and marijuana [see: chloral hydrate; cocaine, crack; marijuana]

**toxy** [see: opium]

**toys** [see: opium]

**tragic magic** crack dipped in PCP [see: cocaine, crack; PCP]

**trank** from "tranquilizer" [see: PCP]

**trikes and bikes; tricycles and bicycles** a combination of Talwin (pentazocine HCl) and PBZ (pyribenzamine), used as a heroin substitute [see: Talwin; pentazocine HCl; tripelennamine]

**trip** [see: LSD; alpha-ethyltryptamine]

**trippers** [see: LSD]

**tropp** [see: cocaine, crack]

**truck drivers** a reference to their use of amphetamines during long-distance runs [see: amphetamines]

**T's and blues; tees and blues; tease and blues** a combination of Talwin (pentazocine HCl) and PBZ (pyribenzamine), used as a heroin substitute [see: Talwin; pentazocine HCl; tripelennamine]

**T's and B's; tees and bees; tease and bees** a combination of Talwin (pentazocine HCl) and PBZ (pyribenzamine), used as a heroin substitute [see: Talwin; pentazocine HCl; tripelennamine]

**T's and P's; tees and pees; tease and peas** a combination of Talwin (pentazocine HCl) and PBZ (pyribenzamine), used as a heroin substitute [see: Talwin; pentazocine HCl; tripelennamine]

**tuie; tooey; twoie** [see: Tuinal; amobarbital sodium; secobarbital sodium]

**turbo** a combination of crack and marijuana [see: cocaine, crack; marijuana]

**turkey** [see: cocaine; amphetamines]
**turnabout; turnarounds** *a reference to truckers' use of amphetamines for long-distance runs* [see: amphetamines]
**turp** *an elixir of terpin hydrate and codeine (disapproved in 1991)* [see: terpin hydrate; codeine]
**tutti-frutti** *a flavored cocaine developed in Brazil* [see: cocaine]
**tweek** *a methamphetamine-like substance* [see: methamphetamine HCl; amphetamines]
**tweeker** [see: methcathinone]
**twenty-five** [see: LSD]
**twist; twistum** *a marijuana cigarette* [see: marijuana]
**twoie; tuie; tooey** [see: Tuinal; amobarbital sodium; secobarbital sodium]
**ultimate** [see: cocaine, crack]
**Uncle Miltie; Uncle Milty** [see: Miltown; meprobamate]
**unkie** [see: morphine]
**uppers; uppies** [see: amphetamines]
**Utopiates** *various hallucinogens*
**Uzi** [see: cocaine, crack]
**video head cleaner** [see: butyl nitrite]
**vitamin Q** *Quaalude (methaqualone; discontinued 1983)* [see: methaqualone]
**vodka acid** [see: LSD]
**wac; wack** *PCP or marijuana laced with PCP* [see: marijuana; PCP]
**wacky dust** [see: cocaine]
**wacky terbacky; wacky weed** [see: marijuana]
**wafer** [see: LSD]
**wake-ups** [see: amphetamines]
**wallbangers** *Quaalude (methaqualone; discontinued 1983)* [see: methaqualone]
**water** [see: methamphetamine HCl; PCP]
**wave** [see: cocaine, crack]
**weasel dust** [see: cocaine]
**wedding bells** [see: LSD]
**wedge** [see: LSD]
**weed** [see: marijuana; PCP]
**weed tea** *a tea made from marijuana waste* [see: marijuana]
**West Coast turnaround** *a reference to truckers' use of amphetamines for long-distance runs* [see: amphetamines]

**whack** *a combination of PCP and heroin* [see: PCP; heroin]
**wheat** [see: marijuana]
**when-shee** [see: opium]
**whiffenpoppers** [see: amyl nitrite]
**whippets** [see: nitrous oxide]
**white** [see: amphetamines]
**white ball** [see: cocaine, crack]
**white boy** [see: heroin]
**white cross** [see: methamphetamine HCl; amphetamines]
**white dust** [see: LSD]
**white ghost** [see: cocaine, crack]
**white girl** [see: cocaine; heroin]
**white horizon** [see: PCP]
**white horse** [see: cocaine]
**white junk** [see: heroin]
**white lady** [see: cocaine; heroin]
**white lightning** [see: LSD]
**white mosquito** [see: cocaine]
**white nurse** [see: heroin]
**white Owsley; Owsley's acid; Owsley** [see: LSD]
**white powder** [see: cocaine; PCP]
**white stuff** [see: heroin]
**white sugar** [see: cocaine, crack]
**white tornado** [see: cocaine, crack]
**white-haired lady** [see: marijuana]
**whiteout** [see: isobutyl nitrite]
**whites** *Benzedrine (amphetamine sulfate; discontinued 1982) or other amphetamines* [see: amphetamine sulfate; amphetamines]
**whiz bang** *a combination of cocaine and heroin* [see: cocaine; heroin]
**whore pills** *Quaalude (methaqualone; discontinued 1983)* [see: methaqualone]
**wild cat** *a combination of methcathinone and cocaine* [see: methcathinone; cocaine]
**window glass; window pane** [see: LSD]
**wings** [see: heroin; cocaine]
**witch** [see: heroin; cocaine]
**witch hazel** [see: heroin]
**wobble weed** [see: PCP]
**wolf** [see: PCP]
**wollie** *rocks of crack rolled into a marijuana cigarette* [see: cocaine, crack; marijuana]

**wonder star** [see: methcathinone]

**woolah** *a hollowed-out cigar refilled with marijuana and crack* [see: marijuana; cocaine, crack]

**woolas** *a cigarette laced with cocaine or a marijuana cigarette sprinkled with crack* [see: cocaine; cocaine, crack; marijuana]

**woolies; wooly blunts** *PCP or a combination of marijuana and crack* [see: PCP; marijuana; cocaine, crack]

**worm** [see: PCP]

**wrecking crew** [see: cocaine, crack]

**X-ing** *from "ecstasy"* [see: MDMA]

**yahoo; yeaho** [see: cocaine, crack]

**Yale** [see: cocaine, crack]

**yeh** [see: marijuana]

**yellow** [see: LSD]

**yellow bam** [see: methamphetamine HCl]

**yellow dimples** [see: LSD]

**yellow fever** [see: PCP]

**yellow jackets** *a reference to the capsule color* [see: Nembutal Sodium; pentobarbital sodium]

**yellow submarine** *a reference to the Beatles' song* [see: marijuana; Nembutal Sodium; pentobarbital sodium]

**yellow sunshine** [see: LSD]

**yen pok** *an opium pellet (for smoking)* [see: opium]

**yen shen suey** *opium wine* [see: opium]

**yerba** (Spanish for "herb" or "grass") [see: marijuana]

**yerba mala** (Spanish for "bad herb" or "bad grass") *a combination of PCP and marijuana* [see: PCP; marijuana]

**yesca; yesco** (Spanish for "tinder") [see: marijuana]

**yeso** (Spanish for "chalk") [see: cocaine]

**yimyom** [see: cocaine, crack]

**yuppie psychedelic** [see: MDMA]

**Zacatecas purple** ("zacate" is Spanish for "hay") *marijuana from Mexico* [see: marijuana]

**zambi** [see: marijuana]

**zen** [see: LSD]

**zero** [see: opium]

**zigzag man** [see: LSD; marijuana]

**zip** [see: cocaine]

**zol** *a marijuana cigarette* [see: marijuana]

**zombie** [see: PCP]

**zombie weed** *PCP or marijuana laced with PCP* [see: PCP; marijuana]

**zoom** *PCP or marijuana laced with PCP* [see: PCP; marijuana]

# Hazardous Materials

Listed below are 3147 materials that pose a threat to human life and health. These industrial chemicals, poisons, flammable materials, radioactive substances, petroleum products, and biological agents produce a wide variety of adverse effects in the human body. Treatment for such hazardous material (HazMat) exposure also varies widely, depending on the nature of the specific material.

Each entry in this section is in the following format:

**hazardous material** [Hazard category] *Potential adverse effects.* ⏃ sound-alike(s)

A HazMat will often fall into more than one hazard category. In such cases, multiple categories are shown, followed by the potential adverse effects associated with each category. Rarely, a HazMat is unique and therefore will have no category shown—only a list of potential adverse effects. [(n.o.s.) = not otherwise specified]

**Abate** [Organophosphate] *Pulmonary edema, respiratory muscle paralysis, respiratory failure, bradycardia, acetylcholinesterase inhibition, hypotension, pulmonary edema, overstimulation of parasympathetic nervous system, striated muscle, sympathetic ganglia, and CNS.*

**accumulator, pressurized** [Flammable gas] *Respiratory failure, cardiac arrest, arrhythmias.*

**acenaphthene** [Naphthalene] *Delayed-onset acute intravascular hemolysis.*

**acenaphthylene** [Naphthalene] *Delayed-onset acute intravascular hemolysis.*

**acenocoumarol** [Warfarin/hydroxycoumarin/indanedione] *Anticoagulation effect, internal hemorrhage.*

**acephate** [Organophosphate] *Pulmonary edema, respiratory muscle paralysis, respiratory failure, bradycardia, acetylcholinesterase inhibition, hypotension, pulmonary edema, overstimulation of parasympathetic nervous system, striated muscle, sympathetic ganglia, and CNS.*

**acetaldehyde** [Aldehyde] *Seizures, respiratory failure, pulmonary edema.*

**acetaldehyde ammonia** [Ammonia] *Pulmonary edema, hypotension.* [Aldehyde] *Seizures, respiratory failure, pulmonary edema.*

**acetaldehyde oxime** [Flammable/combustible liquid] *CNS depression, respiratory arrest, convulsions, arrhythmias, pulmonary edema.*

**acetamide** [Organic acid] *Pulmonary edema, circulatory collapse, laryngeal edema and spasm, severe chemical burns to skin, mucous membranes, and internal organs, GI tract perforation and hemorrhage, peritonitis.*

**acetic acid** [Organic acid] *Pulmonary edema, circulatory collapse, laryngeal edema and spasm, severe chemical burns to skin, mucous membranes, and internal organs, GI tract perforation and hemorrhage, peritonitis.*

**acetic acid & boron trifluoride complex** [Organic acid] *Pulmonary edema, circulatory collapse, laryngeal edema and spasm, severe chemical burns to skin, mucous membranes, and internal organs, GI tract perforation and hemorrhage, peritonitis.* [Boron] *Respiratory tract irritation, laryngeal*

**HazMat**

spasm and edema, pulmonary edema, severe chemical burns.

**acetic anhydride** [Organic acid] *Pulmonary edema, circulatory collapse, laryngeal edema and spasm, severe chemical burns to skin, mucous membranes, and internal organs, GI tract perforation and hemorrhage, peritonitis.*

**acetone** [Ketone] *Respiratory mucous membrane irritation, pulmonary edema, CNS depression.*

**acetone cyanohydrin** [Cyanide] *Impairment of cellular oxygenation and adenosine triphosphate production, hypoxia, death.*

**acetone oil** [Ketone] *Respiratory mucous membrane irritation, pulmonary edema, CNS depression.*

**acetone thiosemicarbazide** [Hydrazine] *Seizures, hemolysis of red blood cells, pulmonary edema.*

**acetonitrile** [Cyanide] *Impairment of cellular oxygenation and adenosine triphosphate production, hypoxia, death.*

**acetophenone** [Ketone] *Respiratory mucous membrane irritation, pulmonary edema, CNS depression.*

**acetyl** [Aldehyde] *Seizures, respiratory failure, pulmonary edema.*

**acetyl acetone peroxide** [Organic peroxide] *Pulmonary and laryngeal edema, circulatory arrest, hypovolemic shock, chemical burns to skin, mucous membranes, and internal organs.* [Ketone] *Respiratory mucous membrane irritation, pulmonary edema, CNS depression.* [Corrosive] *Upper airway burns and edema, circulatory collapse, severe chemical burns to skin, toxic systemic effects, GI tract perforation and hemorrhage, peritonitis.*

**acetyl ammonia** [Ammonia] *Pulmonary edema, hypotension.* [Aldehyde] *Seizures, respiratory failure, pulmonary edema.*

**acetyl benzoyl peroxide** [Organic peroxide] *Pulmonary and laryngeal edema, circulatory arrest, hypovolemic shock, chemical burns to skin, mucous membranes, and internal organs.*

**acetyl bromide** [Organic acid] *Pulmonary edema, circulatory collapse, laryngeal edema and spasm, severe chemical burns to skin, mucous membranes, and internal organs, GI tract perforation and hemorrhage, peritonitis.*

**acetyl chloride** [Organic acid] *Pulmonary edema, circulatory collapse, laryngeal edema and spasm, severe chemical burns to skin, mucous membranes, and internal organs, GI tract perforation and hemorrhage, peritonitis.*

**acetyl cyclohexane sulfonyl peroxide** [Organic peroxide] *Pulmonary and laryngeal edema, circulatory arrest, hypovolemic shock, chemical burns to skin, mucous membranes, and internal organs.*

**acetyl iodide** [Iodine] *Hypotension, circulatory collapse, pulmonary edema.*

**acetyl methyl carbinol** [Ketone] *Respiratory mucous membrane irritation, pulmonary edema, CNS depression.*

**acetyl peroxide** [Organic peroxide] *Pulmonary and laryngeal edema, circulatory arrest, hypovolemic shock, chemical burns to skin, mucous membranes, and internal organs.*

**2-acetylaminofluorene** [Poison] *Cardiovascular collapse, pulmonary edema, CNS depression, coma, seizures, nausea, vomiting, cardiopulmonary arrest.*

**acetylene** [Aliphatic hydrocarbon] *Arrhythmias, asphyxiation, anesthesia.* [Simple asphyxiant] *Asphyxiation.*

**acetylene dichloride** [Aliphatic hydrocarbon] *Arrhythmias, asphyxiation, anesthesia.* [Simple asphyxiant] *Asphyxiation.*

**acetylene & propylene & ethylene mixture (cryogenic liquid)** [Aliphatic hydrocarbon] *Arrhythmias, asphyxiation, anesthesia.* [Simple asphyxiant] *Asphyxiation.*

**acetylene tetrabromide** [Aliphatic hydrocarbon] *Arrhythmias, asphyxiation, anesthesia.* [Simple asphyxiant] *Asphyxiation.*

**1-acetyl-2-thiourea** [Nitrogen oxide] *Lower respiratory tract symptoms, pulmonary edema, laryngospasm, bronchospasm, asphyxiation.*

**acid, liquid (n.o.s.)** [Inorganic acid] *Pulmonary edema, bronchospasm, circulatory collapse, laryngeal spasm and edema, severe chemical burns to skin, mucous membranes, and internal organs, GI tract perforation and hemorrhage, peritonitis.* [Organic acid] *Pulmonary edema, circulatory collapse, laryngeal edema and spasm, severe chemical burns to skin, mucous membranes, and internal organs, GI tract perforation and hemorrhage, peritonitis.*

**acid butyl phosphate** [Organic acid] *Pulmonary edema, circulatory collapse, laryngeal edema and spasm, severe chemical burns to skin, mucous membranes, and internal organs, GI tract perforation and hemorrhage, peritonitis.*

**acid mixture: hydrofluoric acid & sulfuric acid** [Inorganic acid] *Pulmonary edema, bronchospasm, circulatory collapse, laryngeal spasm and edema, severe chemical burns to skin, mucous membranes, and internal organs, GI tract perforation and hemorrhage, peritonitis.* [Hydrofluoric acid] *Pulmonary and laryngeal edema, circulatory collapse, severe skin burns, GI tract perforation, systemic fluoride poisoning.*

**acid mixture, nitrating** [Inorganic acid] *Pulmonary edema, bronchospasm, circulatory collapse, laryngeal spasm and edema, severe chemical burns to skin, mucous membranes, and internal organs, GI tract perforation and hemorrhage, peritonitis.*

**acid sludge** [Inorganic acid] *Pulmonary edema, bronchospasm, circulatory collapse, laryngeal spasm and edema, severe chemical burns to skin, mucous membranes, and internal organs, GI tract perforation and hemorrhage, peritonitis.*

**acridine** [Aromatic hydrocarbon] *Arrhythmias, respiratory failure, pulmonary edema, paralysis, brain and kidney damage.*

**acrolein; acrolein dimer** [Acrolein] *Severe respiratory tract irritation, pulmonary edema, respiratory failure.*

**acrylamide** [Triorthocresyl phosphate] *Delayed-onset neurotoxicity, ascending paralysis of the extremities.*

**acrylic acid** [Organic acid] *Pulmonary edema, circulatory collapse, laryngeal edema and spasm, severe chemical burns to skin, mucous membranes, and internal organs, GI tract perforation and hemorrhage, peritonitis.*

**acrylonitrile** [Cyanide] *Impairment of cellular oxygenation and adenosine triphosphate production, hypoxia, death.*

**acrylyl chloride** [Irritant] *Severe immediate or delayed upper airway or respiratory tract irritation, pulmonary edema, glottic spasm, airway obstruction.*

**activated carbon** [Irritant] *Severe immediate or delayed upper airway or respiratory tract irritation, pulmonary edema, glottic spasm, airway obstruction.*

**activated charcoal** [Irritant] *Severe immediate or delayed upper airway or respiratory tract irritation, pulmonary edema, glottic spasm, airway obstruction.*

**adhesive (n.o.s.)** [Irritant] *Severe immediate or delayed upper airway or respiratory tract irritation, pulmonary edema, glottic spasm, airway obstruction.*

**adhesive containing flammable liquid** [Flammable/combustible liquid] *CNS depression, respiratory arrest, convulsions, arrhythmias, pulmonary edema.*

**adipic acid** [Organic acid] *Pulmonary edema, circulatory collapse, laryngeal edema and spasm, severe chemical burns to skin, mucous membranes, and internal organs, GI tract perforation and hemorrhage, peritonitis.*

**adiponitrile** [Cyanide] *Impairment of cellular oxygenation and adenosine triphosphate production, hypoxia, death.*

**aerosol (n.o.s.)** [Irritant] *Severe immediate or delayed upper airway or respiratory tract irritation, pulmonary edema, glottic spasm, airway obstruc-*

HazMat

tion. [Poison] *Cardiovascular collapse, pulmonary edema, CNS depression, coma, seizures, nausea, vomiting, cardiopulmonary arrest.*

**air (gas or cryogenic liquid)** [Nonflammable gas] *Pulmonary edema, respiratory failure, asphyxiation.*

**aircraft M86 fuel** [Hydrocarbon mixture] *CNS depression, respiratory arrest, seizures, arrhythmias, pulmonary edema.*

**alcohol (n.o.s.)** [Lower alcohol (1–3 carbons)] *CNS depression, coma, respiratory arrest, arrhythmias.* [Higher alcohol (4+ carbons)] *CNS depression, respiratory failure, arrhythmias.*

**alcohol, beverage** [Lower alcohol (1–3 carbons)] *CNS depression, coma, respiratory arrest, arrhythmias.*

**alcohol, denatured** [Methyl alcohol] *Respiratory failure, circulatory collapse.*

**alcohol, ethyl** [Lower alcohol (1–3 carbons)] *CNS depression, coma, respiratory arrest, arrhythmias.*

**alcoholic beverage** [Lower alcohol (1–3 carbons)] *CNS depression, coma, respiratory arrest, arrhythmias.*

**aldehyde (n.o.s.)** [Aldehyde] *Seizures, respiratory failure, pulmonary edema.*

**aldicarb** [Carbamate] *Acetylcholinesterase inhibition (reversible), bradycardia, hypotension, respiratory muscle paralysis, respiratory arrest, pulmonary edema.*

**aldicarb & dichloromethane mixture** [Halogenated aliphatic hydrocarbon] *CNS depression, respiratory arrest, circulatory collapse.* [Carbamate] *Acetylcholinesterase inhibition (reversible), bradycardia, hypotension, respiratory muscle paralysis, respiratory arrest, pulmonary edema.*

**aldol** [Aldehyde] *Seizures, respiratory failure, pulmonary edema.*

**aldrin; aldrin mixture (n.o.s.)** [Aldrin/dieldrin/endrin] *Seizures, respiratory failure.*

**aliphatic hydrocarbon (n.o.s.)** [Aliphatic hydrocarbon] *Arrhythmias, asphyxiation, anesthesia.*

**aliphatic thiocyanate (n.o.s.)** [Isocyanate/aliphatic thiocyanate] *CNS depression, respiratory arrest, respiratory paralysis, pulmonary edema, cyanide toxicity.*

**alkali metal alloy (n.o.s.); alkaline earth metal alloy (n.o.s.)** [Inorganic base/alkaline corrosive] *Upper airway burns and edema, pulmonary edema, skin burns, circulatory collapse, GI tract perforation and hemorrhage, peritonitis.*

**alkali metal amalgam (n.o.s.); alkaline earth metal amalgam (n.o.s.)** [Inorganic base/alkaline corrosive] *Upper airway burns and edema, pulmonary edema, skin burns, circulatory collapse, GI tract perforation and hemorrhage, peritonitis.*

**alkali metal amide (n.o.s.)** [Inorganic base/alkaline corrosive] *Upper airway burns and edema, pulmonary edema, skin burns, circulatory collapse, GI tract perforation and hemorrhage, peritonitis.*

**alkaline corrosive liquid (n.o.s.)** [Inorganic base/alkaline corrosive] *Upper airway burns and edema, pulmonary edema, skin burns, circulatory collapse, GI tract perforation and hemorrhage, peritonitis.*

**alkaloid, poisonous (n.o.s.); alkaloid salt, poisonous (n.o.s.)** [Organic base/amine] *Pulmonary edema, cardiac depression, seizures.*

**alkane (C5–C8)** [Aliphatic hydrocarbon] *Arrhythmias, asphyxiation, anesthesia.*

**alkane sulfonic acid** [Organic acid] *Pulmonary edema, circulatory collapse, laryngeal edema and spasm, severe chemical burns to skin, mucous membranes, and internal organs, GI tract perforation and hemorrhage, peritonitis.*

**alkyl aluminum** [Poison] *Cardiovascular collapse, pulmonary edema, CNS depression, coma, seizures, nausea, vomiting, cardiopulmonary arrest.*

**alkyl mercuric chloride** [Mercury] *Circulatory collapse, arrhythmias, res-*

piratory failure, pulmonary edema, neurotoxic effects.

**alkyl phenol (n.o.s.)** [Phenol] *Coma, hypotension, arrhythmias, pulmonary edema, respiratory arrest.*

**alkyl sulfonic acid** [Organic acid] *Pulmonary edema, circulatory collapse, laryngeal edema and spasm, severe chemical burns to skin, mucous membranes, and internal organs, GI tract perforation and hemorrhage, peritonitis.*

**alkylamine (n.o.s.)** [Organic base/ amine] *Pulmonary edema, cardiac depression, seizures.*

**allene** [Aliphatic hydrocarbon] *Arrhythmias, asphyxiation, anesthesia.*

**allethrin** [Pyrethrin/pyrethroid] *Respiratory paralysis, convulsions.*

**allyl acetate** [Ester] *CNS depression, respiratory tract irritation, bronchitis, pneumonia.*

**allyl alcohol** [Lower alcohol (1–3 carbons)] *CNS depression, coma, respiratory arrest, arrhythmias.*

**allyl amine** [Organic base/amine] *Pulmonary edema, cardiac depression, seizures.*

**allyl bromide** [Dichloropropane/ dichloropropene] *Pulmonary edema, bronchospasm, alveolar hemorrhage.*

**allyl chloride** [Dichloropropane/ dichloropropene] *Pulmonary edema, bronchospasm, alveolar hemorrhage.* [Chlorine] *Severe respiratory tract irritation, pulmonary edema, irritation of skin, eyes, and mucous membranes.*

**allyl chlorocarbonate** [Organic acid] *Pulmonary edema, circulatory collapse, laryngeal edema and spasm, severe chemical burns to skin, mucous membranes, and internal organs, GI tract perforation and hemorrhage, peritonitis.*

**allyl chloroformate** [Ester] *CNS depression, respiratory tract irritation, bronchitis, pneumonia.*

**allyl ethyl ether** [Ether] *Anesthesia, respiratory arrest.*

**allyl formate** [Ester] *CNS depression, respiratory tract irritation, bronchitis, pneumonia.*

**allyl glycidyl ether** [Ether] *Anesthesia, respiratory arrest.*

**allyl iodide** [Dichloropropane/dichloropropene] *Pulmonary edema, bronchospasm, alveolar hemorrhage.* [Iodine] *Hypotension, circulatory collapse, pulmonary edema.*

**allyl isothiocyanate** [Isocyanate/aliphatic thiocyanate] *CNS depression, respiratory arrest, respiratory paralysis, pulmonary edema, cyanide toxicity.*

**allyl trichlorosilane** [Silane/chlorosilane] *Respiratory tract irritation, pulmonary edema.*

**alpha naphthylthiourea (ANTU)** [Naphthalene] *Delayed-onset acute intravascular hemolysis.*

**alpha-benzene ethanamine; α-benzene ethanamine** [Aniline] *Methemoglobinemia, hypoxia.*

**alpha-dimethyl benzene ethanamine; α-dimethyl benzene ethanamine** [Aniline] *Methemoglobinemia, hypoxia.*

**alpha-endosulfan; α-endosulfan** [Aldrin/dieldrin/endrin] *Seizures, respiratory failure.*

**alpha-methylstyrene; α-methylstyrene** [Aromatic hydrocarbon] *Arrhythmias, respiratory failure, pulmonary edema, paralysis, brain and kidney damage.*

**alpha-pinene; α-pinene** [Turpentine/ terpene] *Respiratory failure, pulmonary edema, tachycardia.*

**alum** [Inorganic acid] *Pulmonary edema, bronchospasm, circulatory collapse, laryngeal spasm and edema, severe chemical burns to skin, mucous membranes, and internal organs, GI tract perforation and hemorrhage, peritonitis.*

**aluminum** [Poison] *Cardiovascular collapse, pulmonary edema, CNS depression, coma, seizures, nausea, vomiting, cardiopulmonary arrest.*

**aluminum alkyl** [Poison] *Cardiovascular collapse, pulmonary edema, CNS depression, coma, seizures, nausea, vomiting, cardiopulmonary arrest.*

HazMat

286

**aluminum alkyl chloride** [Poison]
*Cardiovascular collapse, pulmonary
edema, CNS depression, coma, seizures, nausea, vomiting, cardiopulmonary arrest. [Chlorine] Severe respiratory tract irritation, pulmonary edema,
irritation of skin, eyes, and mucous
membranes.*

**aluminum alkyl halide** [Poison] *Cardiovascular collapse, pulmonary
edema, CNS depression, coma, seizures, nausea, vomiting, cardiopulmonary arrest.*

**aluminum alkyl hydride** [Poison]
*Cardiovascular collapse, pulmonary
edema, CNS depression, coma, seizures, nausea, vomiting, cardiopulmonary arrest.*

**aluminum borohydride** [Boron] *Respiratory tract irritation, laryngeal
spasm and edema, pulmonary edema,
severe chemical burns.*

**aluminum bromide** [Bromine/meth-
ylbromide] *Severe respiratory irritation, pulmonary edema, respiratory
failure, coma, convulsions, death.*

**aluminum carbide** [Poison] *Cardiovascular collapse, pulmonary edema,
CNS depression, coma, seizures, nausea, vomiting, cardiopulmonary arrest.*

**aluminum chloride** [Poison] *Cardiovascular collapse, pulmonary edema,
CNS depression, coma, seizures, nausea, vomiting, cardiopulmonary arrest.
[Chlorine] Severe respiratory tract irritation, pulmonary edema, irritation of
skin, eyes, and mucous membranes.*

**aluminum ferrosilicon** [Iron] *Hypovolemic shock.*

**aluminum hydride** [Poison] *Cardiovascular collapse, pulmonary edema,
CNS depression, coma, seizures, nausea, vomiting, cardiopulmonary arrest.*

**aluminum nitrate** [Nitrate/nitrite]
*Methemoglobinemia, hypotension, cir-
culatory collapse.*

**aluminum oxide** [Poison] *Cardiovascular collapse, pulmonary edema, CNS
depression, coma, seizures, nausea,
vomiting, cardiopulmonary arrest.*

**aluminum phosphate** [Inorganic
acid] *Pulmonary edema, bronchospasm, circulatory collapse, laryngeal
spasm and edema, severe chemical
burns to skin, mucous membranes, and
internal organs, GI tract perforation
and hemorrhage, peritonitis.*

**aluminum phosphide** [Phosphine]
*Severe pulmonary irritation, pulmonary
edema.*

**aluminum powder, pyrophoric**
[Flammable solid] *Shock, severe
chemical and thermal burns, severe respiratory tract irritation, pulmonary
edema, respiratory arrest, ECG
changes, sudden death.*

**aluminum resinate** [Poison] *Cardiovascular collapse, pulmonary edema,
CNS depression, coma, seizures, nausea, vomiting, cardiopulmonary arrest.*

**aluminum silicon** [Poison] *Cardiovascular collapse, pulmonary edema, CNS
depression, coma, seizures, nausea,
vomiting, cardiopulmonary arrest.*

**aluminum sulfate** [Inorganic acid]
*Pulmonary edema, bronchospasm, cir-
culatory collapse, laryngeal spasm and
edema, severe chemical burns to skin,
mucous membranes, and internal
organs, GI tract perforation and hemorrhage, peritonitis.*

**2-aminoanthraquinone** [Poison]
*Cardiovascular collapse, pulmonary
edema, CNS depression, coma, seizures, nausea, vomiting, cardiopulmonary arrest.*

**4-aminoazobenzene** [Aniline] *Methemoglobinemia, hypoxia.*

**4-aminobiphenyl** [Nitrate/nitrite]
*Methemoglobinemia, hypotension, cir-
culatory collapse.*

**Aminocarb** [Carbamate] *Acetylcholinesterase inhibition (reversible), bradycardia,
hypotension, respiratory muscle paralysis, respiratory arrest, pulmonary edema.*

**aminochlorophenol** [Phenol] *Coma,
hypotension, arrhythmias, pulmonary
edema, respiratory arrest.*

**2-amino-5-diethylaminopentane**
[Organic base/amine] *Pulmonary*

edema, cardiac depression, seizures. [Aliphatic hydrocarbon] Arrhythmias, asphyxiation, anesthesia.

**aminodimethylbutyronitrile** [Cyanide] Impairment of cellular oxygenation and adenosine triphosphate production, hypoxia, death.

**aminoethoxyethanol** [Organic base/amine] Pulmonary edema, cardiac depression, seizures. [Lower alcohol (1–3 carbons)] CNS depression, coma, respiratory arrest, arrhythmias.

**2-aminoethylethanolamine** [Organic base/amine] Pulmonary edema, cardiac depression, seizures. [Lower alcohol (1–3 carbons)] CNS depression, coma, respiratory arrest, arrhythmias.

**aminoethylpiperazine** [Organic base/amine] Pulmonary edema, cardiac depression, seizures.

**1-amino-2-methylanthraquinone** [Organic base/amine] Pulmonary edema, cardiac depression, seizures.

**5-(aminomethyl)-3-isoxazolol** [Poison] Cardiovascular collapse, pulmonary edema, CNS depression, coma, seizures, nausea, vomiting, cardiopulmonary arrest.

**4-amino-2-nitrophenol** [Aniline] Methemoglobinemia, hypoxia.

**aminophenol** [Aniline] Methemoglobinemia, hypoxia.

**aminopropyldiethanolamine** [Organic base/amine] Pulmonary edema, cardiac depression, seizures.

**aminopropylmorpholine** [Organic base/amine] Pulmonary edema, cardiac depression, seizures.

**aminopropylpiperazine** [Organic base/amine] Pulmonary edema, cardiac depression, seizures.

**aminopyridine** [Aromatic hydrocarbon] Arrhythmias, respiratory failure, pulmonary edema, paralysis, brain and kidney damage.

**p-aminosalicylic acid** [Organic acid] Pulmonary edema, circulatory collapse, laryngeal edema and spasm, severe chemical burns to skin, mucous membranes, and internal organs, GI tract perforation and hemorrhage, peritonitis.

**Amiton** [Organophosphate] Pulmonary edema, respiratory muscle paralysis, respiratory failure, bradycardia, acetylcholinesterase inhibition, hypotension, pulmonary edema, overstimulation of parasympathetic nervous system, striated muscle, sympathetic ganglia, and CNS.

**Amiton Oxalate** [Organophosphate] Pulmonary edema, respiratory muscle paralysis, respiratory failure, bradycardia, acetylcholinesterase inhibition, hypotension, pulmonary edema, overstimulation of parasympathetic nervous system, striated muscle, sympathetic ganglia, and CNS.

**amitrole** [Poison] Cardiovascular collapse, pulmonary edema, CNS depression, coma, seizures, nausea, vomiting, cardiopulmonary arrest.

**ammonia; ammonium salt (n.o.s.)** [Ammonia] Pulmonary edema, hypotension.

**ammoniated cupric sulfate** [Ammonia] Pulmonary edema, hypotension. [Copper] Respiratory tract irritation and arrest, hemorrhagic gastritis.

**ammoniated mercury** [Mercury] Circulatory collapse, arrhythmias, respiratory failure, pulmonary edema, neurotoxic effects.

**ammonium acetate** [Ammonia] Pulmonary edema, hypotension.

**ammonium arsenate** [Arsenic] Heavy metal toxicity, vomiting, GI bleeding, CNS depression, pulmonary edema, cardiac arrest.

**ammonium benzoate** [Ammonia] Pulmonary edema, hypotension.

**ammonium bicarbonate** [Ammonia] Pulmonary edema, hypotension.

**ammonium bichromate** [Ammonia] Pulmonary edema, hypotension.

**ammonium bifluoride** [Fluorine] CNS depression, respiratory arrest, cardiovascular collapse, shock, arrhythmias.

**ammonium bisulfite** [Ammonia] Pulmonary edema, hypotension. [Sulfur]

**HazMat**

*Respiratory tract irritation, pulmonary edema, anaphylaxis.*

**ammonium bromide** [Bromine/methylbromide] *Severe respiratory irritation, pulmonary edema, respiratory failure, coma, convulsions, death.*

**ammonium carbamate** [Ammonia] *Pulmonary edema, hypotension.*

**ammonium carbonate** [Ammonia] *Pulmonary edema, hypotension.*

**ammonium chloride** [Ammonia] *Pulmonary edema, hypotension.*

**ammonium chromate** [Ammonia] *Pulmonary edema, hypotension.*

**ammonium citrate** [Ammonia] *Pulmonary edema, hypotension.*

**ammonium dichromate** [Ammonia] *Pulmonary edema, hypotension.*

**ammonium dinitro-o-cresolate** [Ammonia] *Pulmonary edema, hypotension.*

**ammonium fluoride** [Fluorine] *CNS depression, respiratory arrest, cardiovascular collapse, shock, arrhythmias.*

**ammonium fluoroborate** [Ammonia] *Pulmonary edema, hypotension.* [Boron] *Respiratory tract irritation, laryngeal spasm and edema, pulmonary edema, severe chemical burns.*

**ammonium fluorosilicate** [Fluorine] *CNS depression, respiratory arrest, cardiovascular collapse, shock, arrhythmias.*

**ammonium hydrogen fluoride** [Fluorine] *CNS depression, respiratory arrest, cardiovascular collapse, shock, arrhythmias.*

**ammonium hydrogen sulfate** [Inorganic acid] *Pulmonary edema, bronchospasm, circulatory collapse, laryngeal spasm and edema, severe chemical burns to skin, mucous membranes, and internal organs, GI tract perforation and hemorrhage, peritonitis.*

**ammonium hydrosulfide** [Ammonia] *Pulmonary edema, hypotension.*

**ammonium hydroxide** [Inorganic base/alkaline corrosive] *Upper airway burns and edema, pulmonary edema, skin burns, circulatory collapse, GI tract perforation and hemorrhage, peritonitis.*

**ammonium metavanadate** [Poison] *Cardiovascular collapse, pulmonary edema, CNS depression, coma, seizures, nausea, vomiting, cardiopulmonary arrest.*

**ammonium nitrate** [Nitrate/nitrite] *Methemoglobinemia, hypotension, circulatory collapse.*

**ammonium nitrate & ammonium phosphate mixture** [Nitrate/nitrite] *Methemoglobinemia, hypotension, circulatory collapse.*

**ammonium nitrate & ammonium sulfate mixture** [Ammonia] *Pulmonary edema, hypotension.* [Nitrate/nitrite] *Methemoglobinemia, hypotension, circulatory collapse.* [Sulfur] *Respiratory tract irritation, pulmonary edema, anaphylaxis.*

**ammonium nitrate & calcium carbonate mixture** [Nitrate/nitrite] *Methemoglobinemia, hypotension, circulatory collapse.*

**ammonium nitrate & [diesel] fuel oil (ANFO) mixture** [Explosive] *Multiple trauma, highly toxic chemical exposure.* [Nitrate/nitrite] *Methemoglobinemia, hypotension, circulatory collapse.*

**ammonium nitrate & potash mixture** [Nitrate/nitrite] *Methemoglobinemia, hypotension, circulatory collapse.*

**ammonium oxalate** [Oxalate] *Cardiovascular collapse, arrhythmias, seizures.* [Ammonia] *Pulmonary edema, hypotension.*

**ammonium perchlorate** [Ammonia] *Pulmonary edema, hypotension.* [Chlorate] *Hemolysis, methemoglobinemia, hypoperfusion, CNS depression, delayed-onset renal failure.*

**ammonium permanganate** [Inorganic acid] *Pulmonary edema, bronchospasm, circulatory collapse, laryngeal spasm and edema, severe chemical burns to skin, mucous membranes, and internal organs, GI tract perforation and hemorrhage, peritonitis.*

**ammonium persulfate** [Inorganic acid] *Pulmonary edema, broncho-*

spasm, circulatory collapse, laryngeal spasm and edema, severe chemical burns to skin, mucous membranes, and internal organs, GI tract perforation and hemorrhage, peritonitis.

**ammonium picrate** [Inorganic acid] Pulmonary edema, bronchospasm, circulatory collapse, laryngeal spasm and edema, severe chemical burns to skin, mucous membranes, and internal organs, GI tract perforation and hemorrhage, peritonitis.

**ammonium polysulfide** [Ammonia] Pulmonary edema, hypotension. [Sulfur] Respiratory tract irritation, pulmonary edema, anaphylaxis.

**ammonium polyvanadate** [Poison] Cardiovascular collapse, pulmonary edema, CNS depression, coma, seizures, nausea, vomiting, cardiopulmonary arrest.

**ammonium salt (n.o.s.)** [Ammonia] Pulmonary edema, hypotension.

**ammonium silicofluoride** [Fluorine] CNS depression, respiratory arrest, cardiovascular collapse, shock, arrhythmias.

**ammonium sulfamate** [Ammonia] Pulmonary edema, hypotension. [Sulfur] Respiratory tract irritation, pulmonary edema, anaphylaxis.

**ammonium sulfate** [Ammonia] Pulmonary edema, hypotension. [Sulfur] Respiratory tract irritation, pulmonary edema, anaphylaxis.

**ammonium sulfate & ammonium nitrate mixture** [Ammonia] Pulmonary edema, hypotension. [Nitrate/nitrite] Methemoglobinemia, hypotension, circulatory collapse. [Sulfur] Respiratory tract irritation, pulmonary edema, anaphylaxis.

**ammonium sulfide** [Ammonia] Pulmonary edema, hypotension. [Sulfur] Respiratory tract irritation, pulmonary edema, anaphylaxis.

**ammonium sulfite** [Ammonia] Pulmonary edema, hypotension. [Sulfur] Respiratory tract irritation, pulmonary edema, anaphylaxis.

**ammonium tartrate** [Organic acid] Pulmonary edema, circulatory collapse, laryngeal edema and spasm, severe chemical burns to skin, mucous membranes, and internal organs, GI tract perforation and hemorrhage, peritonitis.

**ammonium thiocyanate** [Isocyanate/aliphatic thiocyanate] CNS depression, respiratory arrest, respiratory paralysis, pulmonary edema, cyanide toxicity.

**ammonium vanadate** [Poison] Cardiovascular collapse, pulmonary edema, CNS depression, coma, seizures, nausea, vomiting, cardiopulmonary arrest.

**amosite; brown asbestos** [Asbestos] Asbestosis, lung cancer, malignant mesothelioma.

**ammunition, irritant nonexplosive** [Irritant] Severe immediate or delayed upper airway or respiratory tract irritation, pulmonary edema, glottic spasm, airway obstruction.

**ammunition, toxic nonexplosive** [Poison] Cardiovascular collapse, pulmonary edema, CNS depression, coma, seizures, nausea, vomiting, cardiopulmonary arrest.

**amphetamine** [Poison] Cardiovascular collapse, pulmonary edema, CNS depression, coma, seizures, nausea, vomiting, cardiopulmonary arrest.

**amygdalin** [Cyanide] Impairment of cellular oxygenation and adenosine triphosphate production, hypoxia, death.

**amyl acetate (n.o.s.)** [Ester] CNS depression, respiratory tract irritation, bronchitis, pneumonia.

**amyl acid phosphate** [Irritant] Severe immediate or delayed upper airway or respiratory tract irritation, pulmonary edema, glottic spasm, airway obstruction.

**amyl alcohol** [Higher alcohol (4+ carbons)] CNS depression, respiratory failure, arrhythmias.

**amyl aldehyde** [Aldehyde] Seizures, respiratory failure, pulmonary edema.

**amyl butyrate** [Organic acid] Pulmonary edema, circulatory collapse,

**HazMat**

laryngeal edema and spasm, severe chemical burns to skin, mucous membranes, and internal organs, GI tract perforation and hemorrhage, peritonitis.

**amyl chloride** [Halogenated aliphatic hydrocarbon] CNS depression, respiratory arrest, circulatory collapse.

**amyl formate** [Ester] CNS depression, respiratory tract irritation, bronchitis, pneumonia.

**amyl mercaptan** [Sulfur] Respiratory tract irritation, pulmonary edema, anaphylaxis.

**amyl methyl ketone** [Ketone] Respiratory mucous membrane irritation, pulmonary edema, CNS depression.

**amyl nitrate** [Nitrate/nitrite] Methemoglobinemia, hypotension, circulatory collapse.

**amyl phenol** [Phenol] Coma, hypotension, arrhythmias, pulmonary edema, respiratory arrest.

**amylamine** [Organic base/amine] Pulmonary edema, cardiac depression, seizures.

**amylene** [Simple asphyxiant] Asphyxiation.

***tert*-amylhydroperoxide** [Organic peroxide] Pulmonary and laryngeal edema, circulatory arrest, hypovolemic shock, chemical burns to skin, mucous membranes, and internal organs.

***tert*-amylperoxybenzoate** [Organic peroxide] Pulmonary and laryngeal edema, circulatory arrest, hypovolemic shock, chemical burns to skin, mucous membranes, and internal organs. [Organic acid] Pulmonary edema, circulatory collapse, laryngeal edema and spasm, severe chemical burns to skin, mucous membranes, and internal organs, GI tract perforation and hemorrhage, peritonitis.

***tert*-amylperoxy-2-ethyl-hexanoate** [Organic peroxide] Pulmonary and laryngeal edema, circulatory arrest, hypovolemic shock, chemical burns to skin, mucous membranes, and internal organs. [Organic acid] Pulmonary edema, circulatory collapse, laryngeal

edema and spasm, severe chemical burns to skin, mucous membranes, and internal organs, GI tract perforation and hemorrhage, peritonitis.

***tert*-amylperoxy-neodecanoate** [Organic peroxide] Pulmonary and laryngeal edema, circulatory arrest, hypovolemic shock, chemical burns to skin, mucous membranes, and internal organs. [Organic acid] Pulmonary edema, circulatory collapse, laryngeal edema and spasm, severe chemical burns to skin, mucous membranes, and internal organs, GI tract perforation and hemorrhage, peritonitis.

***tert*-amylperoxypivalate** [Organic peroxide] Pulmonary and laryngeal edema, circulatory arrest, hypovolemic shock, chemical burns to skin, mucous membranes, and internal organs. [Organic acid] Pulmonary edema, circulatory collapse, laryngeal edema and spasm, severe chemical burns to skin, mucous membranes, and internal organs, GI tract perforation and hemorrhage, peritonitis.

**amyltrichlorocyclane** [Halogenated aliphatic hydrocarbon] CNS depression, respiratory arrest, circulatory collapse.

**amyltrichlorosilane** [Silane/chlorosilane] Respiratory tract irritation, pulmonary edema.

**anethole** [Aromatic hydrocarbon] Arrhythmias, respiratory failure, pulmonary edema, paralysis, brain and kidney damage.

**ANFO (ammonium nitrate & [diesel] fuel oil mixture)** [Explosive] Multiple trauma, highly toxic chemical exposure. [Nitrate/nitrite] Methemoglobinemia, hypotension, circulatory collapse.

**anhydrous ammonia** [Ammonia] Pulmonary edema, hypotension.

**aniline** [Aniline] Methemoglobinemia, hypoxia.

**aniline HCl** [Aniline] Methemoglobinemia, hypoxia.

**animal fabric with oil (n.o.s.)** [Flammable/combustible liquid] *CNS depression, respiratory arrest, convulsions, arrhythmias, pulmonary edema.*

**animal fiber, burnt (n.o.s.)** [Irritant] *Severe immediate or delayed upper airway or respiratory tract irritation, pulmonary edema, glottic spasm, airway obstruction.*

**animal fiber with oil (n.o.s.)** [Flammable/combustible liquid] *CNS depression, respiratory arrest, convulsions, arrhythmias, pulmonary edema.*

**anisidine; *o*-anisidine HCl** [Benzene] *Arrhythmias, respiratory failure, pulmonary edema, CNS depression, liver and kidney damage.*

**anisindione** [Warfarin/hydroxycoumarin/indanedione] *Anticoagulation effect, internal hemorrhage.*

**anisole** [Aromatic hydrocarbon] *Arrhythmias, respiratory failure, pulmonary edema, paralysis, brain and kidney damage.*

**anisoyl chloride** [Organic acid] *Pulmonary edema, circulatory collapse, laryngeal edema and spasm, severe chemical burns to skin, mucous membranes, and internal organs, GI tract perforation and hemorrhage, peritonitis.*

**anthophyllite** [Asbestos] *Asbestosis, lung cancer, malignant mesothelioma.*

**anthracene** [Aromatic hydrocarbon] *Arrhythmias, respiratory failure, pulmonary edema, paralysis, brain and kidney damage.*

**antifreeze** [Ethylene glycol] *Respiratory failure, pulmonary edema, paralysis, cardiovascular collapse, severe acidosis.*

**antiknock compound** [Lead] *Circulatory collapse, coma, rare seizures.*

**antimony; antimony mixture (n.o.s.); antimony salt (n.o.s.)** [Poison] *Cardiovascular collapse, pulmonary edema, CNS depression, coma, seizures, nausea, vomiting, cardiopulmonary arrest.*

**antimony chloride** [Poison] *Cardiovascular collapse, pulmonary edema,* *CNS depression, coma, seizures, nausea, vomiting, cardiopulmonary arrest.*

**antimony hydride** [Poison] *Cardiovascular collapse, pulmonary edema, CNS depression, coma, seizures, nausea, vomiting, cardiopulmonary arrest.*

**antimony lactate** [Poison] *Cardiovascular collapse, pulmonary edema, CNS depression, coma, seizures, nausea, vomiting, cardiopulmonary arrest.*

**antimony pentachloride** [Poison] *Cardiovascular collapse, pulmonary edema, CNS depression, coma, seizures, nausea, vomiting, cardiopulmonary arrest.*

**antimony pentafluoride** [Fluorine] *CNS depression, respiratory arrest, cardiovascular collapse, shock, arrhythmias.*

**antimony pentasulfide** [Poison] *Cardiovascular collapse, pulmonary edema, CNS depression, coma, seizures, nausea, vomiting, cardiopulmonary arrest.*

**antimony potassium** [Poison] *Cardiovascular collapse, pulmonary edema, CNS depression, coma, seizures, nausea, vomiting, cardiopulmonary arrest.*

**antimony potassium tartrate** [Poison] *Cardiovascular collapse, pulmonary edema, CNS depression, coma, seizures, nausea, vomiting, cardiopulmonary arrest.*

**antimony tribromide** [Bromine/methylbromide] *Severe respiratory irritation, pulmonary edema, respiratory failure, coma, convulsions, death.*

**antimony trichloride** [Poison] *Cardiovascular collapse, pulmonary edema, CNS depression, coma, seizures, nausea, vomiting, cardiopulmonary arrest.*

**antimony trifluoride** [Fluorine] *CNS depression, respiratory arrest, cardiovascular collapse, shock, arrhythmias.*

**antimony trioxide** [Poison] *Cardiovascular collapse, pulmonary edema, CNS depression, coma, seizures, nausea, vomiting, cardiopulmonary arrest.*

**HazMat**

**ANTU (alpha naphthylthiourea)**
[Naphthalene] *Delayed-onset acute intravascular hemolysis.*

**Apl-Luster** [Thiabendazole] *Cardiovascular collapse, respiratory tract irritation.*

**Arbotect** [Thiabendazole] *Cardiovascular collapse, respiratory tract irritation.*

**argon (gas or cryogenic liquid)**
[Simple asphyxiant] *Asphyxiation.*

**aroclor 1016, 1221, 1232, 1242, 1248, 1254, or 1260** Polychlorinated biphenyl/polybrominated biphenyl/polychlorinated [dibenzofuran] *Liver and kidney damage.*

**aromatic extract (n.o.s.)** [Aromatic hydrocarbon] *Arrhythmias, respiratory failure, pulmonary edema, paralysis, brain and kidney damage.*

**aromatic hydrocarbon, polynuclear (n.o.s.)** [Poison] *Cardiovascular collapse, pulmonary edema, CNS depression, coma, seizures, nausea, vomiting, cardiopulmonary arrest.*

**aromatic hydrocarbon solvent (n.o.s.)** [Aromatic hydrocarbon] *Arrhythmias, respiratory failure, pulmonary edema, paralysis, brain and kidney damage.*

**aromatic naphtha solvent** [Naphthalene] *Delayed-onset acute intravascular hemolysis.*

**aromatic nitrogen compound** [Aniline] *Methemoglobinemia, hypoxia.*

**arsanilic acid** [Arsenic] *Heavy metal toxicity, vomiting, GI bleeding, CNS depression, pulmonary edema, cardiac arrest.*

**arsenate (n.o.s.)** [Arsenic] *Heavy metal toxicity, vomiting, GI bleeding, CNS depression, pulmonary edema, cardiac arrest.*

**arsenic** [Arsenic] *Heavy metal toxicity, vomiting, GI bleeding, CNS depression, pulmonary edema, cardiac arrest.*

**arsenic acid** [Arsenic] *Heavy metal toxicity, vomiting, GI bleeding, CNS depression, pulmonary edema, cardiac arrest.*

**arsenic bromide** [Arsenic] *Heavy metal toxicity, vomiting, GI bleeding, CNS depression, pulmonary edema,* *cardiac arrest.* [Bromine/methylbromide] *Severe respiratory irritation, pulmonary edema, respiratory failure, coma, convulsions, death.*

**arsenic chloride** [Arsenic] *Heavy metal toxicity, vomiting, GI bleeding, CNS depression, pulmonary edema, cardiac arrest.* [Chlorine] *Severe respiratory tract irritation, pulmonary edema, irritation of skin, eyes, and mucous membranes.*

**arsenic disulfide** [Arsenic] *Heavy metal toxicity, vomiting, GI bleeding, CNS depression, pulmonary edema, cardiac arrest.*

**arsenic iodide** [Arsenic] *Heavy metal toxicity, vomiting, GI bleeding, CNS depression, pulmonary edema, cardiac arrest.*

**arsenic mixture (n.o.s.)** [Arsenic] *Heavy metal toxicity, vomiting, GI bleeding, CNS depression, pulmonary edema, cardiac arrest.*

**arsenic pentoxide** [Arsenic] *Heavy metal toxicity, vomiting, GI bleeding, CNS depression, pulmonary edema, cardiac arrest.*

**arsenic trichloride** [Arsenic] *Heavy metal toxicity, vomiting, GI bleeding, CNS depression, pulmonary edema, cardiac arrest.* [Chlorine] *Severe respiratory tract irritation, pulmonary edema, irritation of skin, eyes, and mucous membranes.*

**arsenic trihydride** [Arsenic] *Heavy metal toxicity, vomiting, GI bleeding, CNS depression, pulmonary edema, cardiac arrest.*

**arsenic trioxide** [Arsenic] *Heavy metal toxicity, vomiting, GI bleeding, CNS depression, pulmonary edema, cardiac arrest.*

**arsenic trisulfide** [Arsenic] *Heavy metal toxicity, vomiting, GI bleeding, CNS depression, pulmonary edema, cardiac arrest.*

**arsenical flue dust** [Arsenic] *Heavy metal toxicity, vomiting, GI bleeding, CNS depression, pulmonary edema, cardiac arrest.*

**arsenical pesticide (n.o.s.)** [Arsenic] *Heavy metal toxicity, vomiting, GI bleeding, CNS depression, pulmonary edema, cardiac arrest.*

**arsenite (n.o.s.)** [Arsenic] *Heavy metal toxicity, vomiting, GI bleeding, CNS depression, pulmonary edema, cardiac arrest.*

**arsenite, bordeaux** [Arsenic] *Heavy metal toxicity, vomiting, GI bleeding, CNS depression, pulmonary edema, cardiac arrest.* [Copper] *Respiratory tract irritation and arrest, hemorrhagic gastritis.*

**arsenous oxide** [Arsenic] *Heavy metal toxicity, vomiting, GI bleeding, CNS depression, pulmonary edema, cardiac arrest.*

**arsenous trichloride** [Arsenic] *Heavy metal toxicity, vomiting, GI bleeding, CNS depression, pulmonary edema, cardiac arrest.* [Chlorine] *Severe respiratory tract irritation, pulmonary edema, irritation of skin, eyes, and mucous membranes.*

**arsine** [Arsine] *Intravascular hemolysis, pulmonary edema, cardiac and respiratory arrest, delayed-onset jaundice and renal failure.*

**aryl amine** [Aniline] *Methemoglobinemia, hypoxia.*

**aryl sulfonic acid** [Organic acid] *Pulmonary edema, circulatory collapse, laryngeal edema and spasm, severe chemical burns to skin, mucous membranes, and internal organs, GI tract perforation and hemorrhage, peritonitis.*

**asbestos** [Asbestos] *Asbestosis, lung cancer, malignant mesothelioma.*

**asphalt** [Hydrocarbon mixture] *CNS depression, respiratory arrest, seizures, arrhythmias, pulmonary edema.*

**auramine** [Aniline] *Methemoglobinemia, hypoxia.*

**aviation fuel** [Hydrocarbon mixture] *CNS depression, respiratory arrest, seizures, arrhythmias, pulmonary edema.*

**azaserine** [Poison] *Cardiovascular collapse, pulmonary edema, CNS depression, coma, seizures, nausea, vomiting, cardiopulmonary arrest.*

**azinphos-ethyl** [Organophosphate] *Pulmonary edema, respiratory muscle paralysis, respiratory failure, bradycardia, acetylcholinesterase inhibition, hypotension, pulmonary edema, overstimulation of parasympathetic nervous system, striated muscle, sympathetic ganglia, and CNS.*

**azinphos-methyl** [Organophosphate] *Pulmonary edema, respiratory muscle paralysis, respiratory failure, bradycardia, acetylcholinesterase inhibition, hypotension, pulmonary edema, overstimulation of parasympathetic nervous system, striated muscle, sympathetic ganglia, and CNS.*

**aziridine** [Organic base/amine] *Pulmonary edema, cardiac depression, seizures.*

**1-aziridinyl phosphine oxide (tris)** [Poison] *Cardiovascular collapse, pulmonary edema, CNS depression, coma, seizures, nausea, vomiting, cardiopulmonary arrest.*

**azobenzene** [Aniline] *Methemoglobinemia, hypoxia.*

**2,2′-azodi-(2,4-dimethyl-4-methoxyvaleronitrile)** [Poison] *Cardiovascular collapse, pulmonary edema, CNS depression, coma, seizures, nausea, vomiting, cardiopulmonary arrest.*

**2,2′-azodi-(2,4-dimethyl-valeronitrile)** [Poison] *Cardiovascular collapse, pulmonary edema, CNS depression, coma, seizures, nausea, vomiting, cardiopulmonary arrest.*

**1,1′-azodi-(hexahydrobenzonitrile)** [Poison] *Cardiovascular collapse, pulmonary edema, CNS depression, coma, seizures, nausea, vomiting, cardiopulmonary arrest.*

**azodiisobutyronitrile** [Cyanide] *Impairment of cellular oxygenation and adenosine triphosphate production, hypoxia, death.*

**2,2′-azodi-(2-methyl-butyronitrile)** [Poison] *Cardiovascular collapse, pulmonary edema, CNS depression,*

HazMat

*coma, seizures, nausea, vomiting, cardiopulmonary arrest.*

**Bandane** [Chlordane] *Respiratory failure, seizures, exhaustion, death.*

**barium; barium alloy (n.o.s.); barium mixture (n.o.s.); barium salt (n.o.s.)** [Barium] *Hypokalemia, muscle paralysis, arrhythmias, cardiac and respiratory arrest.*

**barium azide** [Barium] *Hypokalemia, muscle paralysis, arrhythmias, cardiac and respiratory arrest.*

**barium bromate** [Barium] *Hypokalemia, muscle paralysis, arrhythmias, cardiac and respiratory arrest.* [Bromate] *CNS and respiratory system depression, delayed-onset renal failure.*

**barium chlorate** [Barium] *Hypokalemia, muscle paralysis, arrhythmias, cardiac and respiratory arrest.* [Chlorate] *Hemolysis, methemoglobinemia, hypoperfusion, CNS depression, delayed-onset renal failure.*

**barium cyanide** [Barium] *Hypokalemia, muscle paralysis, arrhythmias, cardiac and respiratory arrest.* [Cyanide] *Impairment of cellular oxygenation and adenosine triphosphate production, hypoxia, death.*

**barium fluosilicate** [Rotenone] *Respiratory arrest, asphyxia.* [Barium] *Hypokalemia, muscle paralysis, arrhythmias, cardiac and respiratory arrest.*

**barium hypochlorite** [Hypochlorite] *Circulatory collapse, respiratory tract irritation, upper airway obstruction, pulmonary edema.* [Barium] *Hypokalemia, muscle paralysis, arrhythmias, cardiac and respiratory arrest.*

**barium metaborate** [Barium] *Hypokalemia, muscle paralysis, arrhythmias, cardiac and respiratory arrest.* [Boron] *Respiratory tract irritation, laryngeal spasm and edema, pulmonary edema, severe chemical burns.*

**barium nitrate** [Nitrate/nitrite] *Methemoglobinemia, hypotension, circulatory collapse.* [Barium] *Hypokalemia, muscle paralysis, arrhythmias, cardiac and respiratory arrest.*

**barium oxide** [Barium] *Hypokalemia, muscle paralysis, arrhythmias, cardiac and respiratory arrest.*

**barium perchlorate** [Barium] *Hypokalemia, muscle paralysis, arrhythmias, cardiac and respiratory arrest.* [Chlorate] *Hemolysis, methemoglobinemia, hypoperfusion, CNS depression, delayed-onset renal failure.*

**barium permanganate** [Inorganic acid] *Pulmonary edema, bronchospasm, circulatory collapse, laryngeal spasm and edema, severe chemical burns to skin, mucous membranes, and internal organs, GI tract perforation and hemorrhage, peritonitis.* [Barium] *Hypokalemia, muscle paralysis, arrhythmias, cardiac and respiratory arrest.*

**barium peroxide** [Barium] *Hypokalemia, muscle paralysis, arrhythmias, cardiac and respiratory arrest.*

**barium selenate** [Barium] *Hypokalemia, muscle paralysis, arrhythmias, cardiac and respiratory arrest.* [Selenium] *Arrhythmias, pulmonary edema, bronchospasm, seizures, vomiting, GI bleeding.*

**barium selenite** [Barium] *Hypokalemia, muscle paralysis, arrhythmias, cardiac and respiratory arrest.* [Selenium] *Arrhythmias, pulmonary edema, bronchospasm, seizures, vomiting, GI bleeding.*

**barthrin** [Pyrethrin/pyrethroid] *Respiratory paralysis, convulsions.*

**battery (electric), acid-filled** [Inorganic acid] *Pulmonary edema, bronchospasm, circulatory collapse, laryngeal spasm and edema, severe chemical burns to skin, mucous membranes, and internal organs, GI tract perforation and hemorrhage, peritonitis.*

**battery (electric), alkali-filled** [Inorganic base/alkaline corrosive] *Upper airway burns and edema, pulmonary edema, skin burns, circulatory collapse, GI tract perforation and hemorrhage, peritonitis.*

**battery (electric) with potassium hydroxide** [Inorganic base/alkaline corrosive] *Upper airway burns and edema, pulmonary edema, skin burns, circulatory collapse, GI tract perforation and hemorrhage, peritonitis.*

**battery fluid, acid** [Inorganic acid] *Pulmonary edema, bronchospasm, circulatory collapse, laryngeal spasm and edema, severe chemical burns to skin, mucous membranes, and internal organs, GI tract perforation and hemorrhage, peritonitis.*

**battery fluid, alkali** [Inorganic base/alkaline corrosive] *Upper airway burns and edema, pulmonary edema, skin burns, circulatory collapse, GI tract perforation and hemorrhage, peritonitis.*

**Baygon** [Carbamate] *Acetylcholinesterase inhibition (reversible), bradycardia, hypotension, respiratory muscle paralysis, respiratory arrest, pulmonary edema.*

**bendiocarb** [Carbamate] *Acetylcholinesterase inhibition (reversible), bradycardia, hypotension, respiratory muscle paralysis, respiratory arrest, pulmonary edema.*

**benomyl** [Dithiocarbamate] *Hypotension, respiratory failure.*

**bensulfide** [Organophosphate] *Pulmonary edema, respiratory muscle paralysis, respiratory failure, bradycardia, acetylcholinesterase inhibition, hypotension, pulmonary edema, overstimulation of parasympathetic nervous system, striated muscle, sympathetic ganglia, and CNS.*

**benz[c]acridine** [Poison] *Cardiovascular collapse, pulmonary edema, CNS depression, coma, seizures, nausea, vomiting, cardiopulmonary arrest.*

**benzal chloride** [Aromatic hydrocarbon] *Arrhythmias, respiratory failure, pulmonary edema, paralysis, brain and kidney damage.*

**benzaldehyde** [Aldehyde] *Seizures, respiratory failure, pulmonary edema.*

**benzamide** [Organic acid] *Pulmonary edema, circulatory collapse, laryngeal edema and spasm, severe chemical burns to skin, mucous membranes, and internal organs, GI tract perforation and hemorrhage, peritonitis.*

**benz[a]anthracene** [Naphthalene] *Delayed-onset acute intravascular hemolysis.*

**benzenamine, 3-(trifluoromethyl)** [Aniline] *Methemoglobinemia, hypoxia.*

**benzene** [Benzene] *Arrhythmias, respiratory failure, pulmonary edema, CNS depression, liver and kidney damage.* 🔊 benzine

**benzene, chlorinated** [Lindane] *CNS stimulation, seizures, respiratory failure.*

**α-benzene ethanamine; alpha-benzene ethanamine** [Aniline] *Methemoglobinemia, hypoxia.*

**benzene ethanamine, alpha-dimethyl** [Aniline] *Methemoglobinemia, hypoxia.*

**benzene hexachloride** [Lindane] *CNS stimulation, seizures, respiratory failure.*

**benzene phosphorus dichloride** [Phosphorus] *Hypovolemic shock, severe tissue burns, severe respiratory irritation, pulmonary edema, respiratory arrest, arrhythmias, sudden death.*

**benzene phosphorus thiodichloride** [Phosphorus] *Hypovolemic shock, severe tissue burns, severe respiratory irritation, pulmonary edema, respiratory arrest, arrhythmias, sudden death.*

**benzene sulfohydrazide** [Organic acid] *Pulmonary edema, circulatory collapse, laryngeal edema and spasm, severe chemical burns to skin, mucous membranes, and internal organs, GI tract perforation and hemorrhage, peritonitis.*

**benzene sulfonyl chloride** [Organic acid] *Pulmonary edema, circulatory collapse, laryngeal edema and spasm, severe chemical burns to skin, mucous membranes, and internal organs, GI tract perforation and hemorrhage, peritonitis.*

**benzenearsonic acid** [Arsenic] *Heavy metal toxicity, vomiting, GI bleeding, CNS depression, pulmonary edema, cardiac arrest.*

**benzene-1,3-disulfohydrazide** [Aromatic hydrocarbon] *Arrhythmias, res-*

*piratory failure, pulmonary edema, paralysis, brain and kidney damage.*

**benzenethiol** [Aliphatic hydrocarbon] *Arrhythmias, asphyxiation, anesthesia.*

**benzidine** [Aliphatic hydrocarbon] *Arrhythmias, asphyxiation, anesthesia.*

**benzimidazole, 4,5-dichloro-2-(trifluorome)** [Aromatic hydrocarbon] *Arrhythmias, respiratory failure, pulmonary edema, paralysis, brain and kidney damage.*

**benzine** [Benzene] *Arrhythmias, respiratory failure, pulmonary edema, CNS depression, liver and kidney damage.* [Hydrocarbon mixture] *CNS depression, respiratory arrest, seizures, arrhythmias, pulmonary edema.* ⊡ benzene

**benzo[b]fluoranthene** [Aromatic hydrocarbon] *Arrhythmias, respiratory failure, pulmonary edema, paralysis, brain and kidney damage.*

**benzo[k]fluoranthene** [Aromatic hydrocarbon] *Arrhythmias, respiratory failure, pulmonary edema, paralysis, brain and kidney damage.*

**benzoic acid** [Organic acid] *Pulmonary edema, circulatory collapse, laryngeal edema and spasm, severe chemical burns to skin, mucous membranes, and internal organs, GI tract perforation and hemorrhage, peritonitis.*

**benzoic acid derivative pesticide (n.o.s.)** [Organic acid] *Pulmonary edema, circulatory collapse, laryngeal edema and spasm, severe chemical burns to skin, mucous membranes, and internal organs, GI tract perforation and hemorrhage, peritonitis.*

**benzoic trichloride** [Organic acid] *Pulmonary edema, circulatory collapse, laryngeal edema and spasm, severe chemical burns to skin, mucous membranes, and internal organs, GI tract perforation and hemorrhage, peritonitis.*

**benzol** [Benzene] *Arrhythmias, respiratory failure, pulmonary edema, CNS depression, liver and kidney damage.*

**benzonitrile** [Cyanide] *Impairment of cellular oxygenation and adenosine triphosphate production, hypoxia, death.*

**benzo[ghi]perylene** [Aromatic hydrocarbon] *Arrhythmias, respiratory failure, pulmonary edema, paralysis, brain and kidney damage.*

**benzo[a]pyrene** [Aromatic hydrocarbon] *Arrhythmias, respiratory failure, pulmonary edema, paralysis, brain and kidney damage.*

**benzoquinone** [Aromatic hydrocarbon] *Arrhythmias, respiratory failure, pulmonary edema, paralysis, brain and kidney damage.*

**benzotrichloride** [Irritant] *Severe immediate or delayed upper airway or respiratory tract irritation, pulmonary edema, glottic spasm, airway obstruction.* [Aromatic hydrocarbon] *Arrhythmias, respiratory failure, pulmonary edema, paralysis, brain and kidney damage.*

**benzotrifluoride** [Irritant] *Severe immediate or delayed upper airway or respiratory tract irritation, pulmonary edema, glottic spasm, airway obstruction.* [Aromatic hydrocarbon] *Arrhythmias, respiratory failure, pulmonary edema, paralysis, brain and kidney damage.*

**benzoyl chloride** [Irritant] *Severe immediate or delayed upper airway or respiratory tract irritation, pulmonary edema, glottic spasm, airway obstruction.* [Aromatic hydrocarbon] *Arrhythmias, respiratory failure, pulmonary edema, paralysis, brain and kidney damage.*

**benzoyl peroxide** [Organic peroxide] *Pulmonary and laryngeal edema, circulatory arrest, hypovolemic shock, chemical burns to skin, mucous membranes, and internal organs.*

**benzyl bromide** [Aromatic hydrocarbon] *Arrhythmias, respiratory failure, pulmonary edema, paralysis, brain and kidney damage.*

**benzyl chloride** [Aromatic hydrocarbon] *Arrhythmias, respiratory failure, pulmonary edema, paralysis, brain and kidney damage.*

**benzyl chloroformate** [Ester] *CNS depression, respiratory tract irritation, bronchitis, pneumonia.*

**benzyl cyanide** [Cyanide] *Impairment of cellular oxygenation and adenosine triphosphate production, hypoxia, death.*

**benzyl dimethylamine** [Aniline] *Methemoglobinemia, hypoxia.*

**benzyl iodide** [Aromatic hydrocarbon] *Arrhythmias, respiratory failure, pulmonary edema, paralysis, brain and kidney damage.*

**4-(benzyl(ethyl)amino)-3-ethoxybenzenediazonium zinc chloride** [Poison] *Cardiovascular collapse, pulmonary edema, CNS depression, coma, seizures, nausea, vomiting, cardiopulmonary arrest.* [Zinc] *Respiratory tract irritation, metal fume fever, pulmonary edema.*

**benzylidene chloride** [Aromatic hydrocarbon] *Arrhythmias, respiratory failure, pulmonary edema, paralysis, brain and kidney damage.*

**4-(benzyl(methyl)amino)-3-ethoxybenzenediazonium zinc chloride** [Poison] *Cardiovascular collapse, pulmonary edema, CNS depression, coma, seizures, nausea, vomiting, cardiopulmonary arrest.* [Zinc] *Respiratory tract irritation, metal fume fever, pulmonary edema.*

**o-benzyl-p-chlorophenol** [Aromatic hydrocarbon] *Arrhythmias, respiratory failure, pulmonary edema, paralysis, brain and kidney damage.*

**beryllium chloride** [Beryllium] *Pneumonitis, pulmonary edema.*

**beryllium fluoride** [Beryllium] *Pneumonitis, pulmonary edema.*

**beryllium mixture (n.o.s.)** [Beryllium] *Pneumonitis, pulmonary edema.*

**beryllium nitrate** [Beryllium] *Pneumonitis, pulmonary edema.*

**beryllium powder** [Beryllium] *Pneumonitis, pulmonary edema.*

**beta-endosulfan; β-endosulfan** [Aldrin/dieldrin/endrin] *Seizures, respiratory failure.*

**beta-naphthol; β-naphthol** [Phenol] *Coma, hypotension, arrhythmias, pulmonary edema, respiratory arrest.*

**beta-propiolactone; β-propiolactone; β-propionolactone** [Ketone] *Respiratory mucous membrane irritation, pulmonary edema, CNS depression.*

**BHC (alpha-, beta-, or delta-)** [Lindane] *CNS stimulation, seizures, respiratory failure.*

**bhusa** [Poison] *Cardiovascular collapse, pulmonary edema, CNS depression, coma, seizures, nausea, vomiting, cardiopulmonary arrest.*

**Bidrin** [Organophosphate] *Pulmonary edema, respiratory muscle paralysis, respiratory failure, bradycardia, acetylcholinesterase inhibition, hypotension, pulmonary edema, overstimulation of parasympathetic nervous system, striated muscle, sympathetic ganglia, and CNS.*

**bifluoride (n.o.s.)** [Fluorine] *CNS depression, respiratory arrest, cardiovascular collapse, shock, arrhythmias.*

**biological agent (n.o.s.)** *No acute symptoms during incubation period. Physiologic response varies depending on strain of microorganism or toxin.*

**2,2'-bioxirane** [Ether] *Anesthesia, respiratory arrest.*

**biphenyl** [Aromatic hydrocarbon] *Arrhythmias, respiratory failure, pulmonary edema, paralysis, brain and kidney damage.*

**bipyridilium pesticide (n.o.s.)** [Paraquat] *Widespread edema, cardiac damage, circulatory collapse, cerebral hemorrhage or infarcts, death. (Defoliant used in warfare.)*

**bis(aminopropyl) amine** [Organic base/amine] *Pulmonary edema, cardiac depression, seizures.*

**bis(2-chloroethoxy) methane** [Ether] *Anesthesia, respiratory arrest.*

**bis(2-chloroethyl) ether** [Ether] *Anesthesia, respiratory arrest.*

**bis(2-chloroisopropyl) ether** [Ether] *Anesthesia, respiratory arrest.*

**bis(2-chloro-1-methyl(ethyl)) ether** [Ether] *Anesthesia, respiratory arrest.*

**HazMat**

**bis(chloromethyl) ether; bis(2-chloromethyl) ether** [Ether] *Anesthesia, respiratory arrest.*

**bis(chloromethyl) ketone** [Ketone] *Respiratory mucous membrane irritation, pulmonary edema, CNS depression.*

**bis(dimethylamino) ethane** [Aliphatic hydrocarbon] *Arrhythmias, asphyxiation, anesthesia.*

**bis(2-ethyl(hexyl)) adipate** [Organic acid] *Pulmonary edema, circulatory collapse, laryngeal edema and spasm, severe chemical burns to skin, mucous membranes, and internal organs, GI tract perforation and hemorrhage, peritonitis.*

**bis(2-ethylhexyl) phthalate** [Ester] *CNS depression, respiratory tract irritation, bronchitis, pneumonia.*

**bishydroxycoumarin** [Warfarin/hydroxycoumarin/indanedione] *Anticoagulation effect, internal hemorrhage.*

**bismuth subnitrate** [Nitrate/nitrite] *Methemoglobinemia, hypotension, circulatory collapse.*

**bisulfite mixture (n.o.s.)** [Sulfur] *Respiratory tract irritation, pulmonary edema, anaphylaxis.*

**bithionol** [Sulfur] *Respiratory tract irritation, pulmonary edema, anaphylaxis.*

**bitoscanate** [Isocyanate/aliphatic thiocyanate] *CNS depression, respiratory arrest, respiratory paralysis, pulmonary edema, cyanide toxicity.*

**blasting agent (n.o.s.)** [Explosive] *Multiple trauma, highly toxic chemical exposure.*

**bleaching powder** [Hypochlorite] *Circulatory collapse, respiratory tract irritation, upper airway obstruction, pulmonary edema.*

**blue asbestos** [Asbestos] *Asbestosis, lung cancer, malignant mesothelioma.*

**bomb, smoke** [Irritant] *Severe immediate or delayed upper airway or respiratory tract irritation, pulmonary edema, glottic spasm, airway obstruction.* [Corrosive] *Upper airway burns and edema, circulatory collapse, severe chemical burns to skin, toxic systemic effects, GI tract perforation and hemorrhage, peritonitis.*

**bomyl** [Organophosphate] *Pulmonary edema, respiratory muscle paralysis, respiratory failure, bradycardia, acetylcholinesterase inhibition, hypotension, pulmonary edema, overstimulation of parasympathetic nervous system, striated muscle, sympathetic ganglia, and CNS.*

**borate & chlorate mixture** [Boron] *Respiratory tract irritation, laryngeal spasm and edema, pulmonary edema, severe chemical burns.* [Chlorate] *Hemolysis, methemoglobinemia, hypoperfusion, CNS depression, delayed-onset renal failure.*

**bordeaux arsenite** [Arsenic] *Heavy metal toxicity, vomiting, GI bleeding, CNS depression, pulmonary edema, cardiac arrest.* [Copper] *Respiratory tract irritation and arrest, hemorrhagic gastritis.*

**Bordeaux mixture** [Poison] *Cardiovascular collapse, pulmonary edema, CNS depression, coma, seizures, nausea, vomiting, cardiopulmonary arrest.*

**boric acid** [Boron] *Respiratory tract irritation, laryngeal spasm and edema, pulmonary edema, severe chemical burns.*

**borneol** [Camphor] *Status epilepticus, respiratory failure.*

**bornyl chloride** [Camphor] *Status epilepticus, respiratory failure.*

**boron; borate (n.o.s.)** [Boron] *Respiratory tract irritation, laryngeal spasm and edema, pulmonary edema, severe chemical burns.*

**boron oxide** [Boron] *Respiratory tract irritation, laryngeal spasm and edema, pulmonary edema, severe chemical burns.*

**boron tribromide** [Boron] *Respiratory tract irritation, laryngeal spasm and edema, pulmonary edema, severe chemical burns.*

**boron trichloride** [Boron] *Respiratory tract irritation, laryngeal spasm and edema, pulmonary edema, severe chemical burns.*

**boron trifluoride** [Boron] *Respiratory tract irritation, laryngeal spasm and edema, pulmonary edema, severe chemical burns.*

**boron trifluoride & acetic acid complex** [Boron] *Respiratory tract irritation, laryngeal spasm and edema, pulmonary edema, severe chemical burns.*

**boron trifluoride diethyl etherate** [Boron] *Respiratory tract irritation, laryngeal spasm and edema, pulmonary edema, severe chemical burns.*

**boron trifluoride dihydrate** [Boron] *Respiratory tract irritation, laryngeal spasm and edema, pulmonary edema, severe chemical burns.*

**boron trifluoride dimethyl etherate** [Boron] *Respiratory tract irritation, laryngeal spasm and edema, pulmonary edema, severe chemical burns.*

**boron trifluoride & propionic acid complex** [Boron] *Respiratory tract irritation, laryngeal spasm and edema, pulmonary edema, severe chemical burns.*

**Bovizole** [Thiabendazole] *Cardiovascular collapse, respiratory tract irritation.*

**BPMC** [Carbamate] *Acetylcholinesterase inhibition (reversible), bradycardia, hypotension, respiratory muscle paralysis, respiratory arrest, pulmonary edema.*

**brake fluid, hydraulic** [Hydrocarbon mixture] *CNS depression, respiratory arrest, seizures, arrhythmias, pulmonary edema.*

**bromadiolone** [Warfarin/hydroxycoumarin/indanedione] *Anticoagulation effect, internal hemorrhage.*

**bromate (n.o.s.)** [Bromate] *CNS and respiratory system depression, delayed-onset renal failure.*

**bromide, methyl** [Bromine/methylbromide] *Severe respiratory irritation, pulmonary edema, respiratory failure, coma, convulsions, death.*

**bromine** [Bromine/methylbromide] *Severe respiratory irritation, pulmonary edema, respiratory failure, coma, convulsions, death.*

**bromine chloride** [Bromine/methylbromide] *Severe respiratory irritation, pulmonary edema, respiratory failure, coma, convulsions, death.*

**bromine pentafluoride** [Bromine/methylbromide] *Severe respiratory irritation, pulmonary edema, respiratory failure, coma, convulsions, death.*

**bromine trifluoride** [Bromine/methylbromide] *Severe respiratory irritation, pulmonary edema, respiratory failure, coma, convulsions, death.*

**bromoacetic acid** [Bromine/methylbromide] *Severe respiratory irritation, pulmonary edema, respiratory failure, coma, convulsions, death.*

**bromoacetone** [Ketone] *Respiratory mucous membrane irritation, pulmonary edema, CNS depression.* [Bromine/methylbromide] *Severe respiratory irritation, pulmonary edema, respiratory failure, coma, convulsions, death.*

**bromoacetyl bromide** [Bromine/methylbromide] *Severe respiratory irritation, pulmonary edema, respiratory failure, coma, convulsions, death.*

**bromobenzene** [Halogenated aliphatic hydrocarbon] *CNS depression, respiratory arrest, circulatory collapse.*

**bromobenzyl cyanide** [Cyanide] *Impairment of cellular oxygenation and adenosine triphosphate production, hypoxia, death.*

**2-bromobutane** [Halogenated aliphatic hydrocarbon] *CNS depression, respiratory arrest, circulatory collapse.*

**bromochlorodifluoromethane (Halon 1211)** [Chlorinated fluorocarbon] *Asphyxiation, anesthesia, arrhythmias.*

**1-bromo-2-chloroethane** [Chlorinated fluorocarbon] *Asphyxiation, anesthesia, arrhythmias.*

**bromochloromethane** [Chlorinated fluorocarbon] *Asphyxiation, anesthesia, arrhythmias.*

**bromoethyl ethyl ether** [Ether] *Anesthesia, respiratory arrest.*

**bromoethylbutane** [Halogenated aliphatic hydrocarbon] *CNS depression, respiratory arrest, circulatory collapse.*

**bromoethylpropane** [Halogenated aliphatic hydrocarbon] *CNS depression, respiratory arrest, circulatory collapse.*

**bromoform** [Halogenated aliphatic hydrocarbon] *CNS depression, respiratory arrest, circulatory collapse.*

**bromomethane** [Halogenated aliphatic hydrocarbon] *CNS depression, respiratory arrest, circulatory collapse.*

**bromomethylbutane** [Halogenated aliphatic hydrocarbon] *CNS depression, respiratory arrest, circulatory collapse.*

**bromomethylpropane** [Halogenated aliphatic hydrocarbon] *CNS depression, respiratory arrest, circulatory collapse.*

**bromopentane** [Halogenated aliphatic hydrocarbon] *CNS depression, respiratory arrest, circulatory collapse.*

**2-bromo-4-phenyl ether** [Phenol] *Coma, hypotension, arrhythmias, pulmonary edema, respiratory arrest.*

**4-bromophenyl phenyl ether** [Ether] *Anesthesia, respiratory arrest.* [Phenol] *Coma, hypotension, arrhythmias, pulmonary edema, respiratory arrest.*

**bromopropane** [Halogenated aliphatic hydrocarbon] *CNS depression, respiratory arrest, circulatory collapse.*

**bromopropylate** [Poison] *Cardiovascular collapse, pulmonary edema, CNS depression, coma, seizures, nausea, vomiting, cardiopulmonary arrest.* [Organic acid] *Pulmonary edema, circulatory collapse, laryngeal edema and spasm, severe chemical burns to skin, mucous membranes, and internal organs, GI tract perforation and hemorrhage, peritonitis.*

**bromopropyne** [Halogenated aliphatic hydrocarbon] *CNS depression, respiratory arrest, circulatory collapse.*

**bromotrifluoroethylene** [Halogenated aliphatic hydrocarbon] *CNS depression, respiratory arrest, circulatory collapse.*

**bromotrifluoromethane** [Halogenated aliphatic hydrocarbon] *CNS depression, respiratory arrest, circulatory collapse.*

**brown asbestos; amosite** [Asbestos] *Asbestosis, lung cancer, malignant mesothelioma.*

**brucine** [Strychnine] *Convulsions, acidosis, diaphragmatic spasms, respiratory arrest.*

**bufencarb** [Carbamate] *Acetylcholinesterase inhibition (reversible), bradycardia, hypotension, respiratory muscle paralysis, respiratory arrest, pulmonary edema.*

**Bulan** [Lindane] *CNS stimulation, seizures, respiratory failure.*

**butacarb** [Carbamate] *Acetylcholinesterase inhibition (reversible), bradycardia, hypotension, respiratory muscle paralysis, respiratory arrest, pulmonary edema.*

**1,3-butadiene** [Aliphatic hydrocarbon] *Arrhythmias, asphyxiation, anesthesia.* ⊡ butylene

**n-butane** [Aliphatic hydrocarbon] *Arrhythmias, asphyxiation, anesthesia.* ⊡ butene

**1,3-butanediol** [Higher alcohol (4+ carbons)] *CNS depression, respiratory failure, arrhythmias.*

**butanedione** [Ethylene oxide] *Respiratory tract irritation, pulmonary edema.*

**butanethiol** [Aliphatic hydrocarbon] *Arrhythmias, asphyxiation, anesthesia.* [Sulfur] *Respiratory tract irritation, pulmonary edema, anaphylaxis.*

**butanol** [Higher alcohol (4+ carbons)] *CNS depression, respiratory failure, arrhythmias.*

**butene** [Aliphatic hydrocarbon] *Arrhythmias, asphyxiation, anesthesia.* ⊡ butane

**butonate** [Organophosphate] *Pulmonary edema, respiratory muscle paralysis, respiratory failure, bradycardia, acetylcholinesterase inhibition, hypotension, pulmonary edema, overstimulation of parasympathetic nervous system, striated muscle, sympathetic ganglia, and CNS.*

**butoxy polypropylene glycol** [Ethylene glycol] *Respiratory failure, pulmonary edema, paralysis, cardiovascular collapse, severe acidosis.*

**2-butoxyethanol; *n*-butoxyethanol** [Ethylene glycol] *Respiratory failure, pulmonary edema, paralysis, cardiovascular collapse, severe acidosis.*

**butoxyl** [Ester] *CNS depression, respiratory tract irritation, bronchitis, pneumonia.*

**butyl acetate** [Ester] *CNS depression, respiratory tract irritation, bronchitis, pneumonia.*

**butyl acid phosphate** [Organic acid] *Pulmonary edema, circulatory collapse, laryngeal edema and spasm, severe chemical burns to skin, mucous membranes, and internal organs, GI tract perforation and hemorrhage, peritonitis.*

***n*-butyl acrylate** [Ester] *CNS depression, respiratory tract irritation, bronchitis, pneumonia.*

**butyl alcohol** [Higher alcohol (4+ carbons)] *CNS depression, respiratory failure, arrhythmias.*

**butyl aldehyde** [Aldehyde] *Seizures, respiratory failure, pulmonary edema.*

**butyl benzene** [Aromatic hydrocarbon] *Arrhythmias, respiratory failure, pulmonary edema, paralysis, brain and kidney damage.*

**butyl benzyl phthalate** [Ester] *CNS depression, respiratory tract irritation, bronchitis, pneumonia.*

**butyl bromide** [Halogenated aliphatic hydrocarbon] *CNS depression, respiratory arrest, circulatory collapse.*

**butyl carbitol** [Ethylene glycol] *Respiratory failure, pulmonary edema, paralysis, cardiovascular collapse, severe acidosis.*

***n*-butyl chloride** [Halogenated aliphatic hydrocarbon] *CNS depression, respiratory arrest, circulatory collapse.*

**butyl chloroformate; *sec*-butyl chloroformate** [Ester] *CNS depression, respiratory tract irritation, bronchitis, pneumonia.*

***tert*-butyl cumene peroxide** [Organic peroxide] *Pulmonary and laryngeal edema, circulatory arrest, hypovolemic shock, chemical burns to skin, mucous membranes, and internal organs.*

***tert*-butyl cumyl peroxide** [Organic peroxide] *Pulmonary and laryngeal edema, circulatory arrest, hypovolemic shock, chemical burns to skin, mucous membranes, and internal organs.*

**butyl ether** [Ether] *Anesthesia, respiratory arrest.*

**butyl formate** [Ester] *CNS depression, respiratory tract irritation, bronchitis, pneumonia.*

***tert*-butyl hydroperoxide** [Organic peroxide] *Pulmonary and laryngeal edema, circulatory arrest, hypovolemic shock, chemical burns to skin, mucous membranes, and internal organs.*

**butyl hydroxytoluene** [Aromatic hydrocarbon] *Arrhythmias, respiratory failure, pulmonary edema, paralysis, brain and kidney damage.*

**butyl imidazole** [Aliphatic hydrocarbon] *Arrhythmias, asphyxiation, anesthesia.*

***tert*-butyl isocyanate** [Isocyanate/aliphatic thiocyanate] *CNS depression, respiratory arrest, respiratory paralysis, pulmonary edema, cyanide toxicity.*

***n*-butyl isocyanate; *tert*-butyl isocyanate** [Isocyanate/aliphatic thiocyanate] *CNS depression, respiratory arrest, respiratory paralysis, pulmonary edema, cyanide toxicity.*

***tert*-butyl isopropyl benzene hydroperoxide** [Organic peroxide] *Pulmonary and laryngeal edema, circulatory arrest, hypovolemic shock, chemical burns to skin, mucous membranes, and internal organs.*

**butyl lithium** [Lithium] *Chemical burns to respiratory tract, pulmonary edema.*

**butyl mercaptan** [Sulfur] *Respiratory tract irritation, pulmonary edema, anaphylaxis.*

**butyl methacrylate** [Ester] *CNS depression, respiratory tract irritation, bronchitis, pneumonia.*

**butyl methyl ether** [Ether] *Anesthesia, respiratory arrest.*

***tert*-butyl monoperoxy-maleate** [Organic peroxide] *Pulmonary and laryngeal edema, circulatory arrest,*

**HazMat**

*hypovolemic shock, chemical burns to skin, mucous membranes, and internal organs.* [Organic acid] *Pulmonary edema, circulatory collapse, laryngeal edema and spasm, severe chemical burns to skin, mucous membranes, and internal organs, GI tract perforation and hemorrhage, peritonitis.*

**tert-butyl monoperoxy-phthalate** [Organic peroxide] *Pulmonary and laryngeal edema, circulatory arrest, hypovolemic shock, chemical burns to skin, mucous membranes, and internal organs.* [Organic acid] *Pulmonary edema, circulatory collapse, laryngeal edema and spasm, severe chemical burns to skin, mucous membranes, and internal organs, GI tract perforation and hemorrhage, peritonitis.*

**butyl nitrite** [Nitrate/nitrite] *Methemoglobinemia, hypotension, circulatory collapse.*

**butyl perbenzoate** [Organic peroxide] *Pulmonary and laryngeal edema, circulatory arrest, hypovolemic shock, chemical burns to skin, mucous membranes, and internal organs.* [Organic acid] *Pulmonary edema, circulatory collapse, laryngeal edema and spasm, severe chemical burns to skin, mucous membranes, and internal organs, GI tract perforation and hemorrhage, peritonitis.*

**tert-butyl peroxide** [Organic peroxide] *Pulmonary and laryngeal edema, circulatory arrest, hypovolemic shock, chemical burns to skin, mucous membranes, and internal organs.*

**2,2-DL-(tert-butyl peroxy) butane & tert-butyl peroxy-2-ethyl hexanoate mixture** [Organic peroxide] *Pulmonary and laryngeal edema, circulatory arrest, hypovolemic shock, chemical burns to skin, mucous membranes, and internal organs.* [Organic acid] *Pulmonary edema, circulatory collapse, laryngeal edema and spasm, severe chemical burns to skin, mucous membranes, and internal organs, GI tract perforation and hemorrhage, peritonitis.*

**tert-butyl peroxyacetate** [Organic peroxide] *Pulmonary and laryngeal edema, circulatory arrest, hypovolemic shock, chemical burns to skin, mucous membranes, and internal organs.* [Organic acid] *Pulmonary edema, circulatory collapse, laryngeal edema and spasm, severe chemical burns to skin, mucous membranes, and internal organs, GI tract perforation and hemorrhage, peritonitis.*

**tert-butyl peroxybenzoate** [Organic peroxide] *Pulmonary and laryngeal edema, circulatory arrest, hypovolemic shock, chemical burns to skin, mucous membranes, and internal organs.* [Organic acid] *Pulmonary edema, circulatory collapse, laryngeal edema and spasm, severe chemical burns to skin, mucous membranes, and internal organs, GI tract perforation and hemorrhage, peritonitis.*

**tert-butyl peroxybenzoate & tert-butyl peroxydiethylacetate mixture** [Organic peroxide] *Pulmonary and laryngeal edema, circulatory arrest, hypovolemic shock, chemical burns to skin, mucous membranes, and internal organs.* [Organic acid] *Pulmonary edema, circulatory collapse, laryngeal edema and spasm, severe chemical burns to skin, mucous membranes, and internal organs, GI tract perforation and hemorrhage, peritonitis.*

**tert-butyl peroxycrotonate** [Organic peroxide] *Pulmonary and laryngeal edema, circulatory arrest, hypovolemic shock, chemical burns to skin, mucous membranes, and internal organs.* [Organic acid] *Pulmonary edema, circulatory collapse, laryngeal edema and spasm, severe chemical burns to skin, mucous membranes, and internal organs, GI tract perforation and hemorrhage, peritonitis.*

**butyl peroxydicarbonate** [Organic peroxide] *Pulmonary and laryngeal edema, circulatory arrest, hypovolemic shock, chemical burns to skin, mucous membranes, and internal organs.*

[Organic acid] *Pulmonary edema, circulatory collapse, laryngeal edema and spasm, severe chemical burns to skin, mucous membranes, and internal organs, GI tract perforation and hemorrhage, peritonitis.*

**tert-butyl peroxydiethylacetate** [Organic peroxide] *Pulmonary and laryngeal edema, circulatory arrest, hypovolemic shock, chemical burns to skin, mucous membranes, and internal organs.* [Organic acid] *Pulmonary edema, circulatory collapse, laryngeal edema and spasm, severe chemical burns to skin, mucous membranes, and internal organs, GI tract perforation and hemorrhage, peritonitis.*

**tert-butyl peroxydiethylacetate & tert-butyl peroxybenzoate mixture** [Organic peroxide] *Pulmonary and laryngeal edema, circulatory arrest, hypovolemic shock, chemical burns to skin, mucous membranes, and internal organs.* [Organic acid] *Pulmonary edema, circulatory collapse, laryngeal edema and spasm, severe chemical burns to skin, mucous membranes, and internal organs, GI tract perforation and hemorrhage, peritonitis.*

**tert-butyl peroxy-2-ethyl hexanoate** [Organic peroxide] *Pulmonary and laryngeal edema, circulatory arrest, hypovolemic shock, chemical burns to skin, mucous membranes, and internal organs.* [Organic acid] *Pulmonary edema, circulatory collapse, laryngeal edema and spasm, severe chemical burns to skin, mucous membranes, and internal organs, GI tract perforation and hemorrhage, peritonitis.*

**tert-butyl peroxy-2-ethyl hexanoate & 2,2-DL-(tert-butylperoxy) butane mixture** [Organic peroxide] *Pulmonary and laryngeal edema, circulatory arrest, hypovolemic shock, chemical burns to skin, mucous membranes, and internal organs.* [Organic acid] *Pulmonary edema, circulatory collapse, laryngeal edema and spasm, severe chemical burns to skin, mucous mem-*

*branes, and internal organs, GI tract perforation and hemorrhage, peritonitis.*

**tert-butyl peroxyisobutyrate** [Organic peroxide] *Pulmonary and laryngeal edema, circulatory arrest, hypovolemic shock, chemical burns to skin, mucous membranes, and internal organs.* [Organic acid] *Pulmonary edema, circulatory collapse, laryngeal edema and spasm, severe chemical burns to skin, mucous membranes, and internal organs, GI tract perforation and hemorrhage, peritonitis.*

**tert-butyl peroxyisononanoate** [Organic peroxide] *Pulmonary and laryngeal edema, circulatory arrest, hypovolemic shock, chemical burns to skin, mucous membranes, and internal organs.* [Organic acid] *Pulmonary edema, circulatory collapse, laryngeal edema and spasm, severe chemical burns to skin, mucous membranes, and internal organs, GI tract perforation and hemorrhage, peritonitis.*

**tert-butyl peroxyisopropyl carbonate** [Organic peroxide] *Pulmonary and laryngeal edema, circulatory arrest, hypovolemic shock, chemical burns to skin, mucous membranes, and internal organs.* [Organic acid] *Pulmonary edema, circulatory collapse, laryngeal edema and spasm, severe chemical burns to skin, mucous membranes, and internal organs, GI tract perforation and hemorrhage, peritonitis.*

**tert-butyl peroxymaleate** [Organic peroxide] *Pulmonary and laryngeal edema, circulatory arrest, hypovolemic shock, chemical burns to skin, mucous membranes, and internal organs.* [Organic acid] *Pulmonary edema, circulatory collapse, laryngeal edema and spasm, severe chemical burns to skin, mucous membranes, and internal organs, GI tract perforation and hemorrhage, peritonitis.*

**tert-butyl peroxy-neodecanoate** [Organic peroxide] *Pulmonary and laryngeal edema, circulatory arrest, hypovolemic shock, chemical burns to*

HazMat

skin, mucous membranes, and internal organs. [Organic acid] *Pulmonary edema, circulatory collapse, laryngeal edema and spasm, severe chemical burns to skin, mucous membranes, and internal organs, GI tract perforation and hemorrhage, peritonitis.*

**tert-butyl peroxy-3-phenylphthalide** [Organic peroxide] *Pulmonary and laryngeal edema, circulatory arrest, hypovolemic shock, chemical burns to skin, mucous membranes, and internal organs.* [Organic acid] *Pulmonary edema, circulatory collapse, laryngeal edema and spasm, severe chemical burns to skin, mucous membranes, and internal organs, GI tract perforation and hemorrhage, peritonitis.*

**tert-butyl peroxyphthalate** [Organic peroxide] *Pulmonary and laryngeal edema, circulatory arrest, hypovolemic shock, chemical burns to skin, mucous membranes, and internal organs.* [Organic acid] *Pulmonary edema, circulatory collapse, laryngeal edema and spasm, severe chemical burns to skin, mucous membranes, and internal organs, GI tract perforation and hemorrhage, peritonitis.*

**tert-butyl peroxypivalate** [Organic peroxide] *Pulmonary and laryngeal edema, circulatory arrest, hypovolemic shock, chemical burns to skin, mucous membranes, and internal organs.* [Organic acid] *Pulmonary edema, circulatory collapse, laryngeal edema and spasm, severe chemical burns to skin, mucous membranes, and internal organs, GI tract perforation and hemorrhage, peritonitis.*

**tert-butyl peroxystearyl carbonate** [Organic peroxide] *Pulmonary and laryngeal edema, circulatory arrest, hypovolemic shock, chemical burns to skin, mucous membranes, and internal organs.* [Organic acid] *Pulmonary edema, circulatory collapse, laryngeal edema and spasm, severe chemical burns to skin, mucous membranes, and*

internal organs, GI tract perforation and hemorrhage, peritonitis.

**tert-butyl peroxy-3,5,5-trimethylhexanoate** [Organic peroxide] *Pulmonary and laryngeal edema, circulatory arrest, hypovolemic shock, chemical burns to skin, mucous membranes, and internal organs.* [Organic acid] *Pulmonary edema, circulatory collapse, laryngeal edema and spasm, severe chemical burns to skin, mucous membranes, and internal organs, GI tract perforation and hemorrhage, peritonitis.*

**butyl phenol; o-sec-butyl phenol** [Phenol] *Coma, hypotension, arrhythmias, pulmonary edema, respiratory arrest.*

**butyl phosphoric acid** [Organic acid] *Pulmonary edema, circulatory collapse, laryngeal edema and spasm, severe chemical burns to skin, mucous membranes, and internal organs, GI tract perforation and hemorrhage, peritonitis.*

**n-butyl phthalate** [Organic acid] *Pulmonary edema, circulatory collapse, laryngeal edema and spasm, severe chemical burns to skin, mucous membranes, and internal organs, GI tract perforation and hemorrhage, peritonitis.*

**butyl propionate** [Ester] *CNS depression, respiratory tract irritation, bronchitis, pneumonia.*

**butyl toluene** [Aromatic hydrocarbon] *Arrhythmias, respiratory failure, pulmonary edema, paralysis, brain and kidney damage.*

**butyl trichlorosilane** [Silane/chlorosilane] *Respiratory tract irritation, pulmonary edema.*

**tert-butyl 2,4,6-trinitro-m-xylene** [Aromatic hydrocarbon] *Arrhythmias, respiratory failure, pulmonary edema, paralysis, brain and kidney damage.*

**butyl vinyl ether** [Ether] *Anesthesia, respiratory arrest.*

**n-butylamine; tert-butylamine** [Organic base/amine] *Pulmonary edema, cardiac depression, seizures.*

**butylaniline** [Aniline] *Methemoglobinemia, hypoxia.*

**n-butyl-4,4-dl(tert-butyl-peroxy valerate)** [Organic acid] *Pulmonary edema, circulatory collapse, laryngeal edema and spasm, severe chemical burns to skin, mucous membranes, and internal organs, GI tract perforation and hemorrhage, peritonitis.*

**tert-butylcyclohexyl chloroformate** [Ester] *CNS depression, respiratory tract irritation, bronchitis, pneumonia.*

**butylene** [Aliphatic hydrocarbon] *Arrhythmias, asphyxiation, anesthesia.* ▣ butadiene

**1,3-butylene glycol** [Aliphatic hydrocarbon] *Arrhythmias, asphyxiation, anesthesia.*

**butylene oxide; 1,2-butylene oxide** [Ethylene oxide] *Respiratory tract irritation, pulmonary edema.*

**butynediol** [Higher alcohol (4+ carbons)] *CNS depression, respiratory failure, arrhythmias.*

**butyraldehyde** [Aldehyde] *Seizures, respiratory failure, pulmonary edema.*

**butyraldoxime** [Aldehyde] *Seizures, respiratory failure, pulmonary edema.*

**butyric acid** [Organic acid] *Pulmonary edema, circulatory collapse, laryngeal edema and spasm, severe chemical burns to skin, mucous membranes, and internal organs, GI tract perforation and hemorrhage, peritonitis.*

**butyric anhydride** [Organic acid] *Pulmonary edema, circulatory collapse, laryngeal edema and spasm, severe chemical burns to skin, mucous membranes, and internal organs, GI tract perforation and hemorrhage, peritonitis.*

**butyrone** [Ketone] *Respiratory mucous membrane irritation, pulmonary edema, CNS depression.*

**n-butyronitrile** [Cyanide] *Impairment of cellular oxygenation and adenosine triphosphate production, hypoxia, death.*

**butyryl chloride** [Organic acid] *Pulmonary edema, circulatory collapse, laryngeal edema and spasm, severe chemical burns to skin, mucous membranes, and internal organs, GI tract perforation and hemorrhage, peritonitis.*

**cacodylic acid** [Arsenic] *Heavy metal toxicity, vomiting, GI bleeding, CNS depression, pulmonary edema, cardiac arrest.*

**cadmium; cadmium mixture (n.o.s.)** [Cadmium] *Respiratory tract irritation, pulmonary edema.*

**cadmium acetate** [Cadmium] *Respiratory tract irritation, pulmonary edema.*

**cadmium bromide** [Cadmium] *Respiratory tract irritation, pulmonary edema.*

**cadmium chloride** [Cadmium] *Respiratory tract irritation, pulmonary edema.*

**cadmium oxide** [Cadmium] *Respiratory tract irritation, pulmonary edema.*

**cadmium stearate** [Cadmium] *Respiratory tract irritation, pulmonary edema.*

**calcium; calcium alloy (n.o.s.)** [Poison] *Cardiovascular collapse, pulmonary edema, CNS depression, coma, seizures, nausea, vomiting, cardiopulmonary arrest.*

**calcium, pyrophoric; calcium alloy, pyrophoric (n.o.s.)** [Flammable solid] *Shock, severe chemical and thermal burns, severe respiratory tract irritation, pulmonary edema, respiratory arrest, ECG changes, sudden death.* [Poison] *Cardiovascular collapse, pulmonary edema, CNS depression, coma, seizures, nausea, vomiting, cardiopulmonary arrest.*

**calcium arsenate** [Arsenic] *Heavy metal toxicity, vomiting, GI bleeding, CNS depression, pulmonary edema, cardiac arrest.*

**calcium arsenite** [Arsenic] *Heavy metal toxicity, vomiting, GI bleeding, CNS depression, pulmonary edema, cardiac arrest.*

**calcium bisulfite** [Sulfur] *Respiratory tract irritation, pulmonary edema, anaphylaxis.*

**calcium carbide** [Corrosive] *Upper airway burns and edema, circulatory collapse, severe chemical burns to skin, toxic systemic effects, GI tract perforation and hemorrhage, peritonitis.*

**calcium carbonate & ammonium nitrate mixture** [Nitrate/nitrite]

**HazMat**

*Methemoglobinemia, hypotension, circulatory collapse.*

**calcium chlorate** [Chlorate] *Hemolysis, methemoglobinemia, hypoperfusion, CNS depression, delayed-onset renal failure.*

**calcium chlorite** [Chlorine] *Severe respiratory tract irritation, pulmonary edema, irritation of skin, eyes, and mucous membranes.*

**calcium chromate** [Poison] *Cardiovascular collapse, pulmonary edema, CNS depression, coma, seizures, nausea, vomiting, cardiopulmonary arrest.*

**calcium cyanamide** [Poison] *Cardiovascular collapse, pulmonary edema, CNS depression, coma, seizures, nausea, vomiting, cardiopulmonary arrest.*

**calcium cyanide** [Cyanide] *Impairment of cellular oxygenation and adenosine triphosphate production, hypoxia, death.*

**calcium dithionite** [Sulfur] *Respiratory tract irritation, pulmonary edema, anaphylaxis.*

**calcium dodecylbenzene sulfonate** [Organic acid] *Pulmonary edema, circulatory collapse, laryngeal edema and spasm, severe chemical burns to skin, mucous membranes, and internal organs, GI tract perforation and hemorrhage, peritonitis.*

**calcium hydride** [Corrosive] *Upper airway burns and edema, circulatory collapse, severe chemical burns to skin, toxic systemic effects, GI tract perforation and hemorrhage, peritonitis.*

**calcium hydrogen sulfite; calcium hydrosulfite** [Sulfur] *Respiratory tract irritation, pulmonary edema, anaphylaxis.*

**calcium hydroxide** [Inorganic base/ alkaline corrosive] *Upper airway burns and edema, pulmonary edema, skin burns, circulatory collapse, GI tract perforation and hemorrhage, peritonitis.*

**calcium hypochlorite** [Hypochlorite] *Circulatory collapse, respiratory tract irritation, upper airway obstruction, pulmonary edema.*

**calcium manganese silicon** [Manganese] *Respiratory tract irritation, pulmonary edema.*

**calcium nitrate** [Nitrate/nitrite] *Methemoglobinemia, hypotension, circulatory collapse.*

**calcium oxide** [Inorganic base/alkaline corrosive] *Upper airway burns and edema, pulmonary edema, skin burns, circulatory collapse, GI tract perforation and hemorrhage, peritonitis.*

**calcium perchlorate** [Chlorate] *Hemolysis, methemoglobinemia, hypoperfusion, CNS depression, delayed-onset renal failure.*

**calcium permanganate** [Inorganic acid] *Pulmonary edema, bronchospasm, circulatory collapse, laryngeal spasm and edema, severe chemical burns to skin, mucous membranes, and internal organs, GI tract perforation and hemorrhage, peritonitis.*

**calcium peroxide** [Organic peroxide] *Pulmonary and laryngeal edema, circulatory arrest, hypovolemic shock, chemical burns to skin, mucous membranes, and internal organs.*

**calcium phosphide** [Phosphine] *Severe pulmonary irritation, pulmonary edema.*

**calcium polysulfide** [Sulfur] *Respiratory tract irritation, pulmonary edema, anaphylaxis.*

**calcium resinate** [Flammable solid] *Shock, severe chemical and thermal burns, severe respiratory tract irritation, pulmonary edema, respiratory arrest, ECG changes, sudden death.*

**calcium selenate** [Selenium] *Arrhythmias, pulmonary edema, bronchospasm, seizures, vomiting, GI bleeding.*

**calcium silicide** [Flammable solid] *Shock, severe chemical and thermal burns, severe respiratory tract irritation, pulmonary edema, respiratory arrest, ECG changes, sudden death.*

**calcium silicon** [Flammable solid] *Shock, severe chemical and thermal burns, severe respiratory tract irritation, pulmonary edema, respiratory arrest, ECG changes, sudden death.*

**camphechlor** [Toxaphene] *Respiratory failure, seizures, exhaustion, death.*

**camphene** [Camphor] *Status epilepticus, respiratory failure.*

**camphene, chlorinated** [Toxaphene] *Respiratory failure, seizures, exhaustion, death.*

**camphor** [Camphor] *Status epilepticus, respiratory failure.*

**camphor oil** [Camphor] *Status epilepticus, respiratory failure.*

**cantharidin** [Irritant] *Severe immediate or delayed upper airway or respiratory tract irritation, pulmonary edema, glottic spasm, airway obstruction.*

**caproic acid (hexanoic acid)** [Organic acid] *Pulmonary edema, circulatory collapse, laryngeal edema and spasm, severe chemical burns to skin, mucous membranes, and internal organs, GI tract perforation and hemorrhage, peritonitis.*

**caprolactam** [Irritant] *Severe immediate or delayed upper airway or respiratory tract irritation, pulmonary edema, glottic spasm, airway obstruction.* [Poison] *Cardiovascular collapse, pulmonary edema, CNS depression, coma, seizures, nausea, vomiting, cardiopulmonary arrest.*

**caprylic alcohol** [Higher alcohol (4+ carbons)] *CNS depression, respiratory failure, arrhythmias.*

**caprylyl peroxide** [Organic peroxide] *Pulmonary and laryngeal edema, circulatory arrest, hypovolemic shock, chemical burns to skin, mucous membranes, and internal organs.*

**captan** [Dithiocarbamate] *Hypotension, respiratory failure.*

**carbachol chloride** [Carbamate] *Acetylcholinesterase inhibition (reversible), bradycardia, hypotension, respiratory muscle paralysis, respiratory arrest, pulmonary edema.*

**carbamate pesticide (n.o.s.)** [Carbamate] *Acetylcholinesterase inhibition (reversible), bradycardia, hypotension, respiratory muscle paralysis, respiratory arrest, pulmonary edema.*

**carbamic acid, ethyl ester** [Ester] *CNS depression, respiratory tract irritation, bronchitis, pneumonia.*

**carbamic acid, methyl-propoxur** [Carbamate] *Acetylcholinesterase inhibition (reversible), bradycardia, hypotension, respiratory muscle paralysis, respiratory arrest, pulmonary edema.*

**carbanolate** [Carbamate] *Acetylcholinesterase inhibition (reversible), bradycardia, hypotension, respiratory muscle paralysis, respiratory arrest, pulmonary edema.*

**carbaryl** [Carbamate] *Acetylcholinesterase inhibition (reversible), bradycardia, hypotension, respiratory muscle paralysis, respiratory arrest, pulmonary edema.*

**Carbitol** [Ethylene glycol] *Respiratory failure, pulmonary edema, paralysis, cardiovascular collapse, severe acidosis.*

**Carbitol ester** [Ester] *CNS depression, respiratory tract irritation, bronchitis, pneumonia.*

**carbofuran** [Carbamate] *Acetylcholinesterase inhibition (reversible), bradycardia, hypotension, respiratory muscle paralysis, respiratory arrest, pulmonary edema.*

**carbolic acid** [Phenol] *Coma, hypotension, arrhythmias, pulmonary edema, respiratory arrest.*

**carbon (animal or vegetable origin)** [Flammable solid] *Shock, severe chemical and thermal burns, severe respiratory tract irritation, pulmonary edema, respiratory arrest, ECG changes, sudden death.* [Irritant] *Severe immediate or delayed upper airway or respiratory tract irritation, pulmonary edema, glottic spasm, airway obstruction.*

**carbon, activated** [Irritant] *Severe immediate or delayed upper airway or respiratory tract irritation, pulmonary edema, glottic spasm, airway obstruction.*

**carbon bisulfide** *CNS depression, respiratory paralysis and arrest.*

**carbon dioxide (gas, cryogenic liquid, or Dry Ice)** [Simple asphyxiant] *Asphyxiation.*

**carbon dioxide & ethylene oxide mixture** [Simple asphyxiant] *Asphyx-*

**HazMat**

*iation.* [Ethylene oxide] *Respiratory tract irritation, pulmonary edema.*

**carbon dioxide & nitrous oxide mixture** [Simple asphyxiant] *Asphyxiation.*

**carbon dioxide & oxygen mixture** [Simple asphyxiant] *Asphyxiation.*

**carbon disulfide** *CNS depression, respiratory paralysis and arrest.*

**carbon monoxide (gas or cryogenic liquid)** [Carbon monoxide] *Impairment of cellular oxygenation, hypoxia, death.*

**carbon monoxide from methylene chloride** [Carbon monoxide] *Impairment of cellular oxygenation, hypoxia, death.* [Halogenated aliphatic hydrocarbon] *CNS depression, respiratory arrest, circulatory collapse.*

**carbon monoxide & hydrogen mixture** [Carbon monoxide] *Impairment of cellular oxygenation, hypoxia, death.*

**carbon oxysulfide** [Hydrogen sulfide] *Severe respiratory tract irritation, pulmonary edema, respiratory paralysis.*

**carbon remover** [Hydrocarbon mixture] *CNS depression, respiratory arrest, seizures, arrhythmias, pulmonary edema.*

**carbon tetrabromide** [Carbon tetrachloride] *CNS depression, respiratory arrest, circulatory collapse.*

**carbon tetrachloride** [Carbon tetrachloride] *CNS depression, respiratory arrest, circulatory collapse.*

**carbon tetrachloride & sulfur chloride mixture** [Carbon tetrachloride] *CNS depression, respiratory arrest, circulatory collapse.* [Sulfur] *Respiratory tract irritation, pulmonary edema, anaphylaxis.*

**carbonic difluoride** [Fluorine] *CNS depression, respiratory arrest, cardiovascular collapse, shock, arrhythmias.*

**carbonyl chloride** [Phosgene] *Severe respiratory irritation, alveolar damage, pulmonary edema.*

**carbonyl fluoride** [Hydrofluoric acid] *Pulmonary and laryngeal edema, circula-*

*tory collapse, severe skin burns, GI tract perforation, systemic fluoride poisoning.*

**carbonyl sulfide** [Hydrogen sulfide] *Severe respiratory tract irritation, pulmonary edema, respiratory paralysis.*

**carbophenothion** [Organophosphate] *Pulmonary edema, respiratory muscle paralysis, respiratory failure, bradycardia, acetylcholinesterase inhibition, hypotension, pulmonary edema, overstimulation of parasympathetic nervous system, striated muscle, sympathetic ganglia, and CNS.*

**Carbowax** [Ethylene glycol] *Respiratory failure, pulmonary edema, paralysis, cardiovascular collapse, severe acidosis.*

**cartap** [Ester] *CNS depression, respiratory tract irritation, bronchitis, pneumonia.*

**carvacrol** [Phenol] *Coma, hypotension, arrhythmias, pulmonary edema, respiratory arrest.*

**casinghead gasoline** [Hydrocarbon mixture] *CNS depression, respiratory arrest, seizures, arrhythmias, pulmonary edema.*

**castor beans** [Poison] *Cardiovascular collapse, pulmonary edema, CNS depression, coma, seizures, nausea, vomiting, cardiopulmonary arrest.*

**Castrix** [Strychnine] *Convulsions, acidosis, diaphragmatic spasms, respiratory arrest.*

**catechol** [Phenol] *Coma, hypotension, arrhythmias, pulmonary edema, respiratory arrest.*

**caustic alkali liquid (n.o.s.)** [Inorganic base/alkaline corrosive] *Upper airway burns and edema, pulmonary edema, skin burns, circulatory collapse, GI tract perforation and hemorrhage, peritonitis.*

**caustic potash** [Inorganic base/alkaline corrosive] *Upper airway burns and edema, pulmonary edema, skin burns, circulatory collapse, GI tract perforation and hemorrhage, peritonitis*

**caustic soda** [Inorganic base/alkaline corrosive] *Upper airway burns and edema, pulmonary edema, skin burns,* circulatory collapse, GI tract perforation and hemorrhage, peritonitis.

**CBP** [Dichloropropane/dichloropropene] *Pulmonary edema, bronchospasm, alveolar hemorrhage.*

**Cellosolve; cellosolve sulfate** [Ethylene glycol] *Respiratory failure, pulmonary edema, paralysis, cardiovascular collapse, severe acidosis.*

**celluloid** [Flammable solid] *Shock, severe chemical and thermal burns, severe respiratory tract irritation, pulmonary edema, respiratory arrest, ECG changes, sudden death.*

**cement (n.o.s.)** [Inorganic base/alkaline corrosive] *Upper airway burns and edema, pulmonary edema, skin burns, circulatory collapse, GI tract perforation and hemorrhage, peritonitis.*

**cerium** [Poison] *Cardiovascular collapse, pulmonary edema, CNS depression, coma, seizures, nausea, vomiting, cardiopulmonary arrest.*

**cesium** [Flammable solid] *Shock, severe chemical and thermal burns, severe respiratory tract irritation, pulmonary edema, respiratory arrest, ECG changes, sudden death.*

**cesium hydroxide** [Inorganic base/ alkaline corrosive] *Upper airway burns and edema, pulmonary edema, skin burns, circulatory collapse, GI tract perforation and hemorrhage, peritonitis.*

**cesium nitrate** [Inorganic acid] *Pulmonary edema, bronchospasm, circulatory collapse, laryngeal spasm and edema, severe chemical burns to skin, mucous membranes, and internal organs, GI tract perforation and hemorrhage, peritonitis.* [Nitrate/nitrite] *Methemoglobinemia, hypotension, circulatory collapse.*

**cetyl alcohol** [Higher alcohol (4+ carbons)] *CNS depression, respiratory failure, arrhythmias.*

**CFC (chlorofluorocarbon) (n.o.s.)** [Chlorinated fluorocarbon] *Asphyxiation, anesthesia, arrhythmias.*

**charcoal** [Irritant] *Severe immediate or delayed upper airway or respiratory tract irritation, pulmonary edema, glottic spasm, airway obstruction.*

**chemical ammunition, irritant** [Irritant] *Severe immediate or delayed upper airway or respiratory tract irritation, pulmonary edema, glottic spasm, airway obstruction.*

**chemical ammunition, toxic** [Irritant] *Severe immediate or delayed upper airway or respiratory tract irritation, pulmonary edema, glottic spasm, airway obstruction.* [Poison] *Cardiovascular collapse, pulmonary edema, CNS depression, coma, seizures, nausea, vomiting, cardiopulmonary arrest.*

**chemical kit** [Poison] *Cardiovascular collapse, pulmonary edema, CNS depression, coma, seizures, nausea, vomiting, cardiopulmonary arrest.*

**chloral** [Halogenated aliphatic hydrocarbon] *CNS depression, respiratory arrest, circulatory collapse.*

**chloramben** [Organic acid] *Pulmonary edema, circulatory collapse, laryngeal edema and spasm, severe chemical burns to skin, mucous membranes, and internal organs, GI tract perforation and hemorrhage, peritonitis.*

**chlorambucil** [Poison] *Cardiovascular collapse, pulmonary edema, CNS depression, coma, seizures, nausea, vomiting, cardiopulmonary arrest.*

**chloramine (n.o.s.)** [Organic base/ amine] *Pulmonary edema, cardiac depression, seizures.*

**chloramine T** [Hypochlorite] *Circulatory collapse, respiratory tract irritation, upper airway obstruction, pulmonary edema.*

**chlorasol** [Hypochlorite] *Circulatory collapse, respiratory tract irritation, upper airway obstruction, pulmonary edema.*

**chlorate; chlorate salt (n.o.s.)** [Chlorate] *Hemolysis, methemoglobinemia, hypoperfusion, CNS depression, delayed-onset renal failure.*

**chlorate & borate mixture** [Chlorate] *Hemolysis, methemoglobinemia, hypoperfusion, CNS depression, delayed-onset renal failure.* [Boron]

*Respiratory tract irritation, laryngeal spasm and edema, pulmonary edema, severe chemical burns.*

**chlorate & magnesium chloride mixture** [Chlorate] *Hemolysis, methemoglobinemia, hypoperfusion, CNS depression, delayed-onset renal failure.* [Magnesium] *Cardiovascular collapse, respiratory depression.*

**chlorate of potash** [Chlorate] *Hemolysis, methemoglobinemia, hypoperfusion, CNS depression, delayed-onset renal failure.*

**chlorate of soda** [Chlorate] *Hemolysis, methemoglobinemia, hypoperfusion, CNS depression, delayed-onset renal failure.*

**chlordane** [Chlordane] *Respiratory failure, seizures, exhaustion, death.*

**chlordecone** [Lindane] *CNS stimulation, seizures, respiratory failure.*

**chlordimeform** [Aniline] *Methemoglobinemia, hypoxia.*

**chlorfenvinphos** [Organophosphate] *Pulmonary edema, respiratory muscle paralysis, respiratory failure, bradycardia, acetylcholinesterase inhibition, hypotension, pulmonary edema, overstimulation of parasympathetic nervous system, striated muscle, sympathetic ganglia, and CNS.*

**chloric acid** [Inorganic acid] *Pulmonary edema, bronchospasm, circulatory collapse, laryngeal spasm and edema, severe chemical burns to skin, mucous membranes, and internal organs, GI tract perforation and hemorrhage, peritonitis.*

**chloride of phosphorus** [Chlorine] *Severe respiratory tract irritation, pulmonary edema, irritation of skin, eyes, and mucous membranes.* [Phosphorus] *Hypovolemic shock, severe tissue burns, severe respiratory irritation, pulmonary edema, respiratory arrest, arrhythmias, sudden death.*

**chloride of sulfur** [Sulfur] *Respiratory tract irritation, pulmonary edema, anaphylaxis.*

**chlorinated benzene** [Lindane] *CNS stimulation, seizures, respiratory failure.*

**chlorinated camphene** [Toxaphene] *Respiratory failure, seizures, exhaustion, death.*

**chlorinated ethane** [Halogenated aliphatic hydrocarbon] *CNS depression, respiratory arrest, circulatory collapse.*

**chlorinated hydrocarbon** [Halogenated aliphatic hydrocarbon] *CNS depression, respiratory arrest, circulatory collapse.*

**chlorinated lime** [Hypochlorite] *Circulatory collapse, respiratory tract irritation, upper airway obstruction, pulmonary edema.*

**chlorinated naphthalene** [Naphthalene] *Delayed-onset acute intravascular hemolysis.*

**chlorinated phenol** [Phenol] *Coma, hypotension, arrhythmias, pulmonary edema, respiratory arrest.*

**chlorinated solvent (n.o.s.)** [Halogenated aliphatic hydrocarbon] *CNS depression, respiratory arrest, circulatory collapse.*

**chlorinated trisodium phosphate** [Inorganic base/alkaline corrosive] *Upper airway burns and edema, pulmonary edema, skin burns, circulatory collapse, GI tract perforation and hemorrhage, peritonitis.* [Hypochlorite] *Circulatory collapse, respiratory tract irritation, upper airway obstruction, pulmonary edema.*

**chlorine** [Chlorine] *Severe respiratory tract irritation, pulmonary edema, irritation of skin, eyes, and mucous membranes.*

**chlorine dioxide** [Chlorine] *Severe respiratory tract irritation, pulmonary edema, irritation of skin, eyes, and mucous membranes.*

**chlorine dioxide hydrate** [Chlorine] *Severe respiratory tract irritation, pulmonary edema, irritation of skin, eyes, and mucous membranes.*

**chlorine pentafluoride** [Chlorine] *Severe respiratory tract irritation, pulmonary edema, irritation of skin, eyes, and mucous membranes.* [Fluorine]

CNS depression, respiratory arrest, cardiovascular collapse, shock, arrhythmias.

**chlorine trifluoride** [Hydrofluoric acid] *Pulmonary and laryngeal edema, circulatory collapse, severe skin burns, GI tract perforation, systemic fluoride poisoning.* [Chlorine] *Severe respiratory tract irritation, pulmonary edema, irritation of skin, eyes, and mucous membranes.*

**chlorite (n.o.s.)** [Chlorine] *Severe respiratory tract irritation, pulmonary edema, irritation of skin, eyes, and mucous membranes.*

**chlormephos** [Organophosphate] *Pulmonary edema, respiratory muscle paralysis, respiratory failure, bradycardia, acetylcholinesterase inhibition, hypotension, pulmonary edema, overstimulation of parasympathetic nervous system, striated muscle, sympathetic ganglia, and CNS.*

**chlormequat chloride** [Poison] *Cardiovascular collapse, pulmonary edema, CNS depression, coma, seizures, nausea, vomiting, cardiopulmonary arrest.*

**chlornaphazine** [Poison] *Cardiovascular collapse, pulmonary edema, CNS depression, coma, seizures, nausea, vomiting, cardiopulmonary arrest.*

**chloroacetaldehyde** [Aldehyde] *Seizures, respiratory failure, pulmonary edema.*

**chloroacetic acid** [Organic acid] *Pulmonary edema, circulatory collapse, laryngeal edema and spasm, severe chemical burns to skin, mucous membranes, and internal organs, GI tract perforation and hemorrhage, peritonitis.*

**chloroacetone** [Ketone] *Respiratory mucous membrane irritation, pulmonary edema, CNS depression.*

**chloroacetonitrile** [Cyanide] *Impairment of cellular oxygenation and adenosine triphosphate production, hypoxia, death.*

**chloroacetophenone; 2-chloroacetophenone** [Ketone] *Respiratory*

mucous membrane irritation, pulmonary edema, CNS depression.

**chloroacetyl chloride** [Chlorine] *Severe respiratory tract irritation, pulmonary edema, irritation of skin, eyes, and mucous membranes.*

**chloroaniline** [Aniline] *Methemoglobinemia, hypoxia.*

**chloroanisidine** [Aromatic hydrocarbon] *Arrhythmias, respiratory failure, pulmonary edema, paralysis, brain and kidney damage.* [Nitrate/nitrite] *Methemoglobinemia, hypotension, circulatory collapse.*

**chlorobenzene** [Benzene] *Arrhythmias, respiratory failure, pulmonary edema, CNS depression, liver and kidney damage.*

**chlorobenzilate** [Lindane] *CNS stimulation, seizures, respiratory failure.*

**3-chlorobenzoic acid & 3-chloroperoxybenzoic acid mixture** [Organic acid] *Pulmonary edema, circulatory collapse, laryngeal edema and spasm, severe chemical burns to skin, mucous membranes, and internal organs, GI tract perforation and hemorrhage, peritonitis.*

**chlorobenzotrifluoride** [Aromatic hydrocarbon] *Arrhythmias, respiratory failure, pulmonary edema, paralysis, brain and kidney damage.*

**p-chlorobenzoyl peroxide** [Organic peroxide] *Pulmonary and laryngeal edema, circulatory arrest, hypovolemic shock, chemical burns to skin, mucous membranes, and internal organs.*

**chlorobenzyl chloride** [Aromatic hydrocarbon] *Arrhythmias, respiratory failure, pulmonary edema, paralysis, brain and kidney damage.*

**o-chlorobenzylidene malonitrile** [Cyanide] *Impairment of cellular oxygenation and adenosine triphosphate production, hypoxia, death.*

**chlorobromomethane** [Halogenated aliphatic hydrocarbon] *CNS depression, respiratory arrest, circulatory collapse.*

**HazMat**

**chlorobromopropane** [Chlorinated fluorocarbon] *Asphyxiation, anesthesia, arrhythmias.*

**chlorobutane** [Chlorinated fluorocarbon] *Asphyxiation, anesthesia, arrhythmias.*

***p*-chloro-*m*-cresol** [Phenol] *Coma, hypotension, arrhythmias, pulmonary edema, respiratory arrest.*

**4-chloro-2-cyclopentylphenol** [Phenol] *Coma, hypotension, arrhythmias, pulmonary edema, respiratory arrest.*

**chlorodibromomethane** [Halogenated aliphatic hydrocarbon] *CNS depression, respiratory arrest, circulatory collapse.*

**chlorodiethylaluminum** [Flammable solid] *Shock, severe chemical and thermal burns, severe respiratory tract irritation, pulmonary edema, respiratory arrest, ECG changes, sudden death.* [Poison] *Cardiovascular collapse, pulmonary edema, CNS depression, coma, seizures, nausea, vomiting, cardiopulmonary arrest.*

**3-chloro-4-diethylamino-benediazonium zinc chloride** [Zinc] *Respiratory tract irritation, metal fume fever, pulmonary edema.*

**chlorodifluorobromomethane** [Chlorinated fluorocarbon] *Asphyxiation, anesthesia, arrhythmias.*

**chlorodifluoroethane** [Chlorinated fluorocarbon] *Asphyxiation, anesthesia, arrhythmias.*

**chlorodifluoromethane** [Chlorinated fluorocarbon] *Asphyxiation, anesthesia, arrhythmias.*

**chlorodifluoromethane & chloropentafluoroethane mixture** [Chlorinated fluorocarbon] *Asphyxiation, anesthesia, arrhythmias.*

**chlorodifluoromethane & dichlorodifluoromethane mixture** [Chlorinated fluorocarbon] *Asphyxiation, anesthesia, arrhythmias.*

**chlorodifluoromethane & dichlorodifluoromethane & trichlorofluoromethane mixture** [Chlorinated fluorocarbon] *Asphyxiation, anesthesia, arrhythmias.*

**chlorodinitrobenzene; 1-chloro-2,4-dinitrobenzene** [Aromatic hydrocarbon] *Arrhythmias, respiratory failure, pulmonary edema, paralysis, brain and kidney damage.* [Nitrate/nitrite] *Methemoglobinemia, hypotension, circulatory collapse.*

**chlorodiphenyl** Polychlorinated biphenyl/polybrominated biphenyl/polychlorinated [dibenzofuran] *Liver and kidney damage.*

**chloroethane** [Halogenated aliphatic hydrocarbon] *CNS depression, respiratory arrest, circulatory collapse.*

**chloroethanol** [Ether] *Anesthesia, respiratory arrest.*

**chloroethyl chloroformate** [Ester] *CNS depression, respiratory tract irritation, bronchitis, pneumonia.*

**2-chloroethyl vinyl ether** [Chlorinated fluorocarbon] *Asphyxiation, anesthesia, arrhythmias.*

**chlorofluorocarbon (CFC) (n.o.s.)** [Chlorinated fluorocarbon] *Asphyxiation, anesthesia, arrhythmias.*

**chloroform** [Halogenated aliphatic hydrocarbon] *CNS depression, respiratory arrest, circulatory collapse.*

**chloroformate (n.o.s.)** [Ester] *CNS depression, respiratory tract irritation, bronchitis, pneumonia.*

**2-chloro-4(hydroxymercuri)phenol** [Mercury] *Circulatory collapse, arrhythmias, respiratory failure, pulmonary edema, neurotoxic effects.*

**chloromethane** [Halogenated aliphatic hydrocarbon] *CNS depression, respiratory arrest, circulatory collapse.*

**chloromethyl ethyl ether** [Ether] *Anesthesia, respiratory arrest.*

**chloromethyl methyl ether** [Ether] *Anesthesia, respiratory arrest.*

**5-chloro-6-((((methylamino)carbonyl)oxy)imino)-bicyclo(2.2.1)heptane-2-carbonitrile** [Carbamate] *Acetylcholinesterase inhibition (reversible), bradycardia, hypotension,* *respiratory muscle paralysis, respiratory arrest, pulmonary edema.*

**3-chloro-4-methylaniline** [Aniline] *Methemoglobinemia, hypoxia.*

**chloromethylchloroformate** [Ester] *CNS depression, respiratory tract irritation, bronchitis, pneumonia.*

**chloromethyloxypropylmercuric acetate** [Ester] *CNS depression, respiratory tract irritation, bronchitis, pneumonia.*

**chloromethylphenylisocyanate** [Isocyanate/aliphatic thiocyanate] *CNS depression, respiratory arrest, respiratory paralysis, pulmonary edema, cyanide toxicity.*

**3-chloro-2-methyl-1-propene** [Dichloropropane/dichloropropene] *Pulmonary edema, bronchospasm, alveolar hemorrhage.*

**2-chloronaphthalene** [Naphthalene] *Delayed-onset acute intravascular hemolysis.*

**chloronitroaniline** [Aniline] *Methemoglobinemia, hypoxia.*

**chloronitrobenzenes** [Aromatic hydrocarbon] *Arrhythmias, respiratory failure, pulmonary edema, paralysis, brain and kidney damage.* [Nitrate/nitrite] *Methemoglobinemia, hypotension, circulatory collapse.*

**1-chloro-1-nitropropane** [Halogenated aliphatic hydrocarbon] *CNS depression, respiratory arrest, circulatory collapse.* [Nitrate/nitrite] *Methemoglobinemia, hypotension, circulatory collapse.*

**chloronitrotoluene** [Aromatic hydrocarbon] *Arrhythmias, respiratory failure, pulmonary edema, paralysis, brain and kidney damage.*

**chloropentafluoroethane** [Chlorinated fluorocarbon] *Asphyxiation, anesthesia, arrhythmias.*

**chloropentafluoroethane & chlorodifluoromethane mixture** [Chlorinated fluorocarbon] *Asphyxiation, anesthesia, arrhythmias.*

**3-chloroperoxybenzoic acid** [Organic acid] *Pulmonary edema, cir-*

*culatory collapse, laryngeal edema and spasm, severe chemical burns to skin, mucous membranes, and internal organs, GI tract perforation and hemorrhage, peritonitis.*

**3-chloroperoxybenzoic acid & 3-chlorobenzoic acid mixture** [Organic acid] *Pulmonary edema, circulatory collapse, laryngeal edema and spasm, severe chemical burns to skin, mucous membranes, and internal organs, GI tract perforation and hemorrhage, peritonitis.*

**chlorophacinone** [Warfarin/hydroxycoumarin/indanedione] *Anticoagulation effect, internal hemorrhage.*

**chlorophenate** [Phenol] *Coma, hypotension, arrhythmias, pulmonary edema, respiratory arrest.*

**2-chlorophenol** [Phenol] *Coma, hypotension, arrhythmias, pulmonary edema, respiratory arrest.*

**chlorophenol (n.o.s.)** [Phenol] *Coma, hypotension, arrhythmias, pulmonary edema, respiratory arrest.*

*p***-chlorophenoxyacetic acid** [Chlorophenoxy herbicide] *CNS depression, CNS stimulation, respiratory failure, ventricular fibrillation, seizures.*

**4-chlorophenyl phenyl ether** [Ether] *Anesthesia, respiratory arrest.* [Phenol] *Coma, hypotension, arrhythmias, pulmonary edema, respiratory arrest.*

**chlorophenyl trichlorosilane** [Silane/chlorosilane] *Respiratory tract irritation, pulmonary edema.*

**chloro-2-phenylphenol** [Phenol] *Coma, hypotension, arrhythmias, pulmonary edema, respiratory arrest.*

**chloropicrin** [Irritant] *Severe immediate or delayed upper airway or respiratory tract irritation, pulmonary edema, glottic spasm, airway obstruction.* [Halogenated aliphatic hydrocarbon] *CNS depression, respiratory arrest, circulatory collapse.*

**chloropicrin & methyl bromide mixture** [Irritant] *Severe immediate or delayed upper airway or respiratory tract irritation, pulmonary edema, glot-*

HazMat

tic spasm, *airway obstruction.* [Halogenated aliphatic hydrocarbon] *CNS depression, respiratory arrest, circulatory collapse.* [Bromine/methylbromide] *Severe respiratory irritation, pulmonary edema, respiratory failure, coma, convulsions, death.*

**chloropicrin & methyl chloride mixture** [Irritant] *Severe immediate or delayed upper airway or respiratory tract irritation, pulmonary edema, glottic spasm, airway obstruction.* [Halogenated aliphatic hydrocarbon] *CNS depression, respiratory arrest, circulatory collapse.*

**chloropicrin mixture (n.o.s.)** [Irritant] *Severe immediate or delayed upper airway or respiratory tract irritation, pulmonary edema, glottic spasm, airway obstruction.* [Halogenated aliphatic hydrocarbon] *CNS depression, respiratory arrest, circulatory collapse.*

**chloropivaloyl chloride** [Poison] *Cardiovascular collapse, pulmonary edema, CNS depression, coma, seizures, nausea, vomiting, cardiopulmonary arrest.*

**chloroplatinic acid** [Inorganic acid] *Pulmonary edema, bronchospasm, circulatory collapse, laryngeal spasm and edema, severe chemical burns to skin, mucous membranes, and internal organs, GI tract perforation and hemorrhage, peritonitis.*

**chloroprene** [Irritant] *Severe immediate or delayed upper airway or respiratory tract irritation, pulmonary edema, glottic spasm, airway obstruction.* [Aliphatic hydrocarbon] *Arrhythmias, asphyxiation, anesthesia.*

**chloropropane** [Aliphatic hydrocarbon] *Arrhythmias, asphyxiation, anesthesia.* ▣ chloropropene

**chloropropanol; 2-chloro-1-propanol; 3-chloropropanol; 3-chloropropanol-1** [Higher alcohol (4+ carbons)] *CNS depression, respiratory failure, arrhythmias.*

**chloropropene** [Aliphatic hydrocarbon] *Arrhythmias, asphyxiation, anesthesia.* ▣ chloropropane

**chloropropionic acid** [Organic acid] *Pulmonary edema, circulatory collapse, laryngeal edema and spasm, severe chemical burns to skin, mucous membranes, and internal organs, GI tract perforation and hemorrhage, peritonitis.*

**3-chloropropionitrile** [Cyanide] *Impairment of cellular oxygenation and adenosine triphosphate production, hypoxia, death.*

**chloropyridine** [Aromatic hydrocarbon] *Arrhythmias, respiratory failure, pulmonary edema, paralysis, brain and kidney damage.*

**chlorosilane (n.o.s.)** [Silane/chlorosilane] *Respiratory tract irritation, pulmonary edema.*

**N-chlorosuccinimide** [Phenol] *Coma, hypotension, arrhythmias, pulmonary edema, respiratory arrest.*

**chlorosulfonic acid** [Inorganic acid] *Pulmonary edema, bronchospasm, circulatory collapse, laryngeal spasm and edema, severe chemical burns to skin, mucous membranes, and internal organs, GI tract perforation and hemorrhage, peritonitis.*

**chlorosulfonic acid & sulfur trioxide mixture** [Inorganic acid] *Pulmonary edema, bronchospasm, circulatory collapse, laryngeal spasm and edema, severe chemical burns to skin, mucous membranes, and internal organs, GI tract perforation and hemorrhage, peritonitis.* [Sulfur] *Respiratory tract irritation, pulmonary edema, anaphylaxis.*

**chlorotetrafluoroethane** [Chlorinated fluorocarbon] *Asphyxiation, anesthesia, arrhythmias.*

**chlorothalonil** [Poison] *Cardiovascular collapse, pulmonary edema, CNS depression, coma, seizures, nausea, vomiting, cardiopulmonary arrest.*

**Chlorothion** [Organophosphate] *Pulmonary edema, respiratory muscle paralysis, respiratory failure, bradycardia, acetylcholinesterase inhibition,*

hypotension, *pulmonary edema, overstimulation of parasympathetic nervous
system, striated muscle, sympathetic
ganglia, and CNS.*

**chlorothymol** [Phenol] *Coma, hypotension, arrhythmias, pulmonary
edema, respiratory arrest.*

**chlorotoluene; o-chlorotoluene**
[Aromatic hydrocarbon] *Arrhythmias,
respiratory failure, pulmonary edema,
paralysis, brain and kidney damage.*

**chlorotoluidine** [Organic base/amine]
*Pulmonary edema, cardiac depression,
seizures.*

**4-chloro-o-toluidine HCl** [Organic
base/amine] *Pulmonary edema, cardiac depression, seizures.*

**chlorotrifluoroethane** [Chlorinated
fluorocarbon] *Asphyxiation, anesthesia, arrhythmias.*

**chlorotrifluoromethane** [Chlori-
nated fluorocarbon] *Asphyxiation,
anesthesia, arrhythmias.*

**chlorotrifluoromethane & trifluo-
romethane mixture** [Chlorinated
fluorocarbon] *Asphyxiation, anesthesia, arrhythmias.*

**chlorotrifluoropyridine** [Aromatic
hydrocarbon] *Arrhythmias, respiratory
failure, pulmonary edema, paralysis,
brain and kidney damage.*

**chloroxuron** [Poison] *Cardiovascular
collapse, pulmonary edema, CNS
depression, coma, seizures, nausea,
vomiting, cardiopulmonary arrest.*

**4-chloro-3,5-xylenol** [Phenol] *Coma,
hypotension, arrhythmias, pulmonary
edema, respiratory arrest.*

**chlorpyrifos** [Organophosphate] *Pulmonary edema, respiratory muscle
paralysis, respiratory failure, bradycardia, acetylcholinesterase inhibition,
hypotension, pulmonary edema, overstimulation of parasympathetic nervous
system, striated muscle, sympathetic
ganglia, and CNS.*

**chlorthiophos** [Organophosphate]
*Pulmonary edema, respiratory muscle
paralysis, respiratory failure, bradycardia, acetylcholinesterase inhibition,*

hypotension, *pulmonary edema, overstimulation of parasympathetic nervous
system, striated muscle, sympathetic
ganglia, and CNS.*

**chromic acetate** [Inorganic acid] *Pulmonary edema, bronchospasm, circulatory collapse, laryngeal spasm and
edema, severe chemical burns to skin,
mucous membranes, and internal
organs, GI tract perforation and hemorrhage, peritonitis.*

**chromic acid** [Inorganic acid] *Pulmonary edema, bronchospasm, circulatory
collapse, laryngeal spasm and edema,
severe chemical burns to skin, mucous
membranes, and internal organs, GI
tract perforation and hemorrhage, peritonitis.*

**chromic anhydride** [Inorganic acid]
*Pulmonary edema, bronchospasm, cir-
culatory collapse, laryngeal spasm and
edema, severe chemical burns to skin,
mucous membranes, and internal
organs, GI tract perforation and hemorrhage, peritonitis.*

**chromic chloride; chromous chlo-
ride** [Inorganic acid] *Pulmonary
edema, bronchospasm, circulatory collapse, laryngeal spasm and edema, severe
chemical burns to skin, mucous membranes, and internal organs, GI tract
perforation and hemorrhage, peritonitis.*

**chromic fluoride** [Fluorine] *CNS
depression, respiratory arrest, cardiovascular collapse, shock, arrhythmias.*

**chromic sulfate** [Inorganic acid] *Pulmonary edema, bronchospasm, circulatory collapse, laryngeal spasm and
edema, severe chemical burns to skin,
mucous membranes, and internal
organs, GI tract perforation and hemorrhage, peritonitis.*

**chromium; chromate salt (n.o.s.)**
[Inorganic acid] *Pulmonary edema,
bronchospasm, circulatory collapse,
laryngeal spasm and edema, severe
chemical burns to skin, mucous membranes, and internal organs, GI tract
perforation and hemorrhage, peritonitis.*

**chromium nitrate** [Nitrate/nitrite] *Methemoglobinemia, hypotension, circulatory collapse.*

**chromium oxychloride** [Inorganic acid] *Pulmonary edema, bronchospasm, circulatory collapse, laryngeal spasm and edema, severe chemical burns to skin, mucous membranes, and internal organs, GI tract perforation and hemorrhage, peritonitis.*

**chromium trioxide** [Inorganic acid] *Pulmonary edema, bronchospasm, circulatory collapse, laryngeal spasm and edema, severe chemical burns to skin, mucous membranes, and internal organs, GI tract perforation and hemorrhage, peritonitis.*

**chromosulfuric acid** [Inorganic acid] *Pulmonary edema, bronchospasm, circulatory collapse, laryngeal spasm and edema, severe chemical burns to skin, mucous membranes, and internal organs, GI tract perforation and hemorrhage, peritonitis.*

**chromous chloride; chromic chloride** [Inorganic acid] *Pulmonary edema, bronchospasm, circulatory collapse, laryngeal spasm and edema, severe chemical burns to skin, mucous membranes, and internal organs, GI tract perforation and hemorrhage, peritonitis.*

**chrysene** [Naphthalene] *Delayed-onset acute intravascular hemolysis.*

**chrysotile** [Asbestos] *Asbestosis, lung cancer, malignant mesothelioma.*

**cigarette, self-lighting** [Nicotine] *Respiratory and cardiac arrest, CNS stimulation, CNS depression.*

**cigarette lighter; cigarette lighter refills** [Aliphatic hydrocarbon] *Arrhythmias, asphyxiation, anesthesia.*

**cleaning compound** [Inorganic base/alkaline corrosive] *Upper airway burns and edema, pulmonary edema, skin burns, circulatory collapse, GI tract perforation and hemorrhage, peritonitis.*

**coal** [Flammable solid] *Shock, severe chemical and thermal burns, severe respiratory tract irritation, pulmonary edema, respiratory arrest, ECG changes, sudden death.*

**coal gas** [Flammable gas] *Respiratory failure, cardiac arrest, arrhythmias.*

**coal tar creosote** [Aromatic hydrocarbon] *Arrhythmias, respiratory failure, pulmonary edema, paralysis, brain and kidney damage.* [Phenol] *Coma, hypotension, arrhythmias, pulmonary edema, respiratory arrest.*

**coal tar distillate** [Aromatic hydrocarbon] *Arrhythmias, respiratory failure, pulmonary edema, paralysis, brain and kidney damage.* [Benzene] *Arrhythmias, respiratory failure, pulmonary edema, CNS depression, liver and kidney damage.*

**coal tar naphtha** [Hydrocarbon mixture] *CNS depression, respiratory arrest, seizures, arrhythmias, pulmonary edema.* [Naphthalene] *Delayed-onset acute intravascular hemolysis.*

**coal tar oil** [Aromatic hydrocarbon] *Arrhythmias, respiratory failure, pulmonary edema, paralysis, brain and kidney damage.* [Benzene] *Arrhythmias, respiratory failure, pulmonary edema, CNS depression, liver and kidney damage.*

**coating solution** [Poison] *Cardiovascular collapse, pulmonary edema, CNS depression, coma, seizures, nausea, vomiting, cardiopulmonary arrest.*

**cobalt carbonyl** [Cobalt] *Respiratory tract irritation, possible pulmonary edema, fibrosis.*

**cobalt hydrocarbonyl** [Cobalt] *Respiratory tract irritation, possible pulmonary edema, fibrosis.*

**cobalt naphthenate** [Cobalt] *Respiratory tract irritation, possible pulmonary edema, fibrosis.*

**cobalt resinate** [Cobalt] *Respiratory tract irritation, possible pulmonary edema, fibrosis.*

**cobalt salt (n.o.s.)** [Cobalt] *Respiratory tract irritation, possible pulmonary edema, fibrosis.*

**cobaltous bromide** [Cobalt] *Respiratory tract irritation, possible pulmonary* edema, fibrosis. [Bromine/methylbromide] *Severe respiratory irritation, pulmonary edema, respiratory failure, coma, convulsions, death.*

**cobaltous formate** [Cobalt] *Respiratory tract irritation, possible pulmonary edema, fibrosis.*

**cobaltous sulfamate** [Cobalt] *Respiratory tract irritation, possible pulmonary edema, fibrosis.*

**cocculus** [Poison] *Cardiovascular collapse, pulmonary edema, CNS depression, coma, seizures, nausea, vomiting, cardiopulmonary arrest.*

**colchicine** [Poison] *Cardiovascular collapse, pulmonary edema, CNS depression, coma, seizures, nausea, vomiting, cardiopulmonary arrest.*

**collodion** [Lower alcohol (1–3 carbons)] *CNS depression, coma, respiratory arrest, arrhythmias.* [Ether] *Anesthesia, respiratory arrest.*

**combustible liquid (n.o.s.)** [Flammable/combustible liquid] *CNS depression, respiratory arrest, convulsions, arrhythmias, pulmonary edema.*

**compressed gas (n.o.s.)** [Nonflammable gas] *Pulmonary edema, respiratory failure, asphyxiation.*

**compressed gas, flammable (n.o.s.)** [Flammable gas] *Respiratory failure, cardiac arrest, arrhythmias.*

**compressed gas, flammable poison (n.o.s.)** [Flammable gas] *Respiratory failure, cardiac arrest, arrhythmias.* [Poison] *Cardiovascular collapse, pulmonary edema, CNS depression, coma, seizures, nausea, vomiting, cardiopulmonary arrest.*

**compressed gas, poisonous (n.o.s.)** [Poison] *Cardiovascular collapse, pulmonary edema, CNS depression, coma, seizures, nausea, vomiting, cardiopulmonary arrest.*

**copper; copper mixture (n.o.s.)** [Copper] *Respiratory tract irritation and arrest, hemorrhagic gastritis.*

**copper acetoarsenite; cupric acetoarsenite** [Copper] *Respiratory tract irritation and arrest, hemorrhagic gastritis.*

**copper arsenate** [Arsenic] *Heavy metal toxicity, vomiting, GI bleeding, CNS depression, pulmonary edema, cardiac arrest.* [Copper] *Respiratory tract irritation and arrest, hemorrhagic gastritis.*

**copper arsenite; cupric arsenite** [Arsenic] *Heavy metal toxicity, vomiting, GI bleeding, CNS depression, pulmonary edema, cardiac arrest.* [Copper] *Respiratory tract irritation and arrest, hemorrhagic gastritis.*

**copper chlorate** [Copper] *Respiratory tract irritation and arrest, hemorrhagic gastritis.* [Chlorate] *Hemolysis, methemoglobinemia, hypoperfusion, CNS depression, delayed-onset renal failure.*

**copper chloride; cupric chloride; cuprous chloride** [Copper] *Respiratory tract irritation and arrest, hemorrhagic gastritis.*

**copper cyanide** [Copper] *Respiratory tract irritation and arrest, hemorrhagic gastritis.* [Cyanide] *Impairment of cellular oxygenation and adenosine triphosphate production, hypoxia, death.*

**copper naphthenates** [Naphthalene] *Delayed-onset acute intravascular hemolysis.* [Copper] *Respiratory tract irritation and arrest, hemorrhagic gastritis.*

**copper oxychloride sulfate** [Copper] *Respiratory tract irritation and arrest, hemorrhagic gastritis.*

**copper 3-phenyl-salicylate** [Copper] *Respiratory tract irritation and arrest, hemorrhagic gastritis.*

**copper quinolinolate** [Copper] *Respiratory tract irritation and arrest, hemorrhagic gastritis.*

**copper selenate** [Copper] *Respiratory tract irritation and arrest, hemorrhagic gastritis.* [Selenium] *Arrhythmias, pulmonary edema, bronchospasm, seizures, vomiting, GI bleeding.*

**copper selenite** [Copper] *Respiratory tract irritation and arrest, hemorrhagic gastritis.* [Selenium] *Arrhythmias, pulmonary edema, bronchospasm, seizures, vomiting, GI bleeding.*

**HazMat**

**copper sulfate, tribasic** [Copper] *Respiratory tract irritation and arrest, hemorrhagic gastritis.*

**copper-based pesticide (n.o.s.)** [Copper] *Respiratory tract irritation and arrest, hemorrhagic gastritis.*

**copra** [Flammable/combustible liquid] *CNS depression, respiratory arrest, convulsions, arrhythmias, pulmonary edema.*

**corrosive: acid** [Inorganic acid] *Pulmonary edema, bronchospasm, circulatory collapse, laryngeal spasm and edema, severe chemical burns to skin, mucous membranes, and internal organs, GI tract perforation and hemorrhage, peritonitis.* [Organic acid] *Pulmonary edema, circulatory collapse, laryngeal edema and spasm, severe chemical burns to skin, mucous membranes, and internal organs, GI tract perforation and hemorrhage, peritonitis.*

**corrosive: ammonia** [Ammonia] *Pulmonary edema, hypotension.*

**corrosive: ammonium hydroxide** [Ammonia] *Pulmonary edema, hypotension.*

**corrosive liquid, flammable (n.o.s.)** [Flammable/combustible liquid] *CNS depression, respiratory arrest, convulsions, arrhythmias, pulmonary edema.* [Corrosive] *Upper airway burns and edema, circulatory collapse, severe chemical burns to skin, toxic systemic effects, GI tract perforation and hemorrhage, peritonitis.*

**corrosive solid, flammable (n.o.s.)** [Flammable solid] *Shock, severe chemical and thermal burns, severe respiratory tract irritation, pulmonary edema, respiratory arrest, ECG changes, sudden death.* [Corrosive] *Upper airway burns and edema, circulatory collapse, severe chemical burns to skin, toxic systemic effects, GI tract perforation and hemorrhage, peritonitis.*

**corrosive solid, self-heating (n.o.s.)** [Corrosive] *Upper airway burns and edema, circulatory collapse, severe chemical burns to skin, toxic systemic*

*effects, GI tract perforation and hemorrhage, peritonitis.*

**corrosive solid or liquid (n.o.s.)** [Corrosive] *Upper airway burns and edema, circulatory collapse, severe chemical burns to skin, toxic systemic effects, GI tract perforation and hemorrhage, peritonitis.*

**corrosive solid or liquid, flammable in contact with water (n.o.s.)** [Flammable gas] *Respiratory failure, cardiac arrest, arrhythmias.* [Corrosive] *Upper airway burns and edema, circulatory collapse, severe chemical burns to skin, toxic systemic effects, GI tract perforation and hemorrhage, peritonitis.*

**corrosive solid or liquid, oxidizing (n.o.s.)** [Oxidizer] *Pulmonary and laryngeal edema, circulatory arrest, hypovolemic shock, chemical burns of skin, mucous membranes, and internal organs.* [Corrosive] *Upper airway burns and edema, circulatory collapse, severe chemical burns to skin, toxic systemic effects, GI tract perforation and hemorrhage, peritonitis.*

**corrosive solid or liquid, poisonous (n.o.s.)** [Poison] *Cardiovascular collapse, pulmonary edema, CNS depression, coma, seizures, nausea, vomiting, cardiopulmonary arrest.* [Corrosive] *Upper airway burns and edema, circulatory collapse, severe chemical burns to skin, toxic systemic effects, GI tract perforation and hemorrhage, peritonitis.*

**cosmetic, corrosive (n.o.s.)** [Corrosive] *Upper airway burns and edema, circulatory collapse, severe chemical burns to skin, toxic systemic effects, GI tract perforation and hemorrhage, peritonitis.*

**cosmetic, flammable liquid (n.o.s.)** [Flammable/combustible liquid] *CNS depression, respiratory arrest, convulsions, arrhythmias, pulmonary edema.*

**cosmetic, flammable solid (n.o.s.)** [Flammable solid] *Shock, severe chemical and thermal burns, severe respiratory tract irritation, pulmonary* edema, respiratory arrest, ECG changes, sudden death.

**cosmetic, oxidizer (n.o.s.)** [Oxidizer] *Pulmonary and laryngeal edema, circulatory arrest, hypovolemic shock, chemical burns of skin, mucous membranes, and internal organs.*

**cotton** [Irritant] *Severe immediate or delayed upper airway or respiratory tract irritation, pulmonary edema, glottic spasm, airway obstruction.*

**coumachlor** [Warfarin/hydroxycoumarin/indanedione] *Anticoagulation effect, internal hemorrhage.*

**coumafuryl** [Warfarin/hydroxycoumarin/indanedione] *Anticoagulation effect, internal hemorrhage.*

**coumaphos** [Organophosphate] *Pulmonary edema, respiratory muscle paralysis, respiratory failure, bradycardia, acetylcholinesterase inhibition, hypotension, pulmonary edema, overstimulation of parasympathetic nervous system, striated muscle, sympathetic ganglia, and CNS.*

**coumarin derivative pesticide (n.o.s.)** [Ketone] *Respiratory mucous membrane irritation, pulmonary edema, CNS depression.*

**coumatetralyl** [Warfarin/hydroxycoumarin/indanedione] *Anticoagulation effect, internal hemorrhage.*

**Creolin** [Acrolein] *Severe respiratory tract irritation, pulmonary edema, respiratory failure.*

**creosol** [Phenol] *Coma, hypotension, arrhythmias, pulmonary edema, respiratory arrest.*

**creosote, coal tar** [Aromatic hydrocarbon] *Arrhythmias, respiratory failure, pulmonary edema, paralysis, brain and kidney damage.* [Phenol] *Coma, hypotension, arrhythmias, pulmonary edema, respiratory arrest.*

**creosote salt (n.o.s.)** [Phenol] *Coma, hypotension, arrhythmias, pulmonary edema, respiratory arrest.*

**p-cresidine** [Aromatic hydrocarbon] *Arrhythmias, respiratory failure, pulmonary edema, paralysis, brain and kidney damage.*

**cresol; m-cresol; o-cresol; p-cresol** [Phenol] *Coma, hypotension, arrhythmias, pulmonary edema, respiratory arrest.*

**m-cresyl acetate** [Ester] *CNS depression, respiratory tract irritation, bronchitis, pneumonia.*

**cresylic acid** [Phenol] *Coma, hypotension, arrhythmias, pulmonary edema, respiratory arrest.*

**crimidine** [Poison] *Cardiovascular collapse, pulmonary edema, CNS depression, coma, seizures, nausea, vomiting, cardiopulmonary arrest.*

**crotonaldehyde** [Acrolein] *Severe respiratory tract irritation, pulmonary edema, respiratory failure.*

**crotonic acid** [Organic acid] *Pulmonary edema, circulatory collapse, laryngeal edema and spasm, severe chemical burns to skin, mucous membranes, and internal organs, GI tract perforation and hemorrhage, peritonitis.*

**crotonylene** [Aliphatic hydrocarbon] *Arrhythmias, asphyxiation, anesthesia.*

**crufomate** [Organophosphate] *Pulmonary edema, respiratory muscle paralysis, respiratory failure, bradycardia, acetylcholinesterase inhibition, hypotension, pulmonary edema, overstimulation of parasympathetic nervous system, striated muscle, sympathetic ganglia, and CNS.*

**cryolite** [Fluorine] *CNS depression, respiratory arrest, cardiovascular collapse, shock, arrhythmias.*

**cubé** [Rotenone] *Respiratory arrest, asphyxia.*

**cumene** [Aromatic hydrocarbon] *Arrhythmias, respiratory failure, pulmonary edema, paralysis, brain and kidney damage.*

**cumene hydroperoxide** [Organic peroxide] *Pulmonary and laryngeal edema, circulatory arrest, hypovolemic shock, chemical burns to skin, mucous membranes, and internal organs.* [Aromatic hydrocarbon] *Arrhythmias, res-*

HazMat

*piratory failure, pulmonary edema, paralysis, brain and kidney damage.*

**cumyl hydroperoxide** [Organic peroxide] *Pulmonary and laryngeal edema, circulatory arrest, hypovolemic shock, chemical burns to skin, mucous membranes, and internal organs.* [Aromatic hydrocarbon] *Arrhythmias, respiratory failure, pulmonary edema, paralysis, brain and kidney damage.*

**cumyl peroxy-neo-decanoate** [Organic peroxide] *Pulmonary and laryngeal edema, circulatory arrest, hypovolemic shock, chemical burns to skin, mucous membranes, and internal organs.* [Aromatic hydrocarbon] *Arrhythmias, respiratory failure, pulmonary edema, paralysis, brain and kidney damage.*

**cumyl peroxypivalate** [Organic peroxide] *Pulmonary and laryngeal edema, circulatory arrest, hypovolemic shock, chemical burns to skin, mucous membranes, and internal organs.* [Aromatic hydrocarbon] *Arrhythmias, respiratory failure, pulmonary edema, paralysis, brain and kidney damage.*

**cupferron** [Organic base/amine] *Pulmonary edema, cardiac depression, seizures.*

**cupric acetate** [Copper] *Respiratory tract irritation and arrest, hemorrhagic gastritis.*

**cupric acetoarsenite; copper acetoarsenite** [Copper] *Respiratory tract irritation and arrest, hemorrhagic gastritis.*

**cupric arsenite; copper arsenite** [Arsenic] *Heavy metal toxicity, vomiting, GI bleeding, CNS depression, pulmonary edema, cardiac arrest.* [Copper] *Respiratory tract irritation and arrest, hemorrhagic gastritis.*

**cupric chloride; copper chloride; cuprous chloride** [Copper] *Respiratory tract irritation and arrest, hemorrhagic gastritis.*

**cupric nitrate** [Copper] *Respiratory tract irritation and arrest, hemorrhagic gastritis.*

**cupric oxalate** [Copper] *Respiratory tract irritation and arrest, hemorrhagic gastritis.*

**cupric sulfate** [Copper] *Respiratory tract irritation and arrest, hemorrhagic gastritis.*

**cupric tartrate** [Copper] *Respiratory tract irritation and arrest, hemorrhagic gastritis.*

**cupriethylenediamine** [Organic base/amine] *Pulmonary edema, cardiac depression, seizures.* [Copper] *Respiratory tract irritation and arrest, hemorrhagic gastritis.*

**cuprous chloride; copper chloride; cupric chloride** [Copper] *Respiratory tract irritation and arrest, hemorrhagic gastritis.*

**cuprous oxide** [Copper] *Respiratory tract irritation and arrest, hemorrhagic gastritis.*

**cyanic acid** [Isocyanate/aliphatic thiocyanate] *CNS depression, respiratory arrest, respiratory paralysis, pulmonary edema, cyanide toxicity.*

**cyanide; cyanide mixture (n.o.s.)** [Cyanide] *Impairment of cellular oxygenation and adenosine triphosphate production, hypoxia, death.*

**cyanide potassium; potassium cyanide** [Cyanide] *Impairment of cellular oxygenation and adenosine triphosphate production, hypoxia, death.*

**cyanide sodium** [Cyanide] *Impairment of cellular oxygenation and adenosine triphosphate production, hypoxia, death.*

**cyanogen** [Cyanide] *Impairment of cellular oxygenation and adenosine triphosphate production, hypoxia, death.*

**cyanogen bromide** [Cyanide] *Impairment of cellular oxygenation and adenosine triphosphate production, hypoxia, death.*

**cyanogen chloride** [Cyanide] *Impairment of cellular oxygenation and adenosine triphosphate production, hypoxia, death.*

**cyanogen iodide** [Cyanide] *Impairment of cellular oxygenation and adenosine triphosphate production, hypoxia, death.*

**cyano-organic mixture (n.o.s.)** [Cyanide] *Impairment of cellular oxygenation and adenosine triphosphate production, hypoxia, death.*

**cyanophos** [Organophosphate] *Pulmonary edema, respiratory muscle paralysis, respiratory failure, bradycardia, acetylcholinesterase inhibition, hypotension, pulmonary edema, overstimulation of parasympathetic nervous system, striated muscle, sympathetic ganglia, and CNS.*

**cyanuric chloride** [Organic acid] *Pulmonary edema, circulatory collapse, laryngeal edema and spasm, severe chemical burns to skin, mucous membranes, and internal organs, GI tract perforation and hemorrhage, peritonitis.*

**cyanuric fluoride** [Hydrofluoric acid] *Pulmonary and laryngeal edema, circulatory collapse, severe skin burns, GI tract perforation, systemic fluoride poisoning.*

**cyclethrin** [Pyrethrin/pyrethroid] *Respiratory paralysis, convulsions.*

**cyclobutane** [Simple asphyxiant] *Asphyxiation.*

**cyclobutylchloroformate** [Ester] *CNS depression, respiratory tract irritation, bronchitis, pneumonia.*

**cyclocoumarol** [Warfarin/hydroxycoumarin/indanedione] *Anticoagulation effect, internal hemorrhage.*

**cyclododecatriene** [Aliphatic hydrocarbon] *Arrhythmias, asphyxiation, anesthesia.*

**cycloheptane** [Aliphatic hydrocarbon] *Arrhythmias, asphyxiation, anesthesia.*

**cycloheptatriene** [Aliphatic hydrocarbon] *Arrhythmias, asphyxiation, anesthesia.*

**cycloheptene** [Aliphatic hydrocarbon] *Arrhythmias, asphyxiation, anesthesia.*

**cyclohexane** [Aliphatic hydrocarbon] *Arrhythmias, asphyxiation, anesthesia.*

**cyclohexanol** [Higher alcohol (4+ carbons)] *CNS depression, respiratory failure, arrhythmias.*

**cyclohexanone** [Ketone] *Respiratory mucous membrane irritation, pulmonary edema, CNS depression.*

**cyclohexanone peroxide** [Organic peroxide] *Pulmonary and laryngeal edema, circulatory arrest, hypovolemic shock, chemical burns to skin, mucous membranes, and internal organs.* [Ketone] *Respiratory mucous membrane irritation, pulmonary edema, CNS depression.* [Corrosive] *Upper airway burns and edema, circulatory collapse, severe chemical burns to skin, toxic systemic effects, GI tract perforation and hemorrhage, peritonitis.*

**cyclohexene** [Aliphatic hydrocarbon] *Arrhythmias, asphyxiation, anesthesia.*

**cyclohexene & ozone mixture** [Aliphatic hydrocarbon] *Arrhythmias, asphyxiation, anesthesia.* [Ozone] *Pulmonary edema, airway obstruction.*

**cyclohexenyl trichlorosilane** [Silane/chlorosilane] *Respiratory tract irritation, pulmonary edema.*

**cycloheximide** [Irritant] *Severe immediate or delayed upper airway or respiratory tract irritation, pulmonary edema, glottic spasm, airway obstruction.* [Poison] *Cardiovascular collapse, pulmonary edema, CNS depression, coma, seizures, nausea, vomiting, cardiopulmonary arrest.*

**cyclohexyl acetate** [Ester] *CNS depression, respiratory tract irritation, bronchitis, pneumonia.*

**cyclohexyl isocyanate** [Isocyanate/aliphatic thiocyanate] *CNS depression, respiratory arrest, respiratory paralysis, pulmonary edema, cyanide toxicity.*

**cyclohexyl mercaptan** [Sulfur] *Respiratory tract irritation, pulmonary edema, anaphylaxis.*

**cyclohexyl trichlorosilane** [Silane/chlorosilane] *Respiratory tract irritation, pulmonary edema.*

**cyclohexylamine** [Organic base/amine] *Pulmonary edema, cardiac depression, seizures.*

**2-cyclohexyl-4,6-dinitrophenol** [Dinitrophenol] *Respiratory and circulatory collapse, pulmonary edema, hyperthermia.*

**HazMat**

**cyclonite (RDX, T4, or C4)** [Explosive] *Multiple trauma, highly toxic chemical exposure.*

**cyclooctadiene** [Aliphatic hydrocarbon] *Arrhythmias, asphyxiation, anesthesia.*

**cyclooctadiene phosphine** [Phosphine] *Severe pulmonary irritation, pulmonary edema.*

**cyclooctatetraene** [Aliphatic hydrocarbon] *Arrhythmias, asphyxiation, anesthesia.*

**cyclopentane** [Aliphatic hydrocarbon] *Arrhythmias, asphyxiation, anesthesia.*

**cyclopentanol** [Higher alcohol (4+ carbons)] *CNS depression, respiratory failure, arrhythmias.*

**cyclopentanone** [Ketone] *Respiratory mucous membrane irritation, pulmonary edema, CNS depression.*

**cyclopentene** [Aliphatic hydrocarbon] *Arrhythmias, asphyxiation, anesthesia.*

**cyclophosphamide** [Poison] *Cardiovascular collapse, pulmonary edema, CNS depression, coma, seizures, nausea, vomiting, cardiopulmonary arrest.*

**cyclopropane** [Simple asphyxiant] *Asphyxiation.*

**cymene** [Aromatic hydrocarbon] *Arrhythmias, respiratory failure, pulmonary edema, paralysis, brain and kidney damage.*

**2,4-D; 2,4-D ester (n.o.s.); 2,4-D salt (n.o.s.)** [Chlorophenoxy herbicide] *CNS depression, CNS stimulation, respiratory failure, ventricular fibrillation, seizures.*

**daunomycin** [Poison] *Cardiovascular collapse, pulmonary edema, CNS depression, coma, seizures, nausea, vomiting, cardiopulmonary arrest.*

**DBCP** [Dichloropropane/dichloropropene] *Pulmonary edema, bronchospasm, alveolar hemorrhage.*

**DD mixture** [Dichloropropane/dichloropropene] *Pulmonary edema, bronchospasm, alveolar hemorrhage.*

**DDD** [DDT] *CNS disruption, respiratory control center paralysis, ventricular fibrillation, seizures, respiratory arrest.*

**DDE** [DDT] *CNS disruption, respiratory control center paralysis, ventricular fibrillation, seizures, respiratory arrest.*

**DDT (dichlorodiphenyltrichloroethane)** [DDT] *CNS disruption, respiratory control center paralysis, ventricular fibrillation, seizures, respiratory arrest.* [Lindane] *CNS stimulation, seizures, respiratory failure.*

**decaborane** [Boron] *Respiratory tract irritation, laryngeal spasm and edema, pulmonary edema, severe chemical burns.*

**decabromodiphenyl oxide** [Boron] *Respiratory tract irritation, laryngeal spasm and edema, pulmonary edema, severe chemical burns.*

**decahydronaphthalene** [Naphthalene] *Delayed-onset acute intravascular hemolysis.*

**decane** [Aliphatic hydrocarbon] *Arrhythmias, asphyxiation, anesthesia.*

**decanoyl peroxide** [Organic peroxide] *Pulmonary and laryngeal edema, circulatory arrest, hypovolemic shock, chemical burns to skin, mucous membranes, and internal organs.*

**decyl alcohol** [Higher alcohol (4+ carbons)] *CNS depression, respiratory failure, arrhythmias.*

**degreaser** [Hydrocarbon mixture] *CNS depression, respiratory arrest, seizures, arrhythmias, pulmonary edema.*

**DEHP** [Ester] *CNS depression, respiratory tract irritation, bronchitis, pneumonia.*

**dehydrorotenone** [Rotenone] *Respiratory arrest, asphyxia.*

**demeton** [Organophosphate] *Pulmonary edema, respiratory muscle paralysis, respiratory failure, bradycardia, acetylcholinesterase inhibition, hypotension, pulmonary edema, overstimulation of parasympathetic nervous system, striated muscle, sympathetic ganglia, and CNS.*

**demeton-methyl** [Organophosphate] *Pulmonary edema, respiratory muscle paralysis, respiratory failure, bradycardia, acetylcholinesterase inhibition, hypotension, pulmonary edema, overstimulation of parasympathetic nervous*

system, striated muscle, sympathetic ganglia, and CNS.

**denatured alcohol** [Methyl alcohol] Respiratory failure, circulatory collapse.

**Deobase** [Hydrocarbon mixture] CNS depression, respiratory arrest, seizures, arrhythmias, pulmonary edema.

**Derris powder** [Rotenone] Respiratory arrest, asphyxia.

**desmedipham** [Aniline] Methemoglobinemia, hypoxia. [Carbamate] Acetylcholinesterase inhibition (reversible), bradycardia, hypotension, respiratory muscle paralysis, respiratory arrest, pulmonary edema.

**deuterium** [Flammable gas] Respiratory failure, cardiac arrest, arrhythmias. [Simple asphyxiant] Asphyxiation.

**DFDT** [Simple asphyxiant] Asphyxiation.

**DFP** [Organophosphate] Pulmonary edema, respiratory muscle paralysis, respiratory failure, bradycardia, acetylcholinesterase inhibition, hypotension, pulmonary edema, overstimulation of parasympathetic nervous system, striated muscle, sympathetic ganglia, and CNS.

**diacetone alcohol** [Ketone] Respiratory mucous membrane irritation, pulmonary edema, CNS depression.

**diacetone alcohol peroxide** [Organic peroxide] Pulmonary and laryngeal edema, circulatory arrest, hypovolemic shock, chemical burns to skin, mucous membranes, and internal organs. [Ketone] Respiratory mucous membrane irritation, pulmonary edema, CNS depression. [Corrosive] Upper airway burns and edema, circulatory collapse, severe chemical burns to skin, toxic systemic effects, GI tract perforation and hemorrhage, peritonitis.

**diacetyl** [Ketone] Respiratory mucous membrane irritation, pulmonary edema, CNS depression.

**diacetyl peroxide** [Organic peroxide] Pulmonary and laryngeal edema, circulatory arrest, hypovolemic shock, chemical burns to skin, mucous membranes, and internal organs. [Ketone] Respiratory mucous membrane irritation, pul-

monary edema, CNS depression. [Corrosive] Upper airway burns and edema, circulatory collapse, severe chemical burns to skin, toxic systemic effects, GI tract perforation and hemorrhage, peritonitis.

**dialifor; dialiphor** [Organophosphate] Pulmonary edema, respiratory muscle paralysis, respiratory failure, bradycardia, acetylcholinesterase inhibition, hypotension, pulmonary edema, overstimulation of parasympathetic nervous system, striated muscle, sympathetic ganglia, and CNS.

**dialifos; dialiphos** [Organophosphate] Pulmonary edema, respiratory muscle paralysis, respiratory failure, bradycardia, acetylcholinesterase inhibition, hypotension, pulmonary edema, overstimulation of parasympathetic nervous system, striated muscle, sympathetic ganglia, and CNS.

**di-allate** [Dithiocarbamate] Hypotension, respiratory failure.

**diallylamine** [Organic base/amine] Pulmonary edema, cardiac depression, seizures.

**diallylether** [Ether] Anesthesia, respiratory arrest.

**diamidafos** [Organophosphate] Pulmonary edema, respiratory muscle paralysis, respiratory failure, bradycardia, acetylcholinesterase inhibition, hypotension, pulmonary edema, overstimulation of parasympathetic nervous system, striated muscle, sympathetic ganglia, and CNS.

**2,4-diaminoanisole** [Organic base/amine] Pulmonary edema, cardiac depression, seizures.

**2,4-diaminoanisole sulfate** [Organic base/amine] Pulmonary edema, cardiac depression, seizures.

**4,4'-diaminodiphenoyl ether** [Aniline] Methemoglobinemia, hypoxia.

**diaminodiphenyl methane** [Nitrate/ nitrite] Methemoglobinemia, hypotension, circulatory collapse.

**HazMat**

**diaminotoluene; 2,4-diaminotoluene** [Aniline] *Methemoglobinemia, hypoxia.*

**diamylamine** [Organic base/amine] *Pulmonary edema, cardiac depression, seizures.*

**Diazinon** [Organophosphate] *Pulmonary edema, respiratory muscle paralysis, respiratory failure, bradycardia, acetylcholinesterase inhibition, hypotension, pulmonary edema, overstimulation of parasympathetic nervous system, striated muscle, sympathetic ganglia, and CNS.*

**diazomethane** [Phosgene] *Severe respiratory irritation, alveolar damage, pulmonary edema.*

**2-diazo-1-naphthol-4-sulfochloride; 2-diazo-1-naphthol-5-sulfochloride** [Naphthalene] *Delayed-onset acute intravascular hemolysis.*

**dibenz[a,h]anthracene** [Aromatic hydrocarbon] *Arrhythmias, respiratory failure, pulmonary edema, paralysis, brain and kidney damage.*

**dibenzofuran** Polychlorinated biphenyl/polybrominated biphenyl/ polychlorinated [dibenzofuran] *Liver and kidney damage.*

**dibenzoyl peroxide** [Organic peroxide] *Pulmonary and laryngeal edema, circulatory arrest, hypovolemic shock, chemical burns to skin, mucous membranes, and internal organs.*

**dibenz[a,i]pyrine** [Aromatic hydrocarbon] *Arrhythmias, respiratory failure, pulmonary edema, paralysis, brain and kidney damage.*

**dibenzyl peroxy-dicarbonate** [Organic peroxide] *Pulmonary and laryngeal edema, circulatory arrest, hypovolemic shock, chemical burns to skin, mucous membranes, and internal organs.*

**dibenzyldichlorosilane** [Silane/chlorosilane] *Respiratory tract irritation, pulmonary edema.*

**diborane; diborane mixture (n.o.s.)** [Boron] *Respiratory tract irritation, laryngeal spasm and edema, pulmonary edema, severe chemical burns.*

**dibromobenzene** [Aromatic hydrocarbon] *Arrhythmias, respiratory failure, pulmonary edema, paralysis, brain and kidney damage.*

**dibromobutanone** [Ketone] *Respiratory mucous membrane irritation, pulmonary edema, CNS depression.*

**dibromochloropropane; 1,2-dibromo-3-chloropropane** [Dichloropropane/dichloropropene] *Pulmonary edema, bronchospasm, alveolar hemorrhage.*

**dibromodifluoromethane** [Chlorinated fluorocarbon] *Asphyxiation, anesthesia, arrhythmias.*

**dibromoethane; 1,2-dibromoethane** [Chlorinated fluorocarbon] *Asphyxiation, anesthesia, arrhythmias.*

**dibromomethane** [Chlorinated fluorocarbon] *Asphyxiation, anesthesia, arrhythmias.*

**dibromotetrafluoroethane (Halon 2402)** [Chlorinated fluorocarbon] *Asphyxiation, anesthesia, arrhythmias.*

**dibutyl ether** [Ether] *Anesthesia, respiratory arrest.*

**dibutyl peroxide; di-*tert*-butyl peroxide** [Organic peroxide] *Pulmonary and laryngeal edema, circulatory arrest, hypovolemic shock, chemical burns to skin, mucous membranes, and internal organs.*

**dibutyl peroxy-dicarbonate; di-*sec*-butyl peroxy-dicarbonate** [Organic peroxide] *Pulmonary and laryngeal edema, circulatory arrest, hypovolemic shock, chemical burns to skin, mucous membranes, and internal organs.*

**dibutyl phthalate** [Ester] *CNS depression, respiratory tract irritation, bronchitis, pneumonia.*

**dibutylamine** [Organic base/amine] *Pulmonary edema, cardiac depression, seizures.*

**dibutylaminoethanol** [Higher alcohol (4+ carbons)] *CNS depression, respiratory failure, arrhythmias.*

**2,2-di(*tert*-butylperoxy)-butane** [Organic peroxide] *Pulmonary and laryngeal edema, circulatory arrest,* hypovolemic shock, chemical burns to skin, mucous membranes, and internal organs. [Aliphatic hydrocarbon] Arrhythmias, asphyxiation, anesthesia.

**1,1-di(tert-butylperoxy)-cyclohexane; 1,2-di(tert-butylperoxy)-cyclohexane** [Organic peroxide] Pulmonary and laryngeal edema, circulatory arrest, hypovolemic shock, chemical burns to skin, mucous membranes, and internal organs. [Aliphatic hydrocarbon] Arrhythmias, asphyxiation, anesthesia.

**di-(2-tert-butylperoxy-isopropyl) benzene** [Organic peroxide] Pulmonary and laryngeal edema, circulatory arrest, hypovolemic shock, chemical burns to skin, mucous membranes, and internal organs. [Aromatic hydrocarbon] Arrhythmias, respiratory failure, pulmonary edema, paralysis, brain and kidney damage.

**1,3-di(2-tert-butylperoxy-isopropyl) benzene; 1,4-di(2-tert-butylperoxy-isopropyl) benzene** [Organic peroxide] Pulmonary and laryngeal edema, circulatory arrest, hypovolemic shock, chemical burns to skin, mucous membranes, and internal organs. [Aromatic hydrocarbon] Arrhythmias, respiratory failure, pulmonary edema, paralysis, brain and kidney damage.

**di-tert-butylperoxyphthalate** [Ester] CNS depression, respiratory tract irritation, bronchitis, pneumonia.

**2,2-di(tert-butylperoxy)-propane** [Organic peroxide] Pulmonary and laryngeal edema, circulatory arrest, hypovolemic shock, chemical burns to skin, mucous membranes, and internal organs. [Aliphatic hydrocarbon] Arrhythmias, asphyxiation, anesthesia.

**1,1-di(tert-butylperoxy)-3,3,5-trimethylcyclohexane** [Organic peroxide] Pulmonary and laryngeal edema, circulatory arrest, hypovolemic shock, chemical burns to skin, mucous membranes, and internal organs. [Ali-

phatic hydrocarbon] Arrhythmias, asphyxiation, anesthesia.

**dicamba** [Chlorophenoxy herbicide] CNS depression, CNS stimulation, respiratory failure, ventricular fibrillation, seizures.

**dicetyl peroxydicarbonate** [Organic peroxide] Pulmonary and laryngeal edema, circulatory arrest, hypovolemic shock, chemical burns to skin, mucous membranes, and internal organs.

**dichlobenil** [Poison] Cardiovascular collapse, pulmonary edema, CNS depression, coma, seizures, nausea, vomiting, cardiopulmonary arrest.

**dichlofenthion** [Organophosphate] Pulmonary edema, respiratory muscle paralysis, respiratory failure, bradycardia, acetylcholinesterase inhibition, hypotension, pulmonary edema, overstimulation of parasympathetic nervous system, striated muscle, sympathetic ganglia, and CNS.

**dichlone** [Poison] Cardiovascular collapse, pulmonary edema, CNS depression, coma, seizures, nausea, vomiting, cardiopulmonary arrest.

**Dichloran** [Benzene] Arrhythmias, respiratory failure, pulmonary edema, CNS depression, liver and kidney damage.

**dichloro acetylene** [Aliphatic hydrocarbon] Arrhythmias, asphyxiation, anesthesia. [Simple asphyxiant] Asphyxiation.

**dichloroacetic acid** [Organic acid] Pulmonary edema, circulatory collapse, laryngeal edema and spasm, severe chemical burns to skin, mucous membranes, and internal organs, GI tract perforation and hemorrhage, peritonitis.

**1,3-dichloroacetone** [Ketone] Respiratory mucous membrane irritation, pulmonary edema, CNS depression.

**dichloroacetyl chloride** [Organic acid] Pulmonary edema, circulatory collapse, laryngeal edema and spasm, severe chemical burns to skin, mucous membranes, and internal organs, GI tract perforation and hemorrhage, peritonitis.

**dichloroaniline** [Aniline] *Methemoglobinemia, hypoxia.*

**o-dichlorobenzene; p-dichlorobenzene** [Lindane] *CNS stimulation, seizures, respiratory failure.*

**dichlorobenzidine; 3,3'-dichlorobenzidine** [Aniline] *Methemoglobinemia, hypoxia.*

**di-(4-chlorobenzoyl) peroxide; 2,4-dichlorobenzoyl peroxide** [Organic peroxide] *Pulmonary and laryngeal edema, circulatory arrest, hypovolemic shock, chemical burns to skin, mucous membranes, and internal organs.*

**1,1-dichloro-2,2-bis(p-chlorophenyl) ethane** [Lindane] *CNS stimulation, seizures, respiratory failure.*

**dichlorobromomethane** [Chlorinated fluorocarbon] *Asphyxiation, anesthesia, arrhythmias.*

**dichlorobutene; trans-1,4-dichlorobutene** [Chlorinated fluorocarbon] *Asphyxiation, anesthesia, arrhythmias.*

**dichlorodiethyl ether** [Ether] *Anesthesia, respiratory arrest.*

**dichlorodifluoroethylene** [Chlorinated fluorocarbon] *Asphyxiation, anesthesia, arrhythmias.*

**dichlorodifluoromethane (Freon 12)** [Chlorinated fluorocarbon] *Asphyxiation, anesthesia, arrhythmias.*

**dichlorodifluoromethane & chlorodifluoromethane mixture** [Chlorinated fluorocarbon] *Asphyxiation, anesthesia, arrhythmias.*

**dichlorodifluoromethane & dichlorotetrafluoroethane mixture** [Chlorinated fluorocarbon] *Asphyxiation, anesthesia, arrhythmias.*

**dichlorodifluoromethane & difluoroethane mixture** [Chlorinated fluorocarbon] *Asphyxiation, anesthesia, arrhythmias.*

**dichlorodifluoromethane & ethylene oxide mixture** [Chlorinated fluorocarbon] *Asphyxiation, anesthesia, arrhythmias.* [Ethylene oxide] *Respiratory tract irritation, pulmonary edema.*

**dichlorodifluoromethane & trichlorofluoromethane mixture** [Chlorinated fluorocarbon] *Asphyxiation, anesthesia, arrhythmias.*

**dichlorodifluoromethane & trichlorofluoromethane & chlorodifluoromethane mixture** [Chlorinated fluorocarbon] *Asphyxiation, anesthesia, arrhythmias.*

**dichlorodifluoromethane & trichlorotrifluoroethane mixture** [Chlorinated fluorocarbon] *Asphyxiation, anesthesia, arrhythmias.*

**dichlorodimethyl ether** [Ether] *Anesthesia, respiratory arrest.*

**1,3-dichloro-5,5-dimethyl hydantoin** [Poison] *Cardiovascular collapse, pulmonary edema, CNS depression, coma, seizures, nausea, vomiting, cardiopulmonary arrest.*

**3,5-dichloro-N-(1,1-dimethyl-2-propynyl) benzamide** [Lindane] *CNS stimulation, seizures, respiratory failure.*

**dichlorodiphenyltrichloroethane (DDT)** [DDT] *CNS disruption, respiratory control center paralysis, ventricular fibrillation, seizures, respiratory arrest.* [Lindane] *CNS stimulation, seizures, respiratory failure.*

**1,1-dichloroethane; 1,2-dichloroethane** [Chlorinated fluorocarbon] *Asphyxiation, anesthesia, arrhythmias.*

**dichloroethyl ether** [Ether] *Anesthesia, respiratory arrest.*

**dichloroethylene; 1,1-dichloroethylene; 1,2-dichloroethylene** [Chlorinated fluorocarbon] *Asphyxiation, anesthesia, arrhythmias.*

**1,1-dichloro-1-fluoroethane** [Chlorinated fluorocarbon] *Asphyxiation, anesthesia, arrhythmias.*

**dichlorofluoromethane** [Chlorinated fluorocarbon] *Asphyxiation, anesthesia, arrhythmias.*

**dichloroisocyanuric acid; dichloroisocyanuric acid salt (n.o.s.)** [Organic acid] *Pulmonary edema, circulatory collapse, laryngeal edema and spasm, severe chemical burns to skin, mucous membranes, and internal* *organs, GI tract perforation and hemorrhage, peritonitis.*

**dichloroisopropyl ether** [Ether] *Anesthesia, respiratory arrest.*

**dichloromethane** [Chlorinated fluorocarbon] *Asphyxiation, anesthesia, arrhythmias.*

**dichloromethyl ether** [Ether] *Anesthesia, respiratory arrest.*

**dichloromonofluoromethane** [Chlorinated fluorocarbon] *Asphyxiation, anesthesia, arrhythmias.*

**dichloronitroethane; 1,1-dichloro-1-nitroethane** [Chlorinated fluorocarbon] *Asphyxiation, anesthesia, arrhythmias.*

**dichloropentane** [Chlorinated fluorocarbon] *Asphyxiation, anesthesia, arrhythmias.*

**dichlorophen; dichlorophene** [Phenol] *Coma, hypotension, arrhythmias, pulmonary edema, respiratory arrest.*

**2,4-dichlorophenol; 2,6-dichlorophenol** [Phenol] *Coma, hypotension, arrhythmias, pulmonary edema, respiratory arrest.*

**4-(2,4-dichlorophenoxy) butyric acid** [Chlorophenoxy herbicide] *CNS depression, CNS stimulation, respiratory failure, ventricular fibrillation, seizures.*

**2-(2,4-dichlorophenoxy) ethyl sulfate sodium salt (n.o.s.)** [Chlorophenoxy herbicide] *CNS depression, CNS stimulation, respiratory failure, ventricular fibrillation, seizures.*

**2-(2,4-dichlorophenoxy) propionic acid** [Chlorophenoxy herbicide] *CNS depression, CNS stimulation, respiratory failure, ventricular fibrillation, seizures.*

**2,4-dichlorophenoxyacetic acid** [Chlorophenoxy herbicide] *CNS depression, CNS stimulation, respiratory failure, ventricular fibrillation, seizures.*

**di-(p-chlorophenyl) methylcarbinol (DMC)** [DDT] *CNS disruption, respiratory control center paralysis, ventricular fibrillation, seizures, respiratory arrest.*

**dichlorophenylarsine** [Arsine] *Intravascular hemolysis, pulmonary edema, cardiac and respiratory arrest, delayed-onset jaundice and renal failure.*

**dichlorophenylisocyanate** [Isocyanate/aliphatic thiocyanate] *CNS depression, respiratory arrest, respiratory paralysis, pulmonary edema, cyanide toxicity.*

**dichlorophenylsilane** [Silane/chlorosilane] *Respiratory tract irritation, pulmonary edema.*

**dichlorophenyltrichlorosilane** [Silane/chlorosilane] *Respiratory tract irritation, pulmonary edema.*

**dichloropropane; 1,1-dichloropropane; 1,2-dichloropropane; 1,3-dichloropropane** [Dichloropropane/dichloropropene] *Pulmonary edema, bronchospasm, alveolar hemorrhage.*

**dichloropropanol; 1,3-dichloro-2-propanol** [Higher alcohol (4+ carbons)] *CNS depression, respiratory failure, arrhythmias.*

**dichloropropanone** [Ketone] *Respiratory mucous membrane irritation, pulmonary edema, CNS depression.*

**dichloropropene; 1,3-dichloropropene; 2,3-dichloropropene** [Dichloropropane/dichloropropene] *Pulmonary edema, bronchospasm, alveolar hemorrhage.*

**dichloropropene & propylene dichloride mixture** [Dichloropropane/dichloropropene] *Pulmonary edema, bronchospasm, alveolar hemorrhage.*

**dichloropropionic acid; 2,2-dichloropropionic acid** [Organic acid] *Pulmonary edema, circulatory collapse, laryngeal edema and spasm, severe chemical burns to skin, mucous membranes, and internal organs, GI tract perforation and hemorrhage, peritonitis.*

**1,3-dichloropropylene** [Dichloropropane/dichloropropene] *Pulmonary edema, bronchospasm, alveolar hemorrhage.*

**HazMat**

**dichlorosilane** [Silane/chlorosilane] *Respiratory tract irritation, pulmonary edema.*

**dichlorotetrafluoroethane** [Chlorinated fluorocarbon] *Asphyxiation, anesthesia, arrhythmias.*

**dichlorotetrafluoroethane & dichlorodifluoromethane mixture** [Chlorinated fluorocarbon] *Asphyxiation, anesthesia, arrhythmias.*

**dichloro-S-triazinetrione; dichloro-S-triazinetrione salt (n.o.s.)** [Irritant] *Severe immediate or delayed upper airway or respiratory tract irritation, pulmonary edema, glottic spasm, airway obstruction.*

**4,5-dichloro-2-(trifluorome) benzimidazole** [Aromatic hydrocarbon] *Arrhythmias, respiratory failure, pulmonary edema, paralysis, brain and kidney damage.*

**3,5-dichloro-2,4,6-trifluoropyridine** [Aromatic hydrocarbon] *Arrhythmias, respiratory failure, pulmonary edema, paralysis, brain and kidney damage.*

**dichlorvos** [Organophosphate] *Pulmonary edema, respiratory muscle paralysis, respiratory failure, bradycardia, acetylcholinesterase inhibition, hypotension, pulmonary edema, overstimulation of parasympathetic nervous system, striated muscle, sympathetic ganglia, and CNS.*

**dichromate salt (n.o.s.)** [Poison] *Cardiovascular collapse, pulmonary edema, CNS depression, coma, seizures, nausea, vomiting, cardiopulmonary arrest.*

**dicofol** [Chlordane] *Respiratory failure, seizures, exhaustion, death.*

**dicrotophos** [Organophosphate] *Pulmonary edema, respiratory muscle paralysis, respiratory failure, bradycardia, acetylcholinesterase inhibition, hypotension, pulmonary edema, overstimulation of parasympathetic nervous system, striated muscle, sympathetic ganglia, and CNS.*

**dicumyl peroxide** [Organic peroxide] *Pulmonary and laryngeal edema, circu-latory arrest, hypovolemic shock, chemical burns to skin, mucous membranes, and internal organs.*

**dicycloheptadiene** [Aliphatic hydrocarbon] *Arrhythmias, asphyxiation, anesthesia.*

**dicyclohexyl peroxy-dicarbonate** [Organic peroxide] *Pulmonary and laryngeal edema, circulatory arrest, hypovolemic shock, chemical burns to skin, mucous membranes, and internal organs.*

**dicyclohexylamine** [Dinitrophenol] *Respiratory and circulatory collapse, pulmonary edema, hyperthermia.*

**dicyclohexylamine 4,6-dinitro-o-cyclohexylphenolate** [Dinitrophenol] *Respiratory and circulatory collapse, pulmonary edema, hyperthermia.*

**dicyclohexylamine nitrite** [Nitrate/nitrite] *Methemoglobinemia, hypotension, circulatory collapse.* [Dinitrophenol] *Respiratory and circulatory collapse, pulmonary edema, hyperthermia.*

**dicyclohexylammonium nitrite** [Nitrate/nitrite] *Methemoglobinemia, hypotension, circulatory collapse.*

**dicyclopentadiene** [Aliphatic hydrocarbon] *Arrhythmias, asphyxiation, anesthesia.*

**didecanoyl peroxide** [Organic peroxide] *Pulmonary and laryngeal edema, circulatory arrest, hypovolemic shock, chemical burns to skin, mucous membranes, and internal organs.*

**2,2-di(4,4-di-*tert*-butylperoxy cyclohexyl) propane** [Organic peroxide] *Pulmonary and laryngeal edema, circulatory arrest, hypovolemic shock, chemical burns to skin, mucous membranes, and internal organs.*

**di-2,4-dichlorobenzoyl peroxide** [Organic peroxide] *Pulmonary and laryngeal edema, circulatory arrest, hypovolemic shock, chemical burns to skin, mucous membranes, and internal organs.*

**1,2-di-(dimethylamino) ethane** [Aniline] *Methemoglobinemia, hypoxia.* [Aliphatic hydrocarbon] *Arrhythmias, asphyxiation, anesthesia.*

**didymium nitrate** [Nitrate/nitrite] *Methemoglobinemia, hypotension, circulatory collapse.*

**dieldrin** [Aldrin/dieldrin/endrin] *Seizures, respiratory failure.*

**dienochlor** [Chlordane] *Respiratory failure, seizures, exhaustion, death.*

**diepoxybutane** [Ethylene oxide] *Respiratory tract irritation, pulmonary edema.*

**diesel fuel; diesel oil** [Hydrocarbon mixture] *CNS depression, respiratory arrest, seizures, arrhythmias, pulmonary edema.*

**diethanolamine** [Organic base/amine] *Pulmonary edema, cardiac depression, seizures.*

**diethoxyethane** [Ether] *Anesthesia, respiratory arrest.*

**diethoxymentane** [Ether] *Anesthesia, respiratory arrest.*

**2,5-diethoxy-4-morpholinebenzenediazonium zinc chloride** [Poison] *Cardiovascular collapse, pulmonary edema, CNS depression, coma, seizures, nausea, vomiting, cardiopulmonary arrest.*

**diethoxypropene** [Acrolein] *Severe respiratory tract irritation, pulmonary edema, respiratory failure.*

**diethyl aniline** [Aniline] *Methemoglobinemia, hypoxia.*

**diethyl carbonate** [Ester] *CNS depression, respiratory tract irritation, bronchitis, pneumonia.*

**diethyl cellosolve** [Ethylene glycol] *Respiratory failure, pulmonary edema, paralysis, cardiovascular collapse, severe acidosis.*

**diethyl chlorophosphate** [Organophosphate] *Pulmonary edema, respiratory muscle paralysis, respiratory failure, bradycardia, acetylcholinesterase inhibition, hypotension, pulmonary edema, overstimulation of parasympathetic nervous system, striated muscle, sympathetic ganglia, and CNS.*

**diethyl 2-chlorovinyl phosphate** [Organophosphate] *Pulmonary edema, respiratory muscle paralysis, respiratory failure, bradycardia, acetylcholinesterase inhibition, hypotension, pulmonary edema, overstimulation of parasympathetic nervous system, striated muscle, sympathetic ganglia, and CNS.*

**diethyl dichlorosilane** [Silane/chlorosilane] *Respiratory tract irritation, pulmonary edema.*

**diethyl ether** [Ether] *Anesthesia, respiratory arrest.*

**diethyl isopropylthiomethyl dithiophosphate** [Organophosphate] *Pulmonary edema, respiratory muscle paralysis, respiratory failure, bradycardia, acetylcholinesterase inhibition, hypotension, pulmonary edema, overstimulation of parasympathetic nervous system, striated muscle, sympathetic ganglia, and CNS.*

**diethyl ketone** [Ketone] *Respiratory mucous membrane irritation, pulmonary edema, CNS depression.*

**diethyl peroxydicarbonate** [Organic peroxide] *Pulmonary and laryngeal edema, circulatory arrest, hypovolemic shock, chemical burns to skin, mucous membranes, and internal organs.*

**diethyl phthalate** [Ester] *CNS depression, respiratory tract irritation, bronchitis, pneumonia.*

**diethyl propylmethylpyrimidyl thiophosphate** [Organophosphate] *Pulmonary edema, respiratory muscle paralysis, respiratory failure, bradycardia, acetylcholinesterase inhibition, hypotension, pulmonary edema, overstimulation of parasympathetic nervous system, striated muscle, sympathetic ganglia, and CNS.*

**diethyl sulfate** [Sulfur] *Respiratory tract irritation, pulmonary edema, anaphylaxis.*

**diethyl sulfide** [Sulfur] *Respiratory tract irritation, pulmonary edema, anaphylaxis.*

**diethylamine** [Organic base/amine] *Pulmonary edema, cardiac depression, seizures.*

**diethylaminoethanol** [Organic base/amine] *Pulmonary edema, cardiac depression, seizures.*

**diethylaminopropylamine** [Organic base/amine] *Pulmonary edema, cardiac depression, seizures.*

**diethylarsine** [Arsine] *Intravascular hemolysis, pulmonary edema, cardiac and respiratory arrest, delayed-onset jaundice and renal failure.*

**diethylbenzene** [Aromatic hydrocarbon] *Arrhythmias, respiratory failure, pulmonary edema, paralysis, brain and kidney damage.*

**diethylcarbamazine citrate** [Poison] *Cardiovascular collapse, pulmonary edema, CNS depression, coma, seizures, nausea, vomiting, cardiopulmonary arrest.*

**diethylene glycol** [Ethylene glycol] *Respiratory failure, pulmonary edema, paralysis, cardiovascular collapse, severe acidosis.*

**diethylene glycol abietate** [Ethylene glycol] *Respiratory failure, pulmonary edema, paralysis, cardiovascular collapse, severe acidosis.*

**diethylene glycol diester; diethylene glycol monoester** [Ethylene glycol] *Respiratory failure, pulmonary edema, paralysis, cardiovascular collapse, severe acidosis.*

**diethylene triamine** [Organic base/amine] *Pulmonary edema, cardiac depression, seizures.*

**diethylethylene diamine** [Organic base/amine] *Pulmonary edema, cardiac depression, seizures.*

**di-(2-ethylhexyl) peroxy-dicarbonate** [Organic peroxide] *Pulmonary and laryngeal edema, circulatory arrest, hypovolemic shock, chemical burns to skin, mucous membranes, and internal organs.*

**di-(2-ethylhexyl) phosphoric acid** [Organic acid] *Pulmonary edema, circulatory collapse, laryngeal edema and spasm, severe chemical burns to skin, mucous membranes, and internal organs, GI tract perforation and hemorrhage, peritonitis.*

**di-(2-ethylhexyl) phthalate** [Ester] *CNS depression, respiratory tract irritation, bronchitis, pneumonia.*

**diethylmagnesium** [Magnesium] *Cardiovascular collapse, respiratory depression.*

**diethyl-p-nitrophenyl phosphate** [Organophosphate] *Pulmonary edema, respiratory muscle paralysis, respiratory failure, bradycardia, acetylcholinesterase inhibition, hypotension, pulmonary edema, overstimulation of parasympathetic nervous system, striated muscle, sympathetic ganglia, and CNS.*

**O,O-diethyl-O-pyrazinyl phosphorothioate** [Organophosphate] *Pulmonary edema, respiratory muscle paralysis, respiratory failure, bradycardia, acetylcholinesterase inhibition, hypotension, pulmonary edema, overstimulation of parasympathetic nervous system, striated muscle, sympathetic ganglia, and CNS.*

**diethylstilbestrol** [Poison] *Cardiovascular collapse, pulmonary edema, CNS depression, coma, seizures, nausea, vomiting, cardiopulmonary arrest.*

**diethylthiophosphoryl chloride** [Organophosphate] *Pulmonary edema, respiratory muscle paralysis, respiratory failure, bradycardia, acetylcholinesterase inhibition, hypotension, pulmonary edema, overstimulation of parasympathetic nervous system, striated muscle, sympathetic ganglia, and CNS.*

**diethylzinc** [Zinc] *Respiratory tract irritation, metal fume fever, pulmonary edema.*

**difluorochloroethane** [Chlorinated fluorocarbon] *Asphyxiation, anesthesia, arrhythmias.*

**difluoroethane** [Chlorinated fluorocarbon] *Asphyxiation, anesthesia, arrhythmias.*

**difluoroethane & dichlorodifluoromethane mixture** [Chlorinated fluorocarbon] *Asphyxiation, anesthesia, arrhythmias.*

**difluoroethylene; 1,1-difluoroethylene** [Chlorinated fluorocarbon] *Asphyxiation, anesthesia, arrhythmias.*

**difluoromonochloroethane** [Chlorinated fluorocarbon] *Asphyxiation, anesthesia, arrhythmias.*

**difluorophosphoric acid** [Inorganic acid] *Pulmonary edema, bronchospasm, circulatory collapse, laryngeal spasm and edema, severe chemical burns to skin, mucous membranes, and internal organs, GI tract perforation and hemorrhage, peritonitis.*

**digitoxin** [Poison] *Cardiovascular collapse, pulmonary edema, CNS depression, coma, seizures, nausea, vomiting, cardiopulmonary arrest.*

**diglycidyl ether** [Ether] *Anesthesia, respiratory arrest.*

**digoxin** [Poison] *Cardiovascular collapse, pulmonary edema, CNS depression, coma, seizures, nausea, vomiting, cardiopulmonary arrest.*

**2,2-dihydroperoxy propane** [Organic peroxide] *Pulmonary and laryngeal edema, circulatory arrest, hypovolemic shock, chemical burns to skin, mucous membranes, and internal organs.*

**dihydropyran** [Aromatic hydrocarbon] *Arrhythmias, respiratory failure, pulmonary edema, paralysis, brain and kidney damage.*

**dihydrorotenone** [Rotenone] *Respiratory arrest, asphyxia.*

**dihydrosafrole** [Phenol] *Coma, hypotension, arrhythmias, pulmonary edema, respiratory arrest.*

**di-(1-hydroxycyclohexyl) peroxide** [Organic peroxide] *Pulmonary and laryngeal edema, circulatory arrest, hypovolemic shock, chemical burns to skin, mucous membranes, and internal organs.*

**2,6-diiodo-4-nitrophenol** [Dinitrophenol] *Respiratory and circulatory collapse, pulmonary edema, hyperthermia.*

**diisobutyl carbinol** [Higher alcohol (4+ carbons)] *CNS depression, respiratory failure, arrhythmias.*

**diisobutyl ketone** [Ketone] *Respiratory mucous membrane irritation, pulmonary edema, CNS depression.*

**diisobutylamine** [Organic base/amine] *Pulmonary edema, cardiac depression, seizures.*

**diisobutylene** [Aliphatic hydrocarbon] *Arrhythmias, asphyxiation, anesthesia.*

**diisobutyryl peroxide** [Organic peroxide] *Pulmonary and laryngeal edema, circulatory arrest, hypovolemic shock, chemical burns to skin, mucous membranes, and internal organs.*

**diisooctyl acid phosphate** [Organic acid] *Pulmonary edema, circulatory collapse, laryngeal edema and spasm, severe chemical burns to skin, mucous membranes, and internal organs, GI tract perforation and hemorrhage, peritonitis.*

**diisopropyl ether** [Ether] *Anesthesia, respiratory arrest.*

**diisopropyl fluorophosphate** [Organophosphate] *Pulmonary edema, respiratory muscle paralysis, respiratory failure, bradycardia, acetylcholinesterase inhibition, hypotension, pulmonary edema, overstimulation of parasympathetic nervous system, striated muscle, sympathetic ganglia, and CNS.*

**diisopropyl peroxydicarbonate** [Organic peroxide] *Pulmonary and laryngeal edema, circulatory arrest, hypovolemic shock, chemical burns to skin, mucous membranes, and internal organs.*

**diisopropylamine** [Organic base/amine] *Pulmonary edema, cardiac depression, seizures.*

**diisopropylbenzene hydroperoxide** [Organic peroxide] *Pulmonary and laryngeal edema, circulatory arrest, hypovolemic shock, chemical burns to skin, mucous membranes, and internal organs.*

**diisopropylethanolamine** [Organic base/amine] *Pulmonary edema, cardiac depression, seizures.*

**diisotridecylperoxydicarbonate** [Organic peroxide] *Pulmonary and laryngeal edema, circulatory arrest, hypovolemic shock, chemical burns to skin, mucous membranes, and internal organs.*

**diketene** [Ketone] *Respiratory mucous membrane irritation, pulmonary edema, CNS depression.*

**Dilan** [DDT] *CNS disruption, respiratory control center paralysis, ventricular fibrillation, seizures, respiratory arrest.*

**dilauroyl peroxide** [Organic peroxide] *Pulmonary and laryngeal edema, circulatory arrest, hypovolemic shock, chemical burns to skin, mucous membranes, and internal organs.*

**dimefox** [Organophosphate] *Pulmonary edema, respiratory muscle paralysis, respiratory failure, bradycardia, acetylcholinesterase inhibition, hypotension, pulmonary edema, overstimulation of parasympathetic nervous system, striated muscle, sympathetic ganglia, and CNS.*

**di-1-p-menthene** [Turpentine/terpene] *Respiratory failure, pulmonary edema, tachycardia.*

**Dimetan** [Carbamate] *Acetylcholinesterase inhibition (reversible), bradycardia, hypotension, respiratory muscle paralysis, respiratory arrest, pulmonary edema.*

**dimethoate** [Organophosphate] *Pulmonary edema, respiratory muscle paralysis, respiratory failure, bradycardia, acetylcholinesterase inhibition, hypotension, pulmonary edema, overstimulation of parasympathetic nervous system, striated muscle, sympathetic ganglia, and CNS.*

**3,3'-dimethoxybenzidine** [Aniline] *Methemoglobinemia, hypoxia.*

**dimethoxyethane; 1,1-dimethoxyethane; 1,2-dimethoxyethane** [Ethylene glycol] *Respiratory failure, pulmonary edema, paralysis, cardiovascular collapse, severe acidosis.*

**dimethrin** [Pyrethrin/pyrethroid] *Respiratory paralysis, convulsions.*

**α-dimethyl benzene ethanamine; alpha-dimethyl benzene ethanamine** [Aniline] *Methemoglobinemia, hypoxia.*

**dimethyl carbonate** [Ester] *CNS depression, respiratory tract irritation, bronchitis, pneumonia.*

**dimethyl chlorothiophosphate** [Organophosphate] *Pulmonary edema, respiratory muscle paralysis, respiratory failure, bradycardia, acetylcholinesterase inhibition, hypotension, pulmonary edema, overstimulation of parasympathetic nervous system, striated muscle, sympathetic ganglia, and CNS.*

**dimethyl ether** [Ether] *Anesthesia, respiratory arrest.*

**dimethyl phosphorochloridothioate** [Organophosphate] *Pulmonary edema, respiratory muscle paralysis, respiratory failure, bradycardia, acetylcholinesterase inhibition, hypotension, pulmonary edema, overstimulation of parasympathetic nervous system, striated muscle, sympathetic ganglia, and CNS.*

**dimethyl phthalate** [Ester] *CNS depression, respiratory tract irritation, bronchitis, pneumonia.*

**dimethyl sulfate** [Sulfur] *Respiratory tract irritation, pulmonary edema, anaphylaxis.*

**dimethyl sulfide** [Sulfur] *Respiratory tract irritation, pulmonary edema, anaphylaxis.*

**dimethyl thiophosphoryl chloride** [Organophosphate] *Pulmonary edema, respiratory muscle paralysis, respiratory failure, bradycardia, acetylcholinesterase inhibition, hypotension, pulmonary edema, overstimulation of parasympathetic nervous system, striated muscle, sympathetic ganglia, and CNS.*

**dimethylamine** [Organic base/amine] *Pulmonary edema, cardiac depression, seizures.*

**dimethylaminoacetonitrile** [Cyanide] *Impairment of cellular oxygenation and adenosine triphosphate production, hypoxia, death.*

**dimethylaminoazobenzene; 4-dimethylaminoazobenzene** [Aniline] *Methemoglobinemia, hypoxia.*

**4-dimethylamino-6-(2-di-methylaminoethoxy)toluene-2-diazonium zinc chloride** [Zinc] *Respiratory tract irritation, metal fume fever, pulmonary edema.*

**dimethylaminoethanol** [Organic base/amine] *Pulmonary edema, cardiac depression, seizures.*

**dimethylaminoethyl methacrylate** [Ester] *CNS depression, respiratory tract irritation, bronchitis, pneumonia.*

**dimethylaniline; N,N-dimethylaniline** [Aniline] *Methemoglobinemia, hypoxia.*

**7,12-dimethylbenz[a]anthracene** [Aromatic hydrocarbon] *Arrhythmias, respiratory failure, pulmonary edema, paralysis, brain and kidney damage.*

**3,3′-dimethylbenzidine** [Aniline] *Methemoglobinemia, hypoxia.*

**di-(2-methylbenzoyl) peroxide** [Organic peroxide] *Pulmonary and laryngeal edema, circulatory arrest, hypovolemic shock, chemical burns to skin, mucous membranes, and internal organs.*

**dimethylbutane** [Aliphatic hydrocarbon] *Arrhythmias, asphyxiation, anesthesia.*

**dimethylbutylamine; 1,3-dimethylbutylamine** [Organic base/amine] *Pulmonary edema, cardiac depression, seizures.*

**dimethylcarbamoyl chloride** [Poison] *Cardiovascular collapse, pulmonary edema, CNS depression, coma, seizures, nausea, vomiting, cardiopulmonary arrest.*

**dimethylcyclohexane** [Aliphatic hydrocarbon] *Arrhythmias, asphyxiation, anesthesia.*

**2,3-dimethylcyclohexylamine** [Poison] *Cardiovascular collapse, pulmonary edema, CNS depression, coma, seizures, nausea, vomiting, cardiopulmonary arrest.* [Organic base/amine] *Pulmonary edema, cardiac depression, seizures.*

**2,5-dimethyl-2,5-di-(benzoylperoxy) hexane** [Organic peroxide] *Pulmonary and laryngeal edema, circulatory arrest, hypovolemic shock, chemical burns to skin, mucous membranes, and internal organs.*

**2,5-dimethyl-2,5-di(tert-butylperoxy) hexane** [Organic peroxide]

*Pulmonary and laryngeal edema, circulatory arrest, hypovolemic shock, chemical burns to skin, mucous membranes, and internal organs.*

**2,5-dimethyl-2,5-di(tert-butylperoxy) hexyne-3** [Organic peroxide] *Pulmonary and laryngeal edema, circulatory arrest, hypovolemic shock, chemical burns to skin, mucous membranes, and internal organs.*

**dimethyldichlorosilane** [Silane/chlorosilane] *Respiratory tract irritation, pulmonary edema.*

**dimethyldiethoxysilane** [Silane/chlorosilane] *Respiratory tract irritation, pulmonary edema.*

**2,5-dimethyl-2,5-di(2-ethyl-hexanoylperoxy) hexane** [Organic peroxide] *Pulmonary and laryngeal edema, circulatory arrest, hypovolemic shock, chemical burns to skin, mucous membranes, and internal organs.*

**2,5-dimethyl-2,5-dihydroperoxy hexane** [Organic peroxide] *Pulmonary and laryngeal edema, circulatory arrest, hypovolemic shock, chemical burns to skin, mucous membranes, and internal organs.*

**3,5-dimethyl-3,5-dihydroxydioxolane-1,2** [Ethylene glycol] *Respiratory failure, pulmonary edema, paralysis, cardiovascular collapse, severe acidosis.*

**2,5-dimethyl-2,5-di(iso-nonanopylperoxy) hexane** [Organic peroxide] *Pulmonary and laryngeal edema, circulatory arrest, hypovolemic shock, chemical burns to skin, mucous membranes, and internal organs.*

**dimethyldioxane** [Dioxane] *Pulmonary irritation, respiratory failure, pulmonary edema, CNS depression.*

**dimethyldisulfide** [Sulfur] *Respiratory tract irritation, pulmonary edema, anaphylaxis.*

**2,5-dimethyl-2,5-di(3,5,5-trimethylhexanoylperoxy) hexane** [Organic peroxide] *Pulmonary and laryngeal edema, circulatory arrest, hypovolemic shock, chemical burns to*

HazMat

*skin, mucous membranes, and internal organs.*

**dimethylethanolamine** [Organic base/amine] *Pulmonary edema, cardiac depression, seizures.*

**dimethylformamide** [Poison] *Cardiovascular collapse, pulmonary edema, CNS depression, coma, seizures, nausea, vomiting, cardiopulmonary arrest.*

**N,N-dimethylformamide** [Poison] *Cardiovascular collapse, pulmonary edema, CNS depression, coma, seizures, nausea, vomiting, cardiopulmonary arrest.* [Organic acid] *Pulmonary edema, circulatory collapse, laryngeal edema and spasm, severe chemical burns to skin, mucous membranes, and internal organs, GI tract perforation and hemorrhage, peritonitis.*

**dimethylhydrazine; 1,1-dimethylhydrazine** [Hydrazine] *Seizures, hemolysis of red blood cells, pulmonary edema.*

**dimethylmagnesium** [Magnesium] *Cardiovascular collapse, respiratory depression.*

**dimethyl-p-nitrosoaniline** [Aniline] *Methemoglobinemia, hypoxia.*

**2,4-dimethylphenol** [Phenol] *Coma, hypotension, arrhythmias, pulmonary edema, respiratory arrest.*

**dimethyl-p-phenylenediamine** [Organic base/amine] *Pulmonary edema, cardiac depression, seizures.*

**dimethylpropane** [Aliphatic hydrocarbon] *Arrhythmias, asphyxiation, anesthesia.*

**dimethyl-propylamine** [Organic base/amine] *Pulmonary edema, cardiac depression, seizures.*

**dimethylzinc** [Zinc] *Respiratory tract irritation, metal fume fever, pulmonary edema.*

**dimetilan** [Carbamate] *Acetylcholinesterase inhibition (reversible), bradycardia, hypotension, respiratory muscle paralysis, respiratory arrest, pulmonary edema.*

**dimyristyl peroxy-dicarbonate** [Organic peroxide] *Pulmonary and laryngeal edema, circulatory arrest, hypo-*

*volemic shock, chemical burns to skin, mucous membranes, and internal organs.*

**4,6-dinitro-o-amylphenol** [Dinitrophenol] *Respiratory and circulatory collapse, pulmonary edema, hyperthermia.*

**dinitroaniline** [Aniline] *Methemoglobinemia, hypoxia.*

**dinitrobenzene (n.o.s.)** [Aniline] *Methemoglobinemia, hypoxia.*

**dinitrochlorobenzene** [Aniline] *Methemoglobinemia, hypoxia.*

**dinitro-o-cresol; 4,6-dinitro-o-cresol** [Phenol] *Coma, hypotension, arrhythmias, pulmonary edema, respiratory arrest.*

**4,6-dinitro-o-cresol salt (n.o.s.)** [Phenol] *Coma, hypotension, arrhythmias, pulmonary edema, respiratory arrest.*

**dinitrocyclohexylphenol; 4,6 dinitro-o-cyclohexylphenol** [Dinitrophenol] *Respiratory and circulatory collapse, pulmonary edema, hyperthermia.*

**dinitrogen tetroxide** [Nitrogen oxide] *Lower respiratory tract symptoms, pulmonary edema, laryngospasm, bronchospasm, asphyxiation.*

**dinitrogen tetroxide & nitric oxide mixture** [Nitrogen oxide] *Lower respiratory tract symptoms, pulmonary edema, laryngospasm, bronchospasm, asphyxiation.*

**dinitrophenol; 2,4-dinitrophenol; 2,5-dinitrophenol; 2,6-dinitrophenol** [Dinitrophenol] *Respiratory and circulatory collapse, pulmonary edema, hyperthermia.*

**dinitrophenolate** [Dinitrophenol] *Respiratory and circulatory collapse, pulmonary edema, hyperthermia.*

**dinitroresorcinol** [Dinitrophenol] *Respiratory and circulatory collapse, pulmonary edema, hyperthermia.*

**dinitroso-dimethyl terephthalamide** [Poison] *Cardiovascular collapse, pulmonary edema, CNS depression, coma, seizures, nausea, vomiting, cardiopulmonary arrest.*

**dinitrosopentamethylene tetramine** [Organic base/amine] *Pulmonary edema, cardiac depression, seizures.*

**dinitrotoluene; 2,4-dinitrotoluene; 2,6-dinitrotoluene; 3,4-dinitrotoluene** [Aniline] *Methemoglobinemia, hypoxia.*

**dinocap** [Dinitrophenol] *Respiratory and circulatory collapse, pulmonary edema, hyperthermia.*

**dinonanoyl peroxide** [Organic peroxide] *Pulmonary and laryngeal edema, circulatory arrest, hypovolemic shock, chemical burns to skin, mucous membranes, and internal organs.*

**dinoseb** [Dinitrophenol] *Respiratory and circulatory collapse, pulmonary edema, hyperthermia.*

**dinoterb** [Dinitrophenol] *Respiratory and circulatory collapse, pulmonary edema, hyperthermia.*

**dioctanoyl peroxide** [Organic peroxide] *Pulmonary and laryngeal edema, circulatory arrest, hypovolemic shock, chemical burns to skin, mucous membranes, and internal organs.*

**dioctyl phthalate** [Ester] *CNS depression, respiratory tract irritation, bronchitis, pneumonia.*

**n-dioctylphthalate** [Ester] *CNS depression, respiratory tract irritation, bronchitis, pneumonia.*

**dioxacarb** [Carbamate] *Acetylcholinesterase inhibition (reversible), bradycardia, hypotension, respiratory muscle paralysis, respiratory arrest, pulmonary edema.*

**dioxane; 1,4-dioxane** [Dioxane] *Pulmonary irritation, respiratory failure, pulmonary edema, CNS depression.*

**dioxathion** [Organophosphate] *Pulmonary edema, respiratory muscle paralysis, respiratory failure, bradycardia, acetylcholinesterase inhibition, hypotension, pulmonary edema, overstimulation of parasympathetic nervous system, striated muscle, sympathetic ganglia, and CNS.*

**dioxolane** [Ethylene glycol] *Respiratory failure, pulmonary edema, paralysis, cardiovascular collapse, severe acidosis.*

**dipentene** [Turpentine/terpene] *Respiratory failure, pulmonary edema, tachycardia.*

**diperoxy azelaic acid** [Organic peroxide] *Pulmonary and laryngeal edema, circulatory arrest, hypovolemic shock, chemical burns to skin, mucous membranes, and internal organs.*

**diperoxydodecane diacid & sodium sulfate mixture** [Organic peroxide] *Pulmonary and laryngeal edema, circulatory arrest, hypovolemic shock, chemical burns to skin, mucous membranes, and internal organs.* [Sulfur] *Respiratory tract irritation, pulmonary edema, anaphylaxis.*

**diphacinone** [Warfarin/hydroxycoumarin/indanedione] *Anticoagulation effect, internal hemorrhage.*

**diphenadione** [Warfarin/hydroxycoumarin/indanedione] *Anticoagulation effect, internal hemorrhage.*

**di-(2-phenoxyethyl) peroxydicarbonate** [Organic peroxide] *Pulmonary and laryngeal edema, circulatory arrest, hypovolemic shock, chemical burns to skin, mucous membranes, and internal organs.*

**diphenyl dichlorosilane** [Silane/chlorosilane] *Respiratory tract irritation, pulmonary edema.*

**diphenylamine** [Aniline] *Methemoglobinemia, hypoxia.*

**diphenylaminechloroarsine** [Arsenic] *Heavy metal toxicity, vomiting, GI bleeding, CNS depression, pulmonary edema, cardiac arrest.*

**diphenylchloroarsine** [Arsine] *Intravascular hemolysis, pulmonary edema, cardiac and respiratory arrest, delayed-onset jaundice and renal failure.*

**1,2-diphenylhydrazine** [Hydrazine] *Seizures, hemolysis of red blood cells, pulmonary edema.*

**diphenylmethane-4,4'-diisocyanate (MDI)** [Isocyanate/aliphatic thiocyanate] *CNS depression, respiratory arrest, respiratory paralysis, pulmonary edema, cyanide toxicity.*

**diphenylmethyl bromide** [Bromine/methylbromide] *Severe respiratory irritation, pulmonary edema, respiratory failure, coma, convulsions, death.*

**HazMat**

**diphenyloxide-4,4'-disulfohydrazide**
[Hydrazine] *Seizures, hemolysis of red blood cells, pulmonary edema.*

**diphosphoramide, octamethyl**
[Organophosphate] *Pulmonary edema, respiratory muscle paralysis, respiratory failure, bradycardia, acetylcholinesterase inhibition, hypotension, pulmonary edema, overstimulation of parasympathetic nervous system, striated muscle, sympathetic ganglia, and CNS.*

**dipicryl sulfide** [Nitrate/nitrite] *Methemoglobinemia, hypotension, circulatory collapse.*

**dipropionyl peroxide** [Organic peroxide] *Pulmonary and laryngeal edema, circulatory arrest, hypovolemic shock, chemical burns to skin, mucous membranes, and internal organs.*

**dipropyl ether** [Ether] *Anesthesia, respiratory arrest.*

**dipropyl ketone** [Ketone] *Respiratory mucous membrane irritation, pulmonary edema, CNS depression.*

**dipropyl peroxy-dicarbonate** [Organic peroxide] *Pulmonary and laryngeal edema, circulatory arrest, hypovolemic shock, chemical burns to skin, mucous membranes, and internal organs.*

**dipropylamine** [Organic base/amine] *Pulmonary edema, cardiac depression, seizures.*

**4-dipropylaminobenzene-diazonium zinc chloride** [Zinc] *Respiratory tract irritation, metal fume fever, pulmonary edema.*

**dipropylene glycol** [Ethylene glycol] *Respiratory failure, pulmonary edema, paralysis, cardiovascular collapse, severe acidosis.*

**dipropylene triamine** [Organic base/amine] *Pulmonary edema, cardiac depression, seizures.*

**dipropylnitrosamine** [Nitrate/nitrite] *Methemoglobinemia, hypotension, circulatory collapse.*

**diquat** [Paraquat] *Widespread edema, cardiac damage, circulatory collapse, cerebral hemorrhage or infarcts, death. (Defoliant used in warfare.)*

**diquat dibromide** [Paraquat] *Widespread edema, cardiac damage, circulatory collapse, cerebral hemorrhage or infarcts, death. (Defoliant used in warfare.)* [Bromine/methylbromide] *Severe respiratory irritation, pulmonary edema, respiratory failure, coma, convulsions, death.*

**disinfectant, corrosive (n.o.s.)** [Corrosive] *Upper airway burns and edema, circulatory collapse, severe chemical burns to skin, toxic systemic effects, GI tract perforation and hemorrhage, peritonitis.*

**disinfectant, poisonous (n.o.s.)** [Poison] *Cardiovascular collapse, pulmonary edema, CNS depression, coma, seizures, nausea, vomiting, cardiopulmonary arrest.*

**disodium methanearsonate** [Arsenic] *Heavy metal toxicity, vomiting, GI bleeding, CNS depression, pulmonary edema, cardiac arrest.*

**dispersant gas (n.o.s.)** [Nonflammable gas] *Pulmonary edema, respiratory failure, asphyxiation.*

**dispersant gas, flammable (n.o.s.)** [Flammable gas] *Respiratory failure, cardiac arrest, arrhythmias.*

**distearyl peroxy-dicarbonate** [Organic peroxide] *Pulmonary and laryngeal edema, circulatory arrest, hypovolemic shock, chemical burns to skin, mucous membranes, and internal organs.*

**disuccinic acid peroxide** [Organic peroxide] *Pulmonary and laryngeal edema, circulatory arrest, hypovolemic shock, chemical burns to skin, mucous membranes, and internal organs.*

**disulfoton** [Organophosphate] *Pulmonary edema, respiratory muscle paralysis, respiratory failure, bradycardia, acetylcholinesterase inhibition, hypotension, pulmonary edema, overstimulation of parasympathetic nervous system, striated muscle, sympathetic ganglia, and CNS.*

**dithiazanine iodide** [Poison] *Cardiovascular collapse, pulmonary edema,*

CNS depression, coma, seizures, nausea, vomiting, cardiopulmonary arrest.

**dithiobiuret** [Sulfur] *Respiratory tract irritation, pulmonary edema, anaphylaxis.*

**dithiocarbamate pesticide (n.o.s.)** [Dithiocarbamate] *Hypotension, respiratory failure.*

**di(3,5,5-trimethyl-1,2-dioxolanul-3) peroxide** [Organic peroxide] *Pulmonary and laryngeal edema, circulatory arrest, hypovolemic shock, chemical burns to skin, mucous membranes, and internal organs.*

**di(3,5,5-trimethylhexanoyl) peroxide** [Organic peroxide] *Pulmonary and laryngeal edema, circulatory arrest, hypovolemic shock, chemical burns to skin, mucous membranes, and internal organs.*

**diuron** [Poison] *Cardiovascular collapse, pulmonary edema, CNS depression, coma, seizures, nausea, vomiting, cardiopulmonary arrest.*

**divinyl ether** [Ether] *Anesthesia, respiratory arrest.*

**DMC (di-(p-chlorophenyl) methylcarbinol)** [DDT] *CNS disruption, respiratory control center paralysis, ventricular fibrillation, seizures, respiratory arrest.*

**dodecyl trichlorosilane** [Silane/chlorosilane] *Respiratory tract irritation, pulmonary edema.*

**dodecylbenzene-sulfonic acid** [Organic acid] *Pulmonary edema, circulatory collapse, laryngeal edema and spasm, severe chemical burns to skin, mucous membranes, and internal organs, GI tract perforation and hemorrhage, peritonitis.*

**Donovan solution** [Arsenic] *Heavy metal toxicity, vomiting, GI bleeding, CNS depression, pulmonary edema, cardiac arrest.* [Mercury] *Circulatory collapse, arrhythmias, respiratory failure, pulmonary edema, neurotoxic effects.*

**Dowicide (n.o.s.)** [Phenol] *Coma, hypotension, arrhythmias, pulmonary edema, respiratory arrest.*

**drier, paint and varnish (n.o.s.)** [Poison] *Cardiovascular collapse, pulmonary edema, CNS depression, coma, seizures, nausea, vomiting, cardiopulmonary arrest.*

**drug (n.o.s.)** [Poison] *Cardiovascular collapse, pulmonary edema, CNS depression, coma, seizures, nausea, vomiting, cardiopulmonary arrest.*

**Dry Ice** [Simple asphyxiant] *Asphyxiation.*

**di(4-tert-butylcyclohexyl) peroxydicarbonate** [Organic peroxide] *Pulmonary and laryngeal edema, circulatory arrest, hypovolemic shock, chemical burns to skin, mucous membranes, and internal organs.*

**dye, corrosive (n.o.s.)** [Corrosive] *Upper airway burns and edema, circulatory collapse, severe chemical burns to skin, toxic systemic effects, GI tract perforation and hemorrhage, peritonitis.*

**dye, poisonous (n.o.s.)** [Poison] *Cardiovascular collapse, pulmonary edema, CNS depression, coma, seizures, nausea, vomiting, cardiopulmonary arrest.*

**EDE** [Carbon tetrachloride] *CNS depression, respiratory arrest, circulatory collapse.*

**EDTA (ethylenediamine tetraacetic acid)** [Organic base/amine] *Pulmonary edema, cardiac depression, seizures.*

**electrolyte, acid** [Inorganic acid] *Pulmonary edema, bronchospasm, circulatory collapse, laryngeal spasm and edema, severe chemical burns to skin, mucous membranes, and internal organs, GI tract perforation and hemorrhage, peritonitis.*

**electrolyte, alkaline** [Inorganic base/alkaline corrosive] *Upper airway burns and edema, pulmonary edema, skin burns, circulatory collapse, GI tract perforation and hemorrhage, peritonitis.*

**electrolyte, battery fluid acid** [Poison] *Cardiovascular collapse, pulmonary edema, CNS depression, coma, seizures, nausea, vomiting, cardiopulmonary arrest.* [Corrosive] *Upper air-*

**HazMat**

way burns and edema, circulatory collapse, severe chemical burns to skin, toxic systemic effects, GI tract perforation and hemorrhage, peritonitis.

**emetine dihydrochloride** [Poison] Cardiovascular collapse, pulmonary edema, CNS depression, coma, seizures, nausea, vomiting, cardiopulmonary arrest.

**EMMI** [Mercury] Circulatory collapse, arrhythmias, respiratory failure, pulmonary edema, neurotoxic effects.

**enamel** [Poison] Cardiovascular collapse, pulmonary edema, CNS depression, coma, seizures, nausea, vomiting, cardiopulmonary arrest. [Hydrocarbon mixture] CNS depression, respiratory arrest, seizures, arrhythmias, pulmonary edema.

**endosulfan; α-endosulfan (alpha-endosulfan); β-endosulfan (beta-endosulfan)** [Aldrin/dieldrin/endrin] Seizures, respiratory failure.

**endosulfan sulfate** [Aldrin/dieldrin/endrin] Seizures, respiratory failure.

**endothal; endothall** [Dithiocarbamate] Hypotension, respiratory failure.

**endothion** [Organophosphate] Pulmonary edema, respiratory muscle paralysis, respiratory failure, bradycardia, acetylcholinesterase inhibition, hypotension, pulmonary edema, overstimulation of parasympathetic nervous system, striated muscle, sympathetic ganglia, and CNS.

**endrin aldehyde** [Aldrin/dieldrin/endrin] Seizures, respiratory failure.

**endrin mixture (n.o.s.)** [Aldrin/dieldrin/endrin] Seizures, respiratory failure.

**engine-starting fluid** [Hydrocarbon mixture] CNS depression, respiratory arrest, seizures, arrhythmias, pulmonary edema.

**enviromentally hazardous substance (n.o.s.)** [Poison] Cardiovascular collapse, pulmonary edema, CNS depression, coma, seizures, nausea, vomiting, cardiopulmonary arrest.

**epibromohydrin** [Dichloropropane/dichloropropene] Pulmonary edema, bronchospasm, alveolar hemorrhage.

**epichlorohydrin** [Dichloropropane/dichloropropene] Pulmonary edema, bronchospasm, alveolar hemorrhage.

**epinephrine** [Poison] Cardiovascular collapse, pulmonary edema, CNS depression, coma, seizures, nausea, vomiting, cardiopulmonary arrest.

**EPN** [Organophosphate] Pulmonary edema, respiratory muscle paralysis, respiratory failure, bradycardia, acetylcholinesterase inhibition, hypotension, pulmonary edema, overstimulation of parasympathetic nervous system, striated muscle, sympathetic ganglia, and CNS.

**epoxyethane** [Ethylene oxide] Respiratory tract irritation, pulmonary edema.

**epoxyethoxypropane; 1,2-epoxy-3-ethoxypropane** [Ether] Anesthesia, respiratory arrest.

**1,2-epoxy-3-ethyloxypropane** [Ether] Anesthesia, respiratory arrest.

**EPTC** [Dithiocarbamate] Hypotension, respiratory failure.

**eradicator, paint and grease** [Flammable/combustible liquid] CNS depression, respiratory arrest, convulsions, arrhythmias, pulmonary edema.

**erbon** [Chlorophenoxy herbicide] CNS depression, CNS stimulation, respiratory failure, ventricular fibrillation, seizures.

**ergocalciferol** [Poison] Cardiovascular collapse, pulmonary edema, CNS depression, coma, seizures, nausea, vomiting, cardiopulmonary arrest.

**ergotamine tartrate** [Poison] Cardiovascular collapse, pulmonary edema, CNS depression, coma, seizures, nausea, vomiting, cardiopulmonary arrest.

**ET-15** [Organophosphate] Pulmonary edema, respiratory muscle paralysis, respiratory failure, bradycardia, acetylcholinesterase inhibition, hypotension, pulmonary edema, overstimulation of parasympathetic nervous system, striated muscle, sympathetic ganglia, and CNS.

**etching acid** [Inorganic acid] *Pulmonary edema, bronchospasm, circulatory collapse, laryngeal spasm and edema, severe chemical burns to skin, mucous membranes, and internal organs, GI tract perforation and hemorrhage, peritonitis.* [Hydrofluoric acid] *Pulmonary and laryngeal edema, circulatory collapse, severe skin burns, GI tract perforation, systemic fluoride poisoning.*

**ethane (gas or cryogenic liquid)** [Aliphatic hydrocarbon] *Arrhythmias, asphyxiation, anesthesia.*

**ethane, chlorinated** [Halogenated aliphatic hydrocarbon] *CNS depression, respiratory arrest, circulatory collapse.*

**ethane & propane mixture (cryogenic liquid)** [Aliphatic hydrocarbon] *Arrhythmias, asphyxiation, anesthesia.*

**ethanesulfonyl chloride** [Halogenated aliphatic hydrocarbon] *CNS depression, respiratory arrest, circulatory collapse.*

**ethanol; ethanol mixture (n.o.s.)** [Lower alcohol (1–3 carbons)] *CNS depression, coma, respiratory arrest, arrhythmias.*

**ethanolamine; ethanolamine mixture (n.o.s.)** [Organic base/amine] *Pulmonary edema, cardiac depression, seizures.*

**ether** [Ether] *Anesthesia, respiratory arrest.*

**ethiofencarb** [Carbamate] *Acetylcholinesterase inhibition (reversible), bradycardia, hypotension, respiratory muscle paralysis, respiratory arrest, pulmonary edema.*

**ethion** [Organophosphate] *Pulmonary edema, respiratory muscle paralysis, respiratory failure, bradycardia, acetylcholinesterase inhibition, hypotension, pulmonary edema, overstimulation of parasympathetic nervous system, striated muscle, sympathetic ganglia, and CNS.*

**ethoxyethanol; 2-ethoxyethanol** [Ethylene glycol] *Respiratory failure, pulmonary edema, paralysis, cardiovascular collapse, severe acidosis.*

**ethoxyethyl acetate; 2-ethoxyethyl acetate** [Ethylene glycol] *Respiratory failure, pulmonary edema, paralysis, cardiovascular collapse, severe acidosis.*

**ethoxypropane** [Ether] *Anesthesia, respiratory arrest.*

**ethyl acetate** [Ester] *CNS depression, respiratory tract irritation, bronchitis, pneumonia.*

**ethyl acetylene** [Aliphatic hydrocarbon] *Arrhythmias, asphyxiation, anesthesia.* [Simple asphyxiant] *Asphyxiation.*

**ethyl acrylate** [Ester] *CNS depression, respiratory tract irritation, bronchitis, pneumonia.*

**ethyl alcohol** [Lower alcohol (1–3 carbons)] *CNS depression, coma, respiratory arrest, arrhythmias.*

**ethyl aluminum dichloride** [Poison] *Cardiovascular collapse, pulmonary edema, CNS depression, coma, seizures, nausea, vomiting, cardiopulmonary arrest.*

**ethyl aluminum sesquichloride** [Poison] *Cardiovascular collapse, pulmonary edema, CNS depression, coma, seizures, nausea, vomiting, cardiopulmonary arrest.*

**ethyl amyl ketone** [Ketone] *Respiratory mucous membrane irritation, pulmonary edema, CNS depression.*

**ethyl biscoumacetate** [Warfarin/hydroxycoumarin/indanedione] *Anticoagulation effect, internal hemorrhage.*

**ethyl borate** [Boron] *Respiratory tract irritation, laryngeal spasm and edema, pulmonary edema, severe chemical burns.*

**ethyl bromide** [Bromine/methylbromide] *Severe respiratory irritation, pulmonary edema, respiratory failure, coma, convulsions, death.*

**ethyl bromoacetate** [Bromate] *CNS and respiratory system depression, delayed-onset renal failure.*

**ethyl butyl ether** [Ether] *Anesthesia, respiratory arrest.*

HazMat

**ethyl butyraldehyde** [Aldehyde] *Seizures, respiratory failure, pulmonary edema.*

**ethyl butyrate** [Ester] *CNS depression, respiratory tract irritation, bronchitis, pneumonia.*

**ethyl chloride** [Halogenated aliphatic hydrocarbon] *CNS depression, respiratory arrest, circulatory collapse.*

**ethyl chloroacetate** [Ester] *CNS depression, respiratory tract irritation, bronchitis, pneumonia.*

**ethyl chloroformate** [Ester] *CNS depression, respiratory tract irritation, bronchitis, pneumonia.*

**ethyl chloropropionate** [Ester] *CNS depression, respiratory tract irritation, bronchitis, pneumonia.*

**ethyl chlorothioformate** [Ester] *CNS depression, respiratory tract irritation, bronchitis, pneumonia.*

**ethyl crotonate** [Ester] *CNS depression, respiratory tract irritation, bronchitis, pneumonia.*

**ethyl cyanoacetate** [Ester] *CNS depression, respiratory tract irritation, bronchitis, pneumonia.*

**ethyl 3,3-di(*tert*-butylperoxy) butyrate** [Organic peroxide] *Pulmonary and laryngeal edema, circulatory arrest, hypovolemic shock, chemical burns to skin, mucous membranes, and internal organs.*

**ethyl dichloroarsine** [Arsine] *Intravascular hemolysis, pulmonary edema, cardiac and respiratory arrest, delayed-onset jaundice and renal failure.*

**O-ethyl S,S-dipropyl phosphorodithioate** [Organophosphate] *Pulmonary edema, respiratory muscle paralysis, respiratory failure, bradycardia, acetylcholinesterase inhibition, hypotension, pulmonary edema, overstimulation of parasympathetic nervous system, striated muscle, sympathetic ganglia, and CNS.*

**ethyl ether** [Ether] *Anesthesia, respiratory arrest.*

**ethyl ether & methyl magnesium bromide mixture** [Ether] *Anesthesia, respiratory arrest.* [Bromine/methylbromide] *Severe respiratory irritation, pulmonary edema, respiratory failure, coma, convulsions, death.*

**ethyl fluid** [Aliphatic hydrocarbon] *Arrhythmias, asphyxiation, anesthesia.*

**ethyl fluoride** [Chlorinated fluorocarbon] *Asphyxiation, anesthesia, arrhythmias.*

**ethyl formate** [Ester] *CNS depression, respiratory tract irritation, bronchitis, pneumonia.*

**ethyl hexaldehyde; 2-ethyl hexaldehyde** [Aldehyde] *Seizures, respiratory failure, pulmonary edema.*

**ethyl hexylamine** [Organic base/amine] *Pulmonary edema, cardiac depression, seizures.*

**ethyl hexylchloroformate** [Ester] *CNS depression, respiratory tract irritation, bronchitis, pneumonia.*

**ethyl isobutyrate** [Ester] *CNS depression, respiratory tract irritation, bronchitis, pneumonia.*

**ethyl isocyanate** [Isocyanate/aliphatic thiocyanate] *CNS depression, respiratory arrest, respiratory paralysis, pulmonary edema, cyanide toxicity.*

**ethyl lactate** [Ester] *CNS depression, respiratory tract irritation, bronchitis, pneumonia.*

**ethyl mercaptan** [Sulfur] *Respiratory tract irritation, pulmonary edema, anaphylaxis.*

**ethyl mercuric chloride** [Mercury] *Circulatory collapse, arrhythmias, respiratory failure, pulmonary edema, neurotoxic effects.*

**ethyl mercuri-2,3-dihydroxypropylmercaptide** [Mercury] *Circulatory collapse, arrhythmias, respiratory failure, pulmonary edema, neurotoxic effects.*

**N-ethyl mercuri-*p*-toluene sulfonanilide** [Mercury] *Circulatory collapse, arrhythmias, respiratory failure, pulmonary edema, neurotoxic effects.*

**ethyl mercury phosphate** [Mercury] *Circulatory collapse, arrhythmias, res-*

piratory failure, *pulmonary edema, neurotoxic effects.*

**ethyl methacrylate** [Ester] *CNS depression, respiratory tract irritation, bronchitis, pneumonia.*

**ethyl methyl ether** [Ether] *Anesthesia, respiratory arrest.*

**ethyl methyl ketone** [Ketone] *Respiratory mucous membrane irritation, pulmonary edema, CNS depression.*

**ethyl methyl ketone peroxide** [Organic peroxide] *Pulmonary and laryngeal edema, circulatory arrest, hypovolemic shock, chemical burns to skin, mucous membranes, and internal organs.* [Ketone] *Respiratory mucous membrane irritation, pulmonary edema, CNS depression.* [Corrosive] *Upper airway burns and edema, circulatory collapse, severe chemical burns to skin, toxic systemic effects, GI tract perforation and hemorrhage, peritonitis.*

**ethyl nitrate; ethyl nitrate mixture (n.o.s.)** [Nitrate/nitrite] *Methemoglobinemia, hypotension, circulatory collapse.*

**ethyl orthoformate** [Ester] *CNS depression, respiratory tract irritation, bronchitis, pneumonia.*

**ethyl oxalate** [Oxalate] *Cardiovascular collapse, arrhythmias, seizures.*

**ethyl phenyl dichlorosilane** [Silane/chlorosilane] *Respiratory tract irritation, pulmonary edema.*

**ethyl phosphonous dichloride** [Phosphorus] *Hypovolemic shock, severe tissue burns, severe respiratory irritation, pulmonary edema, respiratory arrest, arrhythmias, sudden death.*

**ethyl phosphorodichloridate** [Corrosive] *Upper airway burns and edema, circulatory collapse, severe chemical burns to skin, toxic systemic effects, GI tract perforation and hemorrhage, peritonitis.*

**ethyl piperidine** [Organic base/amine] *Pulmonary edema, cardiac depression, seizures.*

**ethyl propionate** [Ester] *CNS depression, respiratory tract irritation, bronchitis, pneumonia.*

**ethyl propyl ether** [Ether] *Anesthesia, respiratory arrest.*

**ethyl silicate** [Silane/chlorosilane] *Respiratory tract irritation, pulmonary edema.*

**ethyl sulfate** [Organic acid] *Pulmonary edema, circulatory collapse, laryngeal edema and spasm, severe chemical burns to skin, mucous membranes, and internal organs, GI tract perforation and hemorrhage, peritonitis.*

**ethyl sulfuric acid** [Organic acid] *Pulmonary edema, circulatory collapse, laryngeal edema and spasm, severe chemical burns to skin, mucous membranes, and internal organs, GI tract perforation and hemorrhage, peritonitis.*

**ethyl toluidine** [Aniline] *Methemoglobinemia, hypoxia.*

**ethylamine; ethylamine mixture (n.o.s.)** [Organic base/amine] *Pulmonary edema, cardiac depression, seizures.*

**ethylaniline; 2-ethylaniline; N-ethylaniline** [Aniline] *Methemoglobinemia, hypoxia.*

**ethylbenzene** [Aromatic hydrocarbon] *Arrhythmias, respiratory failure, pulmonary edema, paralysis, brain and kidney damage.*

**ethylbenzyl toluidine** [Aniline] *Methemoglobinemia, hypoxia.*

**ethylbenzylaniline** [Aniline] *Methemoglobinemia, hypoxia.*

**ethylbutanol** [Higher alcohol (4+ carbons)] *CNS depression, respiratory failure, arrhythmias.*

**ethylbutyl acetate** [Ester] *CNS depression, respiratory tract irritation, bronchitis, pneumonia.*

**ethyldichlorosilane** [Silane/chlorosilane] *Respiratory tract irritation, pulmonary edema.*

**ethylene (gas or cryogenic liquid)** [Aliphatic hydrocarbon] *Arrhythmias, asphyxiation, anesthesia.* [Simple asphyxiant] *Asphyxiation.*

HazMat

**ethylene & acetylene & propylene mixture (cryogenic liquid)** [Aliphatic hydrocarbon] *Arrhythmias, asphyxiation, anesthesia.* [Simple asphyxiant] *Asphyxiation.*

**ethylene chlorohydrin** [Carbon tetrachloride] *CNS depression, respiratory arrest, circulatory collapse.* [Dichloropropane/dichloropropene] *Pulmonary edema, bronchospasm, alveolar hemorrhage.*

**ethylene dibromide** [Bromine/methylbromide] *Severe respiratory irritation, pulmonary edema, respiratory failure, coma, convulsions, death.*

**ethylene dibromide & methyl bromide mixture** [Bromine/methylbromide] *Severe respiratory irritation, pulmonary edema, respiratory failure, coma, convulsions, death.*

**ethylene dichloride** [Halogenated aliphatic hydrocarbon] *CNS depression, respiratory arrest, circulatory collapse.*

**ethylene fluorohydrin** [Monofluoroacetate] *Ventricular arrhythmias, seizures.*

**ethylene glycol** [Ethylene glycol] *Respiratory failure, pulmonary edema, paralysis, cardiovascular collapse, severe acidosis.*

**ethylene glycol alkyl ester; ethylene glycol aryl ester** [Ethylene glycol] *Respiratory failure, pulmonary edema, paralysis, cardiovascular collapse, severe acidosis.*

**ethylene glycol diethyl ether** [Ethylene glycol] *Respiratory failure, pulmonary edema, paralysis, cardiovascular collapse, severe acidosis.*

**ethylene glycol dinitrate** [Nitrate/nitrite] *Methemoglobinemia, hypotension, circulatory collapse.*

**ethylene glycol monobutyl ether** [Ethylene glycol] *Respiratory failure, pulmonary edema, paralysis, cardiovascular collapse, severe acidosis.*

**ethylene glycol monoethyl ether** [Ethylene glycol] *Respiratory failure, pulmonary edema, paralysis, cardiovascular collapse, severe acidosis.*

**ethylene glycol monoethyl ether acetate** [Ethylene glycol] *Respiratory failure, pulmonary edema, paralysis, cardiovascular collapse, severe acidosis.*

**ethylene glycol monomethyl ether** [Ethylene glycol] *Respiratory failure, pulmonary edema, paralysis, cardiovascular collapse, severe acidosis.*

**ethylene glycol monomethyl ether & acetate mixture** [Ethylene glycol] *Respiratory failure, pulmonary edema, paralysis, cardiovascular collapse, severe acidosis.*

**ethylene oxide (ETO)** [Ethylene oxide] *Respiratory tract irritation, pulmonary edema.*

**ethylene oxide & carbon dioxide mixture** [Ethylene oxide] *Respiratory tract irritation, pulmonary edema.* [Simple asphyxiant] *Asphyxiation.*

**ethylene oxide & dichlorodifluoromethane mixture** [Chlorinated fluorocarbon] *Asphyxiation, anesthesia, arrhythmias.* [Ethylene oxide] *Respiratory tract irritation, pulmonary edema.*

**ethylene oxide & propylene oxide mixture** [Ethylene oxide] *Respiratory tract irritation, pulmonary edema.*

**ethylenediamine** [Organic base/amine] *Pulmonary edema, cardiac depression, seizures.*

**ethylenediamine & lithium acetylide mixture** [Lithium] *Chemical burns to respiratory tract, pulmonary edema.*

**ethylenediamine tetraacetic acid (EDTA)** [Organic base/amine] *Pulmonary edema, cardiac depression, seizures.*

**ethyleneimine** [Organic base/amine] *Pulmonary edema, cardiac depression, seizures.*

**2-ethylhexyl alcohol** [Higher alcohol (4+ carbons)] *CNS depression, respiratory failure, arrhythmias.*

**DL-(2-ethylhexyl) phosphoric acid** [Organic acid] *Pulmonary edema, circulatory collapse, laryngeal edema and spasm, severe chemical burns to skin, mucous membranes, and internal* organs, GI tract perforation and hemorrhage, peritonitis.

**ethylphosphonothioic dichloride** [Corrosive] *Upper airway burns and edema, circulatory collapse, severe chemical burns to skin, toxic systemic effects, GI tract perforation and hemorrhage, peritonitis.*

**2-ethyl-3-propyl acrolein** [Acrolein] *Severe respiratory tract irritation, pulmonary edema, respiratory failure.*

**ethyltrichlorosilane** [Silane/chlorosilane] *Respiratory tract irritation, pulmonary edema.*

**etiologic agent (n.o.s.)** *No acute symptoms during incubation period. Physiologic response varies depending on strain of microorganism or toxin.*

**ETO (ethylene oxide)** [Ethylene oxide] *Respiratory tract irritation, pulmonary edema.*

**eucalyptol** [Camphor] *Status epilepticus, respiratory failure.*

**eugenol** [Phenol] *Coma, hypotension, arrhythmias, pulmonary edema, respiratory arrest.*

**explosive A, B, or C** [Explosive] *Multiple trauma, highly toxic chemical exposure.*

**extract, aromatic (n.o.s.)** [Aromatic hydrocarbon] *Arrhythmias, respiratory failure, pulmonary edema, paralysis, brain and kidney damage.*

**extract, flavoring (n.o.s.)** [Flammable/combustible liquid] *CNS depression, respiratory arrest, convulsions, arrhythmias, pulmonary edema.*

**fabric, animal or vegetable with oil (n.o.s.)** [Flammable/combustible liquid] *CNS depression, respiratory arrest, convulsions, arrhythmias, pulmonary edema.*

**Fenac** [Chlorophenoxy herbicide] *CNS depression, CNS stimulation, respiratory failure, ventricular fibrillation, seizures.*

**fenamiphos** [Organophosphate] *Pulmonary edema, respiratory muscle paralysis, respiratory failure, bradycardia, acetylcholinesterase inhibition,* hypotension, pulmonary edema, overstimulation of parasympathetic nervous system, striated muscle, sympathetic ganglia, and CNS.

**fenitrothion** [Organophosphate] *Pulmonary edema, respiratory muscle paralysis, respiratory failure, bradycardia, acetylcholinesterase inhibition, hypotension, pulmonary edema, overstimulation of parasympathetic nervous system, striated muscle, sympathetic ganglia, and CNS.*

**fensulfothion** [Organophosphate] *Pulmonary edema, respiratory muscle paralysis, respiratory failure, bradycardia, acetylcholinesterase inhibition, hypotension, pulmonary edema, overstimulation of parasympathetic nervous system, striated muscle, sympathetic ganglia, and CNS.*

**fenthion** [Organophosphate] *Pulmonary edema, respiratory muscle paralysis, respiratory failure, bradycardia, acetylcholinesterase inhibition, hypotension, pulmonary edema, overstimulation of parasympathetic nervous system, striated muscle, sympathetic ganglia, and CNS.*

**fenvalerate** [Pyrethrin/pyrethroid] *Respiratory paralysis, convulsions.*

**ferbam** [Dithiocarbamate] *Hypotension, respiratory failure.*

**ferric ammonium citrate** [Iron] *Hypovolemic shock.*

**ferric arsenate; ferrous arsenate** [Arsenic] *Heavy metal toxicity, vomiting, GI bleeding, CNS depression, pulmonary edema, cardiac arrest.* [Iron] *Hypovolemic shock.*

**ferric arsenite** [Arsenic] *Heavy metal toxicity, vomiting, GI bleeding, CNS depression, pulmonary edema, cardiac arrest.* [Iron] *Hypovolemic shock.*

**ferric chloride; ferrous chloride; iron chloride** [Iron] *Hypovolemic shock.*

**ferric cyanide** [Cyanide] *Impairment of cellular oxygenation and adenosine triphosphate production, hypoxia, death.*

**ferric fluoride** [Iron] *Hypovolemic shock.* [Fluorine] *CNS depression, res-*

HazMat

*piratory arrest, cardiovascular collapse, shock, arrhythmias.*

**ferric nitrate** [Nitrate/nitrite] *Methemoglobinemia, hypotension, circulatory collapse.* [Iron] *Hypovolemic shock.*

**ferric salt (n.o.s.); ferrous salt (n.o.s.)** [Iron] *Hypovolemic shock.*

**ferric subsulfate** [Iron] *Hypovolemic shock.*

**ferric sulfate; ferrous sulfate** [Iron] *Hypovolemic shock.*

**ferrocerium** [Iron] *Hypovolemic shock.*

**ferrocholinate** [Iron] *Hypovolemic shock.*

**ferrosilicon** [Iron] *Hypovolemic shock.*

**ferrous arsenate; ferric arsenate** [Arsenic] *Heavy metal toxicity, vomiting, GI bleeding, CNS depression, pulmonary edema, cardiac arrest.* [Iron] *Hypovolemic shock.*

**ferrous chloride; ferric chloride; iron chloride** [Iron] *Hypovolemic shock.*

**ferrous metal; ferrous salt (n.o.s.); ferric salt (n.o.s.)** [Iron] *Hypovolemic shock.*

**ferrous sulfate; ferric sulfate** [Iron] *Hypovolemic shock.*

**fertilizer, ammoniating** [Ammonia] *Pulmonary edema, hypotension.* [Nitrate/nitrite] *Methemoglobinemia, hypotension, circulatory collapse.*

**fiber, animal or vegetable, burnt (n.o.s.)** [Irritant] *Severe immediate or delayed upper airway or respiratory tract irritation, pulmonary edema, glottic spasm, airway obstruction.*

**fiber, animal or vegetable, with oil (n.o.s.)** [Flammable/combustible liquid] *CNS depression, respiratory arrest, convulsions, arrhythmias, pulmonary edema.*

**film, motion picture, nitrocellulose based** [Flammable solid] *Shock, severe chemical and thermal burns, severe respiratory tract irritation, pulmonary edema, respiratory arrest, ECG changes, sudden death.*

**fire extinguisher with compressed or liquefied gas** [Simple asphyxiant] *Asphyxiation.*

**fire extinguisher with corrosive liquid charge** [Corrosive] *Upper airway burns and edema, circulatory collapse, severe chemical burns to skin, toxic systemic effects, GI tract perforation and hemorrhage, peritonitis.*

**fire lighter, solid with flammable liquid** [Aliphatic hydrocarbon] *Arrhythmias, asphyxiation, anesthesia.*

**fish meal and scrap** [Irritant] *Severe immediate or delayed upper airway or respiratory tract irritation, pulmonary edema, glottic spasm, airway obstruction.*

**flammable gas (n.o.s.)** [Flammable gas] *Respiratory failure, cardiac arrest, arrhythmias.*

**flammable gas in cigarette lighter** [Aliphatic hydrocarbon] *Arrhythmias, asphyxiation, anesthesia.*

**flammable liquid (n.o.s.)** [Flammable/combustible liquid] *CNS depression, respiratory arrest, convulsions, arrhythmias, pulmonary edema.*

**flammable liquid, corrosive (n.o.s.)** [Flammable/combustible liquid] *CNS depression, respiratory arrest, convulsions, arrhythmias, pulmonary edema.* [Corrosive] *Upper airway burns and edema, circulatory collapse, severe chemical burns to skin, toxic systemic effects, GI tract perforation and hemorrhage, peritonitis.*

**flammable liquid, poisonous (n.o.s.)** [Flammable/combustible liquid] *CNS depression, respiratory arrest, convulsions, arrhythmias, pulmonary edema.* [Poison] *Cardiovascular collapse, pulmonary edema, CNS depression, coma, seizures, nausea, vomiting, cardiopulmonary arrest.*

**flammable solid (n.o.s.)** [Flammable solid] *Shock, severe chemical and thermal burns, severe respiratory tract irritation, pulmonary edema, respiratory arrest, ECG changes, sudden death.*

**flammable solid, corrosive (n.o.s.)** [Flammable solid] *Shock, severe chemical and thermal burns, severe respiratory tract irritation, pulmonary edema, respiratory arrest, ECG* changes, sudden death. [Corrosive] Upper airway burns and edema, circulatory collapse, severe chemical burns to skin, toxic systemic effects, GI tract perforation and hemorrhage, peritonitis.

**flammable solid, oxidizing (n.o.s.)** [Flammable solid] Shock, severe chemical and thermal burns, severe respiratory tract irritation, pulmonary edema, respiratory arrest, ECG changes, sudden death. [Oxidizer] Pulmonary and laryngeal edema, circulatory arrest, hypovolemic shock, chemical burns of skin, mucous membranes, and internal organs.

**flammable solid, poisonous (n.o.s.)** [Flammable solid] Shock, severe chemical and thermal burns, severe respiratory tract irritation, pulmonary edema, respiratory arrest, ECG changes, sudden death. [Poison] Cardiovascular collapse, pulmonary edema, CNS depression, coma, seizures, nausea, vomiting, cardiopulmonary arrest.

**flavoring extract (n.o.s.)** [Flammable/combustible liquid] CNS depression, respiratory arrest, convulsions, arrhythmias, pulmonary edema.

**flue dust, poisonous** [Poison] Cardiovascular collapse, pulmonary edema, CNS depression, coma, seizures, nausea, vomiting, cardiopulmonary arrest.

**fluoboric acid** [Hydrofluoric acid] Pulmonary and laryngeal edema, circulatory collapse, severe skin burns, GI tract perforation, systemic fluoride poisoning. [Boron] Respiratory tract irritation, laryngeal spasm and edema, pulmonary edema, severe chemical burns.

**fluoric acid** [Hydrofluoric acid] Pulmonary and laryngeal edema, circulatory collapse, severe skin burns, GI tract perforation, systemic fluoride poisoning.

**fluoride (n.o.s.)** [Fluorine] CNS depression, respiratory arrest, cardiovascular collapse, shock, arrhythmias.

**fluorine (gas or cryogenic liquid)** [Fluorine] CNS depression, respiratory

arrest, cardiovascular collapse, shock, arrhythmias.

**fluoroacetamide** [Monofluoroacetate] Ventricular arrhythmias, seizures.

**fluoroacetate; fluroacetate-1080** [Monofluoroacetate] Ventricular arrhythmias, seizures.

**fluoroacetic acid** [Monofluoroacetate] Ventricular arrhythmias, seizures.

**fluoroaniline** [Aniline] Methemoglobinemia, hypoxia.

**fluorobenzene** [Benzene] Arrhythmias, respiratory failure, pulmonary edema, CNS depression, liver and kidney damage.

**fluorophosphoric acid** [Inorganic acid] Pulmonary edema, bronchospasm, circulatory collapse, laryngeal spasm and edema, severe chemical burns to skin, mucous membranes, and internal organs, GI tract perforation and hemorrhage, peritonitis.

**fluorosilicate (n.o.s.)** [Fluorine] CNS depression, respiratory arrest, cardiovascular collapse, shock, arrhythmias.

**fluorosulfonic acid** [Inorganic acid] Pulmonary edema, bronchospasm, circulatory collapse, laryngeal spasm and edema, severe chemical burns to skin, mucous membranes, and internal organs, GI tract perforation and hemorrhage, peritonitis.

**fluorotoluene** [Aromatic hydrocarbon] Arrhythmias, respiratory failure, pulmonary edema, paralysis, brain and kidney damage.

**fluosilicate salt (n.o.s.)** [Fluorine] CNS depression, respiratory arrest, cardiovascular collapse, shock, arrhythmias.

**fluosilicic acid** [Hydrofluoric acid] Pulmonary and laryngeal edema, circulatory collapse, severe skin burns, GI tract perforation, systemic fluoride poisoning.

**formaldehyde solution (formalin)** [Aldehyde] Seizures, respiratory failure, pulmonary edema.

**formetanate** [Carbamate] Acetylcholinesterase inhibition (reversible), bradycardia, hypotension, respiratory muscle paralysis, respiratory arrest, pulmonary edema.

**HazMat**

**formic acid** [Organic acid] *Pulmonary edema, circulatory collapse, laryngeal edema and spasm, severe chemical burns to skin, mucous membranes, and internal organs, GI tract perforation and hemorrhage, peritonitis.*

**Fowler solution** [Arsenic] *Heavy metal toxicity, vomiting, GI bleeding, CNS depression, pulmonary edema, cardiac arrest.*

**Freon (all types)** [Chlorinated fluorocarbon] *Asphyxiation, anesthesia, arrhythmias.*

**fuel, aviation** [Hydrocarbon mixture] *CNS depression, respiratory arrest, seizures, arrhythmias, pulmonary edema.*

**fuel, pyrophoric (n.o.s.)** [Flammable/combustible liquid] *CNS depression, respiratory arrest, convulsions, arrhythmias, pulmonary edema.*

**fuel oil** [Hydrocarbon mixture] *CNS depression, respiratory arrest, seizures, arrhythmias, pulmonary edema.*

**fuel oil & ammonium nitrate (ANFO) mixture** [Explosive] *Multiple trauma, highly toxic chemical exposure.* [Nitrate/nitrite] *Methemoglobinemia, hypotension, circulatory collapse.*

**fumaric acid** [Organic acid] *Pulmonary edema, circulatory collapse, laryngeal edema and spasm, severe chemical burns to skin, mucous membranes, and internal organs, GI tract perforation and hemorrhage, peritonitis.*

**fumaryl chloride** [Organic acid] *Pulmonary edema, circulatory collapse, laryngeal edema and spasm, severe chemical burns to skin, mucous membranes, and internal organs, GI tract perforation and hemorrhage, peritonitis.*

**fumigant (n.o.s.)** [Poison] *Cardiovascular collapse, pulmonary edema, CNS depression, coma, seizures, nausea, vomiting, cardiopulmonary arrest.*

**fungicide, corrosive (n.o.s.)** [Poison] *Cardiovascular collapse, pulmonary edema, CNS depression, coma, seizures, nausea, vomiting, cardiopulmonary arrest.* [Corrosive] *Upper airway burns and edema, circulatory collapse, severe chemical burns to skin, toxic systemic effects, GI tract perforation and hemorrhage, peritonitis.*

**fungicide, poisonous (n.o.s.)** [Poison] *Cardiovascular collapse, pulmonary edema, CNS depression, coma, seizures, nausea, vomiting, cardiopulmonary arrest.*

**furan** [Aliphatic hydrocarbon] *Arrhythmias, asphyxiation, anesthesia.*

**furfural** [Aldehyde] *Seizures, respiratory failure, pulmonary edema.*

**furfuryl alcohol** [Higher alcohol (4+ carbons)] *CNS depression, respiratory failure, arrhythmias.*

**furfurylamine** [Organic base/amine] *Pulmonary edema, cardiac depression, seizures.*

**fusel oil** [Higher alcohol (4+ carbons)] *CNS depression, respiratory failure, arrhythmias.*

**gallic acid** [Organic acid] *Pulmonary edema, circulatory collapse, laryngeal edema and spasm, severe chemical burns to skin, mucous membranes, and internal organs, GI tract perforation and hemorrhage, peritonitis.*

**gallium** [Poison] *Cardiovascular collapse, pulmonary edema, CNS depression, coma, seizures, nausea, vomiting, cardiopulmonary arrest.*

**gas, liquefied** [see: liquefied gas (various types)]

**gas drip, hydrocarbon** [Hydrocarbon mixture] *CNS depression, respiratory arrest, seizures, arrhythmias, pulmonary edema.*

**gas oil** [Hydrocarbon mixture] *CNS depression, respiratory arrest, seizures, arrhythmias, pulmonary edema.*

**gasoline; gasohol** [Hydrocarbon mixture] *CNS depression, respiratory arrest, seizures, arrhythmias, pulmonary edema.*

**germane; germanium hydride** [Arsine] *Intravascular hemolysis, pulmonary edema, cardiac and respiratory arrest, delayed-onset jaundice and renal failure.*

**glifonox** [Glyphosate] *Hypotension, arrhythmias, pulmonary edema.*

**glutaraldehyde** [Aldehyde] *Seizures, respiratory failure, pulmonary edema.*

**glycerol-α-mono-chlorohydrin** [Dichloropropane/dichloropropene] *Pulmonary edema, bronchospasm, alveolar hemorrhage.*

**glyceryl trinitrate** [Explosive] *Multiple trauma, highly toxic chemical exposure.* [Nitrate/nitrite] *Methemoglobinemia, hypotension, circulatory collapse.*

**glycidaldehyde** [Aldehyde] *Seizures, respiratory failure, pulmonary edema.*

**glycofurol** [Ethylene glycol] *Respiratory failure, pulmonary edema, paralysis, cardiovascular collapse, severe acidosis.*

**glycolic acid** [Organic acid] *Pulmonary edema, circulatory collapse, laryngeal edema and spasm, severe chemical burns to skin, mucous membranes, and internal organs, GI tract perforation and hemorrhage, peritonitis.*

**glyphosate** [Glyphosate] *Hypotension, arrhythmias, pulmonary edema.*

**glyphosate isopropylamine salt (n.o.s.); glyphosate mono(isopropylamine) salt (n.o.s.)** [Glyphosate] *Hypotension, arrhythmias, pulmonary edema.*

**gold bronze powder** [Copper] *Respiratory tract irritation and arrest, hemorrhagic gastritis.*

**grease eradicator** [Flammable/combustible liquid] *CNS depression, respiratory arrest, convulsions, arrhythmias, pulmonary edema.*

**grenade, poisonous gas** [Poison] *Cardiovascular collapse, pulmonary edema, CNS depression, coma, seizures, nausea, vomiting, cardiopulmonary arrest.*

**grenade, tear gas** [Irritant] *Severe immediate or delayed upper airway or respiratory tract irritation, pulmonary edema, glottic spasm, airway obstruction.*

**guaiacol** [Phenol] *Coma, hypotension, arrhythmias, pulmonary edema, respiratory arrest.*

**guanidine nitrate** [Organic base/amine] *Pulmonary edema, cardiac depression, seizures.*

**Guthion (azinphos-methyl)** [Organophosphate] *Pulmonary edema, respiratory muscle paralysis, respiratory failure, bradycardia, acetylcholinesterase inhibition, hypotension, pulmonary edema, overstimulation of parasympathetic nervous system, striated muscle, sympathetic ganglia, and CNS.*

**gutta-percha** [Turpentine/terpene] *Respiratory failure, pulmonary edema, tachycardia.*

**hafnium; hafnium mixture (n.o.s.)** [Flammable solid] *Shock, severe chemical and thermal burns, severe respiratory tract irritation, pulmonary edema, respiratory arrest, ECG changes, sudden death.*

**halogenated solvent (n.o.s.)** [Halogenated aliphatic hydrocarbon] *CNS depression, respiratory arrest, circulatory collapse.*

**Halon (all types)** [Chlorinated fluorocarbon] *Asphyxiation, anesthesia, arrhythmias.*

**hay** [Flammable solid] *Shock, severe chemical and thermal burns, severe respiratory tract irritation, pulmonary edema, respiratory arrest, ECG changes, sudden death.*

**hazardous waste (n.o.s.)** [Poison] *Cardiovascular collapse, pulmonary edema, CNS depression, coma, seizures, nausea, vomiting, cardiopulmonary arrest.*

**helium (gas or cryogenic liquid)** [Simple asphyxiant] *Asphyxiation.*

**helium & oxygen mixture** [Simple asphyxiant] *Asphyxiation.*

**hendecane** [Hydrocarbon mixture] *CNS depression, respiratory arrest, seizures, arrhythmias, pulmonary edema.*

**heptachlor** [Chlordane] *Respiratory failure, seizures, exhaustion, death.*

**heptachlor epoxide** [Chlordane] *Respiratory failure, seizures, exhaustion, death.*

HazMat

**n-heptaldehyde** [Aldehyde] *Seizures, respiratory failure, pulmonary edema.*

**heptane; n-heptane** [Aliphatic hydrocarbon] *Arrhythmias, asphyxiation, anesthesia.* ⊉ heptene

**heptene** [Aliphatic hydrocarbon] *Arrhythmias, asphyxiation, anesthesia.* ⊉ heptane

**hexachloroacetone** [Ketone] *Respiratory mucous membrane irritation, pulmonary edema, CNS depression.*

**hexachlorobenzene** [Lindane] *CNS stimulation, seizures, respiratory failure.*

**hexachlorobutadiene; hexachloro-1,3-butadiene** [Halogenated aliphatic hydrocarbon] *CNS depression, respiratory arrest, circulatory collapse.*

**hexachlorocyclohexane** [Lindane] *CNS stimulation, seizures, respiratory failure.*

**hexachlorocyclopentadiene** [Halogenated aliphatic hydrocarbon] *CNS depression, respiratory arrest, circulatory collapse.*

**hexachloro-epoxy-octahydro-dimethanonaphthalene** [Aldrin/dieldrin/endrin] *Seizures, respiratory failure.*

**hexachloroethane** [Halogenated aliphatic hydrocarbon] *CNS depression, respiratory arrest, circulatory collapse.*

**hexachloronaphthalene** [Naphthalene] *Delayed-onset acute intravascular hemolysis.*

**hexachlorophene** [Halogenated aliphatic hydrocarbon] *CNS depression, respiratory arrest, circulatory collapse.* [Phenol] *Coma, hypotension, arrhythmias, pulmonary edema, respiratory arrest.*

**hexachloropropene** [Halogenated aliphatic hydrocarbon] *CNS depression, respiratory arrest, circulatory collapse.*

**hexadecyl alcohol** [Higher alcohol (4+ carbons)] *CNS depression, respiratory failure, arrhythmias.*

**hexadecyl trichlorosilane** [Silane/chlorosilane] *Respiratory tract irritation, pulmonary edema.*

**hexadiene** [Aliphatic hydrocarbon] *Arrhythmias, asphyxiation, anesthesia.*

**hexaethyl tetraphosphate; hexaethyl tetraphosphate mixture (n.o.s.)** [Organophosphate] *Pulmonary edema, respiratory muscle paralysis, respiratory failure, bradycardia, acetylcholinesterase inhibition, hypotension, pulmonary edema, overstimulation of parasympathetic nervous system, striated muscle, sympathetic ganglia, and CNS.*

**hexafluoroacetone** [Ketone] *Respiratory mucous membrane irritation, pulmonary edema, CNS depression.*

**hexafluoroacetone hydrate** [Ketone] *Respiratory mucous membrane irritation, pulmonary edema, CNS depression.*

**hexafluoroethane** [Halogenated aliphatic hydrocarbon] *CNS depression, respiratory arrest, circulatory collapse.*

**hexafluorophosphoric acid** [Inorganic acid] *Pulmonary edema, bronchospasm, circulatory collapse, laryngeal spasm and edema, severe chemical burns to skin, mucous membranes, and internal organs, GI tract perforation and hemorrhage, peritonitis.*

**hexafluoropropylene** [Halogenated aliphatic hydrocarbon] *CNS depression, respiratory arrest, circulatory collapse.*

**hexafluoropropylene oxide** [Halogenated aliphatic hydrocarbon] *CNS depression, respiratory arrest, circulatory collapse.* [Ether] *Anesthesia, respiratory arrest.*

**hexahydrocresol** [Phenol] *Coma, hypotension, arrhythmias, pulmonary edema, respiratory arrest.*

**hexaldehyde** [Aldehyde] *Seizures, respiratory failure, pulmonary edema.*

**hexamethylene diamine** [Organic base/amine] *Pulmonary edema, cardiac depression, seizures.*

**hexamethylene diisocyanate** [Isocyanate/aliphatic thiocyanate] *CNS depression, respiratory arrest, respiratory paralysis, pulmonary edema, cyanide toxicity.*

**hexamethyleneimine** [Organic base/amine] *Pulmonary edema, cardiac depression, seizures.*

**hexamethylenetetramine** [Organic base/amine] *Pulmonary edema, cardiac depression, seizures.*

**hexamethylphosphoramide** [Aliphatic hydrocarbon] *Arrhythmias, asphyxiation, anesthesia.*

**3,3,6,6,9,9-hexamethyl-1,2,4,5-tetraoxocyclononane** [Organic peroxide] *Pulmonary and laryngeal edema, circulatory arrest, hypovolemic shock, chemical burns to skin, mucous membranes, and internal organs.*

**hexamine** [Organic base/amine] *Pulmonary edema, cardiac depression, seizures.*

**hexane; n-hexane** [Aliphatic hydrocarbon] *Arrhythmias, asphyxiation, anesthesia.* ⚇ hexene

**1,2,6-hexanetriol** [Higher alcohol (4+ carbons)] *CNS depression, respiratory failure, arrhythmias.*

**hexanoic acid (caproic acid)** [Organic acid] *Pulmonary edema, circulatory collapse, laryngeal edema and spasm, severe chemical burns to skin, mucous membranes, and internal organs, GI tract perforation and hemorrhage, peritonitis.*

**hexanol** [Higher alcohol (4+ carbons)] *CNS depression, respiratory failure, arrhythmias.*

**hexene; 1-hexene** [Aliphatic hydrocarbon] *Arrhythmias, asphyxiation, anesthesia.* ⚇ hexane

**hexyl alcohol** [Higher alcohol (4+ carbons)] *CNS depression, respiratory failure, arrhythmias.*

**hexyl trichorosilane** [Silane/chlorosilane] *Respiratory tract irritation, pulmonary edema.*

**hexylene glycol** [Ethylene glycol] *Respiratory failure, pulmonary edema, paralysis, cardiovascular collapse, severe acidosis.*

**hexylresorcinol** [Phenol] *Coma, hypotension, arrhythmias, pulmonary edema, respiratory arrest.*

**HF (hydrofluoric acid)** [Hydrofluoric acid] *Pulmonary and laryngeal edema, circulatory collapse, severe skin burns, GI tract perforation, systemic fluoride poisoning.*

**HFC 134A; R134A refrigerant (1,1,1,2-tetrafluoroethane)** [Chlorinated fluorocarbon] *Asphyxiation, anesthesia, arrhythmias.*

**hydrastine** [Acrolein] *Severe respiratory tract irritation, pulmonary edema, respiratory failure.*

**hydraulic fluids (n.o.s.)** [Hydrocarbon mixture] *CNS depression, respiratory arrest, seizures, arrhythmias, pulmonary edema.*

**hydrazine** [Hydrazine] *Seizures, hemolysis of red blood cells, pulmonary edema.*

**hydrazine hydrate** [Hydrazine] *Seizures, hemolysis of red blood cells, pulmonary edema.*

**hydrazine sulfate** [Hydrazine] *Seizures, hemolysis of red blood cells, pulmonary edema.*

**hydrazobenzene** [Hydrazine] *Seizures, hemolysis of red blood cells, pulmonary edema.*

**hydride, metal (n.o.s.)** [Poison] *Cardiovascular collapse, pulmonary edema, CNS depression, coma, seizures, nausea, vomiting, cardiopulmonary arrest.*

**hydriodic acid; hydriodic acid mixture (n.o.s.)** [Inorganic acid] *Pulmonary edema, bronchospasm, circulatory collapse, laryngeal spasm and edema, severe chemical burns to skin, mucous membranes, and internal organs, GI tract perforation and hemorrhage, peritonitis.* [Iodine] *Hypotension, circulatory collapse, pulmonary edema.*

**hydrobromic acid; hydrobromic acid mixture (n.o.s.)** [Bromine/methylbromide] *Severe respiratory irritation, pulmonary edema, respiratory failure, coma, convulsions, death.*

**hydrocarbon, aliphatic (n.o.s.)** [Aliphatic hydrocarbon] *Arrhythmias, asphyxiation, anesthesia.*

HazMat

**hydrocarbon, chlorinated** [Halogenated aliphatic hydrocarbon] *CNS depression, respiratory arrest, circulatory collapse.*

**hydrocarbon gas (n.o.s.)** [Flammable gas] *Respiratory failure, cardiac arrest, arrhythmias.* [Aliphatic hydrocarbon] *Arrhythmias, asphyxiation, anesthesia.*

**hydrocarbon gas drip** [Hydrocarbon mixture] *CNS depression, respiratory arrest, seizures, arrhythmias, pulmonary edema.*

**hydrocarbon solvent (n.o.s.)** [Hydrocarbon mixture] *CNS depression, respiratory arrest, seizures, arrhythmias, pulmonary edema.*

**hydrocarbon solvent, aromatic (n.o.s.)** [Aromatic hydrocarbon] *Arrhythmias, respiratory failure, pulmonary edema, paralysis, brain and kidney damage.*

**hydrochloric acid** [Inorganic acid] *Pulmonary edema, bronchospasm, circulatory collapse, laryngeal spasm and edema, severe chemical burns to skin, mucous membranes, and internal organs, GI tract perforation and hemorrhage, peritonitis.*

**hydrocyanic acid** [Cyanide] *Impairment of cellular oxygenation and adenosine triphosphate production, hypoxia, death.*

**hydrofluoric acid (HF)** [Hydrofluoric acid] *Pulmonary and laryngeal edema, circulatory collapse, severe skin burns, GI tract perforation, systemic fluoride poisoning.*

**hydrofluoric acid & sulfuric acid mixture** [Inorganic acid] *Pulmonary edema, bronchospasm, circulatory collapse, laryngeal spasm and edema, severe chemical burns to skin, mucous membranes, and internal organs, GI tract perforation and hemorrhage, peritonitis.* [Hydrofluoric acid] *Pulmonary and laryngeal edema, circulatory collapse, severe skin burns, GI tract perforation, systemic fluoride poisoning.*

**hydrofluosilicic acid** [Hydrofluoric acid] *Pulmonary and laryngeal edema, circulatory collapse, severe skin burns, GI tract perforation, systemic fluoride poisoning.*

**hydrogen (gas or cryogenic liquid)** [Flammable gas] *Respiratory failure, cardiac arrest, arrhythmias.* [Simple asphyxiant] *Asphyxiation.*

**hydrogen arsenide** [Arsenic] *Heavy metal toxicity, vomiting, GI bleeding, CNS depression, pulmonary edema, cardiac arrest.*

**hydrogen bromide** [Bromine/methylbromide] *Severe respiratory irritation, pulmonary edema, respiratory failure, coma, convulsions, death.*

**hydrogen & carbon monoxide mixture** [Carbon monoxide] *Impairment of cellular oxygenation, hypoxia, death.*

**hydrogen chloride** [Inorganic acid] *Pulmonary edema, bronchospasm, circulatory collapse, laryngeal spasm and edema, severe chemical burns to skin, mucous membranes, and internal organs, GI tract perforation and hemorrhage, peritonitis.*

**hydrogen cyanide** [Cyanide] *Impairment of cellular oxygenation and adenosine triphosphate production, hypoxia, death.*

**hydrogen fluoride** [Hydrofluoric acid] *Pulmonary and laryngeal edema, circulatory collapse, severe skin burns, GI tract perforation, systemic fluoride poisoning.*

**hydrogen iodide** [Iodine] *Hypotension, circulatory collapse, pulmonary edema.*

**hydrogen & methane mixture** [Simple asphyxiant] *Asphyxiation.*

**hydrogen peroxide** [Oxidizer] *Pulmonary and laryngeal edema, circulatory arrest, hypovolemic shock, chemical burns of skin, mucous membranes, and internal organs.*

**hydrogen peroxide & peroxyacetic acid mixture** [Oxidizer] *Pulmonary and laryngeal edema, circulatory arrest, hypovolemic shock, chemical burns of skin, mucous membranes, and internal organs.*

**hydrogen phosphide** [Phosphine] *Severe pulmonary irritation, pulmonary edema.*

**hydrogen selenide** [Selenium] *Arrhythmias, pulmonary edema, bronchospasm, seizures, vomiting, GI bleeding.*

**hydrogen sulfide** [Hydrogen sulfide] *Severe respiratory tract irritation, pulmonary edema, respiratory paralysis.*

**hydroperoxide** [Oxidizer] *Pulmonary and laryngeal edema, circulatory arrest, hypovolemic shock, chemical burns of skin, mucous membranes, and internal organs.*

**hydroquinone** [Aniline] *Methemoglobinemia, hypoxia.* [Phenol] *Coma, hypotension, arrhythmias, pulmonary edema, respiratory arrest.*

**hydroselenic acid** [Inorganic acid] *Pulmonary edema, bronchospasm, circulatory collapse, laryngeal spasm and edema, severe chemical burns to skin, mucous membranes, and internal organs, GI tract perforation and hemorrhage, peritonitis.* [Selenium] *Arrhythmias, pulmonary edema, bronchospasm, seizures, vomiting, GI bleeding.*

**hydrosilicofluoric acid** [Hydrofluoric acid] *Pulmonary and laryngeal edema, circulatory collapse, severe skin burns, GI tract perforation, systemic fluoride poisoning.*

**DL-(1-hydroxycyclohexyl) peroxide** [Organic peroxide] *Pulmonary and laryngeal edema, circulatory arrest, hypovolemic shock, chemical burns to skin, mucous membranes, and internal organs.*

**3-(2-hydroxyethoxy)-4-pyrrolidin-1-ylbenzene-diazonium zinc chloride** [Zinc] *Respiratory tract irritation, metal fume fever, pulmonary edema.*

**1-hydroxy-1'-hydroperoxy dicyclohexyl peroxide** [Organic peroxide] *Pulmonary and laryngeal edema, circulatory arrest, hypovolemic shock, chemical burns to skin, mucous membranes, and internal organs.*

**hydroxylamine** [Organic base/amine] *Pulmonary edema, cardiac depression, seizures.*

**hydroxylamine sulfate** [Organic base/amine] *Pulmonary edema, cardiac depression, seizures.*

**hydroxymercuricresol** [Mercury] *Circulatory collapse, arrhythmias, respiratory failure, pulmonary edema, neurotoxic effects.*

**hydroxymercurinitrophenol** [Nitrate/nitrite] *Methemoglobinemia, hypotension, circulatory collapse.* [Mercury] *Circulatory collapse, arrhythmias, respiratory failure, pulmonary edema, neurotoxic effects.*

**4-hydroxy-3-nitrophenylarsonic acid** [Arsenic] *Heavy metal toxicity, vomiting, GI bleeding, CNS depression, pulmonary edema, cardiac arrest.*

**hydroxyphenylmercurichloride** [Mercury] *Circulatory collapse, arrhythmias, respiratory failure, pulmonary edema, neurotoxic effects.*

**hypochlorite mixture (n.o.s.)** [Hypochlorite] *Circulatory collapse, respiratory tract irritation, upper airway obstruction, pulmonary edema.*

**ido methylpropane** [Halogenated aliphatic hydrocarbon] *CNS depression, respiratory arrest, circulatory collapse.*

**igniter for aircraft propulsion device** [Flammable solid] *Shock, severe chemical and thermal burns, severe respiratory tract irritation, pulmonary edema, respiratory arrest, ECG changes, sudden death.*

**Imidan** [Organophosphate] *Pulmonary edema, respiratory muscle paralysis, respiratory failure, bradycardia, acetylcholinesterase inhibition, hypotension, pulmonary edema, overstimulation of parasympathetic nervous system, striated muscle, sympathetic ganglia, and CNS.*

**iminobispropylamine** [Organic base/amine] *Pulmonary edema, cardiac depression, seizures.*

**iminodipropylamine** [Organic base/amine] *Pulmonary edema, cardiac depression, seizures.*

**indeno(1,2,3-cd)pyrene** [Aromatic hydrocarbon] *Arrhythmias, respiratory*

**HazMat**

*failure, pulmonary edema, paralysis, brain and kidney damage.*

**infectious substance (n.o.s.)** *No acute symptoms during incubation period. Physiologic response varies depending on strain of microorganism or toxin.*

**ink** [Flammable/combustible liquid] *CNS depression, respiratory arrest, convulsions, arrhythmias, pulmonary edema.*

**insecticide (n.o.s.)** [Poison] *Cardiovascular collapse, pulmonary edema, CNS depression, coma, seizures, nausea, vomiting, cardiopulmonary arrest.*

**insecticide gas (n.o.s.)** [Poison] *Cardiovascular collapse, pulmonary edema, CNS depression, coma, seizures, nausea, vomiting, cardiopulmonary arrest.* [Organophosphate] *Pulmonary edema, respiratory muscle paralysis, respiratory failure, bradycardia, acetylcholinesterase inhibition, hypotension, pulmonary edema, overstimulation of parasympathetic nervous system, striated muscle, sympathetic ganglia, and CNS.*

**iodine monochloride** [Iodine] *Hypotension, circulatory collapse, pulmonary edema.*

**iodine pentafluoride** [Hydrofluoric acid] *Pulmonary and laryngeal edema, circulatory collapse, severe skin burns, GI tract perforation, systemic fluoride poisoning.* [Iodine] *Hypotension, circulatory collapse, pulmonary edema.*

**iodo butane** [Halogenated aliphatic hydrocarbon] *CNS depression, respiratory arrest, circulatory collapse.*

**iodo propane** [Halogenated aliphatic hydrocarbon] *CNS depression, respiratory arrest, circulatory collapse.*

**IPDI** [Isocyanate/aliphatic thiocyanate] *CNS depression, respiratory arrest, respiratory paralysis, pulmonary edema, cyanide toxicity.*

**iron carbonyl** [Iron] *Hypovolemic shock.*

**iron chloride; ferric chloride; ferrous chloride** [Iron] *Hypovolemic shock.*

**iron oxide** [Iron] *Hypovolemic shock.*

**iron pentacarbonyl** [Iron] *Hypovolemic shock.*

**iron sponge** [Iron] *Hypovolemic shock.*

**iron swarf** [Iron] *Hypovolemic shock.*

**irritating substance (n.o.s.)** [Irritant] *Severe immediate or delayed upper airway or respiratory tract irritation, pulmonary edema, glottic spasm, airway obstruction.*

**isoamyl acetate** [Ester] *CNS depression, respiratory tract irritation, bronchitis, pneumonia.*

**isoamyl alcohol** [Higher alcohol (4+ carbons)] *CNS depression, respiratory failure, arrhythmias.*

**isobenzan** [Lindane] *CNS stimulation, seizures, respiratory failure.*

**isobutane; isobutane mixture (n.o.s.)** [Simple asphyxiant] *Asphyxiation.*

**isobutanol** [Higher alcohol (4+ carbons)] *CNS depression, respiratory failure, arrhythmias.*

**isobutyl acetate** [Ester] *CNS depression, respiratory tract irritation, bronchitis, pneumonia.*

**isobutyl acrylate** [Ester] *CNS depression, respiratory tract irritation, bronchitis, pneumonia.*

**isobutyl alcohol** [Higher alcohol (4+ carbons)] *CNS depression, respiratory failure, arrhythmias.*

**isobutyl aldehyde** [Aldehyde] *Seizures, respiratory failure, pulmonary edema.*

**isobutyl chloroformate** [Organic acid] *Pulmonary edema, circulatory collapse, laryngeal edema and spasm, severe chemical burns to skin, mucous membranes, and internal organs, GI tract perforation and hemorrhage, peritonitis.*

**isobutyl formate** [Ester] *CNS depression, respiratory tract irritation, bronchitis, pneumonia.*

**isobutyl isobutyrate** [Ester] *CNS depression, respiratory tract irritation, bronchitis, pneumonia.*

**isobutyl isocyanate** [Isocyanate/aliphatic thiocyanate] *CNS depression, respiratory arrest, respiratory paralysis, pulmonary edema, cyanide toxicity.*

**isobutyl methacrylate** [Ester] *CNS depression, respiratory tract irritation, bronchitis, pneumonia.*

**isobutyl methyl ketone peroxide** [Organic peroxide] *Pulmonary and laryngeal edema, circulatory arrest, hypovolemic shock, chemical burns to skin, mucous membranes, and internal organs.* [Ketone] *Respiratory mucous membrane irritation, pulmonary edema, CNS depression.* [Corrosive] *Upper airway burns and edema, circulatory collapse, severe chemical burns to skin, toxic systemic effects, GI tract perforation and hemorrhage, peritonitis.*

**isobutyl propionate** [Ester] *CNS depression, respiratory tract irritation, bronchitis, pneumonia.*

**isobutylamine; DL-isobutylamine** [Organic base/amine] *Pulmonary edema, cardiac depression, seizures.*

**isobutylene** [Aliphatic hydrocarbon] *Arrhythmias, asphyxiation, anesthesia.*

**DL-isobutylene** [Simple asphyxiant] *Asphyxiation.*

**isobutyraldehyde** [Aldehyde] *Seizures, respiratory failure, pulmonary edema.*

**isobutyric acid** [Organic acid] *Pulmonary edema, circulatory collapse, laryngeal edema and spasm, severe chemical burns to skin, mucous membranes, and internal organs, GI tract perforation and hemorrhage, peritonitis.*

**isobutyric anhydride** [Organic acid] *Pulmonary edema, circulatory collapse, laryngeal edema and spasm, severe chemical burns to skin, mucous membranes, and internal organs, GI tract perforation and hemorrhage, peritonitis.*

**isobutyronitrile** [Cyanide] *Impairment of cellular oxygenation and adenosine triphosphate production, hypoxia, death.*

**isobutyryl chloride** [Halogenated aliphatic hydrocarbon] *CNS depression, respiratory arrest, circulatory collapse.*

**isocyanate; isocyanate mixture (n.o.s.)** [Isocyanate/aliphatic thiocyanate] *CNS depression, respiratory arrest, respiratory paralysis, pulmonary edema, cyanide toxicity.*

**isocyanatobenzotrifluoride** [Isocyanate/aliphatic thiocyanate] *CNS depression, respiratory arrest, respiratory paralysis, pulmonary edema, cyanide toxicity.* [Fluorine] *CNS depression, respiratory arrest, cardiovascular collapse, shock, arrhythmias.*

**isocyanic acid** [Isocyanate/aliphatic thiocyanate] *CNS depression, respiratory arrest, respiratory paralysis, pulmonary edema, cyanide toxicity.*

**isocyanuric acid** [Organic acid] *Pulmonary edema, circulatory collapse, laryngeal edema and spasm, severe chemical burns to skin, mucous membranes, and internal organs, GI tract perforation and hemorrhage, peritonitis.*

**isododecane** [Aliphatic hydrocarbon] *Arrhythmias, asphyxiation, anesthesia.*

**isodrin** [Aldrin/dieldrin/endrin] *Seizures, respiratory failure.*

**isofluorphate** [Organophosphate] *Pulmonary edema, respiratory muscle paralysis, respiratory failure, bradycardia, acetylcholinesterase inhibition, hypotension, pulmonary edema, overstimulation of parasympathetic nervous system, striated muscle, sympathetic ganglia, and CNS.*

**isoheptene** [Aliphatic hydrocarbon] *Arrhythmias, asphyxiation, anesthesia.*

**isohexene** [Aliphatic hydrocarbon] *Arrhythmias, asphyxiation, anesthesia.*

**Isolan** [Carbamate] *Acetylcholinesterase inhibition (reversible), bradycardia, hypotension, respiratory muscle paralysis, respiratory arrest, pulmonary edema.*

**isononanoyl peroxide** [Organic peroxide] *Pulmonary and laryngeal edema, circulatory arrest, hypovolemic shock, chemical burns to skin, mucous membranes, and internal organs.*

**isononyl alcohol** [Higher alcohol (4+ carbons)] *CNS depression, respiratory failure, arrhythmias.*

**isooctane** [Aliphatic hydrocarbon] *Arrhythmias, asphyxiation, anesthesia.*

**isooctene** [Aliphatic hydrocarbon] *Arrhythmias, asphyxiation, anesthesia.*

**HazMat**

**isooctyl alcohol** [Higher alcohol (4+ carbons)] *CNS depression, respiratory failure, arrhythmias.*

**isopentane** [Aliphatic hydrocarbon] *Arrhythmias, asphyxiation, anesthesia.* ⊘ isopentene

**isopentanoic acid** [Organic acid] *Pulmonary edema, circulatory collapse, laryngeal edema and spasm, severe chemical burns to skin, mucous membranes, and internal organs, GI tract perforation and hemorrhage, peritonitis.*

**isopentene** [Aliphatic hydrocarbon] *Arrhythmias, asphyxiation, anesthesia.* ⊘ isopentane

**isophorone** [Ketone] *Respiratory mucous membrane irritation, pulmonary edema, CNS depression.*

**isophorone diisocyanate** [Isocyanate/ aliphatic thiocyanate] *CNS depression, respiratory arrest, respiratory paralysis, pulmonary edema, cyanide toxicity.*

**isophoronediamine** [Organic base/ amine] *Pulmonary edema, cardiac depression, seizures.*

**isoprene** [Aliphatic hydrocarbon] *Arrhythmias, asphyxiation, anesthesia.*

**isoprocarb** [Carbamate] *Acetylcholinesterase inhibition (reversible), bradycardia, hypotension, respiratory muscle paralysis, respiratory arrest, pulmonary edema.*

**isopropanol** [Lower alcohol (1–3 carbons)] *CNS depression, coma, respiratory arrest, arrhythmias.*

**isopropanolamine dodecylbenzene sulfonate** [Poison] *Cardiovascular collapse, pulmonary edema, CNS depression, coma, seizures, nausea, vomiting, cardiopulmonary arrest.*

**isopropenyl acetate** [Ester] *CNS depression, respiratory tract irritation, bronchitis, pneumonia.*

**isopropenyl benzene** [Aromatic hydrocarbon] *Arrhythmias, respiratory failure, pulmonary edema, paralysis, brain and kidney damage.*

**isopropyl acetate** [Ester] *CNS depression, respiratory tract irritation, bronchitis, pneumonia.*

**isopropyl acid phosphate** [Ester] · *CNS depression, respiratory tract irritation, bronchitis, pneumonia.*

**isopropyl alcohol** [Lower alcohol (1–3 carbons)] *CNS depression, coma, respiratory arrest, arrhythmias.*

**isopropyl amine** [Organic base/ amine] *Pulmonary edema, cardiac depression, seizures.*

**isopropyl butyrate** [Ester] *CNS depression, respiratory tract irritation, bronchitis, pneumonia.*

**isopropyl chloroacetate** [Ester] *CNS depression, respiratory tract irritation, bronchitis, pneumonia.*

**isopropyl chloroformate** [Ester] *CNS depression, respiratory tract irritation, bronchitis, pneumonia.*

**isopropyl chloropropionate** [Ester] *CNS depression, respiratory tract irritation, bronchitis, pneumonia.*

**isopropyl ether; DL-isopropyl ether** [Ether] *Anesthesia, respiratory arrest.*

**isopropyl formate** [Ester] *CNS depression, respiratory tract irritation, bronchitis, pneumonia.*

**isopropyl isobutyrate** [Ester] *CNS depression, respiratory tract irritation, bronchitis, pneumonia.*

**isopropyl isocyanate** [Isocyanate/aliphatic thiocyanate] *CNS depression, respiratory arrest, respiratory paralysis, pulmonary edema, cyanide toxicity.*

**isopropyl mercaptan** [Sulfur] *Respiratory tract irritation, pulmonary edema, anaphylaxis.*

**isopropyl nitrate** [Nitrate/nitrite] *Methemoglobinemia, hypotension, circulatory collapse.*

**isopropyl peroxydicarbonate** [Organic peroxide] *Pulmonary and laryngeal edema, circulatory arrest, hypovolemic shock, chemical burns to skin, mucous membranes, and internal organs.*

**isopropyl propionate** [Ester] *CNS depression, respiratory tract irritation, bronchitis, pneumonia.*

**isopropylbenzene** [Aromatic hydrocarbon] *Arrhythmias, respiratory fail-*

ure, *pulmonary edema, paralysis, brain and kidney damage.*

**isopropylcumyl hydroperoxide** [Organic peroxide] *Pulmonary and laryngeal edema, circulatory arrest, hypovolemic shock, chemical burns to skin, mucous membranes, and internal organs.* [Aromatic hydrocarbon] *Arrhythmias, respiratory failure, pulmonary edema, paralysis, brain and kidney damage.*

**4,4'-isopropylidene diphenol** [Phenol] *Coma, hypotension, arrhythmias, pulmonary edema, respiratory arrest.*

**isopropylmethylpyrazolyl dimethylcarbamate** [Carbamate] *Acetylcholinesterase inhibition (reversible), bradycardia, hypotension, respiratory muscle paralysis, respiratory arrest, pulmonary edema.*

**isosafrole** [Phenol] *Coma, hypotension, arrhythmias, pulmonary edema, respiratory arrest.*

**isosorbide dinitrate mixture (n.o.s.)** [Nitrate/nitrite] *Methemoglobinemia, hypotension, circulatory collapse.*

**jet fuel** [Hydrocarbon mixture] *CNS depression, respiratory arrest, seizures, arrhythmias, pulmonary edema.*

**kanechlor S** Polychlorinated biphenyl/polybrominated biphenyl/polychlorinated [dibenzofuran] *Liver and kidney damage.*

**Kelthane** [Lindane] *CNS stimulation, seizures, respiratory failure.*

**Kepone** [Lindane] *CNS stimulation, seizures, respiratory failure.*

**kerosene** [Hydrocarbon mixture] *CNS depression, respiratory arrest, seizures, arrhythmias, pulmonary edema.*

**ketene** [Aldehyde] *Seizures, respiratory failure, pulmonary edema.*

**ketone (n.o.s.)** [Ketone] *Respiratory mucous membrane irritation, pulmonary edema, CNS depression.*

**krypton (gas or cryogenic liquid)** [Simple asphyxiant] *Asphyxiation.*

**lacquer** [Hydrocarbon mixture] *CNS depression, respiratory arrest, seizures, arrhythmias, pulmonary edema.*

**lactic acid** [Organic acid] *Pulmonary edema, circulatory collapse, laryngeal edema and spasm, severe chemical burns to skin, mucous membranes, and internal organs, GI tract perforation and hemorrhage, peritonitis.*

**lactonitrile** [Cyanide] *Impairment of cellular oxygenation and adenosine triphosphate production, hypoxia, death.*

**landrin** [Carbamate] *Acetylcholinesterase inhibition (reversible), bradycardia, hypotension, respiratory muscle paralysis, respiratory arrest, pulmonary edema.*

**Lannate** [Carbamate] *Acetylcholinesterase inhibition (reversible), bradycardia, hypotension, respiratory muscle paralysis, respiratory arrest, pulmonary edema.*

**lasiocarpine** [Poison] *Cardiovascular collapse, pulmonary edema, CNS depression, coma, seizures, nausea, vomiting, cardiopulmonary arrest.*

**lauroyl peroxide** [Organic peroxide] *Pulmonary and laryngeal edema, circulatory arrest, hypovolemic shock, chemical burns to skin, mucous membranes, and internal organs.*

**lauryl alcohol** [Higher alcohol (4+ carbons)] *CNS depression, respiratory failure, arrhythmias.*

**lauryl thiocyanate** [Isocyanate/aliphatic thiocyanate] *CNS depression, respiratory arrest, respiratory paralysis, pulmonary edema, cyanide toxicity.*

**lead; lead mixture (n.o.s.)** [Lead] *Circulatory collapse, coma, rare seizures.*

**lead acetate** [Lead] *Circulatory collapse, coma, rare seizures.*

**lead arsenate** [Arsenic] *Heavy metal toxicity, vomiting, GI bleeding, CNS depression, pulmonary edema, cardiac arrest.* [Lead] *Circulatory collapse, coma, rare seizures.*

**lead arsenite** [Arsenic] *Heavy metal toxicity, vomiting, GI bleeding, CNS depression, pulmonary edema, cardiac arrest.* [Lead] *Circulatory collapse, coma, rare seizures.*

**lead chloride** [Lead] *Circulatory collapse, coma, rare seizures.*

HazMat

**lead chromate** [Lead] *Circulatory collapse, coma, rare seizures.*

**lead cyanide** [Lead] *Circulatory collapse, coma, rare seizures.* [Cyanide] *Impairment of cellular oxygenation and adenosine triphosphate production, hypoxia, death.*

**lead dioxide** [Lead] *Circulatory collapse, coma, rare seizures.*

**lead fluoborate** [Lead] *Circulatory collapse, coma, rare seizures.* [Boron] *Respiratory tract irritation, laryngeal spasm and edema, pulmonary edema, severe chemical burns.*

**lead fluoride** [Lead] *Circulatory collapse, coma, rare seizures.* [Fluorine] *CNS depression, respiratory arrest, cardiovascular collapse, shock, arrhythmias.*

**lead iodide** [Lead] *Circulatory collapse, coma, rare seizures.* [Iodine] *Hypotension, circulatory collapse, pulmonary edema.*

**lead nitrate** [Nitrate/nitrite] *Methemoglobinemia, hypotension, circulatory collapse.* [Lead] *Circulatory collapse, coma, rare seizures.*

**lead perchlorate** [Lead] *Circulatory collapse, coma, rare seizures.*

**lead peroxide** [Lead] *Circulatory collapse, coma, rare seizures.*

**lead phosphate** [Lead] *Circulatory collapse, coma, rare seizures.*

**lead phosphite** [Lead] *Circulatory collapse, coma, rare seizures.*

**lead stearate** [Lead] *Circulatory collapse, coma, rare seizures.*

**lead subacetate** [Lead] *Circulatory collapse, coma, rare seizures.*

**lead sulfate** [Lead] *Circulatory collapse, coma, rare seizures.*

**lead sulfide** [Lead] *Circulatory collapse, coma, rare seizures.*

**lead tetraethyl** [Lead] *Circulatory collapse, coma, rare seizures.*

**lead tetramethyl** [Lead] *Circulatory collapse, coma, rare seizures.*

**lead thiocyanate** [Lead] *Circulatory collapse, coma, rare seizures.* [Isocyanate/aliphatic thiocyanate] *CNS depression, respiratory arrest, respiratory paralysis, pulmonary edema, cyanide toxicity.*

**leptophos** [Organophosphate] *Pulmonary edema, respiratory muscle paralysis, respiratory failure, bradycardia, acetylcholinesterase inhibition, hypotension, pulmonary edema, overstimulation of parasympathetic nervous system, striated muscle, sympathetic ganglia, and CNS.*

**Lethane 60** [Isocyanate/aliphatic thiocyanate] *CNS depression, respiratory arrest, respiratory paralysis, pulmonary edema, cyanide toxicity.*

**lewisite** [Arsine] *Intravascular hemolysis, pulmonary edema, cardiac and respiratory arrest, delayed-onset jaundice and renal failure.*

**lewisite (liquid arsenic compound)** [Arsenic] *Heavy metal toxicity, vomiting, GI bleeding, CNS depression, pulmonary edema, cardiac arrest.*

**lighter, cigarette, and refills** [Aliphatic hydrocarbon] *Arrhythmias, asphyxiation, anesthesia.*

**lighter fluid** [Aliphatic hydrocarbon] *Arrhythmias, asphyxiation, anesthesia.*

**lime** [Inorganic base/alkaline corrosive] *Upper airway burns and edema, pulmonary edema, skin burns, circulatory collapse, GI tract perforation and hemorrhage, peritonitis.*

**lime, chlorinated** [Hypochlorite] *Circulatory collapse, respiratory tract irritation, upper airway obstruction, pulmonary edema.*

**limonene** [Turpentine/terpene] *Respiratory failure, pulmonary edema, tachycardia.*

**linamarin** [Cyanide] *Impairment of cellular oxygenation and adenosine triphosphate production, hypoxia, death.*

**lindane** [Lindane] *CNS stimulation, seizures, respiratory failure.*

**liquefied gas (n.o.s.)** [Flammable gas] *Respiratory failure, cardiac arrest, arrhythmias.*

**liquefied gas, flammable poison (n.o.s.)** [Flammable gas] *Respiratory failure, cardiac arrest, arrhythmias.*

[Poison] *Cardiovascular collapse, pulmonary edema, CNS depression, coma, seizures, nausea, vomiting, cardiopulmonary arrest.*

**liquefied gas, nonflammable (nitrogen, carbon dioxide, or air)** [Nonflammable gas] *Pulmonary edema, respiratory failure, asphyxiation.*

**liquefied gas, poisonous (n.o.s.)** [Flammable gas] *Respiratory failure, cardiac arrest, arrhythmias.* [Poison] *Cardiovascular collapse, pulmonary edema, CNS depression, coma, seizures, nausea, vomiting, cardiopulmonary arrest.*

**liquefied natural gas (LNG)** [Aliphatic hydrocarbon] *Arrhythmias, asphyxiation, anesthesia.* [Simple asphyxiant] *Asphyxiation.*

**liquefied petroleum gas (LPG)** [Flammable gas] *Respiratory failure, cardiac arrest, arrhythmias.* [Hydrocarbon mixture] *CNS depression, respiratory arrest, seizures, arrhythmias, pulmonary edema.*

**lithium** [Lithium] *Chemical burns to respiratory tract, pulmonary edema.*

**lithium acetylide & ethylenediamine mixture** [Lithium] *Chemical burns to respiratory tract, pulmonary edema.*

**lithium alkyl** [Lithium] *Chemical burns to respiratory tract, pulmonary edema.*

**lithium aluminum hydride** [Lithium] *Chemical burns to respiratory tract, pulmonary edema.*

**lithium battery** [Lithium] *Chemical burns to respiratory tract, pulmonary edema.*

**lithium borohydride** [Lithium] *Chemical burns to respiratory tract, pulmonary edema.* [Boron] *Respiratory tract irritation, laryngeal spasm and edema, pulmonary edema, severe chemical burns.*

**lithium chromate** [Lithium] *Chemical burns to respiratory tract, pulmonary edema.*

**lithium ferrosilicon** [Lithium] *Chemical burns to respiratory tract, pulmonary edema.*

**lithium hydride** [Lithium] *Chemical burns to respiratory tract, pulmonary edema.*

**lithium hydroxide** [Inorganic base/alkaline corrosive] *Upper airway burns and edema, pulmonary edema, skin burns, circulatory collapse, GI tract perforation and hemorrhage, peritonitis.* [Lithium] *Chemical burns to respiratory tract, pulmonary edema.*

**lithium hypochlorite** [Hypochlorite] *Circulatory collapse, respiratory tract irritation, upper airway obstruction, pulmonary edema.* [Lithium] *Chemical burns to respiratory tract, pulmonary edema.*

**lithium nitrate** [Nitrate/nitrite] *Methemoglobinemia, hypotension, circulatory collapse.* [Lithium] *Chemical burns to respiratory tract, pulmonary edema.*

**lithium nitride** [Nitrate/nitrite] *Methemoglobinemia, hypotension, circulatory collapse.* [Lithium] *Chemical burns to respiratory tract, pulmonary edema.*

**lithium peroxide** [Lithium] *Chemical burns to respiratory tract, pulmonary edema.*

**lithium silicon** [Lithium] *Chemical burns to respiratory tract, pulmonary edema.*

**lithopone** [Barium] *Hypokalemia, muscle paralysis, arrhythmias, cardiac and respiratory arrest.* [Zinc] *Respiratory tract irritation, metal fume fever, pulmonary edema.*

**LNG (liquefied natural gas)** [Aliphatic hydrocarbon] *Arrhythmias, asphyxiation, anesthesia.* [Simple asphyxiant] *Asphyxiation.*

**London purple** [Aniline] *Methemoglobinemia, hypoxia.* [Arsenic] *Heavy metal toxicity, vomiting, GI bleeding, CNS depression, pulmonary edema, cardiac arrest.*

**LPG (liquefied petroleum gas)** [Flammable gas] *Respiratory failure, cardiac arrest, arrhythmias.* [Hydrocarbon mixture] *CNS depression, respiratory arrest, seizures, arrhythmias, pulmonary edema.*

**HazMat**

**lye** [Inorganic base/alkaline corrosive] *Upper airway burns and edema, pulmonary edema, skin burns, circulatory collapse, GI tract perforation and hemorrhage, peritonitis.*

**magnesium; magnesium alloy (n.o.s.)** [Magnesium] *Cardiovascular collapse, respiratory depression.*

**magnesium alkyl** [Magnesium] *Cardiovascular collapse, respiratory depression.*

**magnesium aluminum phosphide** [Magnesium] *Cardiovascular collapse, respiratory depression.* [Phosphine] *Severe pulmonary irritation, pulmonary edema.*

**magnesium arsenate** [Arsenic] *Heavy metal toxicity, vomiting, GI bleeding, CNS depression, pulmonary edema, cardiac arrest.* [Magnesium] *Cardiovascular collapse, respiratory depression.*

**magnesium bisulfite** [Magnesium] *Cardiovascular collapse, respiratory depression.* [Sulfur] *Respiratory tract irritation, pulmonary edema, anaphylaxis.*

**magnesium bromate** [Magnesium] *Cardiovascular collapse, respiratory depression.* [Bromate] *CNS and respiratory system depression, delayed-onset renal failure.*

**magnesium chlorate** [Magnesium] *Cardiovascular collapse, respiratory depression.* [Chlorate] *Hemolysis, methemoglobinemia, hypoperfusion, CNS depression, delayed-onset renal failure.*

**magnesium chloride & chlorate mixture** [Magnesium] *Cardiovascular collapse, respiratory depression.* [Chlorate] *Hemolysis, methemoglobinemia, hypoperfusion, CNS depression, delayed-onset renal failure.*

**magnesium diamide** [Magnesium] *Cardiovascular collapse, respiratory depression.*

**magnesium diphenyl** [Magnesium] *Cardiovascular collapse, respiratory depression.*

**magnesium fluorosilicate** [Magnesium] *Cardiovascular collapse, respiratory depression.* [Fluorine] *CNS*

*depression, respiratory arrest, cardiovascular collapse, shock, arrhythmias.*

**magnesium hydride** [Magnesium] *Cardiovascular collapse, respiratory depression.*

**magnesium nitrate** [Nitrate/nitrite] *Methemoglobinemia, hypotension, circulatory collapse.* [Magnesium] *Cardiovascular collapse, respiratory depression.*

**magnesium perchlorate** [Magnesium] *Cardiovascular collapse, respiratory depression.* [Chlorate] *Hemolysis, methemoglobinemia, hypoperfusion, CNS depression, delayed-onset renal failure.*

**magnesium peroxide** [Magnesium] *Cardiovascular collapse, respiratory depression.*

**magnesium phosphide** [Magnesium] *Cardiovascular collapse, respiratory depression.* [Phosphine] *Severe pulmonary irritation, pulmonary edema.*

**magnesium silicide** [Magnesium] *Cardiovascular collapse, respiratory depression.*

**magnesium silicofluoride** [Magnesium] *Cardiovascular collapse, respiratory depression.* [Fluorine] *CNS depression, respiratory arrest, cardiovascular collapse, shock, arrhythmias.*

**malathion** [Organophosphate] *Pulmonary edema, respiratory muscle paralysis, respiratory failure, bradycardia, acetylcholinesterase inhibition, hypotension, pulmonary edema, overstimulation of parasympathetic nervous system, striated muscle, sympathetic ganglia, and CNS.*

**maleic acid** [Organic acid] *Pulmonary edema, circulatory collapse, laryngeal edema and spasm, severe chemical burns to skin, mucous membranes, and internal organs, GI tract perforation and hemorrhage, peritonitis.*

**maleic anhydride** [Organic acid] *Pulmonary edema, circulatory collapse, laryngeal edema and spasm, severe chemical burns to skin, mucous membranes, and internal organs, GI tract perforation and hemorrhage, peritonitis.*

**maleic hydrazide** [Organic acid] *Pulmonary edema, circulatory collapse, laryngeal edema and spasm, severe chemical burns to skin, mucous membranes, and internal organs, GI tract perforation and hemorrhage, peritonitis.*

**malonic dinitrile** [Cyanide] *Impairment of cellular oxygenation and adenosine triphosphate production, hypoxia, death.*

**malonic ethyl ester nitrile** [Cyanide] *Impairment of cellular oxygenation and adenosine triphosphate production, hypoxia, death.*

**malononitrile** [Cyanide] *Impairment of cellular oxygenation and adenosine triphosphate production, hypoxia, death.*

**mancozeb** [Carbamate] *Acetylcholinesterase inhibition (reversible), bradycardia, hypotension, respiratory muscle paralysis, respiratory arrest, pulmonary edema.*

**maneb; maneb mixture (n.o.s.)** [Dithiocarbamate] *Hypotension, respiratory failure.*

**manganese nitrate** [Nitrate/nitrite] *Methemoglobinemia, hypotension, circulatory collapse.* [Manganese] *Respiratory tract irritation, pulmonary edema.*

**manganese resinate** [Manganese] *Respiratory tract irritation, pulmonary edema.*

**manganese tricarbonyl methylcyclopentadine** [Manganese] *Respiratory tract irritation, pulmonary edema.*

**matches** [Chlorate] *Hemolysis, methemoglobinemia, hypoperfusion, CNS depression, delayed-onset renal failure.*

**MBOCA** [Aniline] *Methemoglobinemia, hypoxia.*

**MCPA** [Chlorophenoxy herbicide] *CNS depression, CNS stimulation, respiratory failure, ventricular fibrillation, seizures.*

**MDI (diphenylmethane-4,4′-diisocyanate)** [Isocyanate/aliphatic thiocyanate] *CNS depression, respiratory arrest, respiratory paralysis, pulmonary edema, cyanide toxicity.*

**MDI (methylene bis(4-phenyl isocyanate))** [Isocyanate/aliphatic thiocyanate] *CNS depression, respiratory arrest, respiratory paralysis, pulmonary edema, cyanide toxicity.*

**mechlorethamine** [Poison] *Cardiovascular collapse, pulmonary edema, CNS depression, coma, seizures, nausea, vomiting, cardiopulmonary arrest.*

**mecoprop** [Chlorophenoxy herbicide] *CNS depression, CNS stimulation, respiratory failure, ventricular fibrillation, seizures.*

**medication (n.o.s.)** [Poison] *Cardiovascular collapse, pulmonary edema, CNS depression, coma, seizures, nausea, vomiting, cardiopulmonary arrest.*

**melphalan** [Poison] *Cardiovascular collapse, pulmonary edema, CNS depression, coma, seizures, nausea, vomiting, cardiopulmonary arrest.*

**p-menthane hydroperoxide** [Organic peroxide] *Pulmonary and laryngeal edema, circulatory arrest, hypovolemic shock, chemical burns to skin, mucous membranes, and internal organs.*

**menthol** [Aromatic hydrocarbon] *Arrhythmias, respiratory failure, pulmonary edema, paralysis, brain and kidney damage.*

**p-menthyl hydroperoxide** [Organic peroxide] *Pulmonary and laryngeal edema, circulatory arrest, hypovolemic shock, chemical burns to skin, mucous membranes, and internal organs.*

**mercaptan; mercaptan mixture (n.o.s.)** [Sulfur] *Respiratory tract irritation, pulmonary edema, anaphylaxis.*

**mercaptodimethur** [Carbamate] *Acetylcholinesterase inhibition (reversible), bradycardia, hypotension, respiratory muscle paralysis, respiratory arrest, pulmonary edema.*

**mercuric acetate; mercurous acetate; mercury acetate** [Mercury] *Circulatory collapse, arrhythmias, respiratory failure, pulmonary edema, neurotoxic effects.*

**mercuric arsenate** [Arsenic] *Heavy metal toxicity, vomiting, GI bleeding, CNS depression, pulmonary edema, cardiac arrest.* [Mercury] *Circulatory collapse, arrhythmias, respiratory fail-*

**HazMat**

*ure, pulmonary edema, neurotoxic effects.*

**mercuric bromide; mercurous bromide; mercury bromide** [Mercury] *Circulatory collapse, arrhythmias, respiratory failure, pulmonary edema, neurotoxic effects.* [Bromine/methylbromide] *Severe respiratory irritation, pulmonary edema, respiratory failure, coma, convulsions, death.*

**mercuric chloride; mercurous chloride** [Mercury] *Circulatory collapse, arrhythmias, respiratory failure, pulmonary edema, neurotoxic effects.*

**mercuric cyanide; mercury cyanide** [Mercury] *Circulatory collapse, arrhythmias, respiratory failure, pulmonary edema, neurotoxic effects.* [Cyanide] *Impairment of cellular oxygenation and adenosine triphosphate production, hypoxia, death.*

**mercuric nitrate; mercurous nitrate** [Nitrate/nitrite] *Methemoglobinemia, hypotension, circulatory collapse.* [Mercury] *Circulatory collapse, arrhythmias, respiratory failure, pulmonary edema, neurotoxic effects.*

**mercuric oxide; mercury oxide** [Mercury] *Circulatory collapse, arrhythmias, respiratory failure, pulmonary edema, neurotoxic effects.*

**mercuric oxycyanide; mercury oxycyanide** [Mercury] *Circulatory collapse, arrhythmias, respiratory failure, pulmonary edema, neurotoxic effects.* [Cyanide] *Impairment of cellular oxygenation and adenosine triphosphate production, hypoxia, death.*

**mercuric potassium cyanide** [Mercury] *Circulatory collapse, arrhythmias, respiratory failure, pulmonary edema, neurotoxic effects.* [Cyanide] *Impairment of cellular oxygenation and adenosine triphosphate production, hypoxia, death.*

**mercuric sulfate; mercurous sulfate; mercury sulfate** [Mercury] *Circulatory collapse, arrhythmias, respiratory failure, pulmonary edema, neurotoxic effects.*

**mercuric thiocyanate; mercury thiocyanate** [Mercury] *Circulatory collapse, arrhythmias, respiratory failure, pulmonary edema, neurotoxic effects.* [Isocyanate/aliphatic thiocyanate] *CNS depression, respiratory arrest, respiratory paralysis, pulmonary edema, cyanide toxicity.*

**mercurol** [Mercury] *Circulatory collapse, arrhythmias, respiratory failure, pulmonary edema, neurotoxic effects.*

**mercurous acetate; mercuric acetate; mercury acetate** [Mercury] *Circulatory collapse, arrhythmias, respiratory failure, pulmonary edema, neurotoxic effects.*

**mercurous bromide; mercuric bromide; mercury bromide** [Mercury] *Circulatory collapse, arrhythmias, respiratory failure, pulmonary edema, neurotoxic effects.* [Bromine/methylbromide] *Severe respiratory irritation, pulmonary edema, respiratory failure, coma, convulsions, death.*

**mercurous chloride; mercuric chloride** [Mercury] *Circulatory collapse, arrhythmias, respiratory failure, pulmonary edema, neurotoxic effects.*

**mercurous nitrate; mercuric nitrate** [Nitrate/nitrite] *Methemoglobinemia, hypotension, circulatory collapse.* [Mercury] *Circulatory collapse, arrhythmias, respiratory failure, pulmonary edema, neurotoxic effects.*

**mercurous sulfate; mercuric sulfate; mercury sulfate** [Mercury] *Circulatory collapse, arrhythmias, respiratory failure, pulmonary edema, neurotoxic effects.*

**mercury; mercury mixture (n.o.s.)** [Mercury] *Circulatory collapse, arrhythmias, respiratory failure, pulmonary edema, neurotoxic effects.*

**mercury acetate; mercuric acetate; mercurous acetate** [Mercury] *Circulatory collapse, arrhythmias, respiratory failure, pulmonary edema, neurotoxic effects.*

**mercury ammonium chloride** [Mercury] *Circulatory collapse, arrhyth-*

mias, *respiratory failure, pulmonary edema, neurotoxic effects.*

**mercury benzoate** [Mercury] *Circulatory collapse, arrhythmias, respiratory failure, pulmonary edema, neurotoxic effects.*

**mercury bisulfate** [Mercury] *Circulatory collapse, arrhythmias, respiratory failure, pulmonary edema, neurotoxic effects.*

**mercury bromide; mercuric bromide; mercurous bromide** [Mercury] *Circulatory collapse, arrhythmias, respiratory failure, pulmonary edema, neurotoxic effects.* [Bromine/methylbromide] *Severe respiratory irritation, pulmonary edema, respiratory failure, coma, convulsions, death.*

**mercury cyanide; mercuric cyanide** [Mercury] *Circulatory collapse, arrhythmias, respiratory failure, pulmonary edema, neurotoxic effects.* [Cyanide] *Impairment of cellular oxygenation and adenosine triphosphate production, hypoxia, death.*

**mercury fulminate** [Mercury] *Circulatory collapse, arrhythmias, respiratory failure, pulmonary edema, neurotoxic effects.*

**mercury gluconate** [Mercury] *Circulatory collapse, arrhythmias, respiratory failure, pulmonary edema, neurotoxic effects.*

**mercury iodide** [Mercury] *Circulatory collapse, arrhythmias, respiratory failure, pulmonary edema, neurotoxic effects.* [Iodine] *Hypotension, circulatory collapse, pulmonary edema.*

**mercury nucleate** [Mercury] *Circulatory collapse, arrhythmias, respiratory failure, pulmonary edema, neurotoxic effects.*

**mercury oleate** [Mercury] *Circulatory collapse, arrhythmias, respiratory failure, pulmonary edema, neurotoxic effects.*

**mercury oxide; mercuric oxide** [Mercury] *Circulatory collapse, arrhythmias, respiratory failure, pulmonary edema, neurotoxic effects.*

**mercury oxycyanide; mercuric oxycyanide** [Mercury] *Circulatory collapse, arrhythmias, respiratory failure, pulmonary edema, neurotoxic effects.* [Cyanide] *Impairment of cellular oxygenation and adenosine triphosphate production, hypoxia, death.*

**mercury potassium iodide** [Mercury] *Circulatory collapse, arrhythmias, respiratory failure, pulmonary edema, neurotoxic effects.* [Iodine] *Hypotension, circulatory collapse, pulmonary edema.*

**mercury salicylate** [Mercury] *Circulatory collapse, arrhythmias, respiratory failure, pulmonary edema, neurotoxic effects.*

**mercury sulfate; mercuric sulfate; mercurous sulfate** [Mercury] *Circulatory collapse, arrhythmias, respiratory failure, pulmonary edema, neurotoxic effects.*

**mercury thiocyanate; mercuric thiocyanate** [Mercury] *Circulatory collapse, arrhythmias, respiratory failure, pulmonary edema, neurotoxic effects.* [Isocyanate/aliphatic thiocyanate] *CNS depression, respiratory arrest, respiratory paralysis, pulmonary edema, cyanide toxicity.*

**mercury-based pesticide (n.o.s.)** [Mercury] *Circulatory collapse, arrhythmias, respiratory failure, pulmonary edema, neurotoxic effects.*

**Merodicein** [Mercury] *Circulatory collapse, arrhythmias, respiratory failure, pulmonary edema, neurotoxic effects.*

**Mertect; Mertect 160** [Thiabendazole] *Cardiovascular collapse, respiratory tract irritation.*

**mesityl oxide** [Ketone] *Respiratory mucous membrane irritation, pulmonary edema, CNS depression.*

**mesitylene** [Aromatic hydrocarbon] *Arrhythmias, respiratory failure, pulmonary edema, paralysis, brain and kidney damage.*

**metal alkyl; metal alkyl halide (n.o.s.); metal alkyl hydride (n.o.s.)** [Poison] *Cardiovascular collapse, pulmonary edema, CNS depres-*

sion, coma, seizures, nausea, vomiting, cardiopulmonary arrest.

**metal catalyst** [Poison] *Cardiovascular collapse, pulmonary edema, CNS depression, coma, seizures, nausea, vomiting, cardiopulmonary arrest.*

**metal hydride (n.o.s.)** [Poison] *Cardiovascular collapse, pulmonary edema, CNS depression, coma, seizures, nausea, vomiting, cardiopulmonary arrest.*

**metal powder, flammable (n.o.s.)** [Flammable solid] *Shock, severe chemical and thermal burns, severe respiratory tract irritation, pulmonary edema, respiratory arrest, ECG changes, sudden death.* [Poison] *Cardiovascular collapse, pulmonary edema, CNS depression, coma, seizures, nausea, vomiting, cardiopulmonary arrest.*

**metaldehyde** [Aldehyde] *Seizures, respiratory failure, pulmonary edema.*

**Meta-Systox** [Organophosphate] *Pulmonary edema, respiratory muscle paralysis, respiratory failure, bradycardia, acetylcholinesterase inhibition, hypotension, pulmonary edema, overstimulation of parasympathetic nervous system, striated muscle, sympathetic ganglia, and CNS.*

**methacrolein diacetate** [Poison] *Cardiovascular collapse, pulmonary edema, CNS depression, coma, seizures, nausea, vomiting, cardiopulmonary arrest.*

**methacrylaldehyde** [Aldehyde] *Seizures, respiratory failure, pulmonary edema.*

**methacrylic acid** [Organic acid] *Pulmonary edema, circulatory collapse, laryngeal edema and spasm, severe chemical burns to skin, mucous membranes, and internal organs, GI tract perforation and hemorrhage, peritonitis.*

**methacrylic anhydride** [Organic acid] *Pulmonary edema, circulatory collapse, laryngeal edema and spasm, severe chemical burns to skin, mucous mem-*

branes, and internal organs, GI tract perforation and hemorrhage, peritonitis.

**methacrylonitrile** [Cyanide] *Impairment of cellular oxygenation and adenosine triphosphate production, hypoxia, death.*

**methacryloyl chloride** [Poison] *Cardiovascular collapse, pulmonary edema, CNS depression, coma, seizures, nausea, vomiting, cardiopulmonary arrest.*

**methacryloyloxyethyl isocyanate** [Isocyanate/aliphatic thiocyanate] *CNS depression, respiratory arrest, respiratory paralysis, pulmonary edema, cyanide toxicity.*

**methallyl alcohol** [Higher alcohol (4+ carbons)] *CNS depression, respiratory failure, arrhythmias.*

**methamidophos** [Organophosphate] *Pulmonary edema, respiratory muscle paralysis, respiratory failure, bradycardia, acetylcholinesterase inhibition, hypotension, pulmonary edema, overstimulation of parasympathetic nervous system, striated muscle, sympathetic ganglia, and CNS.*

**methanamine** [Organic base/amine] *Pulmonary edema, cardiac depression, seizures.* ⊡ methenamine

**methane (gas or cryogenic liquid)** [Aliphatic hydrocarbon] *Arrhythmias, asphyxiation, anesthesia.* [Simple asphyxiant] *Asphyxiation.*

**methane & hydrogen mixture** [Simple asphyxiant] *Asphyxiation.*

**methanesulfonyl chloride** [Organophosphate] *Pulmonary edema, respiratory muscle paralysis, respiratory failure, bradycardia, acetylcholinesterase inhibition, hypotension, pulmonary edema, overstimulation of parasympathetic nervous system, striated muscle, sympathetic ganglia, and CNS.*

**methanesulfonyl fluoride** [Organophosphate] *Pulmonary edema, respiratory muscle paralysis, respiratory failure, bradycardia, acetylcholinesterase inhibition, hypotension, pulmonary edema, overstimulation of parasympa-*

thetic nervous system, striated muscle, sympathetic ganglia, and CNS.

**methanol** [Methyl alcohol] *Respiratory failure, circulatory collapse.*

**methapyrilene** [Poison] *Cardiovascular collapse, pulmonary edema, CNS depression, coma, seizures, nausea, vomiting, cardiopulmonary arrest.*

**methenamine** [Aldehyde] *Seizures, respiratory failure, pulmonary edema.*

**methidathion** [Organophosphate] *Pulmonary edema, respiratory muscle paralysis, respiratory failure, bradycardia, acetylcholinesterase inhibition, hypotension, pulmonary edema, overstimulation of parasympathetic nervous system, striated muscle, sympathetic ganglia, and CNS.*

**methiocarb** [Carbamate] *Acetylcholinesterase inhibition (reversible), bradycardia, hypotension, respiratory muscle paralysis, respiratory arrest, pulmonary edema.*

**methomyl** [Carbamate] *Acetylcholinesterase inhibition (reversible), bradycardia, hypotension, respiratory muscle paralysis, respiratory arrest, pulmonary edema.*

**methoxychlor** [Aldrin/dieldrin/endrin] *Seizures, respiratory failure.*

**2-methoxyethanol** [Ethylene glycol] *Respiratory failure, pulmonary edema, paralysis, cardiovascular collapse, severe acidosis.*

**methoxyethylmercuric acetate** [Mercury] *Circulatory collapse, arrhythmias, respiratory failure, pulmonary edema, neurotoxic effects.*

**methoxyethylmercuric chloride** [Mercury] *Circulatory collapse, arrhythmias, respiratory failure, pulmonary edema, neurotoxic effects.*

**methoxymethyl isocyanate** [Isocyanate/aliphatic thiocyanate] *CNS depression, respiratory arrest, respiratory paralysis, pulmonary edema, cyanide toxicity.*

**methoxymethylpentanone** [Aliphatic hydrocarbon] *Arrhythmias, asphyxiation, anesthesia.* [Simple asphyxiant] *Asphyxiation.*

**4-methoxyphenol** [Phenol] *Coma, hypotension, arrhythmias, pulmonary edema, respiratory arrest.*

**1-methoxy-2-propanol** [Ethylene glycol] *Respiratory failure, pulmonary edema, paralysis, cardiovascular collapse, severe acidosis.*

**methyl acetate** [Methyl alcohol] *Respiratory failure, circulatory collapse.*

**methyl acetone** [Ketone] *Respiratory mucous membrane irritation, pulmonary edema, CNS depression.*

**methyl acetylene & propadiene mixture** [Hydrocarbon mixture] *CNS depression, respiratory arrest, seizures, arrhythmias, pulmonary edema.*

**methyl acrylonitrile** [Cyanide] *Impairment of cellular oxygenation and adenosine triphosphate production, hypoxia, death.*

**methyl alcohol** [Methyl alcohol] *Respiratory failure, circulatory collapse.*

**methyl allyl chloride** [Dichloropropane/dichloropropene] *Pulmonary edema, bronchospasm, alveolar hemorrhage.*

**methyl aluminum sesquibromide** [Bromine/methylbromide] *Severe respiratory irritation, pulmonary edema, respiratory failure, coma, convulsions, death.*

**methyl aluminum sesquichloride** [Chlorine] *Severe respiratory tract irritation, pulmonary edema, irritation of skin, eyes, and mucous membranes.*

**methyl amyl acetate** [Ester] *CNS depression, respiratory tract irritation, bronchitis, pneumonia.*

**methyl amyl alcohol** [Higher alcohol (4+ carbons)] *CNS depression, respiratory failure, arrhythmias.*

**methyl amyl ketone** [Ketone] *Respiratory mucous membrane irritation, pulmonary edema, CNS depression.*

**2-methyl aziridine** [Organic base/amine] *Pulmonary edema, cardiac depression, seizures.*

**methyl benzoate** [Organic acid] *Pulmonary edema, circulatory collapse, laryngeal edema and spasm, severe chemical burns to skin, mucous mem-*

branes, and internal organs, GI tract perforation and hemorrhage, peritonitis.

**methyl bromide** [Bromine/methylbromide] *Severe respiratory irritation, pulmonary edema, respiratory failure, coma, convulsions, death.*

**methyl bromide & chloropicrin mixture** [Halogenated aliphatic hydrocarbon] *CNS depression, respiratory arrest, circulatory collapse.* [Bromine/methylbromide] *Severe respiratory irritation, pulmonary edema, respiratory failure, coma, convulsions, death.*

**methyl bromide & ethylene dibromide mixture** [Bromine/methylbromide] *Severe respiratory irritation, pulmonary edema, respiratory failure, coma, convulsions, death.*

**methyl bromide & nonflammable compressed gas mixture** [Bromine/methylbromide] *Severe respiratory irritation, pulmonary edema, respiratory failure, coma, convulsions, death.*

**methyl bromoacetate** [Bromine/methylbromide] *Severe respiratory irritation, pulmonary edema, respiratory failure, coma, convulsions, death.*

**methyl butanone** [Ketone] *Respiratory mucous membrane irritation, pulmonary edema, CNS depression.*

**methyl tert-butyl ether (MTBE)** [Ether] *Anesthesia, respiratory arrest.*

**methyl n-butyl ketone** [Ketone] *Respiratory mucous membrane irritation, pulmonary edema, CNS depression.*

**methyl butyrate** [Ester] *CNS depression, respiratory tract irritation, bronchitis, pneumonia.*

**Methyl Cellosolve Acetate** [Ethylene glycol] *Respiratory failure, pulmonary edema, paralysis, cardiovascular collapse, severe acidosis.*

**methyl chloride** [Halogenated aliphatic hydrocarbon] *CNS depression, respiratory arrest, circulatory collapse.*

**methyl chloride & chloropicrin mixture** [Irritant] *Severe immediate or delayed upper airway or respiratory tract irritation, pulmonary edema, glottic spasm, airway obstruction.* [Halogenated aliphatic hydrocarbon] *CNS depression, respiratory arrest, circulatory collapse.*

**methyl chloride & methylene chloride mixture** [Halogenated aliphatic hydrocarbon] *CNS depression, respiratory arrest, circulatory collapse.* [Carbon monoxide] *Impairment of cellular oxygenation, hypoxia, death.*

**methyl chloroacetate** [Ester] *CNS depression, respiratory tract irritation, bronchitis, pneumonia.*

**methyl 2-chloroacrylate** [Ester] *CNS depression, respiratory tract irritation, bronchitis, pneumonia.*

**methyl chlorocarbonate** [Halogenated aliphatic hydrocarbon] *CNS depression, respiratory arrest, circulatory collapse.*

**methyl chloroform** [Halogenated aliphatic hydrocarbon] *CNS depression, respiratory arrest, circulatory collapse.*

**methyl chloroformate** [Halogenated aliphatic hydrocarbon] *CNS depression, respiratory arrest, circulatory collapse.*

**methyl chloromethyl ether** [Halogenated aliphatic hydrocarbon] *CNS depression, respiratory arrest, circulatory collapse.* [Ether] *Anesthesia, respiratory arrest.*

**methyl chloropropionate** [Halogenated aliphatic hydrocarbon] *CNS depression, respiratory arrest, circulatory collapse.*

**methyl cyanide** [Cyanide] *Impairment of cellular oxygenation and adenosine triphosphate production, hypoxia, death.*

**methyl cyclohexanone peroxide** [Organic peroxide] *Pulmonary and laryngeal edema, circulatory arrest, hypovolemic shock, chemical burns to skin, mucous membranes, and internal organs.* [Ketone] *Respiratory mucous membrane irritation, pulmonary edema, CNS depression.* [Corrosive] *Upper airway burns and edema, circulatory collapse, severe chemical burns to skin, toxic systemic effects, GI tract perforation and hemorrhage, peritonitis.*

**methyl cyclopentane** [Aliphatic hydrocarbon] *Arrhythmias, asphyxiation, anesthesia.*

**methyl demeton** [Organophosphate] *Pulmonary edema, respiratory muscle paralysis, respiratory failure, bradycardia, acetylcholinesterase inhibition, hypotension, pulmonary edema, overstimulation of parasympathetic nervous system, striated muscle, sympathetic ganglia, and CNS.*

**methyl dichloroacetate** [Ester] *CNS depression, respiratory tract irritation, bronchitis, pneumonia.*

**methyl dichloroarsine** [Arsine] *Intravascular hemolysis, pulmonary edema, cardiac and respiratory arrest, delayed-onset jaundice and renal failure.*

**methyl dichlorosilane** [Silane/chlorosilane] *Respiratory tract irritation, pulmonary edema.*

**methyl ethyl ether** [Ether] *Anesthesia, respiratory arrest.*

**methyl ethyl ketone** [Ketone] *Respiratory mucous membrane irritation, pulmonary edema, CNS depression.*

**methyl ethyl ketone peroxide** [Organic peroxide] *Pulmonary and laryngeal edema, circulatory arrest, hypovolemic shock, chemical burns to skin, mucous membranes, and internal organs.* [Ketone] *Respiratory mucous membrane irritation, pulmonary edema, CNS depression.* [Corrosive] *Upper airway burns and edema, circulatory collapse, severe chemical burns to skin, toxic systemic effects, GI tract perforation and hemorrhage, peritonitis.*

**methyl ethyl pyridine; 2-methyl-5-ethyl pyridine** [Aromatic hydrocarbon] *Arrhythmias, respiratory failure, pulmonary edema, paralysis, brain and kidney damage.*

**methyl fluoride** [Chlorinated fluorocarbon] *Asphyxiation, anesthesia, arrhythmias.*

**methyl fluoroacetete** [Monofluoroacetate] *Ventricular arrhythmias, seizures.*

**methyl fluorosulfate** [Halogenated aliphatic hydrocarbon] *CNS depression, respiratory arrest, circulatory collapse.*

**methyl formate** [Methyl alcohol] *Respiratory failure, circulatory collapse.*

**methyl iodide** [Pyrethrin/pyrethroid] *Respiratory paralysis, convulsions.*

**methyl isoamyl ketone** [Ketone] *Respiratory mucous membrane irritation, pulmonary edema, CNS depression.*

**methyl isobutyl carbinol** [Higher alcohol (4+ carbons)] *CNS depression, respiratory failure, arrhythmias.*

**methyl isobutyl ketone** [Ketone] *Respiratory mucous membrane irritation, pulmonary edema, CNS depression.*

**methyl isobutyl ketone peroxide** [Organic peroxide] *Pulmonary and laryngeal edema, circulatory arrest, hypovolemic shock, chemical burns to skin, mucous membranes, and internal organs.* [Ketone] *Respiratory mucous membrane irritation, pulmonary edema, CNS depression.* [Corrosive] *Upper airway burns and edema, circulatory collapse, severe chemical burns to skin, toxic systemic effects, GI tract perforation and hemorrhage, peritonitis.*

**methyl isocyanate** [Isocyanate/aliphatic thiocyanate] *CNS depression, respiratory arrest, respiratory paralysis, pulmonary edema, cyanide toxicity.*

**methyl isopropenyl ketone** [Ketone] *Respiratory mucous membrane irritation, pulmonary edema, CNS depression.*

**methyl isopropyl ketone** [Ketone] *Respiratory mucous membrane irritation, pulmonary edema, CNS depression.*

**methyl isothiocyanate** [Isocyanate/aliphatic thiocyanate] *CNS depression, respiratory arrest, respiratory paralysis, pulmonary edema, cyanide toxicity.*

**methyl isovalerate** [Ester] *CNS depression, respiratory tract irritation, bronchitis, pneumonia.*

**methyl magnesium bromide & ethyl ether mixture** [Ether] *Anesthesia, respiratory arrest.* [Bromine/methylbromide] *Severe respiratory*

**HazMat**

*irritation, pulmonary edema, respiratory failure, coma, convulsions, death.*

**methyl mercaptan** [Sulfur] *Respiratory tract irritation, pulmonary edema, anaphylaxis.*

**methyl methacrylate** [Ester] *CNS depression, respiratory tract irritation, bronchitis, pneumonia.*

**methyl naphthalene** [Naphthalene] *Delayed-onset acute intravascular hemolysis.*

**methyl nitrite** [Nitrate/nitrite] *Methemoglobinemia, hypotension, circulatory collapse.*

**methyl orthosilicate** [Silane/chlorosilane] *Respiratory tract irritation, pulmonary edema.*

**methyl parathion** [Organophosphate] *Pulmonary edema, respiratory muscle paralysis, respiratory failure, bradycardia, acetylcholinesterase inhibition, hypotension, pulmonary edema, overstimulation of parasympathetic nervous system, striated muscle, sympathetic ganglia, and CNS.*

**methyl parathion & compressed gas mixture** [Organophosphate] *Pulmonary edema, respiratory muscle paralysis, respiratory failure, bradycardia, acetylcholinesterase inhibition, hypotension, pulmonary edema, overstimulation of parasympathetic nervous system, striated muscle, sympathetic ganglia, and CNS.*

**methyl phenkapton** [Organophosphate] *Pulmonary edema, respiratory muscle paralysis, respiratory failure, bradycardia, acetylcholinesterase inhibition, hypotension, pulmonary edema, overstimulation of parasympathetic nervous system, striated muscle, sympathetic ganglia, and CNS.*

**methyl phosphonic dichloride** [Phosphorus] *Hypovolemic shock, severe tissue burns, severe respiratory irritation, pulmonary edema, respiratory arrest, arrhythmias, sudden death.*

**methyl phosphonothioic dichloride** [Phosphorus] *Hypovolemic shock, severe tissue burns, severe respiratory*

*irritation, pulmonary edema, respiratory arrest, arrhythmias, sudden death.*

**methyl phosphonous dichloride** [Phosphorus] *Hypovolemic shock, severe tissue burns, severe respiratory irritation, pulmonary edema, respiratory arrest, arrhythmias, sudden death.*

**methyl propionate** [Ester] *CNS depression, respiratory tract irritation, bronchitis, pneumonia.*

**methyl propyl benzene** [Aromatic hydrocarbon] *Arrhythmias, respiratory failure, pulmonary edema, paralysis, brain and kidney damage.*

**methyl propyl ether** [Ether] *Anesthesia, respiratory arrest.*

**methyl propyl ketone** [Ketone] *Respiratory mucous membrane irritation, pulmonary edema, CNS depression.*

**methyl silicate** [Silane/chlorosilane] *Respiratory tract irritation, pulmonary edema.*

**methyl styrene** [Aromatic hydrocarbon] *Arrhythmias, respiratory failure, pulmonary edema, paralysis, brain and kidney damage.*

**methyl sulfate** [Sulfur] *Respiratory tract irritation, pulmonary edema, anaphylaxis.*

**methyl sulfide** [Sulfur] *Respiratory tract irritation, pulmonary edema, anaphylaxis.*

**methyl tetrahydrofuran** [Ether] *Anesthesia, respiratory arrest.*

**methyl thiocyanate** [Isocyanate/aliphatic thiocyanate] *CNS depression, respiratory arrest, respiratory paralysis, pulmonary edema, cyanide toxicity.*

**methyl trichloroacetate** [Ester] *CNS depression, respiratory tract irritation, bronchitis, pneumonia.*

**methyl trichlorosilane** [Silane/chlorosilane] *Respiratory tract irritation, pulmonary edema.*

**Methyl Trithion** [Organophosphate] *Pulmonary edema, respiratory muscle paralysis, respiratory failure, bradycardia, acetylcholinesterase inhibition, hypotension, pulmonary edema, overstimulation of parasympathetic nervous*

system, striated muscle, sympathetic ganglia, and CNS.

**methyl valeraldehyde** [Organophosphate] *Pulmonary edema, respiratory muscle paralysis, respiratory failure, bradycardia, acetylcholinesterase inhibition, hypotension, pulmonary edema, overstimulation of parasympathetic nervous system, striated muscle, sympathetic ganglia, and CNS.*

**methyl vinyl ketone** [Ketone] *Respiratory mucous membrane irritation, pulmonary edema, CNS depression.*

**methylacrylate** [Ester] *CNS depression, respiratory tract irritation, bronchitis, pneumonia.*

**methylal** [Ether] *Anesthesia, respiratory arrest.*

**methylamine** [Organic base/amine] *Pulmonary edema, cardiac depression, seizures.*

**p-methylaminophenol sulfate** [Aniline] *Methemoglobinemia, hypoxia.* [Phenol] *Coma, hypotension, arrhythmias, pulmonary edema, respiratory arrest.*

**methylaniline** [Aniline] *Methemoglobinemia, hypoxia.*

**methylbenzyl alcohol** [Higher alcohol (4+ carbons)] *CNS depression, respiratory failure, arrhythmias.*

**methylbutene; 2-methyl-1-butene; 2-methyl-2-butene; 3-methyl-1-butene** [Aliphatic hydrocarbon] *Arrhythmias, asphyxiation, anesthesia.*

**methyl-tert-butyl ether** [Ether] *Anesthesia, respiratory arrest.*

**methylbutylamine** [Organic base/amine] *Pulmonary edema, cardiac depression, seizures.*

**4-(2-methyl-4-chlorophenoxy) butyric acid** [Chlorophenoxy herbicide] *CNS depression, CNS stimulation, respiratory failure, ventricular fibrillation, seizures.*

**methylchlorosilane** [Silane/chlorosilane] *Respiratory tract irritation, pulmonary edema.*

**3-methylcholanthrene** [Aromatic hydrocarbon] *Arrhythmias, respiratory*

failure, pulmonary edema, paralysis, brain and kidney damage.

**methylcyclohexane** [Aliphatic hydrocarbon] *Arrhythmias, asphyxiation, anesthesia.*

**methylcyclohexanol** [Higher alcohol (4+ carbons)] *CNS depression, respiratory failure, arrhythmias.*

**2-methylcyclohexanone** [Ketone] *Respiratory mucous membrane irritation, pulmonary edema, CNS depression.*

**4,4'-methylene bis(2-chloroaniline)** [Aniline] *Methemoglobinemia, hypoxia.*

**4,4'-methylene bis(N,N-dimethyl) benzenamine** [Poison] *Cardiovascular collapse, pulmonary edema, CNS depression, coma, seizures, nausea, vomiting, cardiopulmonary arrest.*

**methylene bis(4-phenyl isocyanate) (MDI)** [Isocyanate/aliphatic thiocyanate] *CNS depression, respiratory arrest, respiratory paralysis, pulmonary edema, cyanide toxicity.*

**methylene bromide** [Bromine/methylbromide] *Severe respiratory irritation, pulmonary edema, respiratory failure, coma, convulsions, death.*

**methylene chloride** [Halogenated aliphatic hydrocarbon] *CNS depression, respiratory arrest, circulatory collapse.* [Carbon monoxide] *Impairment of cellular oxygenation, hypoxia, death.*

**methylene chloride & methyl chloride mixture** [Halogenated aliphatic hydrocarbon] *CNS depression, respiratory arrest, circulatory collapse.* [Carbon monoxide] *Impairment of cellular oxygenation, hypoxia, death.*

**methylene iodide** [Iodine] *Hypotension, circulatory collapse, pulmonary edema.*

**4,4'-methylenedianiline** [Aniline] *Methemoglobinemia, hypoxia.*

**methylfuran** [Aliphatic hydrocarbon] *Arrhythmias, asphyxiation, anesthesia.*

**5-methyl-3-heptanone** [Ketone] *Respiratory mucous membrane irritation, pulmonary edema, CNS depression.*

HazMat

**methylhexanone** [Ketone] *Respiratory mucous membrane irritation, pulmonary edema, CNS depression.*

**methylhydrazine** [Hydrazine] *Seizures, hemolysis of red blood cells, pulmonary edema.*

**methylmercuric dicyanamide** [Mercury] *Circulatory collapse, arrhythmias, respiratory failure, pulmonary edema, neurotoxic effects.*

**methylmorpholine** [Organic base/amine] *Pulmonary edema, cardiac depression, seizures.*

**methylpentadiene** [Aliphatic hydrocarbon] *Arrhythmias, asphyxiation, anesthesia.*

**methylpentane** [Aliphatic hydrocarbon] *Arrhythmias, asphyxiation, anesthesia.*

**methylpentanol** [Higher alcohol (4+ carbons)] *CNS depression, respiratory failure, arrhythmias.*

**methylphenyldichlorosilane** [Silane/chlorosilane] *Respiratory tract irritation, pulmonary edema.*

**methylphosphonic difluoride** [Phosphorus] *Hypovolemic shock, severe tissue burns, severe respiratory irritation, pulmonary edema, respiratory arrest, arrhythmias, sudden death.*

**methylpiperidine** [Organic base/amine] *Pulmonary edema, cardiac depression, seizures.*

**α-methylstyrene; alpha-methylstyrene** [Aromatic hydrocarbon] *Arrhythmias, respiratory failure, pulmonary edema, paralysis, brain and kidney damage.*

**methylthiouracil** [Poison] *Cardiovascular collapse, pulmonary edema, CNS depression, coma, seizures, nausea, vomiting, cardiopulmonary arrest.*

**metolcarb** [Carbamate] *Acetylcholinesterase inhibition (reversible), bradycardia, hypotension, respiratory muscle paralysis, respiratory arrest, pulmonary edema.*

**mevinphos** [Organophosphate] *Pulmonary edema, respiratory muscle paralysis, respiratory failure, bradycardia, acetylcholinesterase inhibition,* hypotension, pulmonary edema, overstimulation of parasympathetic nervous system, striated muscle, sympathetic ganglia, and CNS.

**mexacarbate** [Carbamate] *Acetylcholinesterase inhibition (reversible), bradycardia, hypotension, respiratory muscle paralysis, respiratory arrest, pulmonary edema.*

**MGK 264** [Poison] *Cardiovascular collapse, pulmonary edema, CNS depression, coma, seizures, nausea, vomiting, cardiopulmonary arrest.*

**MIBC** [Higher alcohol (4+ carbons)] *CNS depression, respiratory failure, arrhythmias.*

**Michler's ketone** [Ketone] *Respiratory mucous membrane irritation, pulmonary edema, CNS depression.*

**mineral seal oil** [Hydrocarbon mixture] *CNS depression, respiratory arrest, seizures, arrhythmias, pulmonary edema.*

**mineral spirits** [Hydrocarbon mixture] *CNS depression, respiratory arrest, seizures, arrhythmias, pulmonary edema.*

**mining reagent** [Hydrocarbon mixture] *CNS depression, respiratory arrest, seizures, arrhythmias, pulmonary edema.*

**mintezol** [Thiabendazole] *Cardiovascular collapse, respiratory tract irritation.*

**mipafox** [Organophosphate] *Pulmonary edema, respiratory muscle paralysis, respiratory failure, bradycardia, acetylcholinesterase inhibition, hypotension, pulmonary edema, overstimulation of parasympathetic nervous system, striated muscle, sympathetic ganglia, and CNS.*

**mirex** [Lindane] *CNS stimulation, seizures, respiratory failure.*

**misch metal (powder)** [Flammable solid] *Shock, severe chemical and thermal burns, severe respiratory tract irritation, pulmonary edema, respiratory arrest, ECG changes, sudden death.* [Poison] *Cardiovascular collapse, pulmonary edema, CNS depression,* coma, seizures, nausea, vomiting, cardiopulmonary arrest.

**mitomycin C** [Poison] Cardiovascular collapse, pulmonary edema, CNS depression, coma, seizures, nausea, vomiting, cardiopulmonary arrest.

**mixed acids (n.o.s.)** [Inorganic acid] Pulmonary edema, bronchospasm, circulatory collapse, laryngeal spasm and edema, severe chemical burns to skin, mucous membranes, and internal organs, GI tract perforation and hemorrhage, peritonitis.

**Moban** [Carbamate] Acetylcholinesterase inhibition (reversible), bradycardia, hypotension, respiratory muscle paralysis, respiratory arrest, pulmonary edema.

**MOCA** [Aniline] Methemoglobinemia, hypoxia.

**molybdenum disulfide** [Poison] Cardiovascular collapse, pulmonary edema, CNS depression, coma, seizures, nausea, vomiting, cardiopulmonary arrest.

**molybdenum pentachloride** [Poison] Cardiovascular collapse, pulmonary edema, CNS depression, coma, seizures, nausea, vomiting, cardiopulmonary arrest.

**molybdenum trioxide** [Poison] Cardiovascular collapse, pulmonary edema, CNS depression, coma, seizures, nausea, vomiting, cardiopulmonary arrest.

**Monitor** [Organophosphate] Pulmonary edema, respiratory muscle paralysis, respiratory failure, bradycardia, acetylcholinesterase inhibition, hypotension, pulmonary edema, overstimulation of parasympathetic nervous system, striated muscle, sympathetic ganglia, and CNS.

**monobromotrifluoromethane** [Chlorinated fluorocarbon] Asphyxiation, anesthesia, arrhythmias.

**monochloroacetic acid** [Organic acid] Pulmonary edema, circulatory collapse, laryngeal edema and spasm, severe chemical burns to skin, mucous membranes, and internal organs, GI tract perforation and hemorrhage, peritonitis.

**monochloroacetone** [Ketone] Respiratory mucous membrane irritation, pulmonary edema, CNS depression.

**monochloroethylene** [Halogenated aliphatic hydrocarbon] CNS depression, respiratory arrest, circulatory collapse.

**monochloropentafluorethane** [Chlorinated fluorocarbon] Asphyxiation, anesthesia, arrhythmias.

**monochlorotetrafluoroethane** [Chlorinated fluorocarbon] Asphyxiation, anesthesia, arrhythmias.

**monochlorotrifluoromethane** [Chlorinated fluorocarbon] Asphyxiation, anesthesia, arrhythmias.

**monocrotophos** [Organophosphate] Pulmonary edema, respiratory muscle paralysis, respiratory failure, bradycardia, acetylcholinesterase inhibition, hypotension, pulmonary edema, overstimulation of parasympathetic nervous system, striated muscle, sympathetic ganglia, and CNS.

**monoethanolamine** [Organic base/amine] Pulmonary edema, cardiac depression, seizures.

**monoethylamine** [Organic base/amine] Pulmonary edema, cardiac depression, seizures.

**monofluorophosphoric acid** [Inorganic acid] Pulmonary edema, bronchospasm, circulatory collapse, laryngeal spasm and edema, severe chemical burns to skin, mucous membranes, and internal organs, GI tract perforation and hemorrhage, peritonitis.

**monomethylamine** [Organic base/amine] Pulmonary edema, cardiac depression, seizures.

**monomethylhydrazine** [Hydrazine] Seizures, hemolysis of red blood cells, pulmonary edema.

**monopropylamine** [Organic base/amine] Pulmonary edema, cardiac depression, seizures.

**mono-(trichloro)-tetra-(monopotassium dichloro)-penta-S-triazetri-**

**one** [Irritant] *Severe immediate or delayed upper airway or respiratory tract irritation, pulmonary edema, glottic spasm, airway obstruction.*

**morpholine; morpholine mixture (n.o.s.)** [Organic base/amine] *Pulmonary edema, cardiac depression, seizures.*

**motion picture film, nitrocellulose-based** [Flammable solid] *Shock, severe chemical and thermal burns, severe respiratory tract irritation, pulmonary edema, respiratory arrest, ECG changes, sudden death.*

**motor fuel (n.o.s.)** [Hydrocarbon mixture] *CNS depression, respiratory arrest, seizures, arrhythmias, pulmonary edema.*

**motor fuel anti-knock compound** [Hydrocarbon mixture] *CNS depression, respiratory arrest, seizures, arrhythmias, pulmonary edema.* [Lead] *Circulatory collapse, coma, rare seizures.*

**motor spirit** [Hydrocarbon mixture] *CNS depression, respiratory arrest, seizures, arrhythmias, pulmonary edema.*

**MPMC** [Carbamate] *Acetylcholinesterase inhibition (reversible), bradycardia, hypotension, respiratory muscle paralysis, respiratory arrest, pulmonary edema.*

**MTBE (methyl *tert*-butyl ether)** [Ether] *Anesthesia, respiratory arrest.*

**muriatic acid** [Inorganic acid] *Pulmonary edema, bronchospasm, circulatory collapse, laryngeal spasm and edema, severe chemical burns to skin, mucous membranes, and internal organs, GI tract perforation and hemorrhage, peritonitis.*

**muscimol** [Poison] *Cardiovascular collapse, pulmonary edema, CNS depression, coma, seizures, nausea, vomiting, cardiopulmonary arrest.*

**musk xylene** [Aromatic hydrocarbon] *Arrhythmias, respiratory failure, pulmonary edema, paralysis, brain and kidney damage.*

**mustard gas** [Sulfur] *Respiratory tract irritation, pulmonary edema, anaphylaxis.*

**nabam** [Dithiocarbamate] *Hypotension, respiratory failure.*

**naled** [Organophosphate] *Pulmonary edema, respiratory muscle paralysis, respiratory failure, bradycardia, acetylcholinesterase inhibition, hypotension, pulmonary edema, overstimulation of parasympathetic nervous system, striated muscle, sympathetic ganglia, and CNS.*

**naphtha** [Hydrocarbon mixture] *CNS depression, respiratory arrest, seizures, arrhythmias, pulmonary edema.* [Naphthalene] *Delayed-onset acute intravascular hemolysis.*

**naphtha solvent, aromatic** [Naphthalene] *Delayed-onset acute intravascular hemolysis.*

**naphthalene** [Naphthalene] *Delayed-onset acute intravascular hemolysis.*

**naphthalene, chlorinated** [Naphthalene] *Delayed-onset acute intravascular hemolysis.*

**naphthenic acid** [Organic acid] *Pulmonary edema, circulatory collapse, laryngeal edema and spasm, severe chemical burns to skin, mucous membranes, and internal organs, GI tract perforation and hemorrhage, peritonitis.*

**β-naphthol; beta-naphthol** [Phenol] *Coma, hypotension, arrhythmias, pulmonary edema, respiratory arrest.*

**1,4-naphthoquinone** [Phenol] *Coma, hypotension, arrhythmias, pulmonary edema, respiratory arrest.*

**naphthylamine (alpha or beta)** [Organic base/amine] *Pulmonary edema, cardiac depression, seizures.*

**naphthylthiourea** [Naphthalene] *Delayed-onset acute intravascular hemolysis.*

**naphthylurea** [Naphthalene] *Delayed-onset acute intravascular hemolysis.*

**natural gas (gas or cryogenic liquid)** [Aliphatic hydrocarbon] *Arrhythmias, asphyxiation, anesthesia.* [Simple asphyxiant] *Asphyxiation.*

**natural gasoline** [Hydrocarbon mixture] *CNS depression, respiratory arrest, seizures, arrhythmias, pulmonary edema.*

**Navadel** [Organophosphate] *Pulmonary edema, respiratory muscle paralysis, respiratory failure, bradycardia, acetylcholinesterase inhibition, hypotension, pulmonary edema, overstimulation of parasympathetic nervous system, striated muscle, sympathetic ganglia, and CNS.*

**neohexane** [Aliphatic hydrocarbon] *Arrhythmias, asphyxiation, anesthesia.*

**neon (gas or cryogenic liquid)** [Simple asphyxiant] *Asphyxiation.*

**neopentane** [Aliphatic hydrocarbon] *Arrhythmias, asphyxiation, anesthesia.*

**Neotran** [Chlorophenoxy herbicide] *CNS depression, CNS stimulation, respiratory failure, ventricular fibrillation, seizures.*

**nickel; soluble nickel mixture (n.o.s.)** [Nickel] *Respiratory failure, cerebral edema, allergic reactions.*

**nickel ammonium sulfate** [Nickel] *Respiratory failure, cerebral edema, allergic reactions.*

**nickel carbonyl** [Nickel] *Respiratory failure, cerebral edema, allergic reactions.*

**nickel catalyst** [Nickel] *Respiratory failure, cerebral edema, allergic reactions.*

**nickel chloride** [Nickel] *Respiratory failure, cerebral edema, allergic reactions.*

**nickel cyanide** [Nickel] *Respiratory failure, cerebral edema, allergic reactions.* [Cyanide] *Impairment of cellular oxygenation and adenosine triphosphate production, hypoxia, death.*

**nickel hydroxide** [Nickel] *Respiratory failure, cerebral edema, allergic reactions.*

**nickel nitrate** [Nitrate/nitrite] *Methemoglobinemia, hypotension, circulatory collapse.* [Nickel] *Respiratory failure, cerebral edema, allergic reactions.*

**nickel nitrite** [Nitrate/nitrite] *Methemoglobinemia, hypotension, circulatory collapse.* [Nickel] *Respiratory failure, cerebral edema, allergic reactions.*

**nickel sulfate** [Nickel] *Respiratory failure, cerebral edema, allergic reactions.*

**nicotine; nicotine mixture (n.o.s.)** [Nicotine] *Respiratory and cardiac arrest, CNS stimulation, CNS depression.*

**nicotine HCl; nicotine HCl mixture (n.o.s.)** [Nicotine] *Respiratory and cardiac arrest, CNS stimulation, CNS depression.*

**nicotine salicylate** [Nicotine] *Respiratory and cardiac arrest, CNS stimulation, CNS depression.*

**nicotine sulfate** [Nicotine] *Respiratory and cardiac arrest, CNS stimulation, CNS depression.*

**nicotine tartrate** [Nicotine] *Respiratory and cardiac arrest, CNS stimulation, CNS depression.*

**nitrate (n.o.s.); nitrate salt (n.o.s.)** [Nitrate/nitrite] *Methemoglobinemia, hypotension, circulatory collapse.*

**nitrate of sodium & potash mixture** [Nitrate/nitrite] *Methemoglobinemia, hypotension, circulatory collapse.*

**nitrating acid; nitrating acid mixture (n.o.s.)** [Nitrate/nitrite] *Methemoglobinemia, hypotension, circulatory collapse.*

**nitric acid** [Inorganic acid] *Pulmonary edema, bronchospasm, circulatory collapse, laryngeal spasm and edema, severe chemical burns to skin, mucous membranes, and internal organs, GI tract perforation and hemorrhage, peritonitis.*

**nitric oxide** [Nitrogen oxide] *Lower respiratory tract symptoms, pulmonary edema, laryngospasm, bronchospasm, asphyxiation.*

**nitric oxide & dinitrogen tetroxide mixture** [Nitrogen oxide] *Lower respiratory tract symptoms, pulmonary edema, laryngospasm, bronchospasm, asphyxiation.*

**nitric oxide & nitrogen dioxide mixture** [Nitrogen oxide] *Lower respiratory tract symptoms, pulmonary edema, laryngospasm, bronchospasm, asphyxiation.*

**nitric oxide & nitrogen tetroxide mixture** [Nitrogen oxide] *Lower respiratory tract symptoms, pulmonary edema, laryngospasm, bronchospasm, asphyxiation.*

**nitrilotriacetic acid** [Organic acid] *Pulmonary edema, circulatory collapse, laryngeal edema and spasm, severe chemical burns to skin, mucous membranes, and internal organs, GI tract perforation and hemorrhage, peritonitis.*

**nitrite (n.o.s.)** [Nitrate/nitrite] *Methemoglobinemia, hypotension, circulatory collapse.*

**nitro mixture (n.o.s.)** [Nitrate/nitrite] *Methemoglobinemia, hypotension, circulatory collapse.*

**p-nitroaniline** [Aniline] *Methemoglobinemia, hypoxia.*

**nitroanisole** [Aromatic hydrocarbon] *Arrhythmias, respiratory failure, pulmonary edema, paralysis, brain and kidney damage.* [Nitrate/nitrite] *Methemoglobinemia, hypotension, circulatory collapse.*

**nitrobenzene** [Aromatic hydrocarbon] *Arrhythmias, respiratory failure, pulmonary edema, paralysis, brain and kidney damage.* [Nitrate/nitrite] *Methemoglobinemia, hypotension, circulatory collapse.*

**nitrobenzenesulfonic acid** [Organic acid] *Pulmonary edema, circulatory collapse, laryngeal edema and spasm, severe chemical burns to skin, mucous membranes, and internal organs, GI tract perforation and hemorrhage, peritonitis.*

**nitrobenzotrifluoride** [Aromatic hydrocarbon] *Arrhythmias, respiratory failure, pulmonary edema, paralysis, brain and kidney damage.* [Nitrate/nitrite] *Methemoglobinemia, hypotension, circulatory collapse.*

**4-nitrobiphenyl** [Phenol] *Coma, hypotension, arrhythmias, pulmonary edema, respiratory arrest.* [Nitrate/nitrite] *Methemoglobinemia, hypotension, circulatory collapse.*

**nitrobromobenzene** [Nitrate/nitrite] *Methemoglobinemia, hypotension, circulatory collapse.* [Bromine/methylbromide] *Severe respiratory irritation, pulmonary edema, respiratory failure, coma, convulsions, death.*

**nitrocellulose** [Flammable/combustible liquid] *CNS depression, respiratory arrest, convulsions, arrhythmias, pulmonary edema.*

**nitrocellulose, with plasticizing substance** [Flammable solid] *Shock, severe chemical and thermal burns, severe respiratory tract irritation, pulmonary edema, respiratory arrest, ECG changes, sudden death.* [Poison] *Cardiovascular collapse, pulmonary edema, CNS depression, coma, seizures, nausea, vomiting, cardiopulmonary arrest.*

**nitrocellulose, with 20%+ water** [Flammable solid] *Shock, severe chemical and thermal burns, severe respiratory tract irritation, pulmonary edema, respiratory arrest, ECG changes, sudden death.*

**nitrochlorobenzene; O-nitrochlorobenzene; p-nitrochlorobenzene** [Aromatic hydrocarbon] *Arrhythmias, respiratory failure, pulmonary edema, paralysis, brain and kidney damage.* [Nitrate/nitrite] *Methemoglobinemia, hypotension, circulatory collapse.*

**nitrochlorobenzotrifluoride** [Aromatic hydrocarbon] *Arrhythmias, respiratory failure, pulmonary edema, paralysis, brain and kidney damage.* [Nitrate/nitrite] *Methemoglobinemia, hypotension, circulatory collapse.*

**nitrocresol** [Phenol] *Coma, hypotension, arrhythmias, pulmonary edema, respiratory arrest.* [Nitrate/nitrite] *Methemoglobinemia, hypotension, circulatory collapse.*

**nitrocyclohexane** [Aliphatic hydrocarbon] *Arrhythmias, asphyxiation, anesthesia.* [Nitrate/nitrite] *Methemoglobinemia, hypotension, circulatory collapse.*

**nitroethane** [Aliphatic hydrocarbon] *Arrhythmias, asphyxiation, anesthesia.* [Nitrate/nitrite] *Methemoglobinemia, hypotension, circulatory collapse.*

**nitrofen** [Aromatic hydrocarbon] *Arrhythmias, respiratory failure, pulmonary edema, paralysis, brain and* *kidney damage.* [Nitrate/nitrite] *Methemoglobinemia, hypotension, circulatory collapse.*

**nitrogen (gas or cryogenic liquid)** [Simple asphyxiant] *Asphyxiation.*

**nitrogen compound, aromatic** [Aniline] *Methemoglobinemia, hypoxia.*

**nitrogen dioxide** [Nitrogen oxide] *Lower respiratory tract symptoms, pulmonary edema, laryngospasm, bronchospasm, asphyxiation.*

**nitrogen dioxide & nitric oxide mixture** [Nitrogen oxide] *Lower respiratory tract symptoms, pulmonary edema, laryngospasm, bronchospasm, asphyxiation.*

**nitrogen fluoride oxide** [Nitrogen oxide] *Lower respiratory tract symptoms, pulmonary edema, laryngospasm, bronchospasm, asphyxiation.* [Fluorine] *CNS depression, respiratory arrest, cardiovascular collapse, shock, arrhythmias.*

**nitrogen mustard** [Organic base/amine] *Pulmonary edema, cardiac depression, seizures.*

**nitrogen oxide (n.o.s.)** [Nitrogen oxide] *Lower respiratory tract symptoms, pulmonary edema, laryngospasm, bronchospasm, asphyxiation.*

**nitrogen oxide & ozone mixture** [Nitrogen oxide] *Lower respiratory tract symptoms, pulmonary edema, laryngospasm, bronchospasm, asphyxiation.* [Ozone] *Pulmonary edema, airway obstruction.*

**nitrogen peroxide** [Nitrogen oxide] *Lower respiratory tract symptoms, pulmonary edema, laryngospasm, bronchospasm, asphyxiation.*

**nitrogen & rare gas mixture** [Poison] *Cardiovascular collapse, pulmonary edema, CNS depression, coma, seizures, nausea, vomiting, cardiopulmonary arrest.* [Simple asphyxiant] *Asphyxiation.*

**nitrogen tetroxide** [Nitrogen oxide] *Lower respiratory tract symptoms, pulmonary edema, laryngospasm, bronchospasm, asphyxiation.*

**nitrogen tetroxide & nitric oxide mixture** [Nitrogen oxide] *Lower respiratory tract symptoms, pulmonary edema, laryngospasm, bronchospasm, asphyxiation.*

**nitrogen trifluoride** [Fluorine] *CNS depression, respiratory arrest, cardiovascular collapse, shock, arrhythmias.*

**nitrogen trioxide** [Nitrogen oxide] *Lower respiratory tract symptoms, pulmonary edema, laryngospasm, bronchospasm, asphyxiation.*

**nitroglycerin** [Nitrate/nitrite] *Methemoglobinemia, hypotension, circulatory collapse.*

**nitroglycerin in alcohol** [Lower alcohol (1–3 carbons)] *CNS depression, coma, respiratory arrest, arrhythmias.* [Nitrate/nitrite] *Methemoglobinemia, hypotension, circulatory collapse.*

**nitroguanidine** [Dinitrophenol] *Respiratory and circulatory collapse, pulmonary edema, hyperthermia.*

**nitrohydrochloric acid** [Inorganic acid] *Pulmonary edema, bronchospasm, circulatory collapse, laryngeal spasm and edema, severe chemical burns to skin, mucous membranes, and internal organs, GI tract perforation and hemorrhage, peritonitis.*

**nitroludine** [Aromatic hydrocarbon] *Arrhythmias, respiratory failure, pulmonary edema, paralysis, brain and kidney damage.* [Nitrate/nitrite] *Methemoglobinemia, hypotension, circulatory collapse.*

**nitromethane** [Nitrate/nitrite] *Methemoglobinemia, hypotension, circulatory collapse.*

**nitromuriatic acid** [Inorganic acid] *Pulmonary edema, bronchospasm, circulatory collapse, laryngeal spasm and edema, severe chemical burns to skin, mucous membranes, and internal organs, GI tract perforation and hemorrhage, peritonitis.*

**nitronaphthalene** [Naphthalene] *Delayed-onset acute intravascular hemolysis.*

**HazMat**

**N-nitro-N-methylurethane** [Nitrate/ nitrite] *Methemoglobinemia, hypotension, circulatory collapse.* [Isocyanate/ aliphatic thiocyanate] *CNS depression, respiratory arrest, respiratory paralysis, pulmonary edema, cyanide toxicity.*

**nitrophenol; p-nitrophenol** [Dinitrophenol] *Respiratory and circulatory collapse, pulmonary edema, hyperthermia.*

**nitropropane; 2-nitropropane** [Nitrate/nitrite] *Methemoglobinemia, hypotension, circulatory collapse.*

**nitroprusside salt (n.o.s.)** [Cyanide] *Impairment of cellular oxygenation and adenosine triphosphate production, hypoxia, death.*

**N-nitrosodibutylamine** [Organic base/amine] *Pulmonary edema, cardiac depression, seizures.* [Nitrate/ nitrite] *Methemoglobinemia, hypotension, circulatory collapse.*

**N-nitrosodiethanolamine** [Organic base/amine] *Pulmonary edema, cardiac depression, seizures.* [Nitrate/ nitrite] *Methemoglobinemia, hypotension, circulatory collapse.*

**N-nitrosodiethylamine** [Organic base/amine] *Pulmonary edema, cardiac depression, seizures.* [Nitrate/ nitrite] *Methemoglobinemia, hypotension, circulatory collapse.*

**nitrosodimethylamine; N-nitrosodimethylamine** [Organic base/amine] *Pulmonary edema, cardiac depression, seizures.* [Nitrate/nitrite] *Methemoglobinemia, hypotension, circulatory collapse.*

**nitrosodimethylaniline** [Aniline] *Methemoglobinemia, hypoxia.*

**N-nitrosodiphenylamine; p-nitrosodiphenylamine** [Organic base/ amine] *Pulmonary edema, cardiac depression, seizures.* [Nitrate/nitrite] *Methemoglobinemia, hypotension, circulatory collapse.*

**N-nitrosodipropylamine** [Organic base/amine] *Pulmonary edema, cardiac depression, seizures.* [Nitrate/ nitrite] *Methemoglobinemia, hypotension, circulatory collapse.*

**N-nitrosomethylvinylamine** [Organic base/amine] *Pulmonary edema, cardiac depression, seizures.* [Nitrate/nitrite] *Methemoglobinemia, hypotension, circulatory collapse.*

**N-nitrosomorpholine** [Organic base/ amine] *Pulmonary edema, cardiac depression, seizures.* [Nitrate/nitrite] *Methemoglobinemia, hypotension, circulatory collapse.*

**N-nitroso-N-ethylurea** [Nitrate/ nitrite] *Methemoglobinemia, hypotension, circulatory collapse.* [Nitrogen oxide] *Lower respiratory tract symptoms, pulmonary edema, laryngospasm, bronchospasm, asphyxiation.*

**N-nitroso-N-methylurea** [Nitrate/ nitrite] *Methemoglobinemia, hypotension, circulatory collapse.* [Nitrogen oxide] *Lower respiratory tract symptoms, pulmonary edema, laryngospasm, bronchospasm, asphyxiation.*

**N-nitrosonornicotine** [Nicotine] *Respiratory and cardiac arrest, CNS stimulation, CNS depression.*

**N-nitrosopiperidine** [Nitrate/nitrite] *Methemoglobinemia, hypotension, circulatory collapse.*

**N-nitrosopyrrolidine** [Nitrate/nitrite] *Methemoglobinemia, hypotension, circulatory collapse.*

**nitrostarch** [Nitrate/nitrite] *Methemoglobinemia, hypotension, circulatory collapse.*

**nitrosyl chloride** [Inorganic acid] *Pulmonary edema, bronchospasm, circulatory collapse, laryngeal spasm and edema, severe chemical burns to skin, mucous membranes, and internal organs, GI tract perforation and hemorrhage, peritonitis.*

**nitrosylsulfuric acid** [Inorganic acid] *Pulmonary edema, bronchospasm, circulatory collapse, laryngeal spasm and edema, severe chemical burns to skin, mucous membranes, and internal organs, GI tract perforation and hemorrhage, peritonitis.*

**nitrotoluene** [Aromatic hydrocarbon] *Arrhythmias, respiratory failure, pulmonary edema, paralysis, brain and kidney damage.* [Nitrate/nitrite] *Methemoglobinemia, hypotension, circulatory collapse.*

**nitrous oxide (gas or cryogenic liquid)** [Nitrogen oxide] *Lower respiratory tract symptoms, pulmonary edema, laryngospasm, bronchospasm, asphyxiation.*

**nitrous oxide & carbon dioxide mixture** [Simple asphyxiant] *Asphyxiation.*

**nitroxylene** [Aromatic hydrocarbon] *Arrhythmias, respiratory failure, pulmonary edema, paralysis, brain and kidney damage.* [Nitrate/nitrite] *Methemoglobinemia, hypotension, circulatory collapse.*

**nitroxylol** [Phenol] *Coma, hypotension, arrhythmias, pulmonary edema, respiratory arrest.* [Nitrate/nitrite] *Methemoglobinemia, hypotension, circulatory collapse.*

**nonane** [Aliphatic hydrocarbon] *Arrhythmias, asphyxiation, anesthesia.*

**nonflammable gas (n.o.s.)** [Nonflammable gas] *Pulmonary edema, respiratory failure, asphyxiation.*

**nonyl trichlorosilane** [Silane/chlorosilane] *Respiratory tract irritation, pulmonary edema.*

**norbornadiene** [Aliphatic hydrocarbon] *Arrhythmias, asphyxiation, anesthesia.*

**norbromide** [Poison] *Cardiovascular collapse, pulmonary edema, CNS depression, coma, seizures, nausea, vomiting, cardiopulmonary arrest.*

**normal propyl alcohol** [Lower alcohol (1–3 carbons)] *CNS depression, coma, respiratory arrest, arrhythmias.*

**nux vomica** [Strychnine] *Convulsions, acidosis, diaphragmatic spasms, respiratory arrest.*

**octachloronaphthalene** [Naphthalene] *Delayed-onset acute intravascular hemolysis.*

**octadecyl trichlorosilane** [Silane/chlorosilane] *Respiratory tract irritation, pulmonary edema.*

**octadiene** [Aliphatic hydrocarbon] *Arrhythmias, asphyxiation, anesthesia.*

**octafluorobutene** [Halogenated aliphatic hydrocarbon] *CNS depression, respiratory arrest, circulatory collapse.*

**octafluorocyclobutane** [Halogenated aliphatic hydrocarbon] *CNS depression, respiratory arrest, circulatory collapse.*

**octafluoropropane** [Halogenated aliphatic hydrocarbon] *CNS depression, respiratory arrest, circulatory collapse.*

**octamethyl diphosphoramide** [Organophosphate] *Pulmonary edema, respiratory muscle paralysis, respiratory failure, bradycardia, acetylcholinesterase inhibition, hypotension, pulmonary edema, overstimulation of parasympathetic nervous system, striated muscle, sympathetic ganglia, and CNS.*

**octamethyl pyrophosphoramide** [Organophosphate] *Pulmonary edema, respiratory muscle paralysis, respiratory failure, bradycardia, acetylcholinesterase inhibition, hypotension, pulmonary edema, overstimulation of parasympathetic nervous system, striated muscle, sympathetic ganglia, and CNS.*

**octane** [Aliphatic hydrocarbon] *Arrhythmias, asphyxiation, anesthesia.*

**1-octanol** [Higher alcohol (4+ carbons)] *CNS depression, respiratory failure, arrhythmias.*

**octanoyl peroxide** [Organic peroxide] *Pulmonary and laryngeal edema, circulatory arrest, hypovolemic shock, chemical burns to skin, mucous membranes, and internal organs.*

**octyl aldehyde** [Aldehyde] *Seizures, respiratory failure, pulmonary edema.*

**octyl ammonium metharsonate** [Arsenic] *Heavy metal toxicity, vomiting, GI bleeding, CNS depression, pulmonary edema, cardiac arrest.*

**octyl cresols (n.o.s.)** [Phenol] *Coma, hypotension, arrhythmias, pulmonary edema, respiratory arrest.*

HazMat

**tert-octyl hydroperoxide** [Organic peroxide] *Pulmonary and laryngeal edema, circulatory arrest, hypovolemic shock, chemical burns to skin, mucous membranes, and internal organs.*

**tert-octyl mercaptan** [Sulfur] *Respiratory tract irritation, pulmonary edema, anaphylaxis.*

**tert-octyl peroxy-2-ethylhexanoate** [Organic peroxide] *Pulmonary and laryngeal edema, circulatory arrest, hypovolemic shock, chemical burns to skin, mucous membranes, and internal organs.* [Organic acid] *Pulmonary edema, circulatory collapse, laryngeal edema and spasm, severe chemical burns to skin, mucous membranes, and internal organs, GI tract perforation and hemorrhage, peritonitis.*

**octyl trichlorosilane** [Silane/chlorosilane] *Respiratory tract irritation, pulmonary edema.*

**oil, petroleum (n.o.s.)** [Hydrocarbon mixture] *CNS depression, respiratory arrest, seizures, arrhythmias, pulmonary edema.*

**oil gas** [Hydrocarbon mixture] *CNS depression, respiratory arrest, seizures, arrhythmias, pulmonary edema.*

**oleum** [Inorganic acid] *Pulmonary edema, bronchospasm, circulatory collapse, laryngeal spasm and edema, severe chemical burns to skin, mucous membranes, and internal organs, GI tract perforation and hemorrhage, peritonitis.*

**organic peroxide (n.o.s.); organic peroxide mixture (n.o.s.)** [Organic peroxide] *Pulmonary and laryngeal edema, circulatory arrest, hypovolemic shock, chemical burns to skin, mucous membranes, and internal organs.*

**organic peroxide, types B, C, D, E, and F** [Organic peroxide] *Pulmonary and laryngeal edema, circulatory arrest, hypovolemic shock, chemical burns to skin, mucous membranes, and internal organs.*

**organic phosphate compound (poison B)** [Organophosphate] *Pulmonary edema, respiratory muscle paraly-sis, respiratory failure, bradycardia, acetylcholinesterase inhibition, hypotension, pulmonary edema, overstimulation of parasympathetic nervous system, striated muscle, sympathetic ganglia, and CNS.*

**organic phosphorus compound & compressed gas mixture** [Organophosphate] *Pulmonary edema, respiratory muscle paralysis, respiratory failure, bradycardia, acetylcholinesterase inhibition, hypotension, pulmonary edema, overstimulation of parasympathetic nervous system, striated muscle, sympathetic ganglia, and CNS.*

**organic phosphorus pesticide (n.o.s.)** [Organophosphate] *Pulmonary edema, respiratory muscle paralysis, respiratory failure, bradycardia, acetylcholinesterase inhibition, hypotension, pulmonary edema, overstimulation of parasympathetic nervous system, striated muscle, sympathetic ganglia, and CNS.*

**organochlorine pesticide, liquid (n.o.s.)** [Chlordane] *Respiratory failure, seizures, exhaustion, death.*

**organochlorine pesticide, solid (n.o.s.)** [Aldrin/dieldrin/endrin] *Seizures, respiratory failure.*

**organomercury mixture (n.o.s.)** [Mercury] *Circulatory collapse, arrhythmias, respiratory failure, pulmonary edema, neurotoxic effects.*

**organophosphate (n.o.s.)** [Organophosphate] *Pulmonary edema, respiratory muscle paralysis, respiratory failure, bradycardia, acetylcholinesterase inhibition, hypotension, pulmonary edema, overstimulation of parasympathetic nervous system, striated muscle, sympathetic ganglia, and CNS.*

**organophosphorus pesticide (n.o.s.)** [Organophosphate] *Pulmonary edema, respiratory muscle paralysis, respiratory failure, bradycardia, acetylcholinesterase inhibition, hypotension, pulmonary edema, overstimulation of parasympathetic nervous sys-*

tem, striated muscle, sympathetic ganglia, and CNS.

**organotin mixture (n.o.s.)** [Organotin] *Respiratory failure, pulmonary edema, cerebral edema.*

**organotin pesticide (n.o.s.)** [Organotin] *Respiratory failure, pulmonary edema, cerebral edema.*

**ORM-A (n.o.s.); ORM-B (n.o.s.); ORM-E (n.o.s.)** [Poison] *Cardiovascular collapse, pulmonary edema, CNS depression, coma, seizures, nausea, vomiting, cardiopulmonary arrest.*

**osmic acid** [Inorganic acid] *Pulmonary edema, bronchospasm, circulatory collapse, laryngeal spasm and edema, severe chemical burns to skin, mucous membranes, and internal organs, GI tract perforation and hemorrhage, peritonitis.*

**osmium; osmium mixture (n.o.s.)** [Poison] *Cardiovascular collapse, pulmonary edema, CNS depression, coma, seizures, nausea, vomiting, cardiopulmonary arrest.*

**osmium oxide** [Poison] *Cardiovascular collapse, pulmonary edema, CNS depression, coma, seizures, nausea, vomiting, cardiopulmonary arrest.*

**osmium tetroxide** [Poison] *Cardiovascular collapse, pulmonary edema, CNS depression, coma, seizures, nausea, vomiting, cardiopulmonary arrest.*

**ouabain** [Poison] *Cardiovascular collapse, pulmonary edema, CNS depression, coma, seizures, nausea, vomiting, cardiopulmonary arrest.*

**oxalate (n.o.s.)** [Oxalate] *Cardiovascular collapse, arrhythmias, seizures.*

**oxalic acid** [Oxalate] *Cardiovascular collapse, arrhythmias, seizures.*

**oxamyl** [Carbamate] *Acetylcholinesterase inhibition (reversible), bradycardia, hypotension, respiratory muscle paralysis, respiratory arrest, pulmonary edema.*

**oxetane** [Ether] *Anesthesia, respiratory arrest.*

**oxidizer (n.o.s.)** [Oxidizer] *Pulmonary and laryngeal edema, circulatory arrest, hypovolemic shock, chemical*

burns of skin, mucous membranes, and internal organs.

**oxidizer, corrosive (n.o.s.)** [Oxidizer] *Pulmonary and laryngeal edema, circulatory arrest, hypovolemic shock, chemical burns of skin, mucous membranes, and internal organs.* [Corrosive] *Upper airway burns and edema, circulatory collapse, severe chemical burns to skin, toxic systemic effects, GI tract perforation and hemorrhage, peritonitis.*

**oxidizer, flammable solid (n.o.s.)** [Flammable solid] *Shock, severe chemical and thermal burns, severe respiratory tract irritation, pulmonary edema, respiratory arrest, ECG changes, sudden death.* [Oxidizer] *Pulmonary and laryngeal edema, circulatory arrest, hypovolemic shock, chemical burns of skin, mucous membranes, and internal organs.*

**oxidizer, poisonous (n.o.s.)** [Oxidizer] *Pulmonary and laryngeal edema, circulatory arrest, hypovolemic shock, chemical burns of skin, mucous membranes, and internal organs.* [Poison] *Cardiovascular collapse, pulmonary edema, CNS depression, coma, seizures, nausea, vomiting, cardiopulmonary arrest.*

**oxirane** [Ethylene oxide] *Respiratory tract irritation, pulmonary edema.*

**oxydisulfoton** [Organophosphate] *Pulmonary edema, respiratory muscle paralysis, respiratory failure, bradycardia, acetylcholinesterase inhibition, hypotension, pulmonary edema, overstimulation of parasympathetic nervous system, striated muscle, sympathetic ganglia, and CNS.*

**oxygen (gas or cryogenic liquid)** [Oxidizer] *Pulmonary and laryngeal edema, circulatory arrest, hypovolemic shock, chemical burns of skin, mucous membranes, and internal organs.*

**oxygen & carbon dioxide mixture** [Simple asphyxiant] *Asphyxiation.*

**oxygen difluoride** [Fluorine] *CNS depression, respiratory arrest, cardiovascular collapse, shock, arrhythmias.*

HazMat

[Ozone] *Pulmonary edema, airway obstruction.*

**oxygen & helium mixture** [Simple asphyxiant] *Asphyxiation.*

**oxygen & rare gas mixture** [Poison] *Cardiovascular collapse, pulmonary edema, CNS depression, coma, seizures, nausea, vomiting, cardiopulmonary arrest.* [Simple asphyxiant] *Asphyxiation.*

**ozone (O₃)** [Ozone] *Pulmonary edema, airway obstruction.*

**ozone & cyclohexene mixture** [Aliphatic hydrocarbon] *Arrhythmias, asphyxiation, anesthesia.* [Ozone] *Pulmonary edema, airway obstruction.*

**ozone & nitrogen oxide mixture** [Nitrogen oxide] *Lower respiratory tract symptoms, pulmonary edema, laryngospasm, bronchospasm, asphyxiation.* [Ozone] *Pulmonary edema, airway obstruction.*

**ozone & sulfur dioxide mixture** [Ozone] *Pulmonary edema, airway obstruction.* [Sulfur] *Respiratory tract irritation, pulmonary edema, anaphylaxis.*

**paint and paint-related material, corrosive** [Corrosive] *Upper airway burns and edema, circulatory collapse, severe chemical burns to skin, toxic systemic effects, GI tract perforation and hemorrhage, peritonitis.*

**paint and paint-related material, flammable** [Flammable/combustible liquid] *CNS depression, respiratory arrest, convulsions, arrhythmias, pulmonary edema.*

**paint drier (n.o.s.)** [Poison] *Cardiovascular collapse, pulmonary edema, CNS depression, coma, seizures, nausea, vomiting, cardiopulmonary arrest.*

**paint eradicator** [Flammable/combustible liquid] *CNS depression, respiratory arrest, convulsions, arrhythmias, pulmonary edema.*

**paint stripper** [Hydrocarbon mixture] *CNS depression, respiratory arrest, seizures, arrhythmias, pulmonary edema.*

**painters' naphtha** [Hydrocarbon mixture] *CNS depression, respiratory arrest, seizures, arrhythmias, pulmonary edema.*

**paper, unsaturated oil–treated** [Flammable solid] *Shock, severe chemical and thermal burns, severe respiratory tract irritation, pulmonary edema, respiratory arrest, ECG changes, sudden death.*

**paradiaminobenzene** [Aniline] *Methemoglobinemia, hypoxia.*

**paradichlorobenzene** [Lindane] *CNS stimulation, seizures, respiratory failure.*

**paraffin** [Aliphatic hydrocarbon] *Arrhythmias, asphyxiation, anesthesia.*

**paraformaldehyde** [Aldehyde] *Seizures, respiratory failure, pulmonary edema.*

**paraldehyde** [Aldehyde] *Seizures, respiratory failure, pulmonary edema.*

**paramethane hydroperoxide** [Organic peroxide] *Pulmonary and laryngeal edema, circulatory arrest, hypovolemic shock, chemical burns to skin, mucous membranes, and internal organs.*

**Paraoxon (diethyl-p-nitrophenyl phosphate)** [Organophosphate] *Pulmonary edema, respiratory muscle paralysis, respiratory failure, bradycardia, acetylcholinesterase inhibition, hypotension, pulmonary edema, overstimulation of parasympathetic nervous system, striated muscle, sympathetic ganglia, and CNS.*

**paraquat** [Paraquat] *Widespread edema, cardiac damage, circulatory collapse, cerebral hemorrhage or infarcts, death. (Defoliant used in warfare.)*

**paraquat methosulfate** [Paraquat] *Widespread edema, cardiac damage, circulatory collapse, cerebral hemorrhage or infarcts, death. (Defoliant used in warfare.)*

**parathion; parathion mixture (n.o.s.)** [Organophosphate] *Pulmonary edema, respiratory muscle paralysis, respiratory failure, bradycardia, acetylcholinesterase inhibition, hypotension, pulmonary edema, overstimulation of parasympathetic nervous sys-*

tem, *striated muscle, sympathetic ganglia, and CNS.*

**parathion & compressed gas mixture** [Organophosphate] *Pulmonary edema, respiratory muscle paralysis, respiratory failure, bradycardia, acetylcholinesterase inhibition, hypotension, pulmonary edema, overstimulation of parasympathetic nervous system, striated muscle, sympathetic ganglia, and CNS.*

**parathion-methyl** [Organophosphate] *Pulmonary edema, respiratory muscle paralysis, respiratory failure, bradycardia, acetylcholinesterase inhibition, hypotension, pulmonary edema, overstimulation of parasympathetic nervous system, striated muscle, sympathetic ganglia, and CNS.*

**Paris green** [Arsenic] *Heavy metal toxicity, vomiting, GI bleeding, CNS depression, pulmonary edema, cardiac arrest.* [Copper] *Respiratory tract irritation and arrest, hemorrhagic gastritis.*

**PBB (polybrominated biphenyl)** Polychlorinated biphenyl/polybrominated biphenyl/polychlorinated [dibenzofuran] *Liver and kidney damage.*

**PCB (polychlorinated biphenyl)** Polychlorinated biphenyl/polybrominated biphenyl/polychlorinated [dibenzofuran] *Liver and kidney damage.*

**PCDF (polychlorinated dibenzofuran)** Polychlorinated biphenyl/polybrominated biphenyl/polychlorinated [dibenzofuran] *Liver and kidney damage.*

**PCNB** [Pentachlorophenol] *Respiratory and circulatory collapse, severe hyperthermia.*

**PCP (pentachlorophenol)** [Pentachlorophenol] *Respiratory and circulatory collapse, severe hyperthermia.*

**pelargonyl peroxide** [Organic peroxide] *Pulmonary and laryngeal edema, circulatory arrest, hypovolemic shock, chemical burns to skin, mucous membranes, and internal organs.*

**pentaborane** [Boron] *Respiratory tract irritation, laryngeal spasm and edema, pulmonary edema, severe chemical burns.*

**pentachlorobenzene** [Aromatic hydrocarbon] *Arrhythmias, respiratory failure, pulmonary edema, paralysis, brain and kidney damage.*

**pentachloroethane** [Halogenated aliphatic hydrocarbon] *CNS depression, respiratory arrest, circulatory collapse.*

**pentachloronitrobenzene** [Pentachlorophenol] *Respiratory and circulatory collapse, severe hyperthermia.*

**pentachlorophenol (PCP)** [Pentachlorophenol] *Respiratory and circulatory collapse, severe hyperthermia.*

**pentadecylamine** [Organic base/amine] *Pulmonary edema, cardiac depression, seizures.*

**1,3-pentadiene** [Aliphatic hydrocarbon] *Arrhythmias, asphyxiation, anesthesia.*

**pentaerythritol** [Ethylene glycol] *Respiratory failure, pulmonary edema, paralysis, cardiovascular collapse, severe acidosis.*

**pentamethyl heptane** [Aliphatic hydrocarbon] *Arrhythmias, asphyxiation, anesthesia.*

**pentane** [Aliphatic hydrocarbon] *Arrhythmias, asphyxiation, anesthesia.*

**pentane-2,4-dione** [Ketone] *Respiratory mucous membrane irritation, pulmonary edema, CNS depression.*

**pentanoic acid; n-pentanoic acid (valeric acid)** [Organic acid] *Pulmonary edema, circulatory collapse, laryngeal edema and spasm, severe chemical burns to skin, mucous membranes, and internal organs, GI tract perforation and hemorrhage, peritonitis.*

**2-pentanone** [Ketone] *Respiratory mucous membrane irritation, pulmonary edema, CNS depression.*

**1-pentene** [Aliphatic hydrocarbon] *Arrhythmias, asphyxiation, anesthesia.*

**pentol** [Higher alcohol (4+ carbons)] *CNS depression, respiratory failure, arrhythmias.*

**peracetic acid** [Organic peroxide] *Pulmonary and laryngeal edema, circulatory arrest, hypovolemic shock, chemical burns to skin, mucous membranes, and internal organs.* [Organic acid] *Pulmonary edema, circulatory collapse, laryngeal edema and spasm, severe chemical burns to skin, mucous membranes, and internal organs, GI tract perforation and hemorrhage, peritonitis.*

**perc** [Halogenated aliphatic hydrocarbon] *CNS depression, respiratory arrest, circulatory collapse.*

**perchlorate (n.o.s.)** [Chlorate] *Hemolysis, methemoglobinemia, hypoperfusion, CNS depression, delayed-onset renal failure.*

**perchloric acid** [Oxidizer] *Pulmonary and laryngeal edema, circulatory arrest, hypovolemic shock, chemical burns of skin, mucous membranes, and internal organs.* [Inorganic acid] *Pulmonary edema, bronchospasm, circulatory collapse, laryngeal spasm and edema, severe chemical burns to skin, mucous membranes, and internal organs, GI tract perforation and hemorrhage, peritonitis.*

**perchloroethylene** [Halogenated aliphatic hydrocarbon] *CNS depression, respiratory arrest, circulatory collapse.*

**perchloromethyl mercaptan** [Sulfur] *Respiratory tract irritation, pulmonary edema, anaphylaxis.*

**perchloryl fluoride** [Oxidizer] *Pulmonary and laryngeal edema, circulatory arrest, hypovolemic shock, chemical burns of skin, mucous membranes, and internal organs.* [Fluorine] *CNS depression, respiratory arrest, cardiovascular collapse, shock, arrhythmias.*

**perfluoroethylvinyl ether** [Ether] *Anesthesia, respiratory arrest.*

**perfluoromethylvinyl ether** [Ether] *Anesthesia, respiratory arrest.*

**perfluoropropane** [Halogenated aliphatic hydrocarbon] *CNS depression, respiratory arrest, circulatory collapse.*

**perfume, flammable** [Hydrocarbon mixture] *CNS depression, respiratory arrest, seizures, arrhythmias, pulmonary edema.*

**permanganate (n.o.s.)** [Inorganic acid] *Pulmonary edema, bronchospasm, circulatory collapse, laryngeal spasm and edema, severe chemical burns to skin, mucous membranes, and internal organs, GI tract perforation and hemorrhage, peritonitis.*

**permethrin** [Pyrethrin/pyrethroid] *Respiratory paralysis, convulsions.*

**peroxide (n.o.s.)** [Oxidizer] *Pulmonary and laryngeal edema, circulatory arrest, hypovolemic shock, chemical burns of skin, mucous membranes, and internal organs.*

**peroxyacetic acid** [Organic peroxide] *Pulmonary and laryngeal edema, circulatory arrest, hypovolemic shock, chemical burns to skin, mucous membranes, and internal organs.* [Organic acid] *Pulmonary edema, circulatory collapse, laryngeal edema and spasm, severe chemical burns to skin, mucous membranes, and internal organs, GI tract perforation and hemorrhage, peritonitis.*

**peroxyacetic acid & hydrogen peroxide mixture** [Oxidizer] *Pulmonary and laryngeal edema, circulatory arrest, hypovolemic shock, chemical burns of skin, mucous membranes, and internal organs.*

**persulfate salt (n.o.s.)** [Sulfur] *Respiratory tract irritation, pulmonary edema, anaphylaxis.*

**Perthane** [DDT] *CNS disruption, respiratory control center paralysis, ventricular fibrillation, seizures, respiratory arrest.*

**pesticide, benzoic derivative (n.o.s.)** [Organic acid] *Pulmonary edema, circulatory collapse, laryngeal edema and spasm, severe chemical burns to skin, mucous membranes, and internal organs, GI tract perforation and hemorrhage, peritonitis.*

**pesticide, bipyridilium (n.o.s.)** [Paraquat] *Widespread edema, cardiac damage, circulatory collapse, cerebral hemorrhage or infarcts, death. (Defoliant used in warfare.)*

**pesticide, carbamate (n.o.s.)** [Carbamate] *Acetylcholinesterase inhibition (reversible), bradycardia, hypotension, respiratory muscle paralysis, respiratory arrest, pulmonary edema.*

**pesticide, copper-based (n.o.s.)** [Copper] *Respiratory tract irritation and arrest, hemorrhagic gastritis.*

**pesticide, coumarin derivative (n.o.s.)** [Ketone] *Respiratory mucous membrane irritation, pulmonary edema, CNS depression.*

**pesticide, dithiocarbamate (n.o.s.)** [Dithiocarbamate] *Hypotension, respiratory failure.*

**pesticide, flammable poison (n.o.s.)** [Flammable/combustible liquid] *CNS depression, respiratory arrest, convulsions, arrhythmias, pulmonary edema.* [Poison] *Cardiovascular collapse, pulmonary edema, CNS depression, coma, seizures, nausea, vomiting, cardiopulmonary arrest.*

**pesticide, maneb-containing** [Dithiocarbamate] *Hypotension, respiratory failure.*

**pesticide, mercury-based (n.o.s.)** [Mercury] *Circulatory collapse, arrhythmias, respiratory failure, pulmonary edema, neurotoxic effects.*

**pesticide, organophosphate (n.o.s.)** [Organophosphate] *Pulmonary edema, respiratory muscle paralysis, respiratory failure, bradycardia, acetylcholinesterase inhibition, hypotension, pulmonary edema, overstimulation of parasympathetic nervous system, striated muscle, sympathetic ganglia, and CNS.*

**pesticide, phenoxy (n.o.s.)** [Chlorophenoxy herbicide] *CNS depression, CNS stimulation, respiratory failure, ventricular fibrillation, seizures.*

**pesticide, phenylurea (n.o.s.)** [Naphthalene] *Delayed-onset acute intravascular hemolysis.*

**pesticide, phthalimide derivative (n.o.s.)** [Irritant] *Severe immediate or delayed upper airway or respiratory tract irritation, pulmonary edema, glottic spasm, airway obstruction.*

**pesticide, poisonous (n.o.s.)** [Poison] *Cardiovascular collapse, pulmonary edema, CNS depression, coma, seizures, nausea, vomiting, cardiopulmonary arrest.*

**pesticide, substituted nitrophenol (n.o.s.)** [Dinitrophenol] *Respiratory and circulatory collapse, pulmonary edema, hyperthermia.*

**pesticide, triazine (n.o.s.)** [Irritant] *Severe immediate or delayed upper airway or respiratory tract irritation, pulmonary edema, glottic spasm, airway obstruction.*

**petrol** [Hydrocarbon mixture] *CNS depression, respiratory arrest, seizures, arrhythmias, pulmonary edema.*

**petroleum crude oil** [Hydrocarbon mixture] *CNS depression, respiratory arrest, seizures, arrhythmias, pulmonary edema.*

**petroleum distillate (n.o.s.)** [Hydrocarbon mixture] *CNS depression, respiratory arrest, seizures, arrhythmias, pulmonary edema.*

**petroleum ether** [Ether] *Anesthesia, respiratory arrest.*

**petroleum gas, liquefied (LPG)** [Flammable gas] *Respiratory failure, cardiac arrest, arrhythmias.* [Hydrocarbon mixture] *CNS depression, respiratory arrest, seizures, arrhythmias, pulmonary edema.*

**petroleum naphtha** [Hydrocarbon mixture] *CNS depression, respiratory arrest, seizures, arrhythmias, pulmonary edema.*

**petroleum oil** [Hydrocarbon mixture] *CNS depression, respiratory arrest, seizures, arrhythmias, pulmonary edema.*

**petroleum spirit** [Hydrocarbon mixture] *CNS depression, respiratory arrest, seizures, arrhythmias, pulmonary edema.*

**phenacetin** [Aniline] *Methemoglobinemia, hypoxia.*

**phenacyl bromide** [Bromine/methylbromide] *Severe respiratory irritation, pulmonary edema, respiratory failure, coma, convulsions, death.*

HazMat

**phenamiphos** [Organophosphate] *Pulmonary edema, respiratory muscle paralysis, respiratory failure, bradycardia, acetylcholinesterase inhibition, hypotension, pulmonary edema, overstimulation of parasympathetic nervous system, striated muscle, sympathetic ganglia, and CNS.*

**phenanthrene** [Aromatic hydrocarbon] *Arrhythmias, respiratory failure, pulmonary edema, paralysis, brain and kidney damage.*

**phenazopyridine HCl** [Aniline] *Methemoglobinemia, hypoxia.* [Naphthalene] *Delayed-onset acute intravascular hemolysis.*

**phenetidine** [Aniline] *Methemoglobinemia, hypoxia.*

**phenindione** [Warfarin/hydroxycoumarin/indanedione] *Anticoagulation effect, internal hemorrhage.*

**phenol** [Phenol] *Coma, hypotension, arrhythmias, pulmonary edema, respiratory arrest.*

**phenol, chlorinated** [Phenol] *Coma, hypotension, arrhythmias, pulmonary edema, respiratory arrest.*

**phenolsulfonic acid** [Organic acid] *Pulmonary edema, circulatory collapse, laryngeal edema and spasm, severe chemical burns to skin, mucous membranes, and internal organs, GI tract perforation and hemorrhage, peritonitis.* [Phenol] *Coma, hypotension, arrhythmias, pulmonary edema, respiratory arrest.*

**phenoxarsine** [Arsine] *Intravascular hemolysis, pulmonary edema, cardiac and respiratory arrest, delayed-onset jaundice and renal failure.*

**phenoxy pesticide (n.o.s.)** [Chlorophenoxy herbicide] *CNS depression, CNS stimulation, respiratory failure, ventricular fibrillation, seizures.*

**phenprocoumon** [Warfarin/hydroxycoumarin/indanedione] *Anticoagulation effect, internal hemorrhage.*

**Phenyl Cellosolve** [Ethylene glycol] *Respiratory failure, pulmonary edema, paralysis, cardiovascular collapse, severe acidosis.*

**phenyl chloroformate** [Halogenated aliphatic hydrocarbon] *CNS depression, respiratory arrest, circulatory collapse.*

**phenyl isocyanate** [Isocyanate/aliphatic thiocyanate] *CNS depression, respiratory arrest, respiratory paralysis, pulmonary edema, cyanide toxicity.*

**phenyl mercaptan** [Sulfur] *Respiratory tract irritation, pulmonary edema, anaphylaxis.*

**phenyl phosphorous dichloride** [Phosphorus] *Hypovolemic shock, severe tissue burns, severe respiratory irritation, pulmonary edema, respiratory arrest, arrhythmias, sudden death.*

**phenyl phosphorous thiodichloride** [Phosphorus] *Hypovolemic shock, severe tissue burns, severe respiratory irritation, pulmonary edema, respiratory arrest, arrhythmias, sudden death.*

**phenylacetonitrile** [Cyanide] *Impairment of cellular oxygenation and adenosine triphosphate production, hypoxia, death.*

**phenylacetyl chloride** [Aromatic hydrocarbon] *Arrhythmias, respiratory failure, pulmonary edema, paralysis, brain and kidney damage.*

**phenylcarbylamine chloride** [Aniline] *Methemoglobinemia, hypoxia.*

**phenyldichloroarsine** [Arsenic] *Heavy metal toxicity, vomiting, GI bleeding, CNS depression, pulmonary edema, cardiac arrest.* [Arsine] *Intravascular hemolysis, pulmonary edema, cardiac and respiratory arrest, delayed-onset jaundice and renal failure.*

**phenylenediamine** [Organic base/amine] *Pulmonary edema, cardiac depression, seizures.*

**phenylhydrazine** [Hydrazine] *Seizures, hemolysis of red blood cells, pulmonary edema.*

**phenylhydrazine HCl** [Hydrazine] *Seizures, hemolysis of red blood cells, pulmonary edema.*

**phenylmercuric acetate** [Mercury] *Circulatory collapse, arrhythmias, res-*

piratory failure, pulmonary edema, neurotoxic effects.

**phenylmercuric acid salt (n.o.s.)** [Mercury] Circulatory collapse, arrhythmias, respiratory failure, pulmonary edema, neurotoxic effects.

**phenylmercuric hydroxide** [Mercury] Circulatory collapse, arrhythmias, respiratory failure, pulmonary edema, neurotoxic effects.

**phenylmercuric mixture (n.o.s.)** [Mercury] Circulatory collapse, arrhythmias, respiratory failure, pulmonary edema, neurotoxic effects.

**phenylmercuric nitrate** [Nitrate/ nitrite] Methemoglobinemia, hypotension, circulatory collapse. [Mercury] Circulatory collapse, arrhythmias, respiratory failure, pulmonary edema, neurotoxic effects.

**phenylmercuric triethanol ammonium lactate** [Mercury] Circulatory collapse, arrhythmias, respiratory failure, pulmonary edema, neurotoxic effects.

**phenylmercury acetate** [Mercury] Circulatory collapse, arrhythmias, respiratory failure, pulmonary edema, neurotoxic effects.

**phenylphenol** [Phenol] Coma, hypotension, arrhythmias, pulmonary edema, respiratory arrest.

**phenylphosphine** [Phosphine] Severe pulmonary irritation, pulmonary edema.

**phenylsilatrane** [Poison] Cardiovascular collapse, pulmonary edema, CNS depression, coma, seizures, nausea, vomiting, cardiopulmonary arrest.

**phenylthiourea** [Naphthalene] Delayed-onset acute intravascular hemolysis.

**phenyltrichlorosilane** [Silane/chlorosilane] Respiratory tract irritation, pulmonary edema.

**phenylurea pesticide (n.o.s.)** [Naphthalene] Delayed-onset acute intravascular hemolysis.

**phorate** [Organophosphate] Pulmonary edema, respiratory muscle paralysis, respiratory failure, bradycardia, acetylcho-

linesterase inhibition, hypotension, pulmonary edema, overstimulation of parasympathetic nervous system, striated muscle, sympathetic ganglia, and CNS.

**phosacetim** [Organophosphate] Pulmonary edema, respiratory muscle paralysis, respiratory failure, bradycardia, acetylcholinesterase inhibition, hypotension, pulmonary edema, overstimulation of parasympathetic nervous system, striated muscle, sympathetic ganglia, and CNS.

**Phosdrin** [Organophosphate] Pulmonary edema, respiratory muscle paralysis, respiratory failure, bradycardia, acetylcholinesterase inhibition, hypotension, pulmonary edema, overstimulation of parasympathetic nervous system, striated muscle, sympathetic ganglia, and CNS.

**phosfolan** [Organophosphate] Pulmonary edema, respiratory muscle paralysis, respiratory failure, bradycardia, acetylcholinesterase inhibition, hypotension, pulmonary edema, overstimulation of parasympathetic nervous system, striated muscle, sympathetic ganglia, and CNS.

**phosgene** [Phosgene] Severe respiratory irritation, alveolar damage, pulmonary edema.

**phosmet** [Organophosphate] Pulmonary edema, respiratory muscle paralysis, respiratory failure, bradycardia, acetylcholinesterase inhibition, hypotension, pulmonary edema, overstimulation of parasympathetic nervous system, striated muscle, sympathetic ganglia, and CNS.

**phosphabicyclononane** [Poison] Cardiovascular collapse, pulmonary edema, CNS depression, coma, seizures, nausea, vomiting, cardiopulmonary arrest.

**phosphamidon** [Organophosphate] Pulmonary edema, respiratory muscle paralysis, respiratory failure, bradycardia, acetylcholinesterase inhibition, hypotension, pulmonary edema, overstimulation of parasympathetic nervous

**HazMat**

system, striated muscle, sympathetic ganglia, and CNS.

**phosphine** [Phosphine] *Severe pulmonary irritation, pulmonary edema.*

**phosphonothioic acid** [Organophosphate] *Pulmonary edema, respiratory muscle paralysis, respiratory failure, bradycardia, acetylcholinesterase inhibition, hypotension, pulmonary edema, overstimulation of parasympathetic nervous system, striated muscle, sympathetic ganglia, and CNS.*

**phosphoric acid** [Inorganic acid] *Pulmonary edema, bronchospasm, circulatory collapse, laryngeal spasm and edema, severe chemical burns to skin, mucous membranes, and internal organs, GI tract perforation and hemorrhage, peritonitis.*

**phosphoric acid triethyleneimine** [Poison] *Cardiovascular collapse, pulmonary edema, CNS depression, coma, seizures, nausea, vomiting, cardiopulmonary arrest.*

**phosphoric anhydride** [Inorganic acid] *Pulmonary edema, bronchospasm, circulatory collapse, laryngeal spasm and edema, severe chemical burns to skin, mucous membranes, and internal organs, GI tract perforation and hemorrhage, peritonitis.*

**phosphorous acid** [Inorganic acid] *Pulmonary edema, bronchospasm, circulatory collapse, laryngeal spasm and edema, severe chemical burns to skin, mucous membranes, and internal organs, GI tract perforation and hemorrhage, peritonitis.*

**phosphorus (red, white, or yellow)** [Phosphorus] *Hypovolemic shock, severe tissue burns, severe respiratory irritation, pulmonary edema, respiratory arrest, arrhythmias, sudden death.*

**phosphorus heptasulfide** [Sulfur] *Respiratory tract irritation, pulmonary edema, anaphylaxis.* [Phosphorus] *Hypovolemic shock, severe tissue burns, severe respiratory irritation, pulmonary edema, respiratory arrest, arrhythmias, sudden death.*

**phosphorus oxybromide** [Bromine/methylbromide] *Severe respiratory irritation, pulmonary edema, respiratory failure, coma, convulsions, death.* [Phosphorus] *Hypovolemic shock, severe tissue burns, severe respiratory irritation, pulmonary edema, respiratory arrest, arrhythmias, sudden death.*

**phosphorus oxychloride** [Chlorine] *Severe respiratory tract irritation, pulmonary edema, irritation of skin, eyes, and mucous membranes.* [Phosphorus] *Hypovolemic shock, severe tissue burns, severe respiratory irritation, pulmonary edema, respiratory arrest, arrhythmias, sudden death.*

**phosphorus pentabromide** [Bromine/methylbromide] *Severe respiratory irritation, pulmonary edema, respiratory failure, coma, convulsions, death.* [Phosphorus] *Hypovolemic shock, severe tissue burns, severe respiratory irritation, pulmonary edema, respiratory arrest, arrhythmias, sudden death.*

**phosphorus pentachloride** [Chlorine] *Severe respiratory tract irritation, pulmonary edema, irritation of skin, eyes, and mucous membranes.* [Phosphorus] *Hypovolemic shock, severe tissue burns, severe respiratory irritation, pulmonary edema, respiratory arrest, arrhythmias, sudden death.*

**phosphorus pentafluoride** [Fluorine] *CNS depression, respiratory arrest, cardiovascular collapse, shock, arrhythmias.* [Phosphorus] *Hypovolemic shock, severe tissue burns, severe respiratory irritation, pulmonary edema, respiratory arrest, arrhythmias, sudden death.*

**phosphorus pentasulfide** [Sulfur] *Respiratory tract irritation, pulmonary edema, anaphylaxis.* [Phosphorus] *Hypovolemic shock, severe tissue burns, severe respiratory irritation, pulmonary edema, respiratory arrest, arrhythmias, sudden death.*

**phosphorus pentoxide** [Phosphorus] *Hypovolemic shock, severe tissue burns, severe respiratory irritation, pul-*

monary edema, respiratory arrest, arrhythmias, sudden death.

**phosphorus sesquisulfide** [Sulfur] *Respiratory tract irritation, pulmonary edema, anaphylaxis.* [Phosphorus] *Hypovolemic shock, severe tissue burns, severe respiratory irritation, pulmonary edema, respiratory arrest, arrhythmias, sudden death.*

**phosphorus tribromide** [Bromine/ methylbromide] *Severe respiratory irritation, pulmonary edema, respiratory failure, coma, convulsions, death.* [Phosphorus] *Hypovolemic shock, severe tissue burns, severe respiratory irritation, pulmonary edema, respiratory arrest, arrhythmias, sudden death.*

**phosphorus trichloride** [Chlorine] *Severe respiratory tract irritation, pulmonary edema, irritation of skin, eyes, and mucous membranes.* [Phosphorus] *Hypovolemic shock, severe tissue burns, severe respiratory irritation, pulmonary edema, respiratory arrest, arrhythmias, sudden death.*

**phosphorus trifluoride** [Fluorine] *CNS depression, respiratory arrest, cardiovascular collapse, shock, arrhythmias.* [Phosphorus] *Hypovolemic shock, severe tissue burns, severe respiratory irritation, pulmonary edema, respiratory arrest, arrhythmias, sudden death.*

**phosphorus trioxide** [Phosphorus] *Hypovolemic shock, severe tissue burns, severe respiratory irritation, pulmonary edema, respiratory arrest, arrhythmias, sudden death.*

**phosphorus trisulfide** [Sulfur] *Respiratory tract irritation, pulmonary edema, anaphylaxis.* [Phosphorus] *Hypovolemic shock, severe tissue burns, severe respiratory irritation, pulmonary edema, respiratory arrest, arrhythmias, sudden death.*

**phosphoryl chloride** [Chlorine] *Severe respiratory tract irritation, pulmonary edema, irritation of skin, eyes, and mucous membranes.* [Phosphorus] *Hypovolemic shock, severe tissue burns, severe respiratory irritation, pul-*

monary edema, respiratory arrest, arrhythmias, sudden death.

**phostex** [Organophosphate] *Pulmonary edema, respiratory muscle paralysis, respiratory failure, bradycardia, acetylcholinesterase inhibition, hypotension, pulmonary edema, overstimulation of parasympathetic nervous system, striated muscle, sympathetic ganglia, and CNS.*

**phthalic anhydride** [Organic acid] *Pulmonary edema, circulatory collapse, laryngeal edema and spasm, severe chemical burns to skin, mucous membranes, and internal organs, GI tract perforation and hemorrhage, peritonitis.*

**phthalimide derivative pesticide (n.o.s.)** [Irritant] *Severe immediate or delayed upper airway or respiratory tract irritation, pulmonary edema, glottic spasm, airway obstruction.*

**phthalonitrile** [Cyanide] *Impairment of cellular oxygenation and adenosine triphosphate production, hypoxia, death.*

**physostigmine** [Poison] *Cardiovascular collapse, pulmonary edema, CNS depression, coma, seizures, nausea, vomiting, cardiopulmonary arrest.*

**picoline** [Aromatic hydrocarbon] *Arrhythmias, respiratory failure, pulmonary edema, paralysis, brain and kidney damage.*

**picrate** [Dinitrophenol] *Respiratory and circulatory collapse, pulmonary edema, hyperthermia.*

**picric acid** [Dinitrophenol] *Respiratory and circulatory collapse, pulmonary edema, hyperthermia.*

**picrotoxin** [Poison] *Cardiovascular collapse, pulmonary edema, CNS depression, coma, seizures, nausea, vomiting, cardiopulmonary arrest.*

**pinane hydroperoxide** [Organic peroxide] *Pulmonary and laryngeal edema, circulatory arrest, hypovolemic shock, chemical burns to skin, mucous membranes, and internal organs.*

**pinayl hydroperoxide** [Organic peroxide] *Pulmonary and laryngeal edema, circulatory arrest, hypovolemic* *shock, chemical burns to skin, mucous membranes, and internal organs.*

**pindone** [Warfarin/hydroxycoumarin/indanedione] *Anticoagulation effect, internal hemorrhage.*

**pine oil** [Turpentine/terpene] *Respiratory failure, pulmonary edema, tachycardia.*

**α-pinene; alpha-pinene** [Turpentine/terpene] *Respiratory failure, pulmonary edema, tachycardia.*

**piperazine** [Organic base/amine] *Pulmonary edema, cardiac depression, seizures.*

**piperidine** [Organic base/amine] *Pulmonary edema, cardiac depression, seizures.*

**piperonyl butoxide** [Poison] *Cardiovascular collapse, pulmonary edema, CNS depression, coma, seizures, nausea, vomiting, cardiopulmonary arrest.*

**piperonyl cyclonene** [Poison] *Cardiovascular collapse, pulmonary edema, CNS depression, coma, seizures, nausea, vomiting, cardiopulmonary arrest.*

**pirimicarb** [Carbamate] *Acetylcholinesterase inhibition (reversible), bradycardia, hypotension, respiratory muscle paralysis, respiratory arrest, pulmonary edema.*

**pivaloyl chloride** [Halogenated aliphatic hydrocarbon] *CNS depression, respiratory arrest, circulatory collapse.*

**2-pivalyl-1,3-indandione** [Warfarin/hydroxycoumarin/indanedione] *Anticoagulation effect, internal hemorrhage.*

**plastic, nitrocellulose-based, spontaneously combustible (n.o.s.)** [Flammable solid] *Shock, severe chemical and thermal burns, severe respiratory tract irritation, pulmonary edema, respiratory arrest, ECG changes, sudden death.*

**plastic that evolves a flammable vapor (n.o.s.)** [Flammable solid] *Shock, severe chemical and thermal burns, severe respiratory tract irritation, pulmonary edema, respiratory arrest, ECG changes, sudden death.*

**poison B liquid (n.o.s.)** [Poison] *Cardiovascular collapse, pulmonary edema, CNS depression, coma, seizures, nausea, vomiting, cardiopulmonary arrest.*

**poisonous gas, flammable (n.o.s.)** [Flammable gas] *Respiratory failure, cardiac arrest, arrhythmias.* [Poison] *Cardiovascular collapse, pulmonary edema, CNS depression, coma, seizures, nausea, vomiting, cardiopulmonary arrest.*

**poisonous liquid, flammable (n.o.s.)** [Flammable/combustible liquid] *CNS depression, respiratory arrest, convulsions, arrhythmias, pulmonary edema.* [Poison] *Cardiovascular collapse, pulmonary edema, CNS depression, coma, seizures, nausea, vomiting, cardiopulmonary arrest.*

**poisonous solid, flammable (n.o.s.)** [Flammable solid] *Shock, severe chemical and thermal burns, severe respiratory tract irritation, pulmonary edema, respiratory arrest, ECG changes, sudden death.* [Poison] *Cardiovascular collapse, pulmonary edema, CNS depression, coma, seizures, nausea, vomiting, cardiopulmonary arrest.*

**poisonous solid, liquid, or gas (n.o.s.)** [Poison] *Cardiovascular collapse, pulmonary edema, CNS depression, coma, seizures, nausea, vomiting, cardiopulmonary arrest.*

**poisonous solid, self-heating (n.o.s.)** [Poison] *Cardiovascular collapse, pulmonary edema, CNS depression, coma, seizures, nausea, vomiting, cardiopulmonary arrest.*

**poisonous solid or liquid, corrosive (n.o.s.)** [Poison] *Cardiovascular collapse, pulmonary edema, CNS depression, coma, seizures, nausea, vomiting, cardiopulmonary arrest.* [Corrosive] *Upper airway burns and edema, circulatory collapse, severe chemical burns to skin, toxic systemic effects, GI tract perforation and hemorrhage, peritonitis.*

**poisonous solid or liquid, oxidizing (n.o.s.)** [Oxidizer] *Pulmonary and laryngeal edema, circulatory arrest, hypovolemic shock, chemical burns of skin, mucous membranes, and internal organs.* [Poison] *Cardiovascular col-*

lapse, *pulmonary edema, CNS depression, coma, seizures, nausea, vomiting, cardiopulmonary arrest.*

**poisonous solid or liquid that evolves a flammable vapor (n.o.s.)** [Flammable gas] *Respiratory failure, cardiac arrest, arrhythmias.* [Poison] *Cardiovascular collapse, pulmonary edema, CNS depression, coma, seizures, nausea, vomiting, cardiopulmonary arrest.*

**polishing compound** [Poison] *Cardiovascular collapse, pulmonary edema, CNS depression, coma, seizures, nausea, vomiting, cardiopulmonary arrest.*

**polyalkylamine, corrosive (n.o.s.)** [Organic base/amine] *Pulmonary edema, cardiac depression, seizures.*

**polyalkylamine, flammable corrosive (n.o.s.)** [Flammable/combustible liquid] *CNS depression, respiratory arrest, convulsions, arrhythmias, pulmonary edema.* [Organic base/amine] *Pulmonary edema, cardiac depression, seizures.*

**polybrominated biphenyl (PBB)** Polychlorinated biphenyl/polybrominated biphenyl/polychlorinated [dibenzofuran] *Liver and kidney damage.*

**polychlorinated biphenyl (PCB)** Polychlorinated biphenyl/polybrominated biphenyl/polychlorinated [dibenzofuran] *Liver and kidney damage.*

**polychlorinated dibenzofuran (PCDF)** Polychlorinated biphenyl/polybrominated biphenyl/polychlorinated [dibenzofuran] *Liver and kidney damage.*

**polyester resin kit** [Poison] *Cardiovascular collapse, pulmonary edema, CNS depression, coma, seizures, nausea, vomiting, cardiopulmonary arrest.*

**polyethylene glycol** [Ethylene glycol] *Respiratory failure, pulmonary edema, paralysis, cardiovascular collapse, severe acidosis.*

**polyhalogenated biphenyl** Polychlorinated biphenyl/polybrominated biphenyl/polychlorinated [dibenzofuran] *Liver and kidney damage.*

**polyhalogenated terphenyl** Polychlorinated biphenyl/polybrominated biphenyl/polychlorinated [dibenzofuran] *Liver and kidney damage.*

**polynuclear aromatic hydrocarbon (n.o.s.)** [Poison] *Cardiovascular collapse, pulmonary edema, CNS depression, coma, seizures, nausea, vomiting, cardiopulmonary arrest.*

**polyol** [Ethylene glycol] *Respiratory failure, pulmonary edema, paralysis, cardiovascular collapse, severe acidosis.*

**polystyrene, expandable, that evolves a flammable vapor** [Flammable/combustible liquid] *CNS depression, respiratory arrest, convulsions, arrhythmias, pulmonary edema.*

**polytetrafluoroethylene** [Halogenated aliphatic hydrocarbon] *CNS depression, respiratory arrest, circulatory collapse.*

**Portland cement** [Inorganic base/alkaline corrosive] *Upper airway burns and edema, pulmonary edema, skin burns, circulatory collapse, GI tract perforation and hemorrhage, peritonitis.*

**potash liquor** [Inorganic base/alkaline corrosive] *Upper airway burns and edema, pulmonary edema, skin burns, circulatory collapse, GI tract perforation and hemorrhage, peritonitis.*

**potash & sodium nitrate mixture** [Nitrate/nitrite] *Methemoglobinemia, hypotension, circulatory collapse.*

**potassium; potassium alloy (n.o.s.)** [Poison] *Cardiovascular collapse, pulmonary edema, CNS depression, coma, seizures, nausea, vomiting, cardiopulmonary arrest.*

**potassium arsenate** [Arsenic] *Heavy metal toxicity, vomiting, GI bleeding, CNS depression, pulmonary edema, cardiac arrest.*

**potassium arsenite** [Arsenic] *Heavy metal toxicity, vomiting, GI bleeding, CNS depression, pulmonary edema, cardiac arrest.*

HazMat

**potassium bichromate** [Inorganic acid] *Pulmonary edema, bronchospasm, circulatory collapse, laryngeal spasm and edema, severe chemical burns to skin, mucous membranes, and internal organs, GI tract perforation and hemorrhage, peritonitis.*

**potassium bifluoride** [Hydrofluoric acid] *Pulmonary and laryngeal edema, circulatory collapse, severe skin burns, GI tract perforation, systemic fluoride poisoning.*

**potassium biosulfite** [Sulfur] *Respiratory tract irritation, pulmonary edema, anaphylaxis.*

**potassium bisulfate** [Inorganic acid] *Pulmonary edema, bronchospasm, circulatory collapse, laryngeal spasm and edema, severe chemical burns to skin, mucous membranes, and internal organs, GI tract perforation and hemorrhage, peritonitis.*

**potassium borohydride** [Boron] *Respiratory tract irritation, laryngeal spasm and edema, pulmonary edema, severe chemical burns.*

**potassium bromate** [Bromate] *CNS and respiratory system depression, delayed-onset renal failure.*

**potassium chlorate** [Chlorate] *Hemolysis, methemoglobinemia, hypoperfusion, CNS depression, delayed-onset renal failure.*

**potassium chromate** [Inorganic acid] *Pulmonary edema, bronchospasm, circulatory collapse, laryngeal spasm and edema, severe chemical burns to skin, mucous membranes, and internal organs, GI tract perforation and hemorrhage, peritonitis.*

**potassium cuprocyanide** [Cyanide] *Impairment of cellular oxygenation and adenosine triphosphate production, hypoxia, death.*

**potassium cyanide; cyanide potassium** [Cyanide] *Impairment of cellular oxygenation and adenosine triphosphate production, hypoxia, death.*

**potassium dichloroisocyanurate** [Hypochlorite] *Circulatory collapse, respiratory tract irritation, upper airway obstruction, pulmonary edema.*

**potassium dichloro-S-triazinetrione** [Hypochlorite] *Circulatory collapse, respiratory tract irritation, upper airway obstruction, pulmonary edema.*

**potassium dichromate** [Inorganic acid] *Pulmonary edema, bronchospasm, circulatory collapse, laryngeal spasm and edema, severe chemical burns to skin, mucous membranes, and internal organs, GI tract perforation and hemorrhage, peritonitis.*

**potassium dithionite** [Sulfur] *Respiratory tract irritation, pulmonary edema, anaphylaxis.*

**potassium fluoborate** [Fluorine] *CNS depression, respiratory arrest, cardiovascular collapse, shock, arrhythmias.* [Boron] *Respiratory tract irritation, laryngeal spasm and edema, pulmonary edema, severe chemical burns.*

**potassium fluoride** [Hydrofluoric acid] *Pulmonary and laryngeal edema, circulatory collapse, severe skin burns, GI tract perforation, systemic fluoride poisoning.*

**potassium fluoroacetate** [Monofluoroacetate] *Ventricular arrhythmias, seizures.*

**potassium fluorosilicate** [Fluorine] *CNS depression, respiratory arrest, cardiovascular collapse, shock, arrhythmias.*

**potassium hydrogen fluoride** [Hydrofluoric acid] *Pulmonary and laryngeal edema, circulatory collapse, severe skin burns, GI tract perforation, systemic fluoride poisoning.*

**potassium hydrogen sulfate** [Inorganic acid] *Pulmonary edema, bronchospasm, circulatory collapse, laryngeal spasm and edema, severe chemical burns to skin, mucous membranes, and internal organs, GI tract perforation and hemorrhage, peritonitis.*

**potassium hydrosulfite** [Sulfur] *Respiratory tract irritation, pulmonary edema, anaphylaxis.*

**potassium hydroxide** [Inorganic base/alkaline corrosive] *Upper airway burns* and edema, pulmonary edema, skin burns, circulatory collapse, GI tract perforation and hemorrhage, peritonitis.

**potassium hypochlorite** [Hypochlorite] Circulatory collapse, respiratory tract irritation, upper airway obstruction, pulmonary edema.

**potassium metavanadate** [Poison] Cardiovascular collapse, pulmonary edema, CNS depression, coma, seizures, nausea, vomiting, cardiopulmonary arrest.

**potassium monopersulfate** [Irritant] Severe immediate or delayed upper airway or respiratory tract irritation, pulmonary edema, glottic spasm, airway obstruction.

**potassium monoxide** [Inorganic base/ alkaline corrosive] Upper airway burns and edema, pulmonary edema, skin burns, circulatory collapse, GI tract perforation and hemorrhage, peritonitis.

**potassium nitrate** [Nitrate/nitrite] Methemoglobinemia, hypotension, circulatory collapse.

**potassium nitrate & sodium nitrate mixture** [Nitrate/nitrite] Methemoglobinemia, hypotension, circulatory collapse.

**potassium nitrate & sodium nitrite mixture** [Nitrate/nitrite] Methemoglobinemia, hypotension, circulatory collapse.

**potassium nitrite** [Nitrate/nitrite] Methemoglobinemia, hypotension, circulatory collapse.

**potassium oxide** [Inorganic base/alkaline corrosive] Upper airway burns and edema, pulmonary edema, skin burns, circulatory collapse, GI tract perforation and hemorrhage, peritonitis.

**potassium perchlorate** [Chlorate] Hemolysis, methemoglobinemia, hypoperfusion, CNS depression, delayed-onset renal failure.

**potassium permanganate** [Inorganic acid] Pulmonary edema, bronchospasm, circulatory collapse, laryngeal spasm and edema, severe chemical burns to skin, mucous membranes, and

internal organs, GI tract perforation and hemorrhage, peritonitis.

**potassium peroxide** [Oxidizer] Pulmonary and laryngeal edema, circulatory arrest, hypovolemic shock, chemical burns of skin, mucous membranes, and internal organs.

**potassium persulfate** [Irritant] Severe immediate or delayed upper airway or respiratory tract irritation, pulmonary edema, glottic spasm, airway obstruction.

**potassium phosphate** [Inorganic base/ alkaline corrosive] Upper airway burns and edema, pulmonary edema, skin burns, circulatory collapse, GI tract perforation and hemorrhage, peritonitis.

**potassium phosphide** [Phosphine] Severe pulmonary irritation, pulmonary edema.

**potassium selenate** [Selenium] Arrhythmias, pulmonary edema, bronchospasm, seizures, vomiting, GI bleeding.

**potassium selenite** [Selenium] Arrhythmias, pulmonary edema, bronchospasm, seizures, vomiting, GI bleeding.

**potassium silicofluoride** [Fluorine] CNS depression, respiratory arrest, cardiovascular collapse, shock, arrhythmias.

**potassium silver cyanide** [Cyanide] Impairment of cellular oxygenation and adenosine triphosphate production, hypoxia, death.

**potassium sodium alloy (n.o.s.)** [Flammable solid] Shock, severe chemical and thermal burns, severe respiratory tract irritation, pulmonary edema, respiratory arrest, ECG changes, sudden death.

**potassium sulfide** [Inorganic base/ alkaline corrosive] Upper airway burns and edema, pulmonary edema, skin burns, circulatory collapse, GI tract perforation and hemorrhage, peritonitis.

**potassium superoxide** [Poison] Cardiovascular collapse, pulmonary edema, CNS depression, coma, seizures, nausea, vomiting, cardiopulmonary arrest.

HazMat

**pressurized accumulator** [Flammable gas] *Respiratory failure, cardiac arrest, arrhythmias.*

**primifos-ethyl** [Organophosphate] *Pulmonary edema, respiratory muscle paralysis, respiratory failure, bradycardia, acetylcholinesterase inhibition, hypotension, pulmonary edema, overstimulation of parasympathetic nervous system, striated muscle, sympathetic ganglia, and CNS.*

**Prolan** [Lindane] *CNS stimulation, seizures, respiratory failure.*

**promecarb** [Carbamate] *Acetylcholinesterase inhibition (reversible), bradycardia, hypotension, respiratory muscle paralysis, respiratory arrest, pulmonary edema.*

**propadiene** [Aliphatic hydrocarbon] *Arrhythmias, asphyxiation, anesthesia.*

**propadiene & methyl acetylene mixture** [Hydrocarbon mixture] *CNS depression, respiratory arrest, seizures, arrhythmias, pulmonary edema.*

**propane** [Aliphatic hydrocarbon] *Arrhythmias, asphyxiation, anesthesia.*

**propane & ethane mixture (cryogenic liquid)** [Aliphatic hydrocarbon] *Arrhythmias, asphyxiation, anesthesia.*

**propane sulfone** [Organic acid] *Pulmonary edema, circulatory collapse, laryngeal edema and spasm, severe chemical burns to skin, mucous membranes, and internal organs, GI tract perforation and hemorrhage, peritonitis.*

**propanethiol** [Sulfur] *Respiratory tract irritation, pulmonary edema, anaphylaxis.*

**propanil** [Aniline] *Methemoglobinemia, hypoxia.*

**propanoic acid** [Organic acid] *Pulmonary edema, circulatory collapse, laryngeal edema and spasm, severe chemical burns to skin, mucous membranes, and internal organs, GI tract perforation and hemorrhage, peritonitis.*

**propanol** [Lower alcohol (1–3 carbons)] *CNS depression, coma, respiratory arrest, arrhythmias.*

**propargite** [Poison] *Cardiovascular collapse, pulmonary edema, CNS depression, coma, seizures, nausea, vomiting, cardiopulmonary arrest.*

**propargyl alcohol** [Higher alcohol (4+ carbons)] *CNS depression, respiratory failure, arrhythmias.*

**propargyl bromide** [Bromine/methylbromide] *Severe respiratory irritation, pulmonary edema, respiratory failure, coma, convulsions, death.*

**β-propiolactone; beta-propiolactone; β-propionolactone** [Ketone] *Respiratory mucous membrane irritation, pulmonary edema, CNS depression.*

**propionaldehyde** [Aldehyde] *Seizures, respiratory failure, pulmonary edema.*

**propionic acid** [Organic acid] *Pulmonary edema, circulatory collapse, laryngeal edema and spasm, severe chemical burns to skin, mucous membranes, and internal organs, GI tract perforation and hemorrhage, peritonitis.*

**propionic acid & boron trifluoride complex** [Boron] *Respiratory tract irritation, laryngeal spasm and edema, pulmonary edema, severe chemical burns.*

**propionic anhydride** [Organic acid] *Pulmonary edema, circulatory collapse, laryngeal edema and spasm, severe chemical burns to skin, mucous membranes, and internal organs, GI tract perforation and hemorrhage, peritonitis.*

**propionitrile** [Cyanide] *Impairment of cellular oxygenation and adenosine triphosphate production, hypoxia, death.*

**propionyl chloride** [Halogenated aliphatic hydrocarbon] *CNS depression, respiratory arrest, circulatory collapse.*

**propionyl peroxide** [Organic peroxide] *Pulmonary and laryngeal edema, circulatory arrest, hypovolemic shock, chemical burns to skin, mucous membranes, and internal organs.*

**propiophenone** [Phenol] *Coma, hypotension, arrhythmias, pulmonary edema, respiratory arrest.*

**propoxur** [Carbamate] *Acetylcholinesterase inhibition (reversible), bradycardia,* hypotension, *respiratory muscle paralysis, respiratory arrest, pulmonary edema.*

**propyl acetate** [Ester] *CNS depression, respiratory tract irritation, bronchitis, pneumonia.*

**propyl alcohol** [Lower alcohol (1–3 carbons)] *CNS depression, coma, respiratory arrest, arrhythmias.*

**propyl benzene** [Aromatic hydrocarbon] *Arrhythmias, respiratory failure, pulmonary edema, paralysis, brain and kidney damage.*

**propyl chloroformate; n-propyl chloroformate** [Halogenated aliphatic hydrocarbon] *CNS depression, respiratory arrest, circulatory collapse.*

**propyl formate** [Ester] *CNS depression, respiratory tract irritation, bronchitis, pneumonia.*

**n-propyl gallate** [Phenol] *Coma, hypotension, arrhythmias, pulmonary edema, respiratory arrest.*

**propyl isocyanate** [Isocyanate/aliphatic thiocyanate] *CNS depression, respiratory arrest, respiratory paralysis, pulmonary edema, cyanide toxicity.*

**n-propyl isomer** [Naphthalene] *Delayed-onset acute intravascular hemolysis.*

**propyl mercaptan** [Sulfur] *Respiratory tract irritation, pulmonary edema, anaphylaxis.*

**propyl nitrate** [Nitrate/nitrite] *Methemoglobinemia, hypotension, circulatory collapse.*

**propyl peroxydicarbonate** [Organic peroxide] *Pulmonary and laryngeal edema, circulatory arrest, hypovolemic shock, chemical burns to skin, mucous membranes, and internal organs.*

**propyl trichlorosilane** [Silane/chlorosilane] *Respiratory tract irritation, pulmonary edema.*

**propylamine** [Organic base/amine] *Pulmonary edema, cardiac depression, seizures.*

**propylene** [Aliphatic hydrocarbon] *Arrhythmias, asphyxiation, anesthesia.*

**propylene chlorohydrin** [Dichloropropane/dichloropropene] *Pulmonary edema, bronchospasm, alveolar hemorrhage.*

**propylene dichloride** [Dichloropropane/dichloropropene] *Pulmonary edema, bronchospasm, alveolar hemorrhage.*

**propylene dichloride & dichloropropene mixture** [Dichloropropane/dichloropropene] *Pulmonary edema, bronchospasm, alveolar hemorrhage.*

**propylene & ethylene & acetylene mixture (cryogenic liquid)** [Aliphatic hydrocarbon] *Arrhythmias, asphyxiation, anesthesia.* [Simple asphyxiant] *Asphyxiation.*

**propylene glycol** [Ethylene glycol] *Respiratory failure, pulmonary edema, paralysis, cardiovascular collapse, severe acidosis.*

**propylene glycol monomethyl ether** [Ethylene glycol] *Respiratory failure, pulmonary edema, paralysis, cardiovascular collapse, severe acidosis.*

**propylene glycol monostearate** [Ethylene glycol] *Respiratory failure, pulmonary edema, paralysis, cardiovascular collapse, severe acidosis.*

**propylene oxide** [Ether] *Anesthesia, respiratory arrest.*

**propylene oxide & ethylene oxide mixture** [Ethylene oxide] *Respiratory tract irritation, pulmonary edema.*

**propylene tetramer** [Aliphatic hydrocarbon] *Arrhythmias, asphyxiation, anesthesia.*

**propylenediamine** [Organic base/amine] *Pulmonary edema, cardiac depression, seizures.*

**propyleneimine** [Organic base/amine] *Pulmonary edema, cardiac depression, seizures.*

**prothoate** [Organophosphate] *Pulmonary edema, respiratory muscle paralysis, respiratory failure, bradycardia, acetylcholinesterase inhibition, hypotension, pulmonary edema, overstimulation of parasympathetic nervous system, striated muscle, sympathetic ganglia, and CNS.*

HazMat

**pyramat** [Carbamate] *Acetylcholinesterase inhibition (reversible), bradycardia, hypotension, respiratory muscle paralysis, respiratory arrest, pulmonary edema.*

**pyrazothion** [Organophosphate] *Pulmonary edema, respiratory muscle paralysis, respiratory failure, bradycardia, acetylcholinesterase inhibition, hypotension, pulmonary edema, overstimulation of parasympathetic nervous system, striated muscle, sympathetic ganglia, and CNS.*

**Pyrazoxon** [Organophosphate] *Pulmonary edema, respiratory muscle paralysis, respiratory failure, bradycardia, acetylcholinesterase inhibition, hypotension, pulmonary edema, overstimulation of parasympathetic nervous system, striated muscle, sympathetic ganglia, and CNS.*

**pyrene** [Aromatic hydrocarbon] *Arrhythmias, respiratory failure, pulmonary edema, paralysis, brain and kidney damage.*

**pyrenone** [Pyrethrin/pyrethroid] *Respiratory paralysis, convulsions.*

**pyrethrin; pyrethrum** [Pyrethrin/pyrethroid] *Respiratory paralysis, convulsions.*

**pyrethroid (n.o.s.)** [Pyrethrin/pyrethroid] *Respiratory paralysis, convulsions.*

**pyridine** [Aromatic hydrocarbon] *Arrhythmias, respiratory failure, pulmonary edema, paralysis, brain and kidney damage.*

**pyriminil** [Poison] *Cardiovascular collapse, pulmonary edema, CNS depression, coma, seizures, nausea, vomiting, cardiopulmonary arrest.*

**pyrocatechol** [Phenol] *Coma, hypotension, arrhythmias, pulmonary edema, respiratory arrest.*

**pyrogallol** [Phenol] *Coma, hypotension, arrhythmias, pulmonary edema, respiratory arrest.*

**pyrolan** [Carbamate] *Acetylcholinesterase inhibition (reversible), bradycardia, hypotension, respiratory muscle paralysis, respiratory arrest, pulmonary edema.*

**pyrolysis products** [Poison] *Cardiovascular collapse, pulmonary edema, CNS depression, coma, seizures, nausea, vomiting, cardiopulmonary arrest.*

**pyrophoric fuel (n.o.s.); pyrophoric liquid (n.o.s.)** [Flammable/combustible liquid] *CNS depression, respiratory arrest, convulsions, arrhythmias, pulmonary edema.*

**pyrophoric metal (n.o.s.); pyrophoric metal alloy (n.o.s.); pyrophoric solid (n.o.s.)** [Flammable solid] *Shock, severe chemical and thermal burns, severe respiratory tract irritation, pulmonary edema, respiratory arrest, ECG changes, sudden death.*

**pyrosulfuric acid** [Inorganic acid] *Pulmonary edema, bronchospasm, circulatory collapse, laryngeal spasm and edema, severe chemical burns to skin, mucous membranes, and internal organs, GI tract perforation and hemorrhage, peritonitis.*

**pyrosulfuryl chloride** [Inorganic acid] *Pulmonary edema, bronchospasm, circulatory collapse, laryngeal spasm and edema, severe chemical burns to skin, mucous membranes, and internal organs, GI tract perforation and hemorrhage, peritonitis.*

**pyroxylin** [Ether] *Anesthesia, respiratory arrest.*

**pyrrolidine** [Organic base/amine] *Pulmonary edema, cardiac depression, seizures.*

**quinoline** [Aromatic hydrocarbon] *Arrhythmias, respiratory failure, pulmonary edema, paralysis, brain and kidney damage.*

**quinone** [Ketone] *Respiratory mucous membrane irritation, pulmonary edema, CNS depression.*

**quintozene** [Pentachlorophenol] *Respiratory and circulatory collapse, severe hyperthermia.*

**R134A refrigerant (1,1,1,2-tetrafluoroethane)** [Chlorinated fluorocarbon] *Asphyxiation, anesthesia, arrhythmias.*

**radioactive material (n.o.s.)** [Radioactive] *DNA or RNA damage, severe GI or hematologic damage, loss of bone marrow function, immunocompromise, systemic infection, carcinoma.*

**rare gas mixture (n.o.s.)** [Poison] *Cardiovascular collapse, pulmonary edema, CNS depression, coma, seizures, nausea, vomiting, cardiopulmonary arrest.* [Simple asphyxiant] *Asphyxiation.*

**rare gas & nitrogen mixture** [Poison] *Cardiovascular collapse, pulmonary edema, CNS depression, coma, seizures, nausea, vomiting, cardiopulmonary arrest.* [Simple asphyxiant] *Asphyxiation.*

**rare gas & oxygen mixture** [Poison] *Cardiovascular collapse, pulmonary edema, CNS depression, coma, seizures, nausea, vomiting, cardiopulmonary arrest.* [Simple asphyxiant] *Asphyxiation.*

**red phosphorus** [Phosphorus] *Hypovolemic shock, severe tissue burns, severe respiratory irritation, pulmonary edema, respiratory arrest, arrhythmias, sudden death.*

**reducing liquid** [Poison] *Cardiovascular collapse, pulmonary edema, CNS depression, coma, seizures, nausea, vomiting, cardiopulmonary arrest.*

**refrigerant gas (n.o.s.)** [Chlorinated fluorocarbon] *Asphyxiation, anesthesia, arrhythmias.*

**refrigerant gas, flammable (n.o.s.)** [Flammable gas] *Respiratory failure, cardiac arrest, arrhythmias.*

**refrigerant R134A (1,1,1,2-tetrafluoroethane)** [Chlorinated fluorocarbon] *Asphyxiation, anesthesia, arrhythmias.*

**refrigerator with flammable liquefied gas** [Flammable gas] *Respiratory failure, cardiac arrest, arrhythmias.* [Simple asphyxiant] *Asphyxiation.*

**refrigerator with nonflammable liquefied gas** [Nonflammable gas] *Pulmonary edema, respiratory failure, asphyxiation.* [Simple asphyxiant] *Asphyxiation.*

**removing liquid** [Poison] *Cardiovascular collapse, pulmonary edema, CNS depression, coma, seizures, nausea, vomiting, cardiopulmonary arrest.*

**reserpine** [Poison] *Cardiovascular collapse, pulmonary edema, CNS depression, coma, seizures, nausea, vomiting, cardiopulmonary arrest.*

**residual oil** [Hydrocarbon mixture] *CNS depression, respiratory arrest, seizures, arrhythmias, pulmonary edema.*

**resin compound, flammable** [Flammable/combustible liquid] *CNS depression, respiratory arrest, convulsions, arrhythmias, pulmonary edema.*

**resin compound, poisonous** [Poison] *Cardiovascular collapse, pulmonary edema, CNS depression, coma, seizures, nausea, vomiting, cardiopulmonary arrest.*

**resmethrin** [Pyrethrin/pyrethroid] *Respiratory paralysis, convulsions.*

**resorcinol** [Phenol] *Coma, hypotension, arrhythmias, pulmonary edema, respiratory arrest.*

**road asphalt** [Hydrocarbon mixture] *CNS depression, respiratory arrest, seizures, arrhythmias, pulmonary edema.*

**road oil** [Hydrocarbon mixture] *CNS depression, respiratory arrest, seizures, arrhythmias, pulmonary edema.*

**rodenticide (n.o.s.)** [Poison] *Cardiovascular collapse, pulmonary edema, CNS depression, coma, seizures, nausea, vomiting, cardiopulmonary arrest.*

**ronnel** [Organophosphate] *Pulmonary edema, respiratory muscle paralysis, respiratory failure, bradycardia, acetylcholinesterase inhibition, hypotension, pulmonary edema, overstimulation of parasympathetic nervous system, striated muscle, sympathetic ganglia, and CNS.*

**rosin oil** [Poison] *Cardiovascular collapse, pulmonary edema, CNS depression, coma, seizures, nausea, vomiting, cardiopulmonary arrest.*

**rotenoid (n.o.s.)** [Rotenone] *Respiratory arrest, asphyxia.*

HazMat

**rotenone** [Rotenone] *Respiratory arrest, asphyxia.*

**Roundup** [Glyphosate] *Hypotension, arrhythmias, pulmonary edema.*

**rubber scrap, powder, granules, or solution** [Poison] *Cardiovascular collapse, pulmonary edema, CNS depression, coma, seizures, nausea, vomiting, cardiopulmonary arrest.*

**rubber solvent (naphtha)** [Hydrocarbon mixture] *CNS depression, respiratory arrest, seizures, arrhythmias, pulmonary edema.*

**rubidium** [Poison] *Cardiovascular collapse, pulmonary edema, CNS depression, coma, seizures, nausea, vomiting, cardiopulmonary arrest.*

**rubidium hydroxide** [Poison] *Cardiovascular collapse, pulmonary edema, CNS depression, coma, seizures, nausea, vomiting, cardiopulmonary arrest.*

**Ruelene** [Organophosphate] *Pulmonary edema, respiratory muscle paralysis, respiratory failure, bradycardia, acetylcholinesterase inhibition, hypotension, pulmonary edema, overstimulation of parasympathetic nervous system, striated muscle, sympathetic ganglia, and CNS.*

**saccharin; saccharin salt (n.o.s.)** [Poison] *Cardiovascular collapse, pulmonary edema, CNS depression, coma, seizures, nausea, vomiting, cardiopulmonary arrest.*

**safrole** [Phenol] *Coma, hypotension, arrhythmias, pulmonary edema, respiratory arrest.*

**salcomine** [Poison] *Cardiovascular collapse, pulmonary edema, CNS depression, coma, seizures, nausea, vomiting, cardiopulmonary arrest.*

**saltpeter** [Nitrate/nitrite] *Methemoglobinemia, hypotension, circulatory collapse.*

**saprol** [Phenol] *Coma, hypotension, arrhythmias, pulmonary edema, respiratory arrest.*

**sarin** [Organophosphate] *Pulmonary edema, respiratory muscle paralysis, respiratory failure, bradycardia, acetylcholinesterase inhibition, hypotension, pulmonary edema, overstimulation of parasympathetic nervous system, striated muscle, sympathetic ganglia, and CNS.*

**sea coal** [Flammable solid] *Shock, severe chemical and thermal burns, severe respiratory tract irritation, pulmonary edema, respiratory arrest, ECG changes, sudden death.*

**selenate (n.o.s.)** [Selenium] *Arrhythmias, pulmonary edema, bronchospasm, seizures, vomiting, GI bleeding.*

**selenic acid** [Inorganic acid] *Pulmonary edema, bronchospasm, circulatory collapse, laryngeal spasm and edema, severe chemical burns to skin, mucous membranes, and internal organs, GI tract perforation and hemorrhage, peritonitis.* [Selenium] *Arrhythmias, pulmonary edema, bronchospasm, seizures, vomiting, GI bleeding.*

**selenious acid** [Inorganic acid] *Pulmonary edema, bronchospasm, circulatory collapse, laryngeal spasm and edema, severe chemical burns to skin, mucous membranes, and internal organs, GI tract perforation and hemorrhage, peritonitis.* [Selenium] *Arrhythmias, pulmonary edema, bronchospasm, seizures, vomiting, GI bleeding.*

**selenious acid, dithallium (1+) salt** [Selenium] *Arrhythmias, pulmonary edema, bronchospasm, seizures, vomiting, GI bleeding.* [Thallium] *Pulmonary edema, respiratory failure, circulatory collapse, seizures.*

**selenite (n.o.s.)** [Selenium] *Arrhythmias, pulmonary edema, bronchospasm, seizures, vomiting, GI bleeding.*

**selenium** [Selenium] *Arrhythmias, pulmonary edema, bronchospasm, seizures, vomiting, GI bleeding.*

**selenium dioxide** [Selenium] *Arrhythmias, pulmonary edema, bronchospasm, seizures, vomiting, GI bleeding.*

**selenium disulfide** [Selenium] *Arrhythmias, pulmonary edema, bronchospasm, seizures, vomiting, GI bleeding.* [Sulfur] *Respiratory tract irritation, pulmonary edema, anaphylaxis.*

**selenium hexafluoride** [Selenium] *Arrhythmias, pulmonary edema, bronchospasm, seizures, vomiting, GI bleeding.* [Fluorine] *CNS depression, respiratory arrest, cardiovascular collapse, shock, arrhythmias.*

**selenium oxide** [Selenium] *Arrhythmias, pulmonary edema, bronchospasm, seizures, vomiting, GI bleeding.*

**selenium oxychloride** [Selenium] *Arrhythmias, pulmonary edema, bronchospasm, seizures, vomiting, GI bleeding.*

**selenium sulfide** [Selenium] *Arrhythmias, pulmonary edema, bronchospasm, seizures, vomiting, GI bleeding.* [Sulfur] *Respiratory tract irritation, pulmonary edema, anaphylaxis.*

**selenourea** [Selenium] *Arrhythmias, pulmonary edema, bronchospasm, seizures, vomiting, GI bleeding.*

**self-heating substance, corrosive (n.o.s.)** [Corrosive] *Upper airway burns and edema, circulatory collapse, severe chemical burns to skin, toxic systemic effects, GI tract perforation and hemorrhage, peritonitis.*

**self-heating substance, oxidizing (n.o.s.)** [Oxidizer] *Pulmonary and laryngeal edema, circulatory arrest, hypovolemic shock, chemical burns of skin, mucous membranes, and internal organs.*

**self-heating substance, poisonous (n.o.s.)** [Poison] *Cardiovascular collapse, pulmonary edema, CNS depression, coma, seizures, nausea, vomiting, cardiopulmonary arrest.*

**self-reactive substance (n.o.s.)** [Poison] *Cardiovascular collapse, pulmonary edema, CNS depression, coma, seizures, nausea, vomiting, cardiopulmonary arrest.*

**semicarbazide HCl** [Hydrazine] *Seizures, hemolysis of red blood cells, pulmonary edema.*

**shale oil** [Aliphatic hydrocarbon] *Arrhythmias, asphyxiation, anesthesia.*

**shellac** [Hydrocarbon mixture] *CNS depression, respiratory arrest, seizures, arrhythmias, pulmonary edema.*

**silane** [Silane/chlorosilane] *Respiratory tract irritation, pulmonary edema.*

**silicofluoric acid** [Fluorine] *CNS depression, respiratory arrest, cardiovascular collapse, shock, arrhythmias.*

**silicofluoride (n.o.s.)** [Fluorine] *CNS depression, respiratory arrest, cardiovascular collapse, shock, arrhythmias.*

**silicon** [Irritant] *Severe immediate or delayed upper airway or respiratory tract irritation, pulmonary edema, glottic spasm, airway obstruction.*

**silicon chloride** [Chlorine] *Severe respiratory tract irritation, pulmonary edema, irritation of skin, eyes, and mucous membranes.*

**silicon tetrachloride** [Chlorine] *Severe respiratory tract irritation, pulmonary edema, irritation of skin, eyes, and mucous membranes.*

**silicon tetrafluoride** [Fluorine] *CNS depression, respiratory arrest, cardiovascular collapse, shock, arrhythmias.*

**silver** [Poison] *Cardiovascular collapse, pulmonary edema, CNS depression, coma, seizures, nausea, vomiting, cardiopulmonary arrest.*

**silver arsenite** [Arsenic] *Heavy metal toxicity, vomiting, GI bleeding, CNS depression, pulmonary edema, cardiac arrest.*

**silver cyanide** [Cyanide] *Impairment of cellular oxygenation and adenosine triphosphate production, hypoxia, death.*

**silver nitrate** [Nitrate/nitrite] *Methemoglobinemia, hypotension, circulatory collapse.*

**silver picrate** [Poison] *Cardiovascular collapse, pulmonary edema, CNS depression, coma, seizures, nausea, vomiting, cardiopulmonary arrest.*

**silvex** [Chlorophenoxy herbicide] *CNS depression, CNS stimulation, respiratory failure, ventricular fibrillation, seizures.*

**sludge acid** [Poison] *Cardiovascular collapse, pulmonary edema, CNS depression, coma, seizures, nausea, vomiting, cardiopulmonary arrest.*

HazMat

**smoke bomb** [Irritant] *Severe immediate or delayed upper airway or respiratory tract irritation, pulmonary edema, glottic spasm, airway obstruction.* [Corrosive] *Upper airway burns and edema, circulatory collapse, severe chemical burns to skin, toxic systemic effects, GI tract perforation and hemorrhage, peritonitis.*

**smokeless powder** [Explosive] *Multiple trauma, highly toxic chemical exposure.*

**soda lime** [Inorganic base/alkaline corrosive] *Upper airway burns and edema, pulmonary edema, skin burns, circulatory collapse, GI tract perforation and hemorrhage, peritonitis.*

**sodium; sodium alloy (n.o.s.)** [Flammable solid] *Shock, severe chemical and thermal burns, severe respiratory tract irritation, pulmonary edema, respiratory arrest, ECG changes, sudden death.*

**sodium acid sulfate** [Inorganic acid] *Pulmonary edema, bronchospasm, circulatory collapse, laryngeal spasm and edema, severe chemical burns to skin, mucous membranes, and internal organs, GI tract perforation and hemorrhage, peritonitis.*

**sodium aluminate** [Poison] *Cardiovascular collapse, pulmonary edema, CNS depression, coma, seizures, nausea, vomiting, cardiopulmonary arrest.*

**sodium aluminum hydride** [Poison] *Cardiovascular collapse, pulmonary edema, CNS depression, coma, seizures, nausea, vomiting, cardiopulmonary arrest.*

**sodium amalgam** [Mercury] *Circulatory collapse, arrhythmias, respiratory failure, pulmonary edema, neurotoxic effects.*

**sodium amide** [Inorganic base/alkaline corrosive] *Upper airway burns and edema, pulmonary edema, skin burns, circulatory collapse, GI tract perforation and hemorrhage, peritonitis.*

**sodium ammonium vanadate** [Poison] *Cardiovascular collapse, pulmonary edema, CNS depression, coma,*

*seizures, nausea, vomiting, cardiopulmonary arrest.*

**sodium arsanilate** [Arsenic] *Heavy metal toxicity, vomiting, GI bleeding, CNS depression, pulmonary edema, cardiac arrest.*

**sodium arsenate** [Arsenic] *Heavy metal toxicity, vomiting, GI bleeding, CNS depression, pulmonary edema, cardiac arrest.*

**sodium arsenite** [Arsenic] *Heavy metal toxicity, vomiting, GI bleeding, CNS depression, pulmonary edema, cardiac arrest.*

**sodium azide** *Hypotension, arrhythmias, asystole, seizures, coma.*

**sodium bichromate** [Inorganic acid] *Pulmonary edema, bronchospasm, circulatory collapse, laryngeal spasm and edema, severe chemical burns to skin, mucous membranes, and internal organs, GI tract perforation and hemorrhage, peritonitis.*

**sodium bifluoride** [Fluorine] *CNS depression, respiratory arrest, cardiovascular collapse, shock, arrhythmias.*

**sodium binoxalate** [Oxalate] *Cardiovascular collapse, arrhythmias, seizures.*

**sodium bisulfate** [Poison] *Cardiovascular collapse, pulmonary edema, CNS depression, coma, seizures, nausea, vomiting, cardiopulmonary arrest.*

**sodium bisulfite** [Sulfur] *Respiratory tract irritation, pulmonary edema, anaphylaxis.*

**sodium borohydride** [Boron] *Respiratory tract irritation, laryngeal spasm and edema, pulmonary edema, severe chemical burns.*

**sodium bromate** [Bromate] *CNS and respiratory system depression, delayed-onset renal failure.*

**sodium cacodylate** [Arsenic] *Heavy metal toxicity, vomiting, GI bleeding, CNS depression, pulmonary edema, cardiac arrest.*

**sodium carbonate** [Inorganic base/alkaline corrosive] *Upper airway burns and edema, pulmonary edema, skin* burns, circulatory collapse, GI tract perforation and hemorrhage, peritonitis.

**sodium chlorate** [Chlorate] Hemolysis, methemoglobinemia, hypoperfusion, CNS depression, delayed-onset renal failure.

**sodium chlorite** [Hypochlorite] Circulatory collapse, respiratory tract irritation, upper airway obstruction, pulmonary edema.

**sodium chloroacetate** [Ester] CNS depression, respiratory tract irritation, bronchitis, pneumonia.

**sodium chromate** [Poison] Cardiovascular collapse, pulmonary edema, CNS depression, coma, seizures, nausea, vomiting, cardiopulmonary arrest.

**sodium cuprocyanide** [Cyanide] Impairment of cellular oxygenation and adenosine triphosphate production, hypoxia, death.

**sodium cyanide** [Cyanide] Impairment of cellular oxygenation and adenosine triphosphate production, hypoxia, death.

**sodium 2-diazo-1-naphthol-4-sulfonate; sodium 2-diazo-1-naphthol-5-sulfonate** [Phenol] Coma, hypotension, arrhythmias, pulmonary edema, respiratory arrest.

**sodium dichloroisocyanate** [Hypochlorite] Circulatory collapse, respiratory tract irritation, upper airway obstruction, pulmonary edema.

**sodium dichloroisocyanurate** [Hypochlorite] Circulatory collapse, respiratory tract irritation, upper airway obstruction, pulmonary edema.

**sodium dichloro-S-triazinetrione** [Hypochlorite] Circulatory collapse, respiratory tract irritation, upper airway obstruction, pulmonary edema.

**sodium dichromate** [Poison] Cardiovascular collapse, pulmonary edema, CNS depression, coma, seizures, nausea, vomiting, cardiopulmonary arrest.

**sodium dinitro-o-cresolate** [Phenol] Coma, hypotension, arrhythmias, pulmonary edema, respiratory arrest.

**sodium dithionite** [Sulfur] Respiratory tract irritation, pulmonary edema, anaphylaxis.

**sodium dodecylbenzenesulfonate** [Poison] Cardiovascular collapse, pulmonary edema, CNS depression, coma, seizures, nausea, vomiting, cardiopulmonary arrest.

**sodium fluoride** [Hydrofluoric acid] Pulmonary and laryngeal edema, circulatory collapse, severe skin burns, GI tract perforation, systemic fluoride poisoning.

**sodium fluoroacetate** [Monofluoroacetate] Ventricular arrhythmias, seizures.

**sodium fluorosilicate** [Fluorine] CNS depression, respiratory arrest, cardiovascular collapse, shock, arrhythmias.

**sodium hydrate** [Inorganic base/alkaline corrosive] Upper airway burns and edema, pulmonary edema, skin burns, circulatory collapse, GI tract perforation and hemorrhage, peritonitis.

**sodium hydride** [Inorganic base/alkaline corrosive] Upper airway burns and edema, pulmonary edema, skin burns, circulatory collapse, GI tract perforation and hemorrhage, peritonitis.

**sodium hydrogen fluoride** [Hydrofluoric acid] Pulmonary and laryngeal edema, circulatory collapse, severe skin burns, GI tract perforation, systemic fluoride poisoning.

**sodium hydrogen sulfate** [Sulfur] Respiratory tract irritation, pulmonary edema, anaphylaxis.

**sodium hydrosulfide** [Hydrogen sulfide] Severe respiratory tract irritation, pulmonary edema, respiratory paralysis.

**sodium hydrosulfite** [Sulfur] Respiratory tract irritation, pulmonary edema, anaphylaxis.

**sodium hydroxide** [Inorganic base/alkaline corrosive] Upper airway burns and edema, pulmonary edema, skin burns, circulatory collapse, GI tract perforation and hemorrhage, peritonitis.

**sodium hypochlorite** [Hypochlorite] Circulatory collapse, respiratory tract irritation, upper airway obstruction, pulmonary edema.

HazMat

**sodium metasilicate** [Inorganic base/ alkaline corrosive] *Upper airway burns and edema, pulmonary edema, skin burns, circulatory collapse, GI tract perforation and hemorrhage, peritonitis.*

**sodium methylate** [Inorganic base/ alkaline corrosive] *Upper airway burns and edema, pulmonary edema, skin burns, circulatory collapse, GI tract perforation and hemorrhage, peritonitis.* [Methyl alcohol] *Respiratory failure, circulatory collapse.*

**sodium monoxide** [Inorganic base/ alkaline corrosive] *Upper airway burns and edema, pulmonary edema, skin burns, circulatory collapse, GI tract perforation and hemorrhage, peritonitis.*

**sodium nitrate** [Nitrate/nitrite] *Methemoglobinemia, hypotension, circulatory collapse.*

**sodium nitrate & potash mixture** [Nitrate/nitrite] *Methemoglobinemia, hypotension, circulatory collapse.*

**sodium nitrate & potassium nitrate mixture** [Nitrate/nitrite] *Methemoglobinemia, hypotension, circulatory collapse.*

**sodium nitrite** [Nitrate/nitrite] *Methemoglobinemia, hypotension, circulatory collapse.*

**sodium nitrite & potassium nitrate mixture** [Nitrate/nitrite] *Methemoglobinemia, hypotension, circulatory collapse.*

**sodium pentachlorophenate** [Pentachlorophenol] *Respiratory and circulatory collapse, severe hyperthermia.*

**sodium percarbonate** [Oxidizer] *Pulmonary and laryngeal edema, circulatory arrest, hypovolemic shock, chemical burns of skin, mucous membranes, and internal organs.*

**sodium perchlorate** [Chlorate] *Hemolysis, methemoglobinemia, hypoperfusion, CNS depression, delayed-onset renal failure.*

**sodium permanganate** [Inorganic acid] *Pulmonary edema, bronchospasm, circulatory collapse, laryngeal spasm and edema, severe chemical burns to skin, mucous membranes, and internal organs, GI tract perforation and hemorrhage, peritonitis.*

**sodium peroxide** [Oxidizer] *Pulmonary and laryngeal edema, circulatory arrest, hypovolemic shock, chemical burns of skin, mucous membranes, and internal organs.*

**sodium persulfate** [Sulfur] *Respiratory tract irritation, pulmonary edema, anaphylaxis.*

**sodium phenolate** [Phenol] *Coma, hypotension, arrhythmias, pulmonary edema, respiratory arrest.*

**sodium phosphate** [Inorganic acid] *Pulmonary edema, bronchospasm, circulatory collapse, laryngeal spasm and edema, severe chemical burns to skin, mucous membranes, and internal organs, GI tract perforation and hemorrhage, peritonitis.*

**sodium phosphide** [Phosphine] *Severe pulmonary irritation, pulmonary edema.*

**sodium picramate** [Flammable solid] *Shock, severe chemical and thermal burns, severe respiratory tract irritation, pulmonary edema, respiratory arrest, ECG changes, sudden death.*

**sodium–potassium alloy (n.o.s.)** [Flammable solid] *Shock, severe chemical and thermal burns, severe respiratory tract irritation, pulmonary edema, respiratory arrest, ECG changes, sudden death.*

**sodium selenate** [Selenium] *Arrhythmias, pulmonary edema, bronchospasm, seizures, vomiting, GI bleeding.*

**sodium selenite** [Selenium] *Arrhythmias, pulmonary edema, bronchospasm, seizures, vomiting, GI bleeding.*

**sodium sesquicarbonate** [Organic base/amine] *Pulmonary edema, cardiac depression, seizures.*

**sodium silicate** [Inorganic base/alkaline corrosive] *Upper airway burns and edema, pulmonary edema, skin burns, circulatory collapse, GI tract perforation and hemorrhage, peritonitis.*

**sodium silicofluoride** [Fluorine] *CNS depression, respiratory arrest, cardiovascular collapse, shock, arrhythmias.*

**sodium sulfate & diperoxydodecane diacid mixture** [Organic peroxide] *Pulmonary and laryngeal edema, circulatory arrest, hypovolemic shock, chemical burns to skin, mucous membranes, and internal organs.* [Sulfur] *Respiratory tract irritation, pulmonary edema, anaphylaxis.*

**sodium sulfide** [Hydrogen sulfide] *Severe respiratory tract irritation, pulmonary edema, respiratory paralysis.*

**sodium superoxide** [Oxidizer] *Pulmonary and laryngeal edema, circulatory arrest, hypovolemic shock, chemical burns of skin, mucous membranes, and internal organs.*

**sodium tellurite** [Poison] *Cardiovascular collapse, pulmonary edema, CNS depression, coma, seizures, nausea, vomiting, cardiopulmonary arrest.*

**sodium thioglycolate** [Inorganic base/alkaline corrosive] *Upper airway burns and edema, pulmonary edema, skin burns, circulatory collapse, GI tract perforation and hemorrhage, peritonitis.*

**solox** [Higher alcohol (4+ carbons)] *CNS depression, respiratory failure, arrhythmias.* [Hydrocarbon mixture] *CNS depression, respiratory arrest, seizures, arrhythmias, pulmonary edema.*

**solvent, aromatic hydrocarbon (n.o.s.)** [Aromatic hydrocarbon] *Arrhythmias, respiratory failure, pulmonary edema, paralysis, brain and kidney damage.*

**solvent, chlorinated (n.o.s.)** [Halogenated aliphatic hydrocarbon] *CNS depression, respiratory arrest, circulatory collapse.*

**soman** [Organophosphate] *Pulmonary edema, respiratory muscle paralysis, respiratory failure, bradycardia, acetylcholinesterase inhibition, hypotension, pulmonary edema, overstimulation of parasympathetic nervous system, striated muscle, sympathetic ganglia, and CNS.*

**spirit of nitroglycerin** [Nitrate/nitrite] *Methemoglobinemia, hypotension, circulatory collapse.*

**stain (n.o.s.)** [Hydrocarbon mixture] *CNS depression, respiratory arrest, seizures, arrhythmias, pulmonary edema.*

**stannane** [Organotin] *Respiratory failure, pulmonary edema, cerebral edema.*

**stannic chloride** [Inorganic acid] *Pulmonary edema, bronchospasm, circulatory collapse, laryngeal spasm and edema, severe chemical burns to skin, mucous membranes, and internal organs, GI tract perforation and hemorrhage, peritonitis.*

**stannic phosphide** [Phosphine] *Severe pulmonary irritation, pulmonary edema.*

**stannous chloride** [Inorganic acid] *Pulmonary edema, bronchospasm, circulatory collapse, laryngeal spasm and edema, severe chemical burns to skin, mucous membranes, and internal organs, GI tract perforation and hemorrhage, peritonitis.*

**stearyl alcohol** [Higher alcohol (4+ carbons)] *CNS depression, respiratory failure, arrhythmias.*

**steel swarf** [Iron] *Hypovolemic shock.*

**stibine** [Poison] *Cardiovascular collapse, pulmonary edema, CNS depression, coma, seizures, nausea, vomiting, cardiopulmonary arrest.*

**Stoddard solvent** [Hydrocarbon mixture] *CNS depression, respiratory arrest, seizures, arrhythmias, pulmonary edema.*

**straw** [Flammable solid] *Shock, severe chemical and thermal burns, severe respiratory tract irritation, pulmonary edema, respiratory arrest, ECG changes, sudden death.*

**Strobane** [Halogenated aliphatic hydrocarbon] *CNS depression, respiratory arrest, circulatory collapse.*

**strontium; strontium alloy (n.o.s.)** [Poison] *Cardiovascular collapse, pulmonary edema, CNS depression, coma, seizures, nausea, vomiting, cardiopulmonary arrest.*

HazMat

**strontium arsenite** [Arsenic] *Heavy metal toxicity, vomiting, GI bleeding, CNS depression, pulmonary edema, cardiac arrest.*

**strontium chlorate** [Chlorate] *Hemolysis, methemoglobinemia, hypoperfusion, CNS depression, delayed-onset renal failure.*

**strontium chromate** [Poison] *Cardiovascular collapse, pulmonary edema, CNS depression, coma, seizures, nausea, vomiting, cardiopulmonary arrest.*

**strontium nitrate** [Nitrate/nitrite] *Methemoglobinemia, hypotension, circulatory collapse.*

**strontium perchlorate** [Chlorate] *Hemolysis, methemoglobinemia, hypoperfusion, CNS depression, delayed-onset renal failure.*

**strontium peroxide** [Oxidizer] *Pulmonary and laryngeal edema, circulatory arrest, hypovolemic shock, chemical burns of skin, mucous membranes, and internal organs.*

**strontium phosphide** [Phosphine] *Severe pulmonary irritation, pulmonary edema.*

**strontium sulfide** [Chlorate] *Hemolysis, methemoglobinemia, hypoperfusion, CNS depression, delayed-onset renal failure.*

**strychnine; strychnine salt (n.o.s.)** [Strychnine] *Convulsions, acidosis, diaphragmatic spasms, respiratory arrest.*

**styrene** [Aromatic hydrocarbon] *Arrhythmias, respiratory failure, pulmonary edema, paralysis, brain and kidney damage.*

**styrene oxide** [Aromatic hydrocarbon] *Arrhythmias, respiratory failure, pulmonary edema, paralysis, brain and kidney damage.*

**substituted nitrophenol pesticide (n.o.s.)** [Dinitrophenol] *Respiratory and circulatory collapse, pulmonary edema, hyperthermia.*

**succinic acid peroxide** [Organic acid] *Pulmonary edema, circulatory collapse, laryngeal edema and spasm, severe chemical burns to skin, mucous membranes, and internal organs, GI tract perforation and hemorrhage, peritonitis.*

**succinonitrile** [Cyanide] *Impairment of cellular oxygenation and adenosine triphosphate production, hypoxia, death.*

**sulfallate** [Carbamate] *Acetylcholinesterase inhibition (reversible), bradycardia, hypotension, respiratory muscle paralysis, respiratory arrest, pulmonary edema.*

**sulfamic acid** [Inorganic acid] *Pulmonary edema, bronchospasm, circulatory collapse, laryngeal spasm and edema, severe chemical burns to skin, mucous membranes, and internal organs, GI tract perforation and hemorrhage, peritonitis.*

**sulfide (n.o.s.); sulfide salt (n.o.s.)** [Hydrogen sulfide] *Severe respiratory tract irritation, pulmonary edema, respiratory paralysis.*

**sulfotep** [Organophosphate] *Pulmonary edema, respiratory muscle paralysis, respiratory failure, bradycardia, acetylcholinesterase inhibition, hypotension, pulmonary edema, overstimulation of parasympathetic nervous system, striated muscle, sympathetic ganglia, and CNS.*

**sulfoxide** [Sulfur] *Respiratory tract irritation, pulmonary edema, anaphylaxis.*

**sulfur** [Sulfur] *Respiratory tract irritation, pulmonary edema, anaphylaxis.*

**sulfur chloride** [Sulfur] *Respiratory tract irritation, pulmonary edema, anaphylaxis.*

**sulfur chloride & carbon tetrachloride mixture** [Carbon tetrachloride] *CNS depression, respiratory arrest, circulatory collapse.* [Sulfur] *Respiratory tract irritation, pulmonary edema, anaphylaxis.*

**sulfur chloride pentafluoride** [Fluorine] *CNS depression, respiratory arrest, cardiovascular collapse, shock, arrhythmias.* [Sulfur] *Respiratory tract irritation, pulmonary edema, anaphylaxis.*

**sulfur dioxide** [Sulfur] *Respiratory tract irritation, pulmonary edema, anaphylaxis.*

**sulfur dioxide & ozone mixture**
[Ozone] *Pulmonary edema, airway obstruction.* [Sulfur] *Respiratory tract irritation, pulmonary edema, anaphylaxis.*

**sulfur hexafluoride** [Simple asphyxiant] *Asphyxiation.*

**sulfur monochloride** [Sulfur] *Respiratory tract irritation, pulmonary edema, anaphylaxis.*

**sulfur pentafluoride** [Fluorine] *CNS depression, respiratory arrest, cardiovascular collapse, shock, arrhythmias.* [Sulfur] *Respiratory tract irritation, pulmonary edema, anaphylaxis.*

**sulfur phosphide** [Phosphine] *Severe pulmonary irritation, pulmonary edema.*

**sulfur tetrafluoride** [Hydrofluoric acid] *Pulmonary and laryngeal edema, circulatory collapse, severe skin burns, GI tract perforation, systemic fluoride poisoning.* [Sulfur] *Respiratory tract irritation, pulmonary edema, anaphylaxis.*

**sulfur trioxide** [Inorganic acid] *Pulmonary edema, bronchospasm, circulatory collapse, laryngeal spasm and edema, severe chemical burns to skin, mucous membranes, and internal organs, GI tract perforation and hemorrhage, peritonitis.*

**sulfur trioxide & chlorosulfonic acid mixture** [Inorganic acid] *Pulmonary edema, bronchospasm, circulatory collapse, laryngeal spasm and edema, severe chemical burns to skin, mucous membranes, and internal organs, GI tract perforation and hemorrhage, peritonitis.* [Sulfur] *Respiratory tract irritation, pulmonary edema, anaphylaxis.*

**sulfuric acid** [Inorganic acid] *Pulmonary edema, bronchospasm, circulatory collapse, laryngeal spasm and edema, severe chemical burns to skin, mucous membranes, and internal organs, GI tract perforation and hemorrhage, peritonitis.*

**sulfuric acid & hydrofluoric acid mixture** [Inorganic acid] *Pulmonary edema, bronchospasm, circulatory collapse, laryngeal spasm and edema,* severe chemical burns to skin, mucous membranes, and internal organs, GI tract perforation and hemorrhage, peritonitis. [Hydrofluoric acid] *Pulmonary and laryngeal edema, circulatory collapse, severe skin burns, GI tract perforation, systemic fluoride poisoning.*

**sulfuric anhydride** [Inorganic acid] *Pulmonary edema, bronchospasm, circulatory collapse, laryngeal spasm and edema, severe chemical burns to skin, mucous membranes, and internal organs, GI tract perforation and hemorrhage, peritonitis.*

**sulfuric trioxide** [Inorganic acid] *Pulmonary edema, bronchospasm, circulatory collapse, laryngeal spasm and edema, severe chemical burns to skin, mucous membranes, and internal organs, GI tract perforation and hemorrhage, peritonitis.*

**sulfurous acid** [Inorganic acid] *Pulmonary edema, bronchospasm, circulatory collapse, laryngeal spasm and edema, severe chemical burns to skin, mucous membranes, and internal organs, GI tract perforation and hemorrhage, peritonitis.*

**sulfurous acid 2-(p-tert-butylphenoxy)-1-methylethyl-2-chloroethyl ester** [Poison] *Cardiovascular collapse, pulmonary edema, CNS depression, coma, seizures, nausea, vomiting, cardiopulmonary arrest.*

**sulfuryl chloride** [Inorganic acid] *Pulmonary edema, bronchospasm, circulatory collapse, laryngeal spasm and edema, severe chemical burns to skin, mucous membranes, and internal organs, GI tract perforation and hemorrhage, peritonitis.*

**sulfuryl fluoride** [Fluorine] *CNS depression, respiratory arrest, cardiovascular collapse, shock, arrhythmias.* [Sulfur] *Respiratory tract irritation, pulmonary edema, anaphylaxis.*

**superphosphate (n.o.s.)** [Inorganic acid] *Pulmonary edema, bronchospasm, circulatory collapse, laryngeal spasm and edema, severe chemical*

**HazMat**

*burns to skin, mucous membranes, and internal organs, GI tract perforation and hemorrhage, peritonitis.*

**2,4,5-T** [Chlorophenoxy herbicide] *CNS depression, CNS stimulation, respiratory failure, ventricular fibrillation, seizures.*

**2,4,5-T acid** [Chlorophenoxy herbicide] *CNS depression, CNS stimulation, respiratory failure, ventricular fibrillation, seizures.*

**2,4,5-T amine (n.o.s.); 2,4,5-T ester (n.o.s.); 2,4,5-T salt (n.o.s.)** [Chlorophenoxy herbicide] *CNS depression, CNS stimulation, respiratory failure, ventricular fibrillation, seizures.*

**tabun** [Organophosphate] *Pulmonary edema, respiratory muscle paralysis, respiratory failure, bradycardia, acetylcholinesterase inhibition, hypotension, pulmonary edema, overstimulation of parasympathetic nervous system, striated muscle, sympathetic ganglia, and CNS.*

**tannic acid** [Organic acid] *Pulmonary edema, circulatory collapse, laryngeal edema and spasm, severe chemical burns to skin, mucous membranes, and internal organs, GI tract perforation and hemorrhage, peritonitis.*

**tar** [Aromatic hydrocarbon] *Arrhythmias, respiratory failure, pulmonary edema, paralysis, brain and kidney damage.* [Benzene] *Arrhythmias, respiratory failure, pulmonary edema, CNS depression, liver and kidney damage.*

**TBZ (thiabendazole)** [Thiabendazole] *Cardiovascular collapse, respiratory tract irritation.*

**TCDD (2,3,7,8-tetrachlorodibenzo-p-dioxin)** [Chlorophenoxy herbicide] *CNS depression, CNS stimulation, respiratory failure, ventricular fibrillation, seizures.*

**TDE (1,1-dichloro-2,2-bis-(p-chlorophenyl) ethane)** [DDT] *CNS disruption, respiratory control center paralysis, ventricular fibrillation, seizures, respiratory arrest.*

**TDI (toluene diisocyanate)** [Isocyanate/aliphatic thiocyanate] *CNS depression, respiratory arrest, respiratory paralysis, pulmonary edema, cyanide toxicity.*

**tear gas** [Irritant] *Severe immediate or delayed upper airway or respiratory tract irritation, pulmonary edema, glottic spasm, airway obstruction.*

**tecto; tecto 60** [Thiabendazole] *Cardiovascular collapse, respiratory tract irritation.*

**tellurium** [Poison] *Cardiovascular collapse, pulmonary edema, CNS depression, coma, seizures, nausea, vomiting, cardiopulmonary arrest.*

**tellurium hexafluoride** [Poison] *Cardiovascular collapse, pulmonary edema, CNS depression, coma, seizures, nausea, vomiting, cardiopulmonary arrest.*

**temephos** [Organophosphate] *Pulmonary edema, respiratory muscle paralysis, respiratory failure, bradycardia, acetylcholinesterase inhibition, hypotension, pulmonary edema, overstimulation of parasympathetic nervous system, striated muscle, sympathetic ganglia, and CNS.*

**TEPP** [Organophosphate] *Pulmonary edema, respiratory muscle paralysis, respiratory failure, bradycardia, acetylcholinesterase inhibition, hypotension, pulmonary edema, overstimulation of parasympathetic nervous system, striated muscle, sympathetic ganglia, and CNS.*

**terbufos** [Organophosphate] *Pulmonary edema, respiratory muscle paralysis, respiratory failure, bradycardia, acetylcholinesterase inhibition, hypotension, pulmonary edema, overstimulation of parasympathetic nervous system, striated muscle, sympathetic ganglia, and CNS.*

**terebene** [Turpentine/terpene] *Respiratory failure, pulmonary edema, tachycardia.*

**terpene; terpene hydrocarbon (n.o.s.)** [Turpentine/terpene] *Respiratory failure, pulmonary edema, tachycardia.*

**terphenyl** [Turpentine/terpene] *Respiratory failure, pulmonary edema, tachycardia.*

**terpin hydrate** [Turpentine/terpene] *Respiratory failure, pulmonary edema, tachycardia.*

**terpineol** [Turpentine/terpene] *Respiratory failure, pulmonary edema, tachycardia.*

**terpinolene** [Turpentine/terpene] *Respiratory failure, pulmonary edema, tachycardia.*

**tetrabromo-*o*-cresol** [Phenol] *Coma, hypotension, arrhythmias, pulmonary edema, respiratory arrest.*

**tetrabromoethane; 1,1,2,2-tetrabromoethane** [Halogenated aliphatic hydrocarbon] *CNS depression, respiratory arrest, circulatory collapse.*

**1,2,4,5-tetrachlorobenzene** [Aromatic hydrocarbon] *Arrhythmias, respiratory failure, pulmonary edema, paralysis, brain and kidney damage.*

**2,3,7,8-tetrachlorodibenzo-*p*-dioxin (TCDD)** [Chlorophenoxy herbicide] *CNS depression, CNS stimulation, respiratory failure, ventricular fibrillation, seizures.*

**tetrachlorodifluoroethane** [Chlorinated fluorocarbon] *Asphyxiation, anesthesia, arrhythmias.*

**tetrachloroethane; 1,1,1,2-tetrachloroethane** [Halogenated aliphatic hydrocarbon] *CNS depression, respiratory arrest, circulatory collapse.*

**tetrachloroethylene** [Carbon tetrachloride] *CNS depression, respiratory arrest, circulatory collapse.*

**2,3,4,6-tetrachlorophenol** [Phenol] *Coma, hypotension, arrhythmias, pulmonary edema, respiratory arrest.*

**tetrachlorvinfos; tetrachlorvinphos** [Organophosphate] *Pulmonary edema, respiratory muscle paralysis, respiratory failure, bradycardia, acetylcholinesterase inhibition, hypotension, pulmonary edema, overstimulation of parasympathetic nervous system, striated muscle, sympathetic ganglia, and CNS.*

**tetraethyl dithiopyrophosphate** [Organophosphate] *Pulmonary edema, respiratory muscle paralysis, respiratory failure, bradycardia, acetylcholinesterase inhibition, hypotension, pulmonary edema, overstimulation of parasympathetic nervous system, striated muscle, sympathetic ganglia, and CNS.*

**tetraethyl dithiopyrophosphate & compressed gas mixture** [Organophosphate] *Pulmonary edema, respiratory muscle paralysis, respiratory failure, bradycardia, acetylcholinesterase inhibition, hypotension, pulmonary edema, overstimulation of parasympathetic nervous system, striated muscle, sympathetic ganglia, and CNS.*

**tetraethyl lead** [Lead] *Circulatory collapse, coma, rare seizures.*

**tetraethyl pyrophosphate** [Organophosphate] *Pulmonary edema, respiratory muscle paralysis, respiratory failure, bradycardia, acetylcholinesterase inhibition, hypotension, pulmonary edema, overstimulation of parasympathetic nervous system, striated muscle, sympathetic ganglia, and CNS.*

**tetraethyl pyrophosphate & compressed gas mixture** [Organophosphate] *Pulmonary edema, respiratory muscle paralysis, respiratory failure, bradycardia, acetylcholinesterase inhibition, hypotension, pulmonary edema, overstimulation of parasympathetic nervous system, striated muscle, sympathetic ganglia, and CNS.*

**tetraethyl silicate** [Silane/chlorosilane] *Respiratory tract irritation, pulmonary edema.*

**tetraethyl tin** [Organotin] *Respiratory failure, pulmonary edema, cerebral edema.*

**tetraethylammonium perchlorate** [Chlorate] *Hemolysis, methemoglobinemia, hypoperfusion, CNS depression, delayed-onset renal failure.*

**tetraethylenepentamine** [Organic base/amine] *Pulmonary edema, cardiac depression, seizures.*

**HazMat**

**1,1,1,2-tetrafluoroethane (R134A refrigerant)** [Chlorinated fluorocarbon] *Asphyxiation, anesthesia, arrhythmias.*

**tetrafluoroethylene** [Halogenated aliphatic hydrocarbon] *CNS depression, respiratory arrest, circulatory collapse.*

**tetrafluorohydrazine** [Hydrazine] *Seizures, hemolysis of red blood cells, pulmonary edema.*

**tetrafluoromethane** [Chlorinated fluorocarbon] *Asphyxiation, anesthesia, arrhythmias.*

**tetrahydrobenzaldehyde** [Aldehyde] *Seizures, respiratory failure, pulmonary edema.*

**tetrahydrofuran** [Ether] *Anesthesia, respiratory arrest.*

**tetrahydrofurfurylamine** [Organic base/amine] *Pulmonary edema, cardiac depression, seizures.*

**tetrahydronaphthalene** [Naphthalene] *Delayed-onset acute intravascular hemolysis.*

**tetrahydronaphthyl hydroperoxide** [Organic peroxide] *Pulmonary and laryngeal edema, circulatory arrest, hypovolemic shock, chemical burns to skin, mucous membranes, and internal organs.* [Naphthalene] *Delayed-onset acute intravascular hemolysis.*

**tetrahydrophthalic anhydride** [Organic acid] *Pulmonary edema, circulatory collapse, laryngeal edema and spasm, severe chemical burns to skin, mucous membranes, and internal organs, GI tract perforation and hemorrhage, peritonitis.*

**tetrahydropyridine** [Aromatic hydrocarbon] *Arrhythmias, respiratory failure, pulmonary edema, paralysis, brain and kidney damage.*

**tetrahydrothiophene** [Sulfur] *Respiratory tract irritation, pulmonary edema, anaphylaxis.*

**tetralin hydroperoxide** [Organic peroxide] *Pulmonary and laryngeal edema, circulatory arrest, hypovolemic shock, chemical burns to skin, mucous membranes, and internal organs.*

[Naphthalene] *Delayed-onset acute intravascular hemolysis.*

**Tetram** [Organophosphate] *Pulmonary edema, respiratory muscle paralysis, respiratory failure, bradycardia, acetylcholinesterase inhibition, hypotension, pulmonary edema, overstimulation of parasympathetic nervous system, striated muscle, sympathetic ganglia, and CNS.*

**tetramethoxysilane** [Silane/chlorosilane] *Respiratory tract irritation, pulmonary edema.*

**tetramethrin** [Pyrethrin/pyrethroid] *Respiratory paralysis, convulsions.*

**tetramethyl ammonium hydroxide** [Organic base/amine] *Pulmonary edema, cardiac depression, seizures.*

**tetramethyl lead** [Lead] *Circulatory collapse, coma, rare seizures.*

**tetramethyl silane** [Silane/chlorosilane] *Respiratory tract irritation, pulmonary edema.*

**1,1,3,3-tetramethylbutyl hydroxide** [Organic peroxide] *Pulmonary and laryngeal edema, circulatory arrest, hypovolemic shock, chemical burns to skin, mucous membranes, and internal organs.*

**1,1,3,3-tetramethylbutylperoxy-2-ethyl hexanoate** [Organic peroxide] *Pulmonary and laryngeal edema, circulatory arrest, hypovolemic shock, chemical burns to skin, mucous membranes, and internal organs.*

**tetramethylmethylenediamine** [Organic base/amine] *Pulmonary edema, cardiac depression, seizures.*

**tetranitromethane** [Nitrate/nitrite] *Methemoglobinemia, hypotension, circulatory collapse.*

**tetrapropyl dithionopyrophosphate** [Organophosphate] *Pulmonary edema, respiratory muscle paralysis, respiratory failure, bradycardia, acetylcholinesterase inhibition, hypotension, pulmonary edema, overstimulation of parasympathetic nervous system, striated muscle, sympathetic ganglia, and CNS.*

**tetrapropyl-o-titanate** [Poison] *Cardiovascular collapse, pulmonary edema, CNS depression, coma, sei-*

zures, nausea, vomiting, cardiopulmonary arrest.

**Tetryl** [Naphthalene] *Delayed-onset acute intravascular hemolysis.*

**textile waste (n.o.s.)** [see also: animal fabric with oil; vegetable fabric with oil] [Thallium] *Pulmonary edema, respiratory failure, circulatory collapse, seizures.* [Chlorate] *Hemolysis, methemoglobinemia, hypoperfusion, CNS depression, delayed-onset renal failure.*

**textile-treating compound** [Poison] *Cardiovascular collapse, pulmonary edema, CNS depression, coma, seizures, nausea, vomiting, cardiopulmonary arrest.*

**thallic oxide** [Thallium] *Pulmonary edema, respiratory failure, circulatory collapse, seizures.*

**thallium acetate** [Thallium] *Pulmonary edema, respiratory failure, circulatory collapse, seizures.*

**thallium carbonate; thallous carbonate** [Thallium] *Pulmonary edema, respiratory failure, circulatory collapse, seizures.*

**thallium chlorate** [Thallium] *Pulmonary edema, respiratory failure, circulatory collapse, seizures.* [Chlorate] *Hemolysis, methemoglobinemia, hypoperfusion, CNS depression, delayed-onset renal failure.*

**thallium chloride; thallous chloride** [Thallium] *Pulmonary edema, respiratory failure, circulatory collapse, seizures.*

**thallium mixture (n.o.s.); thallium salt (n.o.s.)** [Thallium] *Pulmonary edema, respiratory failure, circulatory collapse, seizures.*

**thallium nitrate** [Nitrate/nitrite] *Methemoglobinemia, hypotension, circulatory collapse.* [Thallium] *Pulmonary edema, respiratory failure, circulatory collapse, seizures.*

**thallium sulfate; thallous sulfate** [Thallium] *Pulmonary edema, respiratory failure, circulatory collapse, seizures.*

**thallous carbonate; thallium carbonate** [Thallium] *Pulmonary*

edema, respiratory failure, circulatory collapse, seizures.

**thallous chloride; thallium chloride** [Thallium] *Pulmonary edema, respiratory failure, circulatory collapse, seizures.*

**thallous malonate** [Thallium] *Pulmonary edema, respiratory failure, circulatory collapse, seizures.*

**thallous sulfate; thallium sulfate** [Thallium] *Pulmonary edema, respiratory failure, circulatory collapse, seizures.*

**thanite** [Isocyanate/aliphatic thiocyanate] *CNS depression, respiratory arrest, respiratory paralysis, pulmonary edema, cyanide toxicity.*

**thiabendazole** [Thiabendazole] *Cardiovascular collapse, respiratory tract irritation.*

**thiapentanal** [Poison] *Cardiovascular collapse, pulmonary edema, CNS depression, coma, seizures, nausea, vomiting, cardiopulmonary arrest.*

**2-(4-thiazolyl) benzimidazole** [Thiabendazole] *Cardiovascular collapse, respiratory tract irritation.*

**Thibenzole** [Thiabendazole] *Cardiovascular collapse, respiratory tract irritation.*

**thimerosal** [Mercury] *Circulatory collapse, arrhythmias, respiratory failure, pulmonary edema, neurotoxic effects.*

**thinner, paint and varnish** [Hydrocarbon mixture] *CNS depression, respiratory arrest, seizures, arrhythmias, pulmonary edema.*

**thioacetamide** [Sulfur] *Respiratory tract irritation, pulmonary edema, anaphylaxis.*

**thioacetic acid** [Organic acid] *Pulmonary edema, circulatory collapse, laryngeal edema and spasm, severe chemical burns to skin, mucous membranes, and internal organs, GI tract perforation and hemorrhage, peritonitis.* [Sulfur] *Respiratory tract irritation, pulmonary edema, anaphylaxis.*

**thiocarbazide** [Hydrazine] *Seizures, hemolysis of red blood cells, pulmonary edema.*

**thiocyanates, aliphatic (n.o.s.)** [Isocyanate/aliphatic thiocyanate] *CNS*

**HazMat**

*depression, respiratory arrest, respiratory paralysis, pulmonary edema, cyanide toxicity.*

**Thiodan** [Aldrin/dieldrin/endrin] *Seizures, respiratory failure.*

**4,4'-thiodianiline** [Aniline] *Methemoglobinemia, hypoxia.*

**thiofanox** [Carbamate] *Acetylcholinesterase inhibition (reversible), bradycardia, hypotension, respiratory muscle paralysis, respiratory arrest, pulmonary edema.*

**thioglycol** [Sulfur] *Respiratory tract irritation, pulmonary edema, anaphylaxis.*

**thioglycolate salt (n.o.s.)** [Organic acid] *Pulmonary edema, circulatory collapse, laryngeal edema and spasm, severe chemical burns to skin, mucous membranes, and internal organs, GI tract perforation and hemorrhage, peritonitis.*

**thioglycolic acid** [Organic acid] *Pulmonary edema, circulatory collapse, laryngeal edema and spasm, severe chemical burns to skin, mucous membranes, and internal organs, GI tract perforation and hemorrhage, peritonitis.*

**thiolactic acid** [Organic acid] *Pulmonary edema, circulatory collapse, laryngeal edema and spasm, severe chemical burns to skin, mucous membranes, and internal organs, GI tract perforation and hemorrhage, peritonitis.*

**thiomethanol** [Sulfur] *Respiratory tract irritation, pulmonary edema, anaphylaxis.*

**thionazin** [Organophosphate] *Pulmonary edema, respiratory muscle paralysis, respiratory failure, bradycardia, acetylcholinesterase inhibition, hypotension, pulmonary edema, overstimulation of parasympathetic nervous system, striated muscle, sympathetic ganglia, and CNS.*

**thionyl chloride** [Sulfur] *Respiratory tract irritation, pulmonary edema, anaphylaxis.*

**thiophene** [Sulfur] *Respiratory tract irritation, pulmonary edema, anaphylaxis.*

**thiophenol** [Sulfur] *Respiratory tract irritation, pulmonary edema, anaphylaxis.*

**thiophosgene** [Phosgene] *Severe respiratory irritation, alveolar damage, pulmonary edema.*

**thiophosphoryl chloride** [Phosphorus] *Hypovolemic shock, severe tissue burns, severe respiratory irritation, pulmonary edema, respiratory arrest, arrhythmias, sudden death.*

**thiosemicarbazide** [Hydrazine] *Seizures, hemolysis of red blood cells, pulmonary edema.*

**thiourea** [Naphthalene] *Delayed-onset acute intravascular hemolysis.*

**thiram** [Dithiocarbamate] *Hypotension, respiratory failure.*

**thorium; thorium mixture (n.o.s.)** [Flammable solid] *Shock, severe chemical and thermal burns, severe respiratory tract irritation, pulmonary edema, respiratory arrest, ECG changes, sudden death.* [Poison] *Cardiovascular collapse, pulmonary edema, CNS depression, coma, seizures, nausea, vomiting, cardiopulmonary arrest.*

**thorium dioxide** [Poison] *Cardiovascular collapse, pulmonary edema, CNS depression, coma, seizures, nausea, vomiting, cardiopulmonary arrest.*

**thorium nitrate** [Nitrate/nitrite] *Methemoglobinemia, hypotension, circulatory collapse.*

**thymol** [Phenol] *Coma, hypotension, arrhythmias, pulmonary edema, respiratory arrest.*

**tin; tin mixture (n.o.s.)** [Poison] *Cardiovascular collapse, pulmonary edema, CNS depression, coma, seizures, nausea, vomiting, cardiopulmonary arrest.*

**tin chloride** [Poison] *Cardiovascular collapse, pulmonary edema, CNS depression, coma, seizures, nausea, vomiting, cardiopulmonary arrest.*

**tin tetrachloride** [Poison] *Cardiovascular collapse, pulmonary edema, CNS depression, coma, seizures, nausea, vomiting, cardiopulmonary arrest.*

**tincture, medicinal (n.o.s.)** [Poison] *Cardiovascular collapse, pulmonary* edema, CNS depression, coma, seizures, nausea, vomiting, cardiopulmonary arrest.

**titanium** [Poison] Cardiovascular collapse, pulmonary edema, CNS depression, coma, seizures, nausea, vomiting, cardiopulmonary arrest.

**titanium hydride** [Poison] Cardiovascular collapse, pulmonary edema, CNS depression, coma, seizures, nausea, vomiting, cardiopulmonary arrest.

**titanium sulfate** [Poison] Cardiovascular collapse, pulmonary edema, CNS depression, coma, seizures, nausea, vomiting, cardiopulmonary arrest.

**titanium tetrachloride** [Poison] Cardiovascular collapse, pulmonary edema, CNS depression, coma, seizures, nausea, vomiting, cardiopulmonary arrest.

**titanium tetrachloride & vanadium oxytrichloride mixture** [Poison] Cardiovascular collapse, pulmonary edema, CNS depression, coma, seizures, nausea, vomiting, cardiopulmonary arrest.

**titanium trichloride; titanium trichloride mixture (n.o.s.)** [Poison] Cardiovascular collapse, pulmonary edema, CNS depression, coma, seizures, nausea, vomiting, cardiopulmonary arrest.

**Toe Puffs, nitrocellulose-based** [Flammable solid] Shock, severe chemical and thermal burns, severe respiratory tract irritation, pulmonary edema, respiratory arrest, ECG changes, sudden death.

*o*-**tolidine** [Aniline] Methemoglobinemia, hypoxia.

**toluene** [Aromatic hydrocarbon] Arrhythmias, respiratory failure, pulmonary edema, paralysis, brain and kidney damage.

**toluene diisocyanate (TDI)** [Isocyanate/aliphatic thiocyanate] CNS depression, respiratory arrest, respiratory paralysis, pulmonary edema, cyanide toxicity.

**toluene sulfonic acid** [Organic acid] Pulmonary edema, circulatory collapse, laryngeal edema and spasm, severe chemical burns to skin, mucous membranes, and internal organs, GI tract perforation and hemorrhage, peritonitis.

**toluenediamine** [Aniline] Methemoglobinemia, hypoxia.

*m*-**toluidine;** *o*-**toluidine;** *p*-**toluidine** [Aniline] Methemoglobinemia, hypoxia.

*o*-**toluidine HCl** [Aniline] Methemoglobinemia, hypoxia.

**toluol** [Aromatic hydrocarbon] Arrhythmias, respiratory failure, pulmonary edema, paralysis, brain and kidney damage. [Phenol] Coma, hypotension, arrhythmias, pulmonary edema, respiratory arrest.

**toluylenediamine** [Aniline] Methemoglobinemia, hypoxia.

**N-*m*-tolylphthalamic acid** [Aniline] Methemoglobinemia, hypoxia.

**toxaphene** [Toxaphene] Respiratory failure, seizures, exhaustion, death.

**2,4,5-TP** [Chlorophenoxy herbicide] CNS depression, CNS stimulation, respiratory failure, ventricular fibrillation, seizures.

**tree-killing compound, corrosive** [Poison] Cardiovascular collapse, pulmonary edema, CNS depression, coma, seizures, nausea, vomiting, cardiopulmonary arrest. [Corrosive] Upper airway burns and edema, circulatory collapse, severe chemical burns to skin, toxic systemic effects, GI tract perforation and hemorrhage, peritonitis.

**tree-killing compound, flammable** [Flammable/combustible liquid] CNS depression, respiratory arrest, convulsions, arrhythmias, pulmonary edema. [Poison] Cardiovascular collapse, pulmonary edema, CNS depression, coma, seizures, nausea, vomiting, cardiopulmonary arrest.

**tremolite** [Asbestos] Asbestosis, lung cancer, malignant mesothelioma.

**triallyl borate** [Boron] Respiratory tract irritation, laryngeal spasm and edema, *pulmonary edema, severe chemical burns.*

**triallylamine** [Organic base/amine] *Pulmonary edema, cardiac depression, seizures.*

**triamiphos** [Organophosphate] *Pulmonary edema, respiratory muscle paralysis, respiratory failure, bradycardia, acetylcholinesterase inhibition, hypotension, pulmonary edema, overstimulation of parasympathetic nervous system, striated muscle, sympathetic ganglia, and CNS.*

**triatomic oxygen** [Ozone] *Pulmonary edema, airway obstruction.*

**triazine pesticide (n.o.s.)** [Irritant] *Severe immediate or delayed upper airway or respiratory tract irritation, pulmonary edema, glottic spasm, airway obstruction.*

**triaziquone** [Poison] *Cardiovascular collapse, pulmonary edema, CNS depression, coma, seizures, nausea, vomiting, cardiopulmonary arrest.*

**tri(1-aziridinyl)phosphine oxide** [Poison] *Cardiovascular collapse, pulmonary edema, CNS depression, coma, seizures, nausea, vomiting, cardiopulmonary arrest.*

**triazofos** [Organophosphate] *Pulmonary edema, respiratory muscle paralysis, respiratory failure, bradycardia, acetylcholinesterase inhibition, hypotension, pulmonary edema, overstimulation of parasympathetic nervous system, striated muscle, sympathetic ganglia, and CNS.*

**tribasic copper sulfate** [Copper] *Respiratory tract irritation and arrest, hemorrhagic gastritis.*

**tribromomethane** [Chlorinated fluorocarbon] *Asphyxiation, anesthesia, arrhythmias.*

**tributyl aluminum** [Poison] *Cardiovascular collapse, pulmonary edema, CNS depression, coma, seizures, nausea, vomiting, cardiopulmonary arrest.*

**S,S,S-tributyl phosphorotrithiolate** [Organophosphate] *Pulmonary edema, respiratory muscle paralysis, respiratory failure, bradycardia, acetylcholinesterase inhibition, hypotension, pulmonary edema, overstimulation of parasympathetic nervous system, striated muscle, sympathetic ganglia, and CNS.*

**tributylamine** [Organic base/amine] *Pulmonary edema, cardiac depression, seizures.*

**trichlorfon** [Organophosphate] *Pulmonary edema, respiratory muscle paralysis, respiratory failure, bradycardia, acetylcholinesterase inhibition, hypotension, pulmonary edema, overstimulation of parasympathetic nervous system, striated muscle, sympathetic ganglia, and CNS.*

**trichloroacetic acid** [Organic acid] *Pulmonary edema, circulatory collapse, laryngeal edema and spasm, severe chemical burns to skin, mucous membranes, and internal organs, GI tract perforation and hemorrhage, peritonitis.*

**trichloroacetyl chloride** [Halogenated aliphatic hydrocarbon] *CNS depression, respiratory arrest, circulatory collapse.*

**trichlorobenzene; 1,2,4-trichlorobenzene** [Aromatic hydrocarbon] *Arrhythmias, respiratory failure, pulmonary edema, paralysis, brain and kidney damage.*

**trichlorobutene** [Halogenated aliphatic hydrocarbon] *CNS depression, respiratory arrest, circulatory collapse.*

**trichloro(chloromethyl)silane** [Silane/chlorosilane] *Respiratory tract irritation, pulmonary edema.*

**trichloro(dichlorophenyl)silane** [Silane/chlorosilane] *Respiratory tract irritation, pulmonary edema.*

**trichloroethane; 1,1,1-trichloroethane; 1,1,2-trichloroethane** [Halogenated aliphatic hydrocarbon] *CNS depression, respiratory arrest, circulatory collapse.*

**trichloroethylene** [Carbon tetrachloride] *CNS depression, respiratory arrest, circulatory collapse.*

**trichloroethylsilane** [Silane/chlorosilane] *Respiratory tract irritation, pulmonary edema.*

**trichlorofluoromethane (Freon 11)** [Chlorinated fluorocarbon] *Asphyxiation, anesthesia, arrhythmias.*

**trichlorofluoromethane & chlorodifluoromethane & dichlorodifluoromethane mixture** [Chlorinated fluorocarbon] *Asphyxiation, anesthesia, arrhythmias.*

**trichlorofluoromethane & dichlorodifluoromethane mixture** [Chlorinated fluorocarbon] *Asphyxiation, anesthesia, arrhythmias.*

**trichloroisocyanuric acid** [Hypochlorite] *Circulatory collapse, respiratory tract irritation, upper airway obstruction, pulmonary edema.*

**trichloromethanesulfenyl chloride** [Sulfur] *Respiratory tract irritation, pulmonary edema, anaphylaxis.*

**trichloromonofluoromethane** [Chlorinated fluorocarbon] *Asphyxiation, anesthesia, arrhythmias.*

**trichloronate** [Organophosphate] *Pulmonary edema, respiratory muscle paralysis, respiratory failure, bradycardia, acetylcholinesterase inhibition, hypotension, pulmonary edema, overstimulation of parasympathetic nervous system, striated muscle, sympathetic ganglia, and CNS.*

**trichlorophenol** [Phenol] *Coma, hypotension, arrhythmias, pulmonary edema, respiratory arrest.*

**trichlorophenoxy ethyl sulfate sodium salt (n.o.s.)** [Chlorophenoxy herbicide] *CNS depression, CNS stimulation, respiratory failure, ventricular fibrillation, seizures.*

**trichlorophenoxyacetic acid; 2,4,5-trichlorophenoxyacetic acid** [Chlorophenoxy herbicide] *CNS depression, CNS stimulation, respiratory failure, ventricular fibrillation, seizures.*

**2,4,5-trichlorophenoxypropionic acid** [Chlorophenoxy herbicide] *CNS depression, CNS stimulation,*

*respiratory failure, ventricular fibrillation, seizures.*

**trichlorophenylsilane** [Silane/chlorosilane] *Respiratory tract irritation, pulmonary edema.*

**trichlorosilane** [Silane/chlorosilane] *Respiratory tract irritation, pulmonary edema.*

**trichloro-S-triazinetrione; trichloro-S-triazinetrione salt (n.o.s.)** [Hypochlorite] *Circulatory collapse, respiratory tract irritation, upper airway obstruction, pulmonary edema.*

**trichlorotrifluorethane (Freon 13)** [Chlorinated fluorocarbon] *Asphyxiation, anesthesia, arrhythmias.*

**trichlorotrifluoroethane & dichlorodifluoromethane mixture** [Chlorinated fluorocarbon] *Asphyxiation, anesthesia, arrhythmias.*

**tricresyl phosphate; tri-o-cresyl phosphate** [Triorthocresyl phosphate] *Delayed-onset neurotoxicity, ascending paralysis of the extremities.*

**triethanolamine dodecylbenzene sulfonate** [Poison] *Cardiovascular collapse, pulmonary edema, CNS depression, coma, seizures, nausea, vomiting, cardiopulmonary arrest.*

**triethoxysilane** [Silane/chlorosilane] *Respiratory tract irritation, pulmonary edema.*

**triethyl phosphite** [Phosphorus] *Hypovolemic shock, severe tissue burns, severe respiratory irritation, pulmonary edema, respiratory arrest, arrhythmias, sudden death.*

**O,O,O-triethyl phosphorothioate** [Organophosphate] *Pulmonary edema, respiratory muscle paralysis, respiratory failure, bradycardia, acetylcholinesterase inhibition, hypotension, pulmonary edema, overstimulation of parasympathetic nervous system, striated muscle, sympathetic ganglia, and CNS.*

**tricthylamine** [Organic base/amine] *Pulmonary edema, cardiac depression, seizures.*

**triethylene glycol** [Ethylene glycol] *Respiratory failure, pulmonary edema,*

HazMat

*paralysis, cardiovascular collapse, severe acidosis.*

**triethylene tetramine** [Poison] *Cardiovascular collapse, pulmonary edema, CNS depression, coma, seizures, nausea, vomiting, cardiopulmonary arrest.*

**trifluoroacetic acid** [Organic acid] *Pulmonary edema, circulatory collapse, laryngeal edema and spasm, severe chemical burns to skin, mucous membranes, and internal organs, GI tract perforation and hemorrhage, peritonitis.*

**trifluoroacetyl chloride** [Organic acid] *Pulmonary edema, circulatory collapse, laryngeal edema and spasm, severe chemical burns to skin, mucous membranes, and internal organs, GI tract perforation and hemorrhage, peritonitis.*

**trifluoroamine oxide** [Fluorine] *CNS depression, respiratory arrest, cardiovascular collapse, shock, arrhythmias.*

**trifluorobromomethane** [Chlorinated fluorocarbon] *Asphyxiation, anesthesia, arrhythmias.*

**trifluorochloroethylene** [Chlorinated fluorocarbon] *Asphyxiation, anesthesia, arrhythmias.*

**trifluorochloromethane** [Chlorinated fluorocarbon] *Asphyxiation, anesthesia, arrhythmias.*

**trifluoroethane** [Chlorinated fluorocarbon] *Asphyxiation, anesthesia, arrhythmias.*

**trifluoromethane (gas or cryogenic liquid)** [Chlorinated fluorocarbon] *Asphyxiation, anesthesia, arrhythmias.*

**3-(trifluoromethyl) benzenamine** [Aniline] *Methemoglobinemia, hypoxia.*

**2-trifluoromethylaniline; 3-trifluoromethylaniline** [Aniline] *Methemoglobinemia, hypoxia.*

**3-trifluoromethylphenylisocyanate** [Isocyanate/aliphatic thiocyanate] *CNS depression, respiratory arrest, respiratory paralysis, pulmonary edema, cyanide toxicity.*

**trifluralin** [Irritant] *Severe immediate or delayed upper airway or respiratory tract irritation, pulmonary edema, glottic spasm, airway obstruction.*

**triisobutyl aluminum** [Poison] *Cardiovascular collapse, pulmonary edema, CNS depression, coma, seizures, nausea, vomiting, cardiopulmonary arrest.*

**triisobutylene** [Aliphatic hydrocarbon] *Arrhythmias, asphyxiation, anesthesia.*

**triisocyanatoisocyanurate of isophoronediisocyanate** [Poison] *Cardiovascular collapse, pulmonary edema, CNS depression, coma, seizures, nausea, vomiting, cardiopulmonary arrest.*

**triisopropyl borate** [Boron] *Respiratory tract irritation, laryngeal spasm and edema, pulmonary edema, severe chemical burns.*

**trimethoxysilane** [Silane/chlorosilane] *Respiratory tract irritation, pulmonary edema.*

**trimethyl aluminum** [Poison] *Cardiovascular collapse, pulmonary edema, CNS depression, coma, seizures, nausea, vomiting, cardiopulmonary arrest.*

**trimethyl norpinanyl hydroperoxide** [Aromatic hydrocarbon] *Arrhythmias, respiratory failure, pulmonary edema, paralysis, brain and kidney damage.*

**trimethyl phosphite** [Phosphorus] *Hypovolemic shock, severe tissue burns, severe respiratory irritation, pulmonary edema, respiratory arrest, arrhythmias, sudden death.*

**trimethylacetyl chloride** [Organic acid] *Pulmonary edema, circulatory collapse, laryngeal edema and spasm, severe chemical burns to skin, mucous membranes, and internal organs, GI tract perforation and hemorrhage, peritonitis.*

**trimethylamine** [Organic base/amine] *Pulmonary edema, cardiac depression, seizures.*

**trimethylbenzene** [Aromatic hydrocarbon] *Arrhythmias, respiratory failure, pulmonary edema, paralysis, brain and kidney damage.*

**trimethylborate** [Boron] *Respiratory tract irritation, laryngeal spasm and edema, pulmonary edema, severe chemical burns.*

**trimethylchlorosilane** [Silane/chlorosilane] *Respiratory tract irritation, pulmonary edema.*

**trimethylcyclohexylamine** [Organic base/amine] *Pulmonary edema, cardiac depression, seizures.*

**trimethylene chlorohydrin** [Dichloropropane/dichloropropene] *Pulmonary edema, bronchospasm, alveolar hemorrhage.*

**trimethylhexamethylene diisocyanate** [Isocyanate/aliphatic thiocyanate] *CNS depression, respiratory arrest, respiratory paralysis, pulmonary edema, cyanide toxicity.*

**trimethylhexamethylenediamine** [Organic base/amine] *Pulmonary edema, cardiac depression, seizures.*

**trimethylolpropane phosphite** [Poison] *Cardiovascular collapse, pulmonary edema, CNS depression, coma, seizures, nausea, vomiting, cardiopulmonary arrest.*

**trimethyloxysilane** [Silane/chlorosilane] *Respiratory tract irritation, pulmonary edema.*

**2,2,4-trimethylpentane** [Aliphatic hydrocarbon] *Arrhythmias, asphyxiation, anesthesia.*

**2,4,4-trimethylpentyl-2-peroxyphenoxyacetate** [Ester] *CNS depression, respiratory tract irritation, bronchitis, pneumonia.*

**trimethyltin chloride** [Organotin] *Respiratory failure, pulmonary edema, cerebral edema.*

**trinitrobenzene** [Aromatic hydrocarbon] *Arrhythmias, respiratory failure, pulmonary edema, paralysis, brain and kidney damage.* [Nitrate/nitrite] *Methemoglobinemia, hypotension, circulatory collapse.*

**trinitrobenzoic acid** [Organic acid] *Pulmonary edema, circulatory collapse, laryngeal edema and spasm, severe chemical burns to skin, mucous membranes, and internal organs, GI tract perforation and hemorrhage, peritonitis.* [Nitrate/nitrite] *Methemoglobinemia, hypotension, circulatory collapse.*

**trinitrophenol** [Dinitrophenol] *Respiratory and circulatory collapse, pulmonary edema, hyperthermia.*

**trinitrotoluene; 2,4,6-trinitrotoluene** [Aromatic hydrocarbon] *Arrhythmias, respiratory failure, pulmonary edema, paralysis, brain and kidney damage.* [Nitrate/nitrite] *Methemoglobinemia, hypotension, circulatory collapse.*

**triphenyl phosphate** [Triorthocresyl phosphate] *Delayed-onset neurotoxicity, ascending paralysis of the extremities.*

**triphenyltin chloride** [Organotin] *Respiratory failure, pulmonary edema, cerebral edema.*

**tripropylaluminum** [Poison] *Cardiovascular collapse, pulmonary edema, CNS depression, coma, seizures, nausea, vomiting, cardiopulmonary arrest.*

**tripropylamine** [Organic base/amine] *Pulmonary edema, cardiac depression, seizures.*

**tripropylene** [Aliphatic hydrocarbon] *Arrhythmias, asphyxiation, anesthesia.*

**tris(1-aziridinyl)phosphine oxide** [Poison] *Cardiovascular collapse, pulmonary edema, CNS depression, coma, seizures, nausea, vomiting, cardiopulmonary arrest.*

**tris(2-chloroethyl)amine** [Organic base/amine] *Pulmonary edema, cardiac depression, seizures.*

**tris(2,3-dibromopropyl)phosphate** [Phosphorus] *Hypovolemic shock, severe tissue burns, severe respiratory irritation, pulmonary edema, respiratory arrest, arrhythmias, sudden death.*

**trisodium phosphate** [Inorganic base/alkaline corrosive] *Upper airway burns and edema, pulmonary edema, skin burns, circulatory collapse, GI tract perforation and hemorrhage, peritonitis.*

**trisodium phosphate, chlorinated** [Inorganic base/alkaline corrosive] *Upper airway burns and edema, pul-*

HazMat

monary edema, skin burns, circulatory collapse, GI tract perforation and hemorrhage, peritonitis. [Hypochlorite] Circulatory collapse, respiratory tract irritation, upper airway obstruction, pulmonary edema.

**trypan blue** [Naphthalene] Delayed-onset acute intravascular hemolysis.

**tungsten hexafluoride** [Fluorine] CNS depression, respiratory arrest, cardiovascular collapse, shock, arrhythmias.

**turpentine; turpentine substitute** [Turpentine/terpene] Respiratory failure, pulmonary edema, tachycardia.

**undecane** [Aliphatic hydrocarbon] Arrhythmias, asphyxiation, anesthesia.

**uracil mustard** [Poison] Cardiovascular collapse, pulmonary edema, CNS depression, coma, seizures, nausea, vomiting, cardiopulmonary arrest.

**uranium** [Radioactive] DNA or RNA damage, severe GI or hematologic damage, loss of bone marrow function, immunocompromise, systemic infection, carcinoma.

**uranium acetate** [Radioactive] DNA or RNA damage, severe GI or hematologic damage, loss of bone marrow function, immunocompromise, systemic infection, carcinoma. [Ester] CNS depression, respiratory tract irritation, bronchitis, pneumonia.

**uranium hexafluoride** [Radioactive] DNA or RNA damage, severe GI or hematologic damage, loss of bone marrow function, immunocompromise, systemic infection, carcinoma. [Fluorine] CNS depression, respiratory arrest, cardiovascular collapse, shock, arrhythmias.

**uranium nitrate hexahydrate** [Radioactive] DNA or RNA damage, severe GI or hematologic damage, loss of bone marrow function, immunocompromise, systemic infection, carcinoma. [Nitrate/nitrite] Methemoglobinemia, hypotension, circulatory collapse.

**uranyl acetate** [Radioactive] DNA or RNA damage, severe GI or hematologic damage, loss of bone marrow

function, immunocompromise, systemic infection, carcinoma. [Ester] CNS depression, respiratory tract irritation, bronchitis, pneumonia.

**uranyl nitrate** [Radioactive] DNA or RNA damage, severe GI or hematologic damage, loss of bone marrow function, immunocompromise, systemic infection, carcinoma. [Nitrate/nitrite] Methemoglobinemia, hypotension, circulatory collapse.

**urea hydrogen peroxide** [Organic peroxide] Pulmonary and laryngeal edema, circulatory arrest, hypovolemic shock, chemical burns to skin, mucous membranes, and internal organs.

**urea nitrate** [Nitrate/nitrite] Methemoglobinemia, hypotension, circulatory collapse.

**urea peroxide** [Organic peroxide] Pulmonary and laryngeal edema, circulatory arrest, hypovolemic shock, chemical burns to skin, mucous membranes, and internal organs.

**urethane** [Isocyanate/aliphatic thiocyanate] CNS depression, respiratory arrest, respiratory paralysis, pulmonary edema, cyanide toxicity.

**valeraldehyde** [Aldehyde] Seizures, respiratory failure, pulmonary edema.

**valeric acid (n-pentanoic acid)** [Organic acid] Pulmonary edema, circulatory collapse, laryngeal edema and spasm, severe chemical burns to skin, mucous membranes, and internal organs, GI tract perforation and hemorrhage, peritonitis.

**valeryl chloride** [Organic acid] Pulmonary edema, circulatory collapse, laryngeal edema and spasm, severe chemical burns to skin, mucous membranes, and internal organs, GI tract perforation and hemorrhage, peritonitis.

**valinomycin** [Poison] Cardiovascular collapse, pulmonary edema, CNS depression, coma, seizures, nausea, vomiting, cardiopulmonary arrest.

**Valone** [Warfarin/hydroxycoumarin/indanedione] Anticoagulation effect, internal hemorrhage.

**vanadium oxytrichloride** [Poison] *Cardiovascular collapse, pulmonary edema, CNS depression, coma, seizures, nausea, vomiting, cardiopulmonary arrest.*

**vanadium oxytrichloride & titanium tetrachloride mixture** [Poison] *Cardiovascular collapse, pulmonary edema, CNS depression, coma, seizures, nausea, vomiting, cardiopulmonary arrest.*

**vanadium pentoxide** [Poison] *Cardiovascular collapse, pulmonary edema, CNS depression, coma, seizures, nausea, vomiting, cardiopulmonary arrest.*

**vanadium tetrachloride** [Poison] *Cardiovascular collapse, pulmonary edema, CNS depression, coma, seizures, nausea, vomiting, cardiopulmonary arrest.*

**vanadium trioxide** [Poison] *Cardiovascular collapse, pulmonary edema, CNS depression, coma, seizures, nausea, vomiting, cardiopulmonary arrest.*

**vanadyl sulfate** [Poison] *Cardiovascular collapse, pulmonary edema, CNS depression, coma, seizures, nausea, vomiting, cardiopulmonary arrest.*

**vanillin** [Phenol] *Coma, hypotension, arrhythmias, pulmonary edema, respiratory arrest.*

**varnish** [Hydrocarbon mixture] *CNS depression, respiratory arrest, seizures, arrhythmias, pulmonary edema.*

**varnish drier (n.o.s.)** [Poison] *Cardiovascular collapse, pulmonary edema, CNS depression, coma, seizures, nausea, vomiting, cardiopulmonary arrest.*

**vegetable fabric with oil (n.o.s.)** [Flammable/combustible liquid] *CNS depression, respiratory arrest, convulsions, arrhythmias, pulmonary edema.*

**vegetable fiber, burnt (n.o.s.)** [Irritant] *Severe immediate or delayed upper airway or respiratory tract irritation, pulmonary edema, glottic spasm, airway obstruction.*

**vegetable fiber with oil (n.o.s.)** [Flammable/combustible liquid] *CNS depression, respiratory arrest, convulsions, arrhythmias, pulmonary edema.*

**vinyl acetate** [Ester] *CNS depression, respiratory tract irritation, bronchitis, pneumonia.*

**vinyl bromide** [Bromine/methylbromide] *Severe respiratory irritation, pulmonary edema, respiratory failure, coma, convulsions, death.*

**vinyl butyl ether** [Ether] *Anesthesia, respiratory arrest.*

**vinyl butyrate** [Ester] *CNS depression, respiratory tract irritation, bronchitis, pneumonia.*

**vinyl chloride** [Carbon tetrachloride] *CNS depression, respiratory arrest, circulatory collapse.*

**vinyl chloroacetate** [Ester] *CNS depression, respiratory tract irritation, bronchitis, pneumonia.*

**vinyl ether** [Ether] *Anesthesia, respiratory arrest.*

**vinyl ethyl ether** [Ether] *Anesthesia, respiratory arrest.*

**vinyl fluoride** [Halogenated aliphatic hydrocarbon] *CNS depression, respiratory arrest, circulatory collapse.*

**vinyl isobutyl ether** [Ether] *Anesthesia, respiratory arrest.*

**vinyl methyl ether** [Ether] *Anesthesia, respiratory arrest.*

**vinyl pyridine** [Aromatic hydrocarbon] *Arrhythmias, respiratory failure, pulmonary edema, paralysis, brain and kidney damage.*

**vinyl toluene** [Aromatic hydrocarbon] *Arrhythmias, respiratory failure, pulmonary edema, paralysis, brain and kidney damage.*

**vinyl trichlorosilane** [Silane/chlorosilane] *Respiratory tract irritation, pulmonary edema.*

**vinylidene chloride** [Halogenated aliphatic hydrocarbon] *CNS depression, respiratory arrest, circulatory collapse.*

**vinylidene fluoride** [Halogenated aliphatic hydrocarbon] *CNS depression, respiratory arrest, circulatory collapse.*

**VM&P naphtha** [Hydrocarbon mixture] *CNS depression, respiratory*

HazMat

*arrest, seizures, arrhythmias, pulmonary edema.*

**warfarin; warfarin salt (n.o.s.)** [Warfarin/hydroxycoumarin/indanedione] *Anticoagulation effect, internal hemorrhage.*

**warfarin sodium** [Warfarin/hydroxycoumarin/indanedione] *Anticoagulation effect, internal hemorrhage.*

**water-reactive solid (n.o.s.)** [Flammable solid] *Shock, severe chemical and thermal burns, severe respiratory tract irritation, pulmonary edema, respiratory arrest, ECG changes, sudden death.*

**wax** [Aliphatic hydrocarbon] *Arrhythmias, asphyxiation, anesthesia.*

**weed-killing compound, corrosive** [Poison] *Cardiovascular collapse, pulmonary edema, CNS depression, coma, seizures, nausea, vomiting, cardiopulmonary arrest.* [Corrosive] *Upper airway burns and edema, circulatory collapse, severe chemical burns to skin, toxic systemic effects, GI tract perforation and hemorrhage, peritonitis.*

**weed-killing compound, flammable** [Flammable/combustible liquid] *CNS depression, respiratory arrest, convulsions, arrhythmias, pulmonary edema.* [Poison] *Cardiovascular collapse, pulmonary edema, CNS depression, coma, seizures, nausea, vomiting, cardiopulmonary arrest.*

**white asbestos** [Asbestos] *Asbestosis, lung cancer, malignant mesothelioma.*

**white phosphorus** [Phosphorus] *Hypovolemic shock, severe tissue burns, severe respiratory irritation, pulmonary edema, respiratory arrest, arrhythmias, sudden death.*

**wood alcohol** [Methyl alcohol] *Respiratory failure, circulatory collapse.*

**wood filler** [Hydrocarbon mixture] *CNS depression, respiratory arrest, seizures, arrhythmias, pulmonary edema.*

**wood preservative** [Hydrocarbon mixture] *CNS depression, respiratory arrest, seizures, arrhythmias, pulmonary edema.*

**wool waste** [Irritant] *Severe immediate or delayed upper airway or respiratory tract irritation, pulmonary edema, glottic spasm, airway obstruction.*

**xenon (gas or cryogenic liquid)** [Simple asphyxiant] *Asphyxiation.*

**xylene (xylol)** [Aromatic hydrocarbon] *Arrhythmias, respiratory failure, pulmonary edema, paralysis, brain and kidney damage.*

**xylenol** [Aromatic hydrocarbon] *Arrhythmias, respiratory failure, pulmonary edema, paralysis, brain and kidney damage.* [Phenol] *Coma, hypotension, arrhythmias, pulmonary edema, respiratory arrest.*

**xylidine** [Aromatic hydrocarbon] *Arrhythmias, respiratory failure, pulmonary edema, paralysis, brain and kidney damage.*

**xylol (xylene)** [Aromatic hydrocarbon] *Arrhythmias, respiratory failure, pulmonary edema, paralysis, brain and kidney damage.*

**xylyl bromide** [Aromatic hydrocarbon] *Arrhythmias, respiratory failure, pulmonary edema, paralysis, brain and kidney damage.* [Bromine/methylbromide] *Severe respiratory irritation, pulmonary edema, respiratory failure, coma, convulsions, death.*

**xylylene dichloride** [Aromatic hydrocarbon] *Arrhythmias, respiratory failure, pulmonary edema, paralysis, brain and kidney damage.*

**yellow phosphorus** [Phosphorus] *Hypovolemic shock, severe tissue burns, severe respiratory irritation, pulmonary edema, respiratory arrest, arrhythmias, sudden death.*

**zinc; zinc salt (n.o.s.)** [Zinc] *Respiratory tract irritation, metal fume fever, pulmonary edema.*

**zinc acetate** [Zinc] *Respiratory tract irritation, metal fume fever, pulmonary edema.*

**zinc ammonium chloride** [Zinc] *Respiratory tract irritation, metal fume fever, pulmonary edema.*

**zinc ammonium nitrate** [Nitrate/nitrite] *Methemoglobinemia, hypotension, circulatory collapse.* [Zinc] *Respiratory tract irritation, metal fume fever, pulmonary edema.*

**zinc arsenate** [Arsenic] *Heavy metal toxicity, vomiting, GI bleeding, CNS depression, pulmonary edema, cardiac arrest.* [Zinc] *Respiratory tract irritation, metal fume fever, pulmonary edema.*

**zinc arsenate & zinc arsenite mixture** [Arsenic] *Heavy metal toxicity, vomiting, GI bleeding, CNS depression, pulmonary edema, cardiac arrest.* [Zinc] *Respiratory tract irritation, metal fume fever, pulmonary edema.*

**zinc arsenite** [Arsenic] *Heavy metal toxicity, vomiting, GI bleeding, CNS depression, pulmonary edema, cardiac arrest.* [Zinc] *Respiratory tract irritation, metal fume fever, pulmonary edema.*

**zinc arsenite & zinc arsenate mixture** [Arsenic] *Heavy metal toxicity, vomiting, GI bleeding, CNS depression, pulmonary edema, cardiac arrest.* [Zinc] *Respiratory tract irritation, metal fume fever, pulmonary edema.*

**zinc bisulfite** [Zinc] *Respiratory tract irritation, metal fume fever, pulmonary edema.* [Sulfur] *Respiratory tract irritation, pulmonary edema, anaphylaxis.*

**zinc borate** [Zinc] *Respiratory tract irritation, metal fume fever, pulmonary edema.* [Boron] *Respiratory tract irritation, laryngeal spasm and edema, pulmonary edema, severe chemical burns.*

**zinc bromate** [Zinc] *Respiratory tract irritation, metal fume fever, pulmonary edema.* [Bromate] *CNS and respiratory system depression, delayed-onset renal failure.*

**zinc bromide** [Zinc] *Respiratory tract irritation, metal fume fever, pulmonary edema.* [Bromine/methylbromide] *Severe respiratory irritation, pulmonary edema, respiratory failure, coma, convulsions, death.*

**zinc carbonate** [Zinc] *Respiratory tract irritation, metal fume fever, pulmonary edema.*

**zinc chlorate** [Zinc] *Respiratory tract irritation, metal fume fever, pulmonary edema.* [Chlorate] *Hemolysis, methemoglobinemia, hypoperfusion, CNS depression, delayed-onset renal failure.*

**zinc chloride** [Zinc] *Respiratory tract irritation, metal fume fever, pulmonary edema.*

**zinc chromate** [Zinc] *Respiratory tract irritation, metal fume fever, pulmonary edema.*

**zinc cyanide** [Zinc] *Respiratory tract irritation, metal fume fever, pulmonary edema.* [Cyanide] *Impairment of cellular oxygenation and adenosine triphosphate production, hypoxia, death.*

**zinc dithionite** [Zinc] *Respiratory tract irritation, metal fume fever, pulmonary edema.*

**zinc fluoride** [Zinc] *Respiratory tract irritation, metal fume fever, pulmonary edema.* [Fluorine] *CNS depression, respiratory arrest, cardiovascular collapse, shock, arrhythmias.*

**zinc fluorosilicate** [Zinc] *Respiratory tract irritation, metal fume fever, pulmonary edema.* [Fluorine] *CNS depression, respiratory arrest, cardiovascular collapse, shock, arrhythmias.*

**zinc formate** [Zinc] *Respiratory tract irritation, metal fume fever, pulmonary edema.*

**zinc hydrosulfite** [Zinc] *Respiratory tract irritation, metal fume fever, pulmonary edema.* [Sulfur] *Respiratory tract irritation, pulmonary edema, anaphylaxis.*

**zinc nitrate** [Nitrate/nitrite] *Methemoglobinemia, hypotension, circulatory collapse.* [Zinc] *Respiratory tract irritation, metal fume fever, pulmonary edema.*

**zinc permanganate** [Inorganic acid] *Pulmonary edema, bronchospasm, circulatory collapse, laryngeal spasm and edema, severe chemical burns to skin, mucous membranes, and internal organs, GI tract perforation and hemorrhage, peritonitis.* [Zinc] *Respiratory tract irritation, metal fume fever, pulmonary edema.*

**HazMat**

**zinc peroxide** [Zinc] *Respiratory tract irritation, metal fume fever, pulmonary edema.*

**zinc phenolsulfonate** [Zinc] *Respiratory tract irritation, metal fume fever, pulmonary edema.* [Sulfur] *Respiratory tract irritation, pulmonary edema, anaphylaxis.*

**zinc phosphide** [Zinc] *Respiratory tract irritation, metal fume fever, pulmonary edema.* [Phosphine] *Severe pulmonary irritation, pulmonary edema.*

**zinc resinate** [Zinc] *Respiratory tract irritation, metal fume fever, pulmonary edema.*

**zinc selenate** [Selenium] *Arrhythmias, pulmonary edema, bronchospasm, seizures, vomiting, GI bleeding.* [Zinc] *Respiratory tract irritation, metal fume fever, pulmonary edema.*

**zinc selenite** [Selenium] *Arrhythmias, pulmonary edema, bronchospasm, seizures, vomiting, GI bleeding.* [Zinc] *Respiratory tract irritation, metal fume fever, pulmonary edema.*

**zinc silicofluoride** [Zinc] *Respiratory tract irritation, metal fume fever, pulmonary edema.* [Fluorine] *CNS depression, respiratory arrest, cardiovascular collapse, shock, arrhythmias.*

**zinc sulfate** [Zinc] *Respiratory tract irritation, metal fume fever, pulmonary edema.*

**zineb** [Dithiocarbamate] *Hypotension, respiratory failure.*

**ziram** [Dithiocarbamate] *Hypotension, respiratory failure.*

**zirconium** [Poison] *Cardiovascular collapse, pulmonary edema, CNS depression, coma, seizures, nausea, vomiting, cardiopulmonary arrest.*

**zirconium hydride** [Poison] *Cardiovascular collapse, pulmonary edema, CNS depression, coma, seizures, nausea, vomiting, cardiopulmonary arrest.*

**zirconium nitrate** [Nitrate/nitrite] *Methemoglobinemia, hypotension, circulatory collapse.*

**zirconium picramate** [Flammable solid] *Shock, severe chemical and thermal burns, severe respiratory tract irritation, pulmonary edema, respiratory arrest, ECG changes, sudden death.* [Poison] *Cardiovascular collapse, pulmonary edema, CNS depression, coma, seizures, nausea, vomiting, cardiopulmonary arrest.*

**zirconium potassium fluoride** [Fluorine] *CNS depression, respiratory arrest, cardiovascular collapse, shock, arrhythmias.*

**zirconium sulfate** [Poison] *Cardiovascular collapse, pulmonary edema, CNS depression, coma, seizures, nausea, vomiting, cardiopulmonary arrest.*

**zirconium tetrachloride** [Poison] *Cardiovascular collapse, pulmonary edema, CNS depression, coma, seizures, nausea, vomiting, cardiopulmonary arrest.*

**Zytron** [Organophosphate] *Pulmonary edema, respiratory muscle paralysis, respiratory failure, bradycardia, acetylcholinesterase inhibition, hypotension, pulmonary edema, overstimulation of parasympathetic nervous system, striated muscle, sympathetic ganglia, and CNS.*